# Medical Dictionary in Six Languages

# OTHER BOOKS BY BERT SPILKER

*Guide to Clinical Studies and Developing Protocols*
(Raven Press, 1984)

*Guide to Clinical Interpretation of Data*
(Raven Press, 1986)

*Guide to Planning and Managing Multiple Clinical Studies*
(Raven Press, 1987)

*Multinational Drug Companies: Issues in Drug Discovery and Development*
(Raven Press, 1989)

*Inside the Drug Industry*
(with Pedro Cuatrecasas, Prous Science Publishers, 1990)

*Quality of Life Assessments in Clinical Trials*
(Edited, Raven Press, 1990)

*Presentation of Clinical Data*
(with John Schoenfelder, Raven Press, 1990)

*Patient Compliance in Medical Practice and Clinical Trials*
(Edited with Joyce A. Cramer, Raven Press, 1991)

*Data Collection Forms in Clinical Trials*
(with John Schoenfelder, Raven Press, 1991)

*Guide to Clinical Trials*
(Raven Press, 1991)

*Patient Recruitment in Clinical Trials*
(with Joyce A. Cramer, Raven Press, 1992)

*Multinational Pharmaceutical Companies: Principles and Practices (Second Edition)*
(Raven Press, 1994)

# Medical Dictionary in Six Languages

Compiled By

## Bert Spilker, Ph.D., M.D.

*President, Orphan Medical Inc.*
*Minnetonka, Minnesota*

*Adjunct Professor of Medicine,*
*Adjunct Professor of Pharmacology, and*
*Clinical Professor of Pharmacy*
*University of North Carolina Schools of Medicine and Pharmacy*
*Chapel Hill, North Carolina*

*Clinical Professor of Pharmacy Practice*
*University of Minnesota School of Pharmacy*
*Minneapolis, Minnesota*

Raven Press 🕮 New York

Raven Press, Ltd., 1185 Avenue of the Americas, New York, New York 10036

Made in the United States of America

Library of Congress Cataloging-in-Publication Data

Spilker, Bert.
   Medical Dictionary in six languages/ compiled by Bert Spilker.
     p.   cm.
   Text in English, French, German, Japanese, Italian, and Spanish.
   Includes indexes.
   ISBN 0-7817-0182-1
   1. Medicine—Dictionaries—Polyglot. I. Title.
   [DNLM: 1. Dictionaries, Medical—Multilingual. W 13 S756m 1995]
   R121.S685 1995   610´.3—dc20
   DNLM/DLC
for Library of Congress             94-30921
                           CIP

9 8 7 6 5 4 3 2 1

Dedicated to all translators whose knowledge and use of words
facilitates and enhances communication among different groups of people.

# Contents

# Preface

Medical professionals often want to translate words that are difficult to find in a dictionary, even in a medical dictionary. This problem is particularly acute when the term to be translated consists of two, three, or four words that cannot be translated word-for-word into another language. These problems frequently arise in conversation, when listening to talks, during patient examinations, and in writing reports and publications.

This book addresses this problem for professionals working in the area of clinical trials by including over 7500 commonly used words and terms. Many of the terms consist of two to four words. The languages included are the major European languages as well as Japanese. Both British and American terms or spellings are noted in many cases where differences exist. In the main section of this book, the words and entries are alphabetized by the American terms and spelling, but readers should be able to translate easily among any of the languages.

# Acknowledgments

The compiler wishes to acknowledge the herculean efforts of DTS Language Services, Inc. (100 Europa Drive, Suite 390, Chapel Hill, NC 27514), without whose help this book could not have been prepared. This project was led creatively by Mr. Henk Ypma, who consistently found new approaches to simplifying the presentation of complex concepts. He was assisted by Mr. Kirk Samuels and Mr. Bill Geschwind, who coordinated the project and participated in the translation work.

The translators and editors for this project, without whose efforts and contributions this project would not have succeeded, were as follows:

*French:*      Dr. Daniel Bossut, Dr. Jean-François Tanguay, and Ms. Patricia Masson
*Spanish:*     Mr. Christian Viveros and Dr. Pablo Gonzalez
*Italian:*     Dr. Valeria Finucci and Dr. Maria Palomba
*German:*      Mr. Kirk Samuels, Mr. Bill Geschwind, and Dr. Nikola Golenhofen
*Japanese:*    Ms. Eiko Murakami, Dr. Masaaki Ikeda, Dr. Koyoshi Ohtani, and Dr. Maki Asamc

# How to Use This Dictionary

This dictionary may be used to find the translation of a medical word or phrase into any of six languages.

♦ When you know the English term, use the first part of the book to look it up alphabetically and find the translation in French, Italian, Spanish, German, or Japanese.

♦ When you know the French, Italian, Spanish, German, or Japanese term, use the second part of the book to look up the entry number of the English term. Then locate that number in the first part of the book to find the translation into the language desired.

# American English and British English

The main list contains spellings in American English. Where the British spelling differs significantly, it is listed in parentheses following the American term.

An alphabetical list of words and terms that differ between British and American English is presented below, and a list of basic spelling rules that differ between American and British English follows.

## British Words and Terms:
### Selected examples with the American term in parentheses

aetiology (etiology)
anaemia (anemia)
anaesthesiology (anesthesiology)
annex (appendix)
caesarian section (cesarian section)
catalogue (catalog)
chemist (druggist)
colour (color)
cot death (sudden infant death syndrome)

Ethics Committee (Institutional Review
　　　　　Board)
fast follower (me-too drug)
fibre (fiber)
flavour (flavor)
foetal (fetal)
full marks (full credit)
gynaecology (gynecology)
haemodialysis (hemodialysis)

hypoxaemia (hypoxemia)
intensive treatment unit (intensive care unit)
ischaemia (ischemia)
manoeuvre (maneuver)
milligramme (milligram)
millimetre (millimeter)
multicentre (multicenter)
oesophagus (esophagus)
oestrogen (estrogen)
oligaemia (oligemia)
operating theatre (operating room)
paediatric (pediatric)
programme (program)
remit (n.) (charge)
surgery (physician's office)
sundry (miscellaneous)
tick (check off)
venue (setting or place)

**Spelling Rules:**

| British English | American English |
| --- | --- |

1. The ending "our" is usually "or" in American:

| | |
| --- | --- |
| colour | color |
| favour | favor |
| labour | labor |
| vapour | vapor |

2. The ending "ence" is usually "ense" in American:

| | |
| --- | --- |
| defence | defense |
| licence | license |
| offence | offense |

"Essence" and "patience" are the same in both languages.

3. The ending "re" in words derived from French is usually "er" in American:

centimetre        centimeter
centre            center
fibre             fiber
litre             liter

4. The letter "l" in words ending in "el" is usually not doubled in American when a suffix is added:

cancelled         canceled
marvellous        marvelous
traveller         traveler

5. The Greek or Latin "oe" and "ae" are both "e" in American:

foetus            fetus
gynaecology       gynecology
haemorrhage       hemorrhage

6. The ending "ise" may be "ize" in American:

authorise         authorize
organise          organize
randomise         randomize
realise           realize

# Abbreviations

The use of abbreviations in reports and publications should be held to an absolute minimum because it slows reading and makes comprehension more difficult. Only universally understood abbreviations should be used. The common use of multiple abbreviations in publications and elsewhere creates confusion and misunderstanding for numerous reasons that will not be discussed here. A list of standard medical abbreviations is presented. Because many, if not most, names of diseases, medicines, and laboratory tests are similar in many languages, few of these words are included in this dictionary.

The basis for confusion with abbreviations includes the following factors: (1) few are universal, (2) the same abbreviation can be used to stand for several different terms, and (3) it is mentally more difficult to read a passage with multiple abbreviations. This may be because the abbreviations are not familiar to the reader, they were made up by the author, or an excessive number is used. Most two-letter and many three-letter abbreviations in medicine could refer to multiple terms. Some examples are:

**AO**     abdominal aorta, acid output, ankle orthosis, anterior oblique

**BB**     beta-blocker, blow bottle, breast biopsy, buffer base, breakthrough bleeding

**CO**     cardiac output, carbon monoxide, castor oil, cervical orthosis

**CP** creatine phosphokinase, cerebral palsy, cleft palate, chest pain, chronic pain

**HCT** hematocrit, hydrocortisone, human chorionic thyrotropin, histamine challenge test

**MAC** maximal allowable concentration, mid-arm circumference, minimum alveolar concentration, macula

**MD** medical doctor, mental deficiency, muscular dystrophy, manic depression, mediodorsal, movement disorder

**NVD** nausea, vomiting, diarrhea; neck vein distension; neovascularization of the disc; neurovesicle dysfunction; number of vessels diseased

**SEM** standard error of the mean, systolic ejection murmur, scanning electron microscopy, semen

**TCA** tricyclic antidepressant, total cholic acid, total circulatory arrest, trichloroacetic acid

Readers who would like to review dictionaries of abbreviations are referred to:

- *Medical Abbreviations: 7000 Conveniences at the Expense of Communication and Safety*, by Neil M. Davis, MS, PharmD (5th ed., 1992). Neil M. Davis Associates, 1143 Wright Drive, Huntingdon Valley, PA 19006; (215) 947–1752.

- *Dictionary of Medical Acronyms & Abbreviations*, by Stanley Jablonski (2nd ed., 1993). Hanley & Belfus Inc., 210 S. 13th St., Philadelphia, PA 19107; (800) 962–1892.

◆ *Stedman's Abbreviations, Acronyms & Symbols* (1992). Practice Management Information Corp.; (800) 633–7467.

# Selected Abbreviations

## Hormones

| | | | | |
|---|---|---|---|---|
| ACTH | adrenocorticotrophic hormone | | GH | growth hormone |
| ADH | antidiuretic hormone | | LH | luteinizing hormone |
| FSH | follicle stimulating hormone | | PTH | parathyroid hormone |

## Chemicals Found in the Body and Medicines

| | | | | |
|---|---|---|---|---|
| Ach | acetylcholine | | GABA | gamma amino butyric acid |
| ATP | adenosine triphosphate | | G-6PD | glucose-6-phosphate dehydrogenase |
| BCG | bacillus Calmette Guérin vaccine | | 5-HT | serotonin (5-hydroxy-tryptamine) |
| DNA | deoxyribonucleic acid | | INH | isoniazid |
| DTP | diphtheria, tetanus, and pertussis vaccine | | $PGE_2$ | prostaglandin $E_2$ |
| 5-FU | 5 fluro-uracil | | RNA | ribonucleic acid |

## Diseases

| | | | |
|---|---|---|---|
| AIDS | acquired immune deficiency syndrome | JRA | juvenile rheumatoid arthritis |
| | | MI | myocardial infarction |
| ALL | acute lymphocytic leukemia | RDS | respiratory distress syndrome |
| CLL | chronic lymphocytic leukemia | TB | tuberculosis |
| | | URI | upper respiratory infection |
| COPD | chronic obstructive pulmonary disease | UTI | urinary tract infection |
| | | VD | venereal disease |

## Routes of Administration

| | | | |
|---|---|---|---|
| ID | intradermal | PO | oral |
| IM | intramuscular | SL | sublingual |
| IP | intraperitoneal | SQ | subcutaneous |
| IV | intravenous | | |

## Frequency of Medicine Administration

| | | | |
|---|---|---|---|
| BID | twice a day | QOD | every other day |
| QD | once a day | TID | three times a day |
| QID | four times a day | | |

## Laboratory Blood Tests

| | |
|---|---|
| ALT | alanine aminotransferase |
| AST | aspartate aminotransferase |
| BUN | blood urea nitrogen |
| CBC | complete blood count |
| CO | carbon monoxide |
| $CO_2$ | carbon dioxide |
| CPK | creatine phosphokinase |
| ESR | erythrocyte sedimentation rate |
| GGT | gamma-glutamyltransferase |
| HDL | high density lipoprotein |
| LDH | lactic dehydrogenase |
| LDL | low density lipoprotein |
| PT | prothrombin time |
| PTT | partial thromboplastin time |
| VLDL | very low density lipoprotein |
| VDRL | Venereal Disease Research Laboratories |

## Laboratory (Non-Blood) Tests

| | |
|---|---|
| CAT | computed axial tomography |
| CSF | cerebrospinal fluid |
| CXR | chest x-ray |
| ECHO | echocardiogram |
| EEG | electroencephalogram |
| EKG | electrocardiogram (also ECG) |
| EMG | electromyogram |
| IVP | intravenous pyelogram |
| NMR | nuclear magnetic resonance |
| PET | positron emission tomography |

## Metric Units of Measure

Note: Many units have multiple abbreviations, e.g., gram may be abbreviated "g" or "gm".

| | | | |
|---|---|---|---|
| C | Celsius | L | liter |
| cc | cubic centimeter | m | meter |
| g | gram | meq | milliequivalent(s) |
| I.U. | international unit(s) | ml | milliliter |
| kg | kilogram | mm | millimeter |
| km | kilometer | | |

## Non-Metric Units of Measure

| | | | |
|---|---|---|---|
| F | Fahrenheit | lb | pound |
| ft | foot | oz | ounce |

## Organizations

| | | | |
|---|---|---|---|
| ABPI | Association of the British Pharmaceutical Industry | DHHS | Department of Health and Human Services (USA) |
| AMA | American Medical Association | DVA | Department of Veterans Affairs (USA) |
| BGA | Bundesgesundheitsamtes (Germany) | EFPIA | European Federation of Pharmaceutical Industries Association |
| CPMP | Committee for Proprietary Medicinal Products | FDA | Food and Drug Administration |
| DoH | Department of Health (UK) | | |

## Organizations (continued)

| | | | |
|---|---|---|---|
| HMO | Health Maintenance Organization | NIH | National Institutes of Health (USA) |
| IFPMA | International Federation of Pharmaceutical Manufacturers Associations | PhrMA | Pharmaceutical Research Manufacturers Association |
| MWH | Ministry of Health and Welfare (Japan) | PPO | Preferred Provider Organization |
| MRC | Medical Research Council (UK) | USP | United States Pharmacopeia |
| | | WHO | World Health Organization |

## Regulatory Submissions and Regulations

| | | | |
|---|---|---|---|
| CTC | clinical trial certificate (UK) | NCE | new chemical entity |
| CTX | clinical trial exemption (UK) | NDA | new drug application (USA, others) |
| GCP | good clinical practices | PLA | product license application (USA, others) |
| GLP | good laboratory practices | SBA | summary basis of approval (USA) |
| GMP | good manufacturing practices | | |
| IND | investigational new drug application (USA, others) | | |

## Physiological Terms and Medical Specialties

| | | | |
|---|---|---|---|
| BMR | basal metabolic rate | Ht | hematocrit |
| BP | blood pressure | LVEDP | left ventricular end diastolic pressure |
| BSA | body surface area | NPO | nothing by mouth |
| CBF | cerebral blood flow | OB-GYN | obstetrics and gynecology |
| CNS | central nervous system | PEEP | positive end-expiratory pressure |
| CO | cardiac output | | |
| ENT | ears, nose, and throat | RBC | red blood cell |
| GFR | glomerular filtration rate | WBC | white blood cell |
| GI | gastrointestinal | | |
| GU | genitourinary | | |
| Hb or Hgb | hemoglobin | | |

## Pharmaceutical Industry/Academic Institution

| | | | |
|---|---|---|---|
| CCU | Coronary Care Unit | ITU | Intensive Treatment Unit (UK) |
| CME | Continuing Medical Education | IRB | Institutional Review Board |
| CRA | Clinical Research Associate | OTC | Over-the-Counter (i.e., sold without a prescription) |
| CRO | Contract Research Organization | PDR | Physicians' Desk Reference |
| ICD-9 | International Classification of Diseases – 9th Revision | SOP | Standard Operating Procedure |
| | | USAN | United States Adopted Names |
| ICU | Intensive Care Unit (USA) | | |
| INN | International Nonproprietary Name | | |

# Medical Dictionary in Six Languages

| English/American | French/Français | Italian/Italiano | Spanish/Español | German/Deutsch | Japanese/日本語 |
|---|---|---|---|---|---|
| 1. abatement - (n) | atténuation; rémission | remissione; attenuazione | atenuación; remisión | Nachlassen; Abgeschlagenheit | (疼痛の) 減退 |
| 2. abbreviation - (n) | abréviation | abbreviazione | abreviación; abreviatura | Abkürzung | 省略 |
| 3. abdomen - (n) | abdomen; ventre | addome; ventre | abdomen; vientre | Bauch; Abdomen | 腹、腹部 |
| 4. abdominal - (a) | abdominal | addominale | abdominal | Bauch-; abdominal | 腹の、腹部の |
| 5. abdominal distension - (n) | distension abdominale | distensione addominale | distensión abdominal | Bauchdehnung | 腹部膨張、膨張 |
| 6. abdominal guarding - (n) | défense abdominale | protezione addominale | defensa abdominal | Bauchabwehrspannung | 腹壁防御 |
| 7. abdominal pain - (n) | douleur abdominale | dolore addominale | dolor abdominal | Bauchschmerzen | 腹痛 |
| 8. abduct - (v) | mettre en abduction | abdurre | abducir | abduzieren | 外転する |
| 9. aberration - (n) | aberration; déviation | aberrazione; deviazione | aberración, desviación | Aberration; Störung | 異常、収差 |
| 10. ability - (n) | capacité; habilité | abilità; capacità | habilidad; capacidad | Fähigkeit; Vermögen | 能力 |
| 11. ablation - (n) | ablation | ablazione | ablación | Ablation | 切除 |
| 12. abnormal - (a) | anormal | anormale | anormal; no normal | abnorm; mißgebildet | 異常の |
| 13. abnormality - (n) | malformation; difformité | anormalità; irregolarità | anormalidad; malformación | Abnormität; Mißbildung | 異常 [性] |
| 14. abortifacient agent - (n) | abortif | abortivo | agente abortante | Abortivum; Abtreibungsmittel | 堕胎薬 |
| 15. abortion - (n) | avortement; fausse couche | aborto | aborto; aborto espontáneo | Abtreibung; Abort | 堕胎、流産 |
| 16. abrade - (v) | écorcher; érafler | scorticare; seccare | raer; raspar | abkratzen; abschürfen | 剥離する、磨耗する |
| 17. abrasion - (n) | écorchure; frottement | abrasione; raschiamento | abrasión; raedura | Abschürfung; Exkoriation | 剥離、擦過傷 |
| 18. abscess - (n) | abcès | ascesso | absceso | Abszeß; Geschwür | 膿瘍 |
| 19. abscissa - (n) | abscisse | ascissa | abscisa | Abszisse | 横座標 |
| 20. absent - (a) | absent; manquant | assente; mancante | ausente | fehlend | 欠けている |
| 21. absolute - (a) | absolu; total | assoluto; totale | absoluto; total | absolut; Total- | 絶対の |

1

| English/American | French/Français | Italian/Italiano | Spanish/Español | German/Deutsch | Japanese/日本語 |
|---|---|---|---|---|---|
| 22. absolute bioavailability - (n) | biodisponibilité absolue | biodisponibilità assoluta | biodisponibilidad absoluta | absolute Bioverfügbarkeit | 絶対的な生物的利用能 |
| 23. absorb - (v) | absorber | assorbire | absorber | absorbieren; aufsaugen | 吸収する |
| 24. absorption - (n) | absorption | assorbimento | absorción | Absorption; Aufnahme | 吸収 |
| 25. abstract - (n) | analyse; extrait | estratto; riassunto | extracto; compendio | Zusammenfassung | 要約 |
| 26. abuse - (n) | abus; mauvais traitement | abuso; maltrattamento | abuso; maltrato | Mißbrauch; Mißhandlung | 乱用、虐待 |
| 27. abuse potential - (n) | potentiel d'abus | potenziale abusivo | potencial de abuso | Mißbrauchspotential | 乱用の可能性 |
| 28. abuser - (n) | personne abusive; usager abusif de drogue | chi abusa | abusador | Mißbraucher | 乱用者、虐待者 |
| 29. acceleration - (n) | accélération | accelerazione | aceleración | Beschleunigung | 促進 |
| 30. acceptance - (n) | acceptation; consentement | accettazione; consentimento | aceptación; consentimiento | Annahme | 受容、承諾 |
| 31. accessibility - (n) | accessibilité | accessibilità | accesibilidad | Zugänglichkeit; Erreichbarkeit | 入手可能 |
| 32. accessory part - (n) | partie accessoire | parte accessoria | parte accesoria | Zubehörteil; Hilfsgerät | 付属品 |
| 33. accident - (n) | accident | accidente | accidente | Unfall | 事故偶発、症候 |
| 34. acclimation, acclimatization - (n) | acclimatation | acclimatazione; acclimatizzazione | aclimatación | Akklimatisierung; Akklimatisation | 順化 |
| 35. accommodation - (n) | accommodation | accomodazione | acomodación | Akkommodation; Anpassung | 調節 |
| 36. accountability - (n) | responsabilité | responsabilità | responsabilidad | Verantwortlichkeit | 責任 |
| 37. accreditation - (n) | accréditation; autorisation | accreditamento; autorizzazione | acreditación; autorización | Akkreditierung | 認定 |
| 38. acculturation - (n) | acculturation | acculturazione | aculturación | Kulturaneignung | 文化受容、順応 |
| 39. accumulation - (n) | accumulation | accumulazione | acumulación | Anhäufung; Kumulation | 蓄積 |
| 40. accuracy - (n) | exactitude; précision | esattezza; precisione | exactitud; precisión | Genauigkeit | 正確性、精度 |

2

| English/American | French/Français | Italian/Italiano | Spanish/Español | German/Deutsch | Japanese/日本語 |
|---|---|---|---|---|---|
| 41. acetabulum - (n) | acétabulum | acetabolo | acetábulo | Azetabulum; Beckenknochenpfanne | 寛骨臼 |
| 42. acetylcholine - (n) | acétylcholine | acetilcolina | acetilcolina | Azetylcholin | アセチルコリン |
| 43. achalasia - (n) | achalasie | acalasia | acalasia | Achalasie | アカラシア |
| 44. ache - (n) | douleur fixe et continue | dolore costante | dolor constante | Schmerz | 痛み |
| 45. achievement - (n) | accomplissement; réalisation | realizzazione; conquista | realización; logro | Leistung; Errungenschaft | 達成 |
| 46. achlorhydria - (n) | anachlorhydrie | acloridria | aclorhydria | Achlorhydrie; Anazidität | 塩酸欠乏症 |
| 47. achondro-plasia - (n) | achondroplasie | acondroplasia | acondroplasia | Achondroplasie; Chondrodystrophie | 軟骨無形成症 |
| 48. acid - (n) | acide | acido | ácido | Säure | 酸 |
| 49. acid-base - (a) | acide-base | acido-base | ácido-base | Säure-Basen- | 酸塩基の |
| 50. acid-base balance - (n) | équilibre acide-base | equilibrio acido-base | equilibrio ácido-base | Säure-Basen-Gleichgewicht | 酸塩基平衡 |
| 51. acid-base status - (n) | état acide-base | stato acido base | estado ácido-base | Zustand des Säure-Basen-Verhältnisses | 酸塩基の状態 |
| 52. acid-fast - (a) | acido-résistant | acido resistente | ácidorresistente | säurebeständig | 抗酸性の |
| 53. acidosis - (n) | acidose | acidosi | acidosis | Azidose | アシドーシス、酸[性]血 |
| 54. acne - (n) | acné | acne | acné | Akne | アクネ、ざ瘡 |
| 55. acneiform - (a) | acnéiforme | acneiforme | acneiforme | akneartig | ざ瘡様の |
| 56. acoustic - (a) | acoustique | acustico | acústico | akustisch | 聴覚の |
| 57. acquired - (a) | acquis | acquisito | adquirido | erworben | 後天性の |
| 58. acquired immuno-deficiency syndrome [abbr] AIDS - (n) | syndrome d'immunodéficience acquise, SIDA | sindrome da immunodeficienza acquisita, SIDA | síndrome de inmunodeficiencia adquirida, SIDA | erworbenes Immundefektsyndrom, AIDS, Aids | 後天性免疫不全症候群、エイズ |
| 59. acromegaly - (n) | acromégalie | acromegalia | acromegalia | Akromegalie | 先端巨大症 |
| 60. acrosome - (n) | acrosome | acrosomo | acrosoma | Akrosom | 先体、アクロゾーム |
| 61. action potential - (n) | potentiel d'action | potenziale di azione | potencial de acción | Aktionspotential | 活動電位 |

3

| English/American | French/Français | Italian/Italiano | Spanish/Español | German/Deutsch | Japanese/日本語 |
|---|---|---|---|---|---|
| 62. activation - (n) | activation | attivazione | activación | Aktivierung | 活性化 |
| 63. activation factor - (n) | facteur d'activation | fattore d'attivazione | factor de activación | Aktivierungsfaktor | 活性化因子 |
| 64. active - (a) | actif | attivo | activo | aktiv; wirksam | 活発な、活性の |
| 65. active control - (n) | contrôle actif | controllo attivo | control activo | aktive Kontrolle | 活性拮抗 |
| 66. active immunity - (n) | immunité active | immunità attiva | inmunidad activa | aktive Immunität | 能動免疫 |
| 67. active ingredient - (n) | ingrédient actif | ingrediente attivo | ingrediente activo | aktiver Bestandteil | 活性成分 |
| 68. active transport - (n) | transport actif | trasporto attivo | transporte activo | aktiver Transport | 能動輸送 |
| 69. activities of daily living [abbr] ADL- (n) | activités de la vie quotidienne | attività quotidiana | actividades de la vida diaria | Aktivitäten des täglichen Lebens | 日常生活動度 |
| 70. activity - (n) | activité | attività | actividad | Aktivität; Tätigkeit | 活動、行動 |
| 71. actuarial analysis - (n) | analyse actuarielle | analisi attuariale | análisis actuarial | versicherungsstatistische Analyse | 保険統計数理分析 |
| 72. acuity - (n) | acuité | acuità | acuidad | Schärfe | 明瞭度 |
| 73. acupuncture - (n) | acupuncture | agopuntura | acupuntura | Akupunktur | 刺鍼法 |
| 74. acute - (a) | aigu | acuto | agudo | akut | 急性の |
| 75. adaptation - (n) | adaptation | adattamento | adaptación | Anpassung; Adaptation | 適応 |
| 76. addict - (n) | toxicomane | tossicomane | toxicómano | Süchtiger | 常習者 |
| 77. addiction - (n) | toxicomanie | tossicomania | toxicomanía; adicción | Sucht; Abhängigkeit | 嗜好、耽溺 |
| 78. additive - (a) | additif | aggiuntivo | aditivo | additiv; zusätzlich | 添加剤の |
| 79. add-on trial - (n) | essai additionnel | prova aggiuntiva | prueba añadida | Zusatzversuch | 付加試験 |
| 80. adduct - (v) | mettre en adduction | addurre | aducir | adduzieren; heranziehen | 内転する |
| 81. adeno-carcinoma - (n) | adenocarcinome | adenocarcinoma | adenocarcinoma | Adenokarzinom; Drüsenkarzinom | 腺癌 |

4

| English/American | French/Français | Italian/Italiano | Spanish/Español | German/Deutsch | Japanese/日本語 |
|---|---|---|---|---|---|
| 82. adenoids - (n) | végétations adénoïdes | adenoidi; vegetazioni adenoidee | vegetaciones adenoideas | Rachenmandel-wucherungen | アデノイド |
| 83. adenoma - (n) | adénome | adenoma | adenoma | Adenom; Drüsengeschwulst | アデノーマ、腺腫 |
| 84. adenopathy - (n) | adénopathie | adenopatia | adenopatía | Adenopathie; Drüsenerkrankung | アデノパシー |
| 85. adherence - (n) | adhérence | aderenza | adherencia | Festhaften; Befolgung | 粘着性、指示順守度 |
| 86. adhesion - (n) | adhésion | adesione | adhesión | Verwachsung; Adhäsion | 粘着、癒着 |
| 87. adhesive - (a) | adhésif | adesivo | adhesivo | anhaftend; adhäsiv | 粘着性の、癒着性の |
| 88. adipose - (a) | adipeux | adiposo | adiposo | fetthaltig; fettig | 脂肪の |
| 89. adjunct - (n) | accessoire; appendice | accessorio; appendice | adjunto; apéndice | Zusatz; Beigabe | 付属物 |
| 90. adjunct - (a) | accessoire; complémentaire | aggiuntivo; complementare | adjunto | verbunden; beigeordnet | 付属した |
| 91. adjust - (v) | ajuster; adapter | aggiustare; regolare | ajustar | einstellen; anpassen | 調整する、適合させる |
| 92. adjustment - (n) | ajustement; adaptation | aggiustamento; regolazione | ajuste; ajustamiento | Einstellung; Anpassen | 調整、適合 |
| 93. adjuvant - (n) | adjuvant | adiuvante | adyuvante | Adjuvans; Hilfsmittel | 補助薬、アジュバント |
| 94. adjuvant - (a) | adjuvant | adiuvante | adyuvante | helfend, förderlich | 補助薬の |
| 95. administration - (n) | administration | amministrazione; somministrazione | administración | Darreichung; Anwendung | 投薬 |
| 96. administrator - (n) | administrateur | amministratore; direttore | administrador | Verwalter | 管理者 |
| 97. admission - (n) | admission | ingresso | ingreso; internación | Aufnahme; Zulassung | 入院 |
| 98. adnexa - (n) | annexes | annessi | adnexa; anexos | Adnexe | 付属器 |
| 99. adolescence - (n) | adolescence | adolescenza | adolescencia | Jugend; Adoleszenz | 青年期 |
| 100. adolescent - (a) | adolescent | adolescente | adolescente | jugendlich; heranwachsend | 青年期の |
| 101. adoption - (n) | adoption | adozione | adopción | Adoption; Annahme | 採用、養一縁組み |
| 102. adrenal - (a) | surrénale | surrenale; adrenale | suprarrenal | adrenal; Nebennieren- | 副腎の |
| 103. adrenal cortex - (n) | corticosurrénale | corteccia surrenale | corteza suprarrenal | Nebennierenrinde | 副腎皮質 |

| English/American | French/Français | Italian/Italiano | Spanish/Español | German/Deutsch | Japanese/日本語 |
|---|---|---|---|---|---|
| 104. adrenal medulla - (n) | médullo-surrénale | midollare surrenale | médula suprarrenal | Nebennierenmark | 副腎髄質 |
| 105. adrenalin - (n) | adrénaline | adrenalina | adrenalina | Adrenalin; Epinephrin | アドレナリン |
| 106. adrenergic - (a) | adrénergique | adrenergico | adrenérgico | adrenergisch | アドレナリン作用性の |
| 107. adrenergic receptor - (n) | récepteur adrénergique | recettore adrenergico | receptor adrenérgico | adrenergischer Rezeptor | アドレナリン作用性受容体 |
| 108. adrenocorticotropic hormone [abbr] ACTH [abbr] | hormone adrénocorticotrope, ACTH | ormone adrenocorticotropo, ACTH | hormona adrenocorticotrópica, ACTH | Adrenotropin, ACTH | 副腎皮質刺激ホルモン |
| 109. adsorb - (v) | adsorber | assorbire | adsorber | adsorbieren | 吸着させる |
| 110. adsorbent - (n) | adsorbant | assorbente | adsorbente | Adsorbens | 吸着剤 |
| 111. adsorption - (n) | adsorption | assorbimento | adsorción | Adsorption | 吸着 |
| 112. adult - (n) | adulte | adulto | adulto | Erwachsene(r) | 成人 |
| 113. advanced case - (n) | cas avancé | caso avanzato | caso avanzado | fortgeschrittener Fall | 進行例 |
| 114. adventitia - (n) | tunique adventice | tunica avventizia | adventicia; túnica adventicia | Adventitia | 外膜 |
| 115. adverse - (a) | défavorable; indésirable | avverso; indesiderato | adverso | nachteilig; ungünstig | 反する、有害な |
| 116. adverse reaction - (n) | réaction indésirable | effetto indesiderato | reacción adversa | ungünstige Reaktion; schädliche Reaktion | 副作用 |
| 117. adverse reaction dictionary - (n) | dictionnaire des réactions indésirables | dizionario degli effetti indesiderati | diccionario de reacciones adversas | Verzeichnis schädlicher Reaktionen | 副作用辞典 |
| 118. advisory committee - (n) | comité consultatif | comitato consultivo | comité asesor | Beratungsausschuß | 諮問委員会 |
| 119. aeration - (n) | aération | aerazione | aeración | Belüftung | 曝気 [化]、通気 |
| 120. aerobe - (n) | aérobie | aerobio | aerobio | Aerobier | 好気性菌、好気性生物 |
| 121. aerobe - (a) | aérobe | aerobio | aerobio | aerob | 好気性生物の |
| 122. aerobic - (a) | aérobique | aerobico | aerobico | aerob | 好気性の |
| 123. aerosol - (n) | aérosol | aerosol | aerosol | Aerosol | 噴霧性物質、エアロゾル |

| English/American | French/Français | Italian/Italiano | Spanish/Español | German/Deutsch | Japanese/日本語 |
|---|---|---|---|---|---|
| 124. aerospace medicine - (n) | médecine aérospatiale | medicina aerospaziale | medicina aeroespacial | (Luft- und) Raumfahrtmedizin | 航空（宇宙）医学 |
| 125. afebrile - (a) | afébrile | afebbrile | afebril | fieberlos | 無熱性の |
| 126. affect - (n) | affect; émotion | affetto; emozione | afecto; emoción | Affekt; Emotion | 情動 |
| 127. affective - (a) | affectif | affettivo | afectivo | affektiv | 情動の |
| 128. affective disorder - (n) | désordre affectif | disordine affettivo | trastorno afectivo | Affektstörung | 情動障害 |
| 129. affective symptoms - (n) | symptômes affectifs | sintomi affettivi | síntomas afectivos | affektive Symptome | 情動症状 |
| 130. afferent - (a) | afférent | afferente | aferente | afferent; zuführend | 求心性の |
| 131. afferent neuron - (n) | neurone afférent | neurone afferente | neurona aferente | afferentes Neuron | 求心性神経 |
| 132. afferent pathway - (n) | voie afférente | via afferente | vía aferente | afferente Bahn | 求心性経路 |
| 133. affinity - (n) | affinité | affinità | afinidad | Affinität | 親和性 |
| 134. affinity chromatography - (n) | chromatographie d'affinité | cromatografia di affinità | cromatografía de afinidad | Affinitätschromatographie | アフィニティークロマトグラフィー |
| 135. affinity label - (n) | étiquette d'affinité; marque d'affinité | marcatore d'affinità | marcador de afinidad | Affinitätsmarkierung | アフィニティーラベル |
| 136. afterbirth - (n) | arrière-faix; délivre | secondine; annessi fetali | secundinas | Nachgeburt | 後産、胎盤 |
| 137. aftercare - (n) | traitement postopératoire | trattamento ulteriore; post-trattamento | tratamiento ulterior; postcura | Nachbehandlung | アフタケア |
| 138. aftereffect - (n) | action tardive | azione tardiva | efecto tardío | Nachwirkung; Spätwirkung | 後［症］作用、後［続］効果 |
| 139. aftertaste - (n) | arrière-goût | gusto residuo | dejo; resabio | Nachgeschmack | 後味 |
| 140. agamma-globulinemia - (n) | agammaglobulinémie | agammaglobulinemia | agammaglobulinemia | Agammaglobulinämie | 無ガンマグロブリン血［症］ |
| 141. agar - (n) | agar | agar | agar | Agar | 寒天、寒天［培地］ |
| 142. age - (n) | âge | età | edad | Alter | 年令 |

| English/American | French/Français | Italian/Italiano | Spanish/Español | German/Deutsch | Japanese/日本語 |
|---|---|---|---|---|---|
| 143. agency - (n) | agence | agenzia | agencia | Agentur | 機関 |
| 144. agenda - (n) | agenda; ordre du jour | agenda; ordine del giorno | agenda; orden del día | Tagesordnung | 予定表、計画表 |
| 145. agent - (n) | agent | agente | agente | Agens; Wirkstoff | [作用] 物質 |
| 146. agglutination - (n) | agglutination | agglutinazione | aglutinación | Agglutination; Zusammenballung | 凝集反応、凝集 [作用] |
| 147. agglutinin - (n) | agglutinine | agglutinina | aglutinina | Agglutinin | 凝集素 |
| 148. aggravate - (v) | aggraver | aggravare | agravar | erschweren; verschlechtern | 悪化させる |
| 149. aggregation - (n) | agrégation | aggregazione | agregación | Anhäufung | 凝集 |
| 150. aggression - (n) | agression | aggressione | agresión | Aggression | 攻撃 [性] |
| 151. aging - (n) | sénescence; vieillissement | senescenza; invecchiamento | senescencia; envejecimiento | Altern; Seneszenz | 老化、加齢 |
| 152. agitation - (n) | agitation | agitazione | agitación | Erregung; Umrühren | 精神興奮、心的動揺 |
| 153. agonist - (n) | agoniste | agonista | agonista | Agonist | 主動筋、作用薬 |
| 154. agonistic behavior - (n) | comportement agoniste; conduite agoniste | comportamento agonistico | conducta agonística | agonistisches Verhalten | 不自然な行動 |
| 155. agranulocytosis - (n) | agranulocytose | agranulocitosi | agranulocitosis | Agranulozytose; maligne Granulozytopenie | 顆粒球減少 [症] |
| 156. AIDS, abbr. of acquired immunodeficiency syndrome - (n) | SIDA | SIDA | SIDA | AIDS; Aids | エイズ |
| 157. AIDS related complex [abbr] ARC - (n) | complexe para-SIDA; complexe parasida | complesso correlato allo SIDA; CCS | complejo relacionado con el SIDA; ARC | AIDS-verwandter Komplex | エイズ関連症候群 |
| 158. aim - (n) | but; objectif | oggetto; scopo | fin; objetivo | Ziel | 目的 |
| 159. air - (n) | air | aria | aire | Luft | 空気 |

| English/American | French/Français | Italian/Italiano | Spanish/Español | German/Deutsch | Japanese/日本語 |
|---|---|---|---|---|---|
| 160. air cell - (n) | alvéole pulmonaire; chambre à air | cellula aerea; alveolo polmonare | célula aérea; cavidad aérea | Lungenbläschen | 肺胞、含気蜂巣 |
| 161. air embolism - (n) | embolie gazeuse | embolia gassosa | embolia gaseosa | Luftembolie | 空気塞栓 [症] |
| 162. air hunger - (n) | respiration de Kussmaul | dispnea acuta; respiro di Kussmaul | respiración de Kussmaul | Lufthunger | 空気飢餓 |
| 163. air passage - (n) | voie aérienne; voie respiratoire | via respiratoria; via aerea | vía respiratoria; vía de aire | Luftweg; Atemweg | 気道 |
| 164. airway - (n) | voie aérienne; voie respiratoire | via respiratoria; via aerea | vía respiratoria; vía de aire | Luftweg; Atemweg | 気道 |
| 165. airway resistance - (n) | résistance de voie respiratoire | resistenza delle vie aere | resistencia de la vía respiratoria | Atemwegswiderstand | 気道抵抗 |
| 166. akathisia - (n) | acathésie; acathisie | acatisia | acatisia | Akathisie; Sitzangst | 正座不能 |
| 167. akinesia - (n) | acinésie | acinesia | acinesia | Akinesie | 運動不能 [症] |
| 168. albinism - (n) | albinisme | albinismo | albinismo | Albinismus | 白色症 |
| 169. albumin - (n) | albumine | albumina | albúm na | Albumin | アルブミン |
| 170. albuminuria - (n) | albuminurie | albuminuria | albuminuria | Albuminurie | 蛋白尿 [症] |
| 171. alcohol - (n) | alcool | alcool | alcohol | Alkohol | アルコール |
| 172. alcoholic - (n) | alcoolique | alcoolico | alcohólico | Alkoholiker | アルコール中毒者 |
| 173. alcoholic psychosis - (n) | psychose alcoolique | psicosi alcoolica | psicosis alcohólica | Alkoholpsychose | アルコール精神病 |
| 174. alcoholism - (n) | alcoolisme | alcoolismo | alcoholismo | Alkoholismus | アルコール中毒 |
| 175. alertness - (n) | vigilance; vivacité | vigilanza; stato di allerta | vivacidad; vigilancia | Wachsamkeit | 油断のないこと |
| 176. algorithm - (n) | algorithme | algoritmo | algoritmo | Algorithmus | アルゴリズム |
| 177. alienation - (n) | aliénation | alienazione | alienación | Entfremdung | 精神異常 |
| 178. alimentary - (adj) | alimentaire | alimentare | alimentario; alimenticio | alimentär; Nahrungs- | 食事の、食物の |
| 179. alimentary canal - (n) | tube digestif; tube alimentaire | canale alimentare | tracto alimentario | Verdauungskanal; Magen-Darm-Kanal | 消化管 |
| 180. alive - (a) | vivant; en vie | vivo; vivente | vivo | lebend; lebendig | 生きている |

| English/American | French/Français | Italian/Italiano | Spanish/Español | German/Deutsch | Japanese/日本語 |
|---|---|---|---|---|---|
| 181. alkali - (n) | alcali | alcali | álcali | Alkali; Laugensalz | アルカリ |
| 182. alkaloid - (n) | alcaloïde | alcaloide | alcaloide | Alkaloid | アルカロイド |
| 183. alkalosis - (n) | alcalose | alcalosi | alcalosis | Alkalose | アルカローシス |
| 184. alkylating agent - (n) | agent d'alcolylation | agente alchilante | agente alkilizante | Alkylierungsmittel; Alkylans | アルキル化剤 |
| 185. allele - (n) | allèle | allele | alelo | Allel | 対立遺伝子 |
| 186. allergen - (n) | allergène | allergene | alergeno | Allergen; Allergiestoff | アレルゲン |
| 187. allergic - (a) | allergique | allergico | alérgico | allergisch | アレルギーの |
| 188. allergic reaction - (n) | réaction allergique | reazione allergica | reacción alérgica | allergische Reaktion | アレルギー反応 |
| 189. allergy - (n) | allergie | allergia | alergia | Allergie | アレルギー |
| 190. alleviate - (v) | alléger; calmer | alleviare | aliviar; calmar | erleichtern; mindern | 和らげる |
| 191. allocation - (n) | allocation; répartition | assegnazione; distribuzione | asignación; distribución | Zuteilung; Zuweisung | 割当 |
| 192. allocation of patients - (n) | allocation des patients; répartition des patients | sistemazione dei pazienti | distribución de pacientes | Patientenzuweisung; -verteilung | 患者の割当 |
| 193. allosteric regulation - (n) | régulation allostérique | regolamento allosterico | regulación alostérica | allosterische Beeinflussung | アロステリック制御 |
| 194. allosteric site - (n) | site allostérique | sito allosterico | sitio alostérico | allosterisches Zentrum | アロステリック部位 |
| 195. allowable dosage level - (n) | dosage admissible; taux sérique admissible | dose permissibile; dosaggio consentito | dosis permitida | zulässige Dosierung | 許容服用量のレベル |
| 196. allowable medicines - (n) | médicaments admissibles | medicamenti permissibile | drogas permitidas | zulässige Arzneimittel | 許容できる医薬品 |
| 197. alloy - (n) | alliage | lega | aleación | Legierung | 合金 |
| 198. alopecia - (n) | alopécie | alopecia | alopecia | Alopecia; Haarausfall | 脱毛症 |
| 199. alpha error - (n) | erreur alpha | errore alpha | error alfa | Alpha-Fehler | α障害 |
| 200. alpha receptor - (n) | récepteur alpha | recettore alpha | receptor alfa | Alpha-Rezeptor | アルファレセプター |
| 201. alpha rhythm - (n) | rythme alpha | ritmo alfa | ritmo alfa | Alpha-Rhythmus | アルファ波 |
| 202. alternate - (a) | alterné; autre | alterno; altro; alternato | alterno; alternativo | abwechselnd | 副の |

10

| English/American | French/Français | Italian/Italiano | Spanish/Español | German/Deutsch | Japanese/日本語 |
|---|---|---|---|---|---|
| 203. alternative - (n) | alternative | alternativa | alternativa | Alternative; Wahl | 二者択一 |
| 204. alternative - (a) | alternatif; alterné | alternativo | alternativo | alternativ; wahlweise | 二者択一の |
| 205. altruism - (n) | altruisme | altruismo | altruismo | Altruismus | 利他主義 |
| 206. aluminum - (n) | aluminium | alluminio | aluminio | Aluminium | アルミニウム |
| 207. alveolar - (a) | alvéolaire | alveolare | alveolar | alveolär | 肺胞の、槽の |
| 208. alveolus - (n) | alvéole | alveolo | alvéolo | Alveole | 肺胞、胃小窩 |
| 209. amalgam - (n) | amalgame | amalgama | amalgama | Amalgam | アマルガム |
| 210. ambidextrous - (a) | ambidextre | ambidestro | ambidextro; ambidiestro | beidhändig | 両手利きの |
| 211. ambiguity - (n) | ambiguïté | ambiguità | ambigüedad | Zweideutigkeit; Vieldeutigkeit | あいまいさ |
| 212. ambivalence - (n) | ambivalence | ambivalenza | ambivalencia | Ambivalenz; Doppelwertigkeit | 両面性、 アンビヴァレンス |
| 213. amblyopia - (n) | amblyopie | ambliopia | ambliopía | Amblyopie; Sehschwäche | 弱視 |
| 214. ambulance - (n) | ambulance | ambulanza | ambulancia | Krankenwagen | 救急車 |
| 215. ambulation - (n) | démarche | deambulazione | ambulación | Mobilisation | 歩行 |
| 216. ambulatory - (a) | ambulatoire | ambulatorio | ambulatorio | ambulant | 歩行の、外来 [通院] の |
| 217. ambulatory care - (n) | soin ambulatoire | assistenza ambulatoriale | tratamiento ambulatorio | ambulante Versorgung | 外来看護 |
| 218. ameba, amoeba - (n) | amibe | ameba | ameba | Amöbe | アメーバ属 |
| 219. amebiasis - (n) | amibiase | amebiasi | amebiasis | Amöbenkrankheit | アメーバ症 |
| 220. amelioration of symptoms - (n) | amélioration des symptômes | miglioramento di sintomi | mejora de los síntomas | Verbesserung der Symptome | 症状の回復 |
| 221. amenorrhea - (n) | aménorrhée | amenorrea | amenorrea | Amenorrhöe | 無月経 |
| 222. amine - (n) | amine | amina | amina | Amin | アミン |
| 223. amino acid - (n) | aminoacide | aminoacido | aminoácido | Aminosäure | アミノ酸 |
| 224. aminoaciduria - (n) | amino-acidurie | aminoaciduria | aminoaciduria | Aminoazidurie | アミノ酸尿 [症] |
| 225. ammonia - (n) | ammoniac | ammoniaca | amoniaco | Ammoniak | アンモニア |

11

| English/American | French/Français | Italian/Italiano | Spanish/Español | German/Deutsch | Japanese/日本語 |
|---|---|---|---|---|---|
| 226. amnesia - (n) | amnésie | amnesia | amnesia | Gedächtnislücke; Amnesie | 健忘 [症] |
| 227. amniocentesis - (n) | amniocentèse | amniocentesi | amniocentesis | Amniozentese | 羊水穿刺 |
| 228. amniotic fluid - (n) | liquide amniotique | liquido amniotico | fluido amniótico; líquido amniótico | Fruchtwasser; Amnionflüssigkeit | 羊水 |
| 229. amorphous - (a) | amorphe | amorfo | amorfo | amorph; formlos | 無定形の、非晶質の |
| 230. amplification - (n) | amplification | amplificazione | amplificación | Erweiterung; Vergrößerung | 増幅 |
| 231. amplifier - (n) | amplificateur | amplificatore | amplificador | Verstärker | 増幅器 |
| 232. ampoule, ampul - (n) | ampoule | ampolla | ampolla | Ampulle | アンプル |
| 233. amputation - (n) | amputation | amputazione | amputación | Amputation; Abnahme | 切断 [術] |
| 234. amylase - (n) | amylase | amilasi | amilasa | Amylase | アミラーゼ |
| 235. amyloid - (a) | amyloïde | amiloide | amiloide | amyloid; stärkeähnlich | アミロイド |
| 236. amyloidosis - (n) | amyloïdose | amiloidosi | amiloidosis | Amyloidose | アミロイドーシス、アミロイド症 |
| 237. anabolic steroids - (n) | stéroïdes anabolisants | steroidi anabolizzanti | esteroides anabólicos | anabole Steroide | 蛋白同化ステロイド |
| 238. anabolism - (n) | anabolisme | anabolismo | anabolismo | Anabolismus; Aufbaustoffwechsel | 同化 [作用]、物質合成代謝 |
| 239. anaerobe - (n) | anaérobe | anaerobio | anaerobio | Anaerobier | 嫌気性菌、嫌気性生物 |
| 240. anaerobic - (a) | anaérobie | anaerobico | anaeróbico | anaerob | 嫌気性の |
| 241. anal - (a) | anal | anale | anal | anal | 肛門の |
| 242. anal sphincter - (n) | sphincter anal | sfintere anale | esfinter anal | Afterschließmuskel; Analsphinkter | 肛門括約筋 |
| 243. analeptic - (a) | analeptique | analettico | analéptico | analeptisch; anregend | 興奮性の、強化する |
| 244. analgesia - (n) | analgésie | analgesia | analgesia | Analgesie; Schmerzlosigkeit | 無痛覚 [症]、痛覚脱失 |

12

| English/American | French/Français | Italian/Italiano | Spanish/Español | German/Deutsch | Japanese日本語 |
|---|---|---|---|---|---|
| 245. analgesic - (n) | analgésique | analgesico | analgésico | Analgetikum; Schmerzstillungsmittel | 鎮痛剤 |
| 246. analog-digital conversion - (n) | conversion analogique-numérique | conversione analogica-numerica | conversión analógica-numérica | Analog-Digital-Umsetzung | アナログ－デジタル変換 |
| 247. analogue (analog) - (n) | analogue | analogo | análogo | Analogon; Analogstoff | 類似物、アナログ |
| 248. analogy - (n) | analogie | analogia | analogía | Analogie; Ähnlichkeit | 相似性 |
| 249. analysis - (n) | analyse | analisi | análisis | Analyse | 分解、分析 |
| 250. analysis of variance - (n) | analyse de la variance | analisi di varianza | análisis de la varianza | Varianzanalyse | 変動分析 |
| 251. analyte - (n) | analyte | analito | analito | Analyt | 分析物 |
| 252. analytical development - (n) | développement analytique | sviluppo analitico | desarrollo analítico | analytische Entwicklung | 分析能力の発育 |
| 253. anamnestic response - (n) | réponse anamnestique | risposta anamnestica | respuesta anamnésica | anamnestische Reaktion | 既往症反応 |
| 254. anaphase - (n) | anaphase | anafase | anafase | Anaphase | 後期、核分裂の後期 |
| 255. anaphylactic reaction - (n) | réaction anaphylactique | reazione anafilattica | reacción anafilactoide; reacción anafiláctica | anaphylaktische Reaktion | アナフィラキシー反応 |
| 256. anaphylaxis - (n) | anaphylaxie | anafilassi | anafilaxia | Anaphylaxie | アナフィラキシー、過敏症 |
| 257. anasarca - (n) | anasarque | anasarca | anasarca | Anasarka; Hautwassersucht | 全身水腫（浮腫） |
| 258. anastomosis - (n) | anastomose | anastomosi | anastomosis | Anastomose | 吻合［術］、交通 |
| 259. anatomical - (a) | anatomique | anatomico | anatómica | anatomisch | 解剖［学］の |
| 260. anatomical terms - (n) | termes anatomiques | termini anatomici | términos anatómicos | anatomische Begriffe | 解剖学用語 |
| 261. anatomy - (n) | anatomie | anatomia | anatomía | Anatomie | 解剖学 |
| 262. ancestor - (n) | ancêtre | antenato; progenitore | antepasado | Vorfahr; Ahne | 先祖 |
| 263. ancillary - (a) | auxiliaire; subordonné | ausiliario; subordinato | auxiliar; subordinado | ergänzend | 補助の |

| English/American | French/Français | Italian/Italiano | Spanish/Español | German/Deutsch | Japanese/日本語 |
|---|---|---|---|---|---|
| 264. androgen - (n) | androgène | androgeno | andrógeno | Androgen; androgener Stoff | 男性ホルモン アンドロゲン |
| 265. anecdotal observation - (n) | observation anecdotique | osservazione aneddotica | observación anecdótica | Zufallsbefund | 逸話（風）の観察 |
| 266. anemia - (n) | anémie | anemia | anemia | Anämie; Blutarmut | 貧血 |
| 267. anencephaly - (n) | anencéphalie | anencefalia | anencefalia | Anenzephalie | 無脳症 |
| 268. anesthesia - (n) | anesthésie; narcose | anestesia; narcosi | anestesia | Anästhesie; Narkose | 麻酔 [法]、感覚（知覚）脱失 |
| 269. anesthesiology - (n) | anesthésiologie | anestesiologia | anestesiología | Anästhesiologie | 麻酔学 |
| 270. anesthetic - (n) | anesthésique | anestetico | anestésico | Betäubungsmittel; Anaesthetikum | 麻酔剤 |
| 271. anesthetic - (a) | anesthésique | anestetico | anestésico | gefühllos; unempfindlich | 麻酔の |
| 272. anesthetist - (n) | anesthésiste | anestesista | anestesista | Narkosearzt | 麻酔士 |
| 273. aneuploidy - (n) | aneuploïdie | aneuploidia | aneuploidía | Aneuploidie | 異数性 |
| 274. aneurysm - (n) | anévrysme; anévrisme | aneurisma | aneurisma | Aneurysma; Schlagaderweiterung | 動脈瘤 |
| 275. anger - (n) | colère | collera; rabbia | cólera; ira | Ärger; Zorn | 怒り |
| 276. angina - (n) | angine | angina | angina | Angina; Halsentzündung | アンギナ、狭心症 |
| 277. angina pectoris - (n) | angine de poitrine | angina pectoris | angina pectoris | Angina pectoris; Stenokardie | 狭心症 |
| 278. angiocardiogram - (n) | angiocardiogramme | angiocardiogramma | angiocardiograma | Angiokardiogramm | 血管心臓撮影 |
| 279. angioedema - (n) | angioedème | angioedema | edema angioneurótico; enfermedad de Quincke | angioneurotisches Ödem | 血管性水腫（浮腫） |
| 280. angiography - (n) | angiographie | angiografia | angiografía | Vasographie; Gefäßdarstellung | 血管撮影法 |
| 281. angioma - (n) | angiome | angioma | angioma | Angiom; Gefäßschwamm | 血管腫 |
| 282. angioneurotic - (a) | angioneurotique | angioneurotico | angioneurótico | angioneurotisch | 血管神経症の |

14

| English/American | French/Français | Italian/Italiano | Spanish/Español | German/Deutsch | Japanese/日本語 |
|---|---|---|---|---|---|
| 283. angiopathy - (n) | angiopathie | angiopatia | angiopatia | Angiopathie | 血管障害, 脈管障害 |
| 284. angioplasty - (n) | angioplastie | angioplastica | plastia vascular; angioplastia | Angioplastie; Gefäßplastik | 血管形成 [術] |
| 285. angle - (n) | angle | angolo | ángulo | Winkel | 角度 |
| 286. animal - (n) | animal | animale | animal | Tier | 動物 |
| 287. animal data - (n) | données animales | dati animali | datos animales | Daten von Tierversuchen | 動物データ |
| 288. animal model - (n) | modèle animal | modello animale | modelo animal | Tiermodell | 動物モデル |
| 289. animal research - (n) | recherche animale | ricerca animale | investigación con animales | Forschung mit Tieren | 動物研究 |
| 290. animal testing - (n) | essai animal; contrôle animal | test su animali | prueba con animales; ensayo con animales | Tierversuchen; Tierversuch | 動物実験 |
| 291. animation - (n) | animation; vivacité | animazione | animación; vivacidad | Belebung; Anregung | 生気 |
| 292. anion - (n) | anion | anione | anión | Anion | 陰イオン、負イオン |
| 293. anisocoria - (n) | anisocorie | anisocoria | anisocoria | Anisokorie; Pupillendifferenz | 瞳孔 [左右] 不同 [症] |
| 294. anisocytosis - (n) | anisocytose | anisocitosi | anisocitosis | Anisozytose | 赤血球 [大小] 不同 [症] |
| 295. ankle - (n) | cheville | caviglia | tobillo | (Fuß)knöchel | 足根関節 |
| 296. ankle edema - (n) | oedème de la cheville | edema della caviglia | edema del tobillo | Knöchelödem | 足根関節浮腫 |
| 297. ankle jerk - (n) | réflexe achilléen | riflesso achilleo | reflejo aquíleo | Achillessehnenreflex | くるぶし反射 |
| 298. ankylosing spondylitis - (n) | spondylite ankylosante | spondilite anchilosante | espondilitis anquilosante | Spondylitis ankylopoietica | 強直性脊椎炎 |
| 299. ankylosis - (n) | ankylose | anchilosi | anquilosis | Gelenkversteifung; Ankylose | 硬直 [症] |
| 300. annual - (a) | annuel | annuale; annuo | anual | jährlich | 年間の |
| 301. annulus - (n) | anneau | anello; annulus | anillo; annulus | Ring; Anulus | 輪 |
| 302. anomaly - (n) | anomalie | anomalia | anomalía | Anomalie | 異常、奇形 |
| 303. anorexia nervosa - (n) | anorexie nerveuse | anoressia nervosa | anorexia nerviosa | Anorexia nervosa; Magersucht | 神経性食欲不振 |

| English/American | French/Français | Italian/Italiano | Spanish/Español | German/Deutsch | Japanese/日本語 |
|---|---|---|---|---|---|
| 304. anosmia - (n) | anosmie | anosmia | anosmia | Anosmie | 無嗅覚［症］、嗅覚脱失（消失） |
| 305. anovulation - (n) | anovulation | anovulazione | anovulación | Ausbleiben der Ovulation | 無排卵 |
| 306. anoxemia - (n) | anoxémie | anossiemia | anoxemia | Anoxämie | 無酸素血［症］ |
| 307. anoxia - (n) | anoxie | anossia | anoxia | Anoxie | 無酸素［症］、酸素欠乏［症］ |
| 308. antacid - (n) | antacide | antiacido | antiácido | Antazidum | 制酸剤 |
| 309. antagonist - (n) | antagoniste | antagonista | antagonista | Antagonist; Gegenmuskel | 抑制剤、拮抗質 |
| 310. antemortem - (a) | antemortem | premorto; ante mortem | antes de la muerte | vor dem Tod; prämortal | 死の前の |
| 311. antenatal - (a) | prénatal | prenatale | prenatal | vor der Geburt; pränatal | 出生前の |
| 312. antepartum - (a) | antepartum | preparto; ante partum | antes del parto | antepartal | 分娩前の |
| 313. anterior - (a) | antérieur | anteriore | anterior | vorder; Vorhergehend | 前方の、前側の |
| 314. anterior chamber of the eye - (n) | chambre antérieure | camera anteriore | cámara anterior | vordere Augenkammer; Augenvorderkammer | 前眼房 |
| 315. anthelmintic - (n) | anthelmintique | antielmintico | antihelmíntico | Wurmmittel; Anthelminthikum | 駆虫剤 |
| 316. anthropology - (n) | anthropologie | antropologia | antropología | Anthropologie | 人類学 |
| 317. anti- - (prefix) | anti-; contre- | anti- | anti- | Anti-; Ant- | 反対の |
| 318. antianginal - (a) | antiangineux | antianginoso | antianginal | antianginös | 抗狭心症の |
| 319. antiarrhythmic - (n) | anti-arythmique | antiaritmico | antiarrítmico | Antiarrhythmikum | 抗不整脈の |
| 320. antiarrhythmic - (a) | antiarythmique | antiaritmia | antiarrítmico | antiarrhythmisch | 抗不整脈［性］の |
| 321. antibacterial - (a) | antibactérien | antibatterico | antibacteriano | antibakteriell | 抗菌［性］の |
| 322. antibiotic - (n) | antibiotique | antibiotico | antibiótico | Antibiotikum | 抗生物質 |
| 323. antibody - (n) | anticorps | anticorpo | anticuerpo | Antikörper; Immunkörper | 抗体 |
| 324. antibody titer (antibody titre) - (n) | titre d'anticorps | titolo anticorpale | título de anticuerpo | Antikörpertiter | 抗体価 |
| 325. antibody-dependent - (a) | dépendant des anticorps | anticorpo-dipendente | dependiente de los anticuerpos | antikörperabhängig | 抗体依存性の |

| English/American | French/Français | Italian/Italiano | Spanish/Español | German/Deutsch | Japanese/日本語 |
|---|---|---|---|---|---|
| 326. anticholinergic - (a) | anticholinergique | anticolinergico | anticolinérgico | anticholinergisch | 抗コリン作用（作動）性の |
| 327. anticoagulant - (n) | anticoagulant | anticoagulante | anticoagulante | Antikoagulans | 抗凝固薬 |
| 328. anticonvulsant - (n) | anticonvulsivant | anticonvulsivo | anticonvulsivante | Antikonvulsivum | 抗痙攣薬 |
| 329. antidepressant - (n) | antidépresseur | antidepressivo | antidepresivo | Antidepressivum | 抗うつ薬 |
| 330. antidiarrheal - (n) | antidiarréique | antidiarroico | antidiarreico | Antidiarrhoikum | 下痢止め薬 |
| 331. antidiuretic - (n) | antidiurétique | antidiuretico | antidiurético | Antidiuretikum | 抗利尿薬 |
| 332. antidote - (n) | antidote | antidoto | antídoto | Gegengift; Gegenmittel | 解毒薬 |
| 333. antiemetic - (n) | antiémétique | antiemetico | antiemético | Antiemetikum | 鎮吐薬 |
| 334. antiepileptic - (n) | antiépileptique | antiepilettico | antiepiléptico | Antiepileptikum | 抗てんかん薬 |
| 335. antifibrinolytic - (n) | antifibrinolytique | antifibrinolitico | antifibrinolítico | Antifibrinolytikum | 抗線維素溶解薬 |
| 336. antifungal - (a) | antifungique | antifungino | antifúngico | pilzhemmend | 抗真菌性の |
| 337. antigen - (n) | antigène | antigene | antígeno | Antigen | 抗原 |
| 338. antihemorrhagic - (a) | antihémorragique | antiemorragico | antihemorrágico | antihämorrhagisch; blutstillend | 抗出血性の |
| 339. antihistamine - (n) | antihistaminique | antistaminico | antihistamínico | Antihistaminstoff; Antihistaminikum | 抗ヒスタミン薬 |
| 340. antihypertensive - (n) | antihypertenseur | agente anti-ipertensivo | antihipertensivo | Antihypertensivum | 抗高血圧［症］薬 |
| 341. anti-infective - (a) | anti-infectieux | antinfettivo | antiinfeccioso | antiinfektiös; infektionsverhütend | 抗伝染性 |
| 342. anti-inflammatory - (n) | anti-inflammatoire | anti-inflammatorio; antiflogistico | antiinflamatorio | Antiphlogistikum; entzündungshemmendes Mittel | 抗炎症性 |
| 343. antilipemic - (n) | antilipémique | antilipemico | antilipemico | Antilipidämikum | 抗脂肪血症 |
| 344. antimalarial - (n) | antimalarique | antimalarico | antimalárico | Antimalariamittel | 抗マラリア薬 |
| 345. antimetabolite - (n) | antimétabolite | antimetabolita | antimetabolito | Antimetabolit | 代謝拮抗物質 |
| 346. antimicrobial - (a) | antimicrobien | antimicrobico | antimicrobiano | antimikrobiell | 抗菌性の |
| 347. antineoplastic - (a) | antinéoplastique | antineoplastico | antineoplásico | antineoplastisch | 抗腫瘍性の |
| 348. antinuclear - (a) | antinucléaire | antinucleare | antinuclear | antinuklear | 抗核の |

17

| English/American | French/Français | Italian/Italiano | Spanish/Español | German/Deutsch | Japanese日本語 |
|---|---|---|---|---|---|
| 349. antioxidant - (n) | antioxydant | antiossidante | antioxidante | Antioxydationsmittel | 抗酸化薬 |
| 350. antipathy - (n) | antipathie | antipatia | antipatía | Antipathie, Abneigung | 嫌悪 |
| 351. antipsychotic - (n) | antipsychotique | antipsicotico | antipsicótico | Antipsychotikum | 抗精神病薬 |
| 352. antipyretic - (n) | antipyrétique | antipiretico | antipirético | Fiebermittel; Antipyretikum | 解熱薬 |
| 353. antisense RNA - (n) | ARN antisense | antisenso ARN | ARN antisenso | Antisense-RNS | アンチセンスRNA |
| 354. antiseptic - (n) | antiseptique | antisettico | antiséptico | Antiseptikum | 防腐薬 |
| 355. antiserum - (n) | antisérum | antisiero | antisuero | Antiserum | 抗血清 |
| 356. antithrombin - (n) | antithrombine | antitrombina | antitrombina | Antithrombin | 抗トロンビン、アンチトロンビン |
| 357. antitoxin - (n) | antitoxine | antitossina | antitoxina | Antitoxin | 抗毒素 |
| 358. antitubercular - (a) | antituberculeux | antitubercolare | antituberculoso | antituberkulös | 抗結核性の |
| 359. antitumor - (n) | antitumoral | antitumorale | antitumoral | Wirkung gegen Tumorwachstum, -ausbreitung | 抗腫瘍 |
| 360. antitussive - (n) | antitussif | antitosse | antitusivo | Antitussivum; Hustenmittel | 鎮咳薬、咳止め |
| 361. antiviral - (a) | antiviral | antivirale | antiviral | antiviral | 抗ウイルス性の |
| 362. antrum - (n) | antre | antro | antro | Antrum; Höhle | 洞 |
| 363. anuresis - (n) | anurèse | anuresi | anuresis | Anurie | 尿閉 |
| 364. anuria - (n) | anurie | anuria | anuria | Anurie; Nierenblockade | 無尿 [症] |
| 365. anus - (n) | anus | ano | ano | After; Anus | 肛門 |
| 366. anxiety - (n) | anxiété; angoisse | ansietà; ansia | ansiedad; angustia | Angst; Beklemmung | 不安 |
| 367. anxiety disorder - (n) | désordre d'anxiété | disturbo ansioso | trastorno de ansiedad | Durch Angst verursachte Störung | 不安障害 |
| 368. anxiolytic - (n) | anxiolytique | ansiolitico | ansiolítico | Angstlösendes Mittel | 抗不安薬 |
| 369. aorta - (n) | aorte | aorta | aorta | Hauptschlagader; Aorta | 大動脈 |
| 370. aortic - (a) | aortique | aortico | aórtico | aortal; Aorten- | 大動脈の |

18

| English/American | French/Français | Italian/Italiano | Spanish/Español | German/Deutsch | Japanese/日本語 |
|---|---|---|---|---|---|
| 371. aortic valve - (n) | valve aortique | valvola aortica | válvula aórtica | Aortenklappe | 大動脈弁 |
| 372. apathy - (n) | apathie | apatia | apatía | Apathie; Gleichgültigkeit | 無関心 |
| 373. aperture - (n) | ouverture; orifice | apertura; orifizio | apertura; orificio | Öffnung; Foramen | 口、開口 |
| 374. apex - (n) | apex; sommet | apice | cima; cumbre | Spitze; Gipfel | 尖 |
| 375. Apgar score - (n) | évaluation Apgar | punteggio di Apgar | puntaje de Apgar | Apgar-Schema | アプガースコア |
| 376. aphasia - (n) | aphasie | afasia | afasia | Aphasie; Sprechstörung | 失語［症］ |
| 377. apheresis - (n) | aphérèse | aferesi | aféresis | Hämapherese | アフェレーシス |
| 378. aphrodisiac - (n) | aphrodisiaque | afrodisiaco | afrodisíaco | Aphrodisiakum | 催淫薬、性欲促進薬 |
| 379. aphthous stomatitis - (a) | stomatite aphteuse | stomatite aftosa | estomatitis aftosa | aphthöse Stomatitis | アフタ性口内炎 |
| 380. aphthous ulcer - (n) | ulcère aphteux | ulcera aftosa | úlcera aftosa | Apthöses Geschwür | アフタ性潰瘍 |
| 381. apical impulse - (n) | impulsion apicale | impulso apicale | impulsión apical | Herzspitzenstoß | 先端刺激 |
| 382. aplastic - (a) | aplasique; aplastique | aplastico | aplástico | aplastisch | 形成不全［性］の |
| 383. aplastic anemia - (n) | anémie aplastique | anemia aplastica | anemia aplástica | aplastische Anämie | 再生不良性貧血 |
| 384. apnea - (n) | apnée | apnea | apnea | Atemstillstand; Atemlosigkeit | 無呼吸 |
| 385. apocrine - (a) | apocrine | apocrino | apocrino | apokrin | アポクリンの |
| 386. apoenzyme - (n) | apoenzyme | apoenzima | apoenzima | Apoenzym | アポ酵素 |
| 387. apolipoprotein - (n) | apolipoprotéine | apolipoproteina | apolipoproteína | Apolipoprotein | アポリポ蛋白 |
| 388. apoplexy - (n) | apoplexie | apoplessia | apoplejia | Gehirnschlag; Schlaganfall | （脳）卒中、出血 |
| 389. apoprotein - (n) | apoprotéine | apoproteina | apoproteína | Apoprotein | アポ蛋白 |
| 390. apparent - (a) | apparent; manifeste | apparente; manifesto | aparente; manifiesto | offenbar; anscheinend | 明らかな、見かけの |
| 391. apparent volume of distribution - (n) | volume de distribution | volume apparente di distribuzione | volumen de distribución | scheinbares Verteilungsvolumen | 分布の明白な容量 |
| 392. appearance - (n) | apparition; aspect | aspetto; apparenza | apariencia; aspecto | Erscheinung; Aussehen | 外観、出現 |
| 393. appendage - (n) | appendice | appendice | apéndice | Fortsatz; Anhang | 付属器、付属体 |
| 394. appendix - (n) | appendice; annexe | appendice; parte aggiunta | apéndice | Blinddarm; Anhang | 虫垂、付録 |

| English/American | French/Français | Italian/Italiano | Spanish/Español | German/Deutsch | Japanese/日本語 |
|---|---|---|---|---|---|
| 395. appetite - (n) | appétit | appetito | apetito | Appetit | 欲求、食欲 |
| 396. application - (n) | application; usage | applicazione; uso | aplicación; solicitud | Anwendung; Antrag | 応用、適用 |
| 397. applied research - (n) | recherche appliquée | ricerca applicata | investigación aplicada | angewandte Forschung | 応用研究 |
| 398. appointment - (n) | rendez-vous; entrevue | appuntamento; carica | cita; nombramiento | Termin | 予約 |
| 399. apprehension - (n) | appréhension | apprensione | aprensión | Befürchtung | 理解 |
| 400. approval time - (n) | temps d'acceptation | tempo di ratifica | tiempo de aprobación | Zulassungszeit; Annahmezeit | 認可時 |
| 401. apraxia - (n) | apraxie | aprassia | apraxia | Apraxie | 失行［症］ |
| 402. aptitude - (n) | aptitude | attitudine; disposizione individuale | aptitud | Eignung; Begabung | 適性 |
| 403. aqueduct - (n) | aqueduc | acquedotto | acueducto | Aquadukt | 水管、水道 |
| 404. aqueous - (a) | aqueux | acqueo | acuoso | wässerig | 水の、水性の |
| 405. aqueous humor - (n) | humeur aqueuse | umore acqueo | humor acuoso | Humor aqueus; Kammerwasser | ［眼］房水 |
| 406. arachnid - (n) | arachnide | aracnide | arácnido | Arachnoide; Spinnentier | クモ類 |
| 407. arachnoid - (n) | arachnoïde | aracnoide | aracnoide | Arachnoidea; Spinngewebehaut | クモ膜 |
| 408. arch - (n) | arc | arco | arco | Bogen | 弓 |
| 409. archive - (n) | archive | archivio | archivo | Archiv | 記録 |
| 410. area - (n) | aire; région | area; regione | área; región | Fläche | 部位、領 |
| 411. area under a curve - (n) | aire sous une courbe | area sotto una curva | área bajo una curva | Fläche unter einer Kurve | 曲線下の部分 |
| 412. areola - (n) | aréole | areola | aréola | Areola; kleiner Hof | 小域、輪 |
| 413. arithmetic scale - (n) | échelle arithmétique | scala aritmetica | escala aritmética | arithmetischer Maßstab | 等差スケール |
| 414. arm - (n) | bras | braccio; ramo | brazo; rama | Arm; Zweig | 腕、アーム |
| 415. arm of treatment - (n) | bras de traitement | ramo di trattamento | rama de tratamiento | Behandlungszweig | 処置（治療）中の腕 |

20

| English/American | French/Français | Italian/Italiano | Spanish/Español | German/Deutsch | Japanese/日本語 |
|---|---|---|---|---|---|
| 416. armpit - (n) | aisselle | ascella | axila; fosa axilar | Achselgrube; Achselhöhle | 腋窩 |
| 417. arousal - (n) | éveil; excitation (sexuelle) | eccitamento; risveglio | excitación (sexual); despertamiento | Erregung; Erwecken | 覚醒 |
| 418. arrhythmia - (n) | arythmie | aritmia | arritmia | Arrhythmie | 不整脈 |
| 419. arrow - (n) | flèche | freccia | flecha | Pfeil | 矢印 |
| 420. art - (n) | art | arte | arte | Kunst | 芸術 |
| 421. arterial - (a) | artériel | arterioso | arterial | arteriell | 動脈 [性] の |
| 422. arterial blood pressure - (n) | pression artérielle | pressione arteriosa | presión arterial | arterieller Blutdruck | 動脈血圧 |
| 423. arterial oxygen saturation - (n) | saturation d'oxygène artériel | saturazione d'ossigeno arterioso | saturación de oxígeno arterial | arterielle Sauerstoffsättigung | 動脈血酸素飽和度 |
| 424. arterial pulse - (n) | pouls artériel | polso arterioso | pulso arterial | arterieller Puls | 動脈拍 |
| 425. arteriogram - (n) | artériogramme | arteriogramma | arteriograma | Arteriogramm | 動脈造影（撮影）図 |
| 426. arteriole - (n) | artériole | arteriola | arteriola | Arteriole | 小動脈、細動脈 |
| 427. arterio-sclerosis - (n) | artériosclérose | arteriosclerosi | arteriosclerosis | Arteriosklerose; Arterienverkalkung | 動脈硬化 [症] |
| 428. arteriospasm - (n) | spasme artériel | arteriospasmo | espasmo arterial | Arteriospasmus | 動脈痙攣 |
| 429. arteriovenous - (a) | artérioveineux | arterovenoso | arteriovenoso | arteriovenös | 動静脈の |
| 430. arteriovenous shunt - (n) | artérioveineuse | anastomosi arterovenosa | arteriovenosa | arteriovenöse Anastomose | 動静脈シャント |
| 431. arteritis - (n) | artérite | arterite | arteritis | Arteritis; Arterienentzündung | 動脈炎 |
| 432. artery - (n) | artère | arteria | arteria | Arterie; Schlagader | 動脈 |
| 433. artery bypass - (n) | pontage artériel | bypass arterioso | bypass arterial; puente arterial | arterielle Überbrückung | 動脈バイパス |
| 434. arthralgia - (n) | arthralgie | artralgia | artralgia | Arthralgie; Gelenkschmerz | 関節痛 |
| 435. arthritis - (n) | arthrite | artrite | artritis | Gelenkentzündung; Arthritis | 関節炎 |

21

| English/American | French/Français | Italian/Italiano | Spanish/Español | German/Deutsch | Japanese/日本語 |
|---|---|---|---|---|---|
| 436. arthrography - (n) | arthrographie | artrografia | artrografía | Arthrographie | 関節造影（撮影）[法] |
| 437. arthroplasty - (n) | arthroplastie | artroplastica | artroplastia | Arthroplastik; Gelenkplastik | 関節形成 [術] |
| 438. arthroscopy - (n) | arthroscopie | artroscopia | artroscopia | Arthroskopie | 関節鏡検査 [法] |
| 439. article - (n) | article; segment | articolo; segmento | artículo; segmento | Posten; Beitrag | 関節間の分節、記事 |
| 440. articular - (a) | articulaire | articolare | articular | artikulär | 関節 [性] の |
| 441. articular cartilage - (n) | cartilage articulaire | cartilagine articolare | cartílago articular | Gelenkknorpel | 間節軟骨 |
| 442. articular ligament - (n) | ligament articulaire | legamento articolare | ligamento articular | Gelenkband | 関節靭帯 |
| 443. articular surface - (n) | surface articulaire | superficie articolare | superficie articular | Gelenkfläche | 関節の表面 |
| 444. articulation - (n) | articulation; jointure | articolazione; giuntura | articulación; juntura | Gelenk; Articulus | 連結、関節 |
| 445. artifact - (n) | artefact | artefatto | artefacto | Artefakt; Kunstprodukt | アーチファクト |
| 446. artificial - (a) | artificiel | artificiale | artificial | künstlich | 人工の |
| 447. artificial insemination - (n) | insémination artificielle | inseminazione artificiale | inseminación artificial | künstliche Befruchtung | 人工授精 |
| 448. artificial intelligence - (n) | intelligence artificielle | intelligenza artificiale | inteligencia artificial | künstliche Intelligenz | 人工知能 |
| 449. asbestos - (n) | asbeste | asbesto; amianto | asbesto | Asbest | アスベスト、石綿 |
| 450. ascending - (a) | ascendant | ascendente | ascendente | aufsteigend | 上昇の |
| 451. ascites - (n) | ascite | ascite | ascitis | Aszites; Bauchwassersucht | 腹水 |
| 452. ascitic fluid - (n) | liquide d'ascite | liquido ascitico | líquido ascítico | Aszitesflüssigkeit; Bauchwasser | 腹水 |
| 453. asepsis - (n) | asepsie | asepsi | asepsia | Asepsis; Keimfreiheit | 無菌 |
| 454. aseptic - (n) | asepsie | asettico | aséptico | Aseptik; Keimfreiheit | 防腐剤 |
| 455. aseptic - (a) | aseptique; stérilisé | asettico | aséptico; estéril | aseptisch; keimfrei | 無菌 [性] の |

22

| English/American | French/Français | Italian/Italiano | Spanish/Español | German/Deutsch | Japanese/日本語 |
|---|---|---|---|---|---|
| 456. aseptic necrosis - (n) | nécrose aseptique | necrosi asettica | necrosis aséptica | aseptische Nekrose | 無菌壊死 |
| 457. asexual - (a) | asexué | asessuale; asessuato | asexua | geschlechtslos; ungeschlechtlich | 無性の、無性欲の |
| 458. asphyxia - (n) | asphyxie | asfissia | asfixia | Asphyxie; Erstickung | 仮死、窒息 |
| 459. aspirate - (v) | aspirer | aspirare | aspirar | einatmen; ansaugen | 吸引する |
| 460. aspiration pneumonia - (n) | pneumonie d'aspiration | polmonite da aspirazione | neumonía por aspiración | Aspirationspneumonie | 吸引性肺炎 |
| 461. assay - (n) | essai; épreuve | assaggio; prova | ensayo; prueba | Probe; Versuch | 分析［法］、アッセイ |
| 462. assay validation - (n) | validation de l'epreuve | conferma della validità della prova | validación del ensayo | Versuchsvalidierung | 分析の妥当性 |
| 463. assessment - (n) | évaluation; estimation | valutazione | evaluación; valoración | Schätzung; Beurteilung | 評価 |
| 464. assigned treatment - (n) | traitement assigné | trattamento stabilito | tratamiento asignado | zugeteilte Therapie (einer Versuchsgruppe) | 指定された治療 |
| 465. assisted - (a) | assisté; aidé | assistito | facilitado | assistiert | 補助された |
| 466. associated - (a) | associé | associato | asociado; relacionado | verbunden | 付随した |
| 467. association - (n) | association | associazione | asociación | Assoziation; Vereinigung | 連合、関連 |
| 468. asterisk - (n) | astérisque | asterisco | asterisis | Sternchen | 星印 |
| 469. asthenia - (n) | asthénie | astenia | astenia | Asthenie; Kraftlosigkeit | 無力［症］ |
| 470. asthma - (n) | asthme | asma | asma | Asthma | ぜん息 |
| 471. astigmatism - (n) | astigmatisme | astigmatismo | astigmatismo | Astigmatismus; Stabsichtigkeit | 乱視 |
| 472. astringent - (n) | astringent | astringente | astringente | Stypikum | 収れん薬 |
| 473. astrocytoma - (n) | astrocytome | astrocitoma | astrocitoma | Astrozytom | ［神経膠］星状細胞腫 |
| 474. asymmetric - (a) | asymétrique | asimmetrico | asimétrico | asymmetrisch | 非対称［性］の |
| 475. asymmetry - (n) | asymétrie | asimmetria | asimetria | Asymmetrie | 非対称 |
| 476. asymptomatic - (a) | asymptomatique | asintomatico | asintomático | asymptomatisch | 無症候［性］の |
| 477. asystole - (n) | asystolie | asistolia | asistolia | Asystolie | 不全収縮［期］ |
| 478. ataxia - (n) | ataxie | atassia | ataxie | Ataxie | 運動失調 |

23

| English/American | French/Français | Italian/Italiano | Spanish/Español | German/Deutsch | Japanese/日本語 |
|---|---|---|---|---|---|
| 479. atelectasis - (n) | atélectasie | atelettasia | atelectasia | Atelektase | 無気肺、アテレクターゼ |
| 480. atherogenic diet - (n) | diète athérogénique | dieta aterogenica | dieta aterogénica | atherogene Kost | 動脈硬化をひきおこす食事 |
| 481. atheroma - (n) | athérome | ateroma | ateroma | Atherom; Belgeschwulst | アテローム、じゅく腫 |
| 482. athero-sclerosis - (n) | athérosclérose | aterosclerosi | aterosclerosis | Atherosklerose | アテローム [性動脈] 硬化 [症] |
| 483. athetosis - (n) | athétose | atetosi | atetosis | Athetose; Hammondsche Krankheit | アテトーシス、無定位運動症 |
| 484. athletic - (a) | athlétique | atletico | atlético | athletisch | 運動の |
| 485. atlanto-axial - (a) | atlanto-axial | atlo-assiale | atlantoaxial | atlanto-axial | 環軸の、環軸間節の |
| 486. atmosphere - (n) | atmosphère; air extérieur | atmosfera; aria esterna | atmósfera; aire exterior | Atmosphäre | 大気 |
| 487. atmospheric - (a) | atmosphérique | atmosferico | atmosférica | atmosphärisch | 大気の |
| 488. atmospheric pressure - (n) | pression atmosphérique | pressione atmosferica | presión atmosférica | Luftdruck | 大気圧 |
| 489. atonia - (n) | atonie | atonia | atonía | Atonie; Schlaffheit | アトニー、無緊張 [症] |
| 490. atonic - (a) | atonique | atonico | atónico | atonisch; schlaff | 無緊張性の、弛緩した |
| 491. atopy - (n) | atopie | atopia | atopia; ectopia | Atopie | アトピー |
| 492. atresia - (n) | atrésie | atresia | atresia | Atresie; Imperforation | 閉鎖 [症] |
| 493. atrial - (a) | auriculaire | atriale; auricolare | auricular; atrial | atrial; Vorhof- | 心房 [性] の |
| 494. atrial fibrillation - (n) | fibrillation auriculaire | fibrillazione atriale | fibrilación auricular | Vorhofflimmern | 心房細動 |
| 495. atrial flutter - (n) | flutter auriculaire | flutter atriale | flutter auricular | Vorhofflattern | 心房粗動 |
| 496. atrial tachycardia - (n) | tachycardie auriculaire | tachicardia atriale | taquicardia auricular | Vorhoftachykardie | 心房頻脈 |
| 497. atrioventricular node - (n) | noeud auriculo-ventriculaire | nodo atrioventricolare | nódulo atrioventricular | Atrioventrikularknoten | 房室結節 |
| 498. atrium - (n) | oreillette | atrio; vestibolo | atrio; aurícula | Vorhof; Atrium | 房 |
| 499. atrophic - (a) | atrophique | atrofico | atrofiado | atrophisch | 萎縮性の |

24

| English/American | French/Français | Italian/Italiano | Spanish, Español | German/Deutsch | Japanese 日本語 |
|---|---|---|---|---|---|
| 500. atrophy - (n) | atrophie | atrofia | atrofia | Atrophie | 萎縮 [症] |
| 501. attachment - (n) | attache; fixation | attaccatura; inserzione | unión; ligación | Befestigung; Zubehörteil | 連結、アタッチメント |
| 502. attack - (n) | attaque | attacco | ataque | Anfall | 発作 |
| 503. attempted suicide | tentative de suicide | tentato suicidio | intento de suicidio | Selbstmordversuch | 自殺未遂 |
| 504. attention - (n) | attention | attenzione | atención | Aufmerksamkeit | 注意 |
| 505. attention deficit disorder - (n) | trouble déficitaire de l'attention | disordine di deficit attentivo | trastorno de falta de atención | Aufmerksamkeitsstörung | 注意欠陥障害 |
| 506. attenuated - (a) | atténué | attenuato | atenuado | abgeschwächt | 減衰の |
| 507. attenuation - (n) | atténuation | attenuazione | atenuación | Abschwächung | 減衰、減衰作用 |
| 508. attitude - (n) | attitude; position | attitudine; posizione | actitud; posición | Einstellung; Haltung | 姿勢、態度 |
| 509. atypical - (a) | atypique | atipico | atipico | atypisch | 異型の |
| 510. audiometry - (n) | audiométrie | audiometria | audiometría | Gehörmessung; Audiometrie | オージオメトリ [一] 、聴力検査 [法] |
| 511. audit - (n) | audit; vérification | controllo; verifica | auditoria | Buchprüfung | 監査、検証 |
| 512. audit trail - (n) | enregistrement témoin | controllo a ritroso | pista de auditoria | Prüfpfad | 監査追跡 |
| 513. auditor - (n) | auditeur; vérificateur | revisore dei conti | auditor; contador | Buchprüfer | 検査官 |
| 514. auditory - (a) | auditif | uditivo | auditiva | akustisch; Gehör- | 聴覚の |
| 515. aura - (n) | aura | aura | aura | Aura | 前兆、アウラ |
| 516. aural - (a) | auriculaire | auricolare; acustico | aural | Ohr- | 耳の、前兆性の |
| 517. auricle - (n) | auricule; pavillon de l'oreille | padiglione auricolare; auricola; orecchietta | auricula; pabellón de la oreja | Ohrmuschel; Auricula | 耳介 |
| 518. auscultation - (n) | auscultation | ascoltazione | auscultación | Auskultation | 聴診 [法] |
| 519. authorities - (n) | autorités | autorità | autoridades | Behörden | 当局 |
| 520. authorship - (n) | paternité | autore; l'essere autore | paternidad | Autorschaft; Urheberschaft | 著述業 |
| 521. autism - (n) | autisme | autismo | autismo | Autismus | 自閉 [症] |
| 522. autistic - (a) | autistique | autistico | autistico | autistisch | 自閉的の |

25

| English/American | French/Français | Italian/Italiano | Spanish/Español | German/Deutsch | Japanese/日本語 |
|---|---|---|---|---|---|
| 523. autoanalysis - (n) | autoanalyse | autoanalisi | autoanálisis | Autoanalyse; Selbstanalyse | 自己分析 |
| 524. autoanalyzer - (n) | auto-analyseur | autoanalizzatore | autoanalizador | Autoanalyzer | 自動分析器 |
| 525. autoantibody - (n) | auto-anticorps | autoanticorpo | autoanticuerpo | Autoantikörper | 自己抗体 |
| 526. autoantigen - (n) | auto-antigène | autoantigene | autoantígeno | Autoantigen | 自己抗原 |
| 527. autobiography - (n) | autobiographie | autobiografia | autobiografía | Autobiographie | 自伝 |
| 528. autoclave - (n) | autoclave | autoclave | autoclave | Autoklav; Druckkessel | オートクレーブ、加圧［蒸気（自己）滅菌器 |
| 529. autograft - (n) | autogreffe | autoinnesto; autotrapianto | autoplastia | Autoplastik | 自家（自己）移植片 |
| 530. autoimmune - (a) | auto-immune | autoimmune | autoinmune | autoimmun | 自己免疫の |
| 531. autoimmunity - (n) | autoimmunité | autoimmunità | autoinmunidad | Autoimmunität | 自己免疫 |
| 532. autologous - (a) | autologue | autologo | autólogo | autolog; von sich selbst | 自己［由来］の、自系の |
| 533. autologous blood - (n) | sang autologue | sangue autologo | sangre autóloga | autologes Blut; Eigenblut | 自己血液 |
| 534. autolysis - (n) | autolyse | autolisi | autólisis | Selbstverdauung; Autolyse | 自己分解、自己溶解 |
| 535. automated data base - (n) | banque de données automatisée | base di dati automatizzata | base de datos automatizada | automatisierte Datenbank | 自動データベース |
| 536. automated DNA sequencing - (n) | séquence d'ADN automatique | sequenza ADN automatizzata | secuencia de ADN automatizada | automatisierte DNS-Sequenzierung | 自動DNAシークエンシング |
| 537. automatic data processing - (n) | traitement des données automatique | elaboratore dati automatizzato | procesamiento de datos automático | automatische Datenverarbeitung | 自動データプロセッシング |
| 538. automaticity - (n) | automaticité | automaticità | automaticidad | Automatie | 自動操作 |
| 539. automation - (n) | automatisation | automazione | automatización | Automatisierung | オートメーション |
| 540. autonomic - (a) | autonome | autonomo | autónomo | autonom; selbständig | 自律の、自律神経［性］の |
| 541. autonomic nervous system - (n) | système nerveux | sistema nervoso | sistema nervioso | autonomes Nervensystem | 自律神経系 |
| 542. autopsy - (n) | autonome autopsie | autonomo autopsia | autónomo autopsia | Leichenschau; Leichenöffnung | 部検、検死 |

| English/American | French/Français | Italian/Italiano | Spanish/Español | German/Deutsch | Japanese/日本語 |
|---|---|---|---|---|---|
| 543. auto-radiography - (n) | autoradiographie | autoradiografia | autorradiografía | Autoradiographie | オートラジオグラフィ |
| 544. autosomal dominant - (a) | autosomal dominant | dominante autosomico | autosómico dominante | autosomal dominant | 常染色体優性 |
| 545. autosomal recessive - (a) | autosomal récessif | recessivo autosomico | autosómico recesivo | autosomal rezessiv | 常染色体劣性 |
| 546. autosome - (n) | autosome | autosoma | autosoma | Autosom | 常染色体 |
| 547. auto-suggestion - (n) | autosuggestion | autosuggestione | autosugestión | Autosuggestion; Selbstsuggestion | 自己暗示 |
| 548. auxiliary - (a) | auxiliaire | ausiliario | auxiliar | zusätzlich | 下位の、二次的な |
| 549. average - (n) | moyenne | valore medio; media | valor promedio | Durchschnitt; Mittelwert | 平均 |
| 550. average - (v) | faire la moyenne de | fare la media di | calcular la media de; calcular el promedio de | den Durchschnitt ermitteln | 平均する |
| 551. average - (a) | moyen | medio | medio | durchschnittlich | 平均の |
| 552. aversion therapy - (n) | thérapie d'aversion | terapia di avversione | terapia de aversión | Aversionstherapie | 嫌悪療法 |
| 553. avitaminosis - (n) | avitaminose | avitaminosi | avitaminosis | Avitaminose | ビタミン欠乏症 |
| 554. avoidance learning - (n) | apprentissage d'évitement | l'imparare a evitare | aprendizaje de evasión | Lernen durch Vermeidung | 回避学習 |
| 555. avulsion - (n) | avulsion; extraction | avulsione; strappamento | avulsión | Absprengung; Abreißung | 剥離、捻除 |
| 556. awareness - (n) | prise de conscience | conoscenza | conciencia; conocimiento | Bewußtsein | 自覚 |
| 557. axilla - (n) | aisselle | ascella | axila | Achsel; Achselhöhle | 腋窩 |
| 558. axis - (n) | axe; axis | asse | axis; eje | Achse | 軸、軸椎 |
| 559. axon - (n) | axone | assone | axón | Axon | 軸索 |
| 560. azotemia - (n) | azotémie | azotemia | azotemia; azoemia | Azotämie | [高] 窒素血 [症] |
| 561. azygous - (a) | azygos; impair | azygos; impari | ázigos; ácigos | unpaarig | 単一の、不対の |

| English/American | French/Français | Italian/Italiano | Spanish/Español | German/Deutsch | Japanese/日本語 |
|---|---|---|---|---|---|
| 562. B lymphocyte - (n) | lymphocyte B | linfocito B | linfocito B | B-Lymphozyt | Bリンパ球 |
| 563. bacillus - (n) | bacille | bacillo | bacilo | Bazillus; Stäbchen | バチルス属 |
| 564. back - (n) | dos | dorso; schiena | espalda | Rücken | 背 |
| 565. back pain - (n) | douleur dorsale | dolore dorsale; dorsalgia | dolor de espalda | Rückenschmerzen | 背部痛 |
| 566. backache - (n) | mal de dos | mal di schiena | dolor de espalda | Rückenschmerzen | 背［部］痛 |
| 567. background - (n) | fond; antécédents | fondo; ambiente | fondo; antecedentes | Hintergrund | バックグラウンド |
| 568. background exposure - (n) | exposition antérieure | esposizione di fondo | exposición de fondo | Vorbelastung | バックグラウンド照射 |
| 569. backup candidate - (n) | candidat supplémentaire | candidato di riserva | candidato de reserva | Ersatzkandidat | 予備の候補 |
| 570. backward displacement - (n) | déplacement vers l'arrière | spostamento all'indietro | desplazamiento hacia atrás | rückwärtige Verdrängung | 後方転位 |
| 571. bacteremia - (n) | bactériémie | batteriemia | bacteremia | Bakteriämie | 菌血［症］ |
| 572. bacterial - (a) | bactérien | batterico | bacteriano | bakteriell; Bakterien- | 細菌［性］の |
| 573. bacterial capsule - (n) | capsule bactérienne | capsula batterica | cápsula bacteriana | Bakterienkapsel | 細菌莢膜 |
| 574. bacterial strain - (n) | souche bactérienne | ceppo batterico | cepa bacteriana | Bakterienstamm | 細菌株 |
| 575. bacterial toxin - (n) | toxine bactérienne | tossina batterica | toxina bacteriana | bakterielles Gift; Bakteriotoxin | 細菌毒素 |
| 576. bactericidal - (a) | bactéricide | battericida | bactericida | bakterizid | 殺菌［性］の |
| 577. bacteriological technique - (n) | technique bactériologique | tecnica batteriologica | técnica bacteriológica | bakteriologisches Verfahren | 細菌学的技術 |
| 578. bacteriology - (n) | bactériologie | batteriologia | bacteriología | Bakteriologie | 細菌学 |
| 579. bacteriophage - (n) | bactériophage | batteriofago | bacteriófago | Bakteriophage | ［バクテリオ］ファージ |
| 580. bacterium - (n) | bactérie | batterio | bacteria | Bakterium; Bakterie | バクテリア，細菌 |
| 581. bad breath - (n) | mauvaise haleine | alitosi | mal aliento; halitosis | Mundgeruch | 悪臭呼気，悪口臭 |
| 582. bad taste in mouth - (n) | goût déplaisant dans la bouche | cattivo sapore in bocca | mal sabor en la boca | übler Nachgeschmack | 口内の悪い味 |
| 583. bag of waters - (n) | sac amniotique | sacco amniotico | bolsa amniótica | Fruchtblase | 卵膜 |

28

| English/American | French/Français | Italian/Italiano | Spanish/Español | German/Deutsch | Japanese/日本語 |
|---|---|---|---|---|---|
| 584. balance - (n) | balance; équilibre | bilancia; equilibrio | balance equilibrio | Gleichgewicht | 平衡 |
| 585. balanced study - (n) | étude équilibrée | studio equilibrato | estudio equilibrado | ausgewogener Versuch | 均衡のとれた研究 |
| 586. bald - (a) | chauve | calvo | calvo | kahlköpfig; unbehaart | はげた |
| 587. baldness - (n) | calvitie | calvizie | calvicie | Kahlheit; Kahlköpfigheit | 禿頭症 |
| 588. ball and socket joint - (n) | articulation par emboîtement réciproque | articolazione sferoidale; enartrosi | articulación esférica y hueca | Kugelgelenk | 球関節 |
| 589. balloon dilatation - (n) | dilatation par ballonnet | dilatazione con palloncino | dilatación con balón | Ballondilatation | バルーン拡張 [法] |
| 590. bandage - (n) | bandage | benda; fascia | vendaje; venda | Binde; Verband | 包帯 |
| 591. bandage - (v) | bander; mettre un bandage sur | bendare; fasciare | vendar | bandagieren; verbinden | 包帯をする |
| 592. banding - (n) | cordelette | bandeggiatura | vendar | Banding; Bändelung | バンディング、染色法 |
| 593. bar code - (n) | code zèbre | codice a barra | código de barras | Bar-Code; Strichkodierung | バーコード |
| 594. bar graph - (n) | graphique en barres | diagramma a colonna | gráfico de barras | Balkendiagramm | 棒グラフ |
| 595. barbiturate - (n) | barbiturique | barbiturato | barbiturato | Barbiturat | バルビツレート |
| 596. barium enema - (n) | lavement baryté | clisma opaco; clisma baritato | enema de bario | Bariumeinlauf | バリウム注腸 |
| 597. barrel chest - (n) | thorax en tonneau | torace a botte | tórax de tonel | Faßthorax | 樽 [状] 胸 |
| 598. barrier - (n) | barrière | barriera | barrera | Barriere; Schranke | 関門, 障壁 |
| 599. basal ganglia - (n) | ganglions de la base du cerveau | gangli basali | gangliones basales | Basalganglien | 脳幹神経節、基底核 |
| 600. basal metabolic rate - (n) | taux métabolique de base | valore metabolico basale | tasa de metabolismo basal | Grundstoffwechselrate | 基礎代謝率 |
| 601. basal metabolism - (n) | métabolisme de base | metabolismo basale | metabolismo basal | Grundstoffwechsel | 基礎代謝 |
| 602. base - (n) | base | base | base | Basis; Grundlage | 基底、基礎 |

| English/American | French/Français | Italian/Italiano | Spanish/Español | German/Deutsch | Japanese/日本語 |
|---|---|---|---|---|---|
| 603. base case - (n) | cas de base | caso base | caso base | als Grundlage genommener Fall | 基本症例 |
| 604. base composition - (n) | composition de bases | composizione delle basi | composición de las bases | grundlegende Zusammensetzung | 塩基組成 |
| 605. base sequence - (n) | séquence de bases | sequenza di basi | secuencia de las bases | Basensequenz | 塩基配列 |
| 606. baseline - (n) | ligne de base; ligne de référence | valore basale; linea di riferimento | línea de base | Grundlinie | 基準線、ベースライン |
| 607. baseline data - (n) | données de base | dati di base | datos de la línea de base | Bezugsdaten | 基準となるデータ |
| 608. baseline examination - (n) | examen de base | esame di base | examen de base | grundlegende Untersuchung | 基準となる試験 |
| 609. baseline risk - (n) | risque de base | rischio di base | riesgo basal | Bezugsrisiko | 基準となるリスク |
| 610. baseline visit - (n) | visite de base | visita di base | visita inicial | Untersuchung zur Ermittlung von Bezugswerten | 基準となる来院 |
| 611. basement membrane - (n) | membrane basale | membrana basale | membrana basal | Basalmembran; Grundmembran | 基底膜 |
| 612. basic research - (n) | recherche fondamentale | ricerca di base | investigación básica | Grundlagenforschung | 基礎研究 |
| 613. basophil - (n) | basophile | cellula basofila | basófilo | Basophile | 好塩基 [性] 細胞 |
| 614. basophilic - (a) | basophile | basofilo | basófilo | basophil | 好塩基 [性] の |
| 615. batch number - (n) | numéro du lot | numero lotto | número del lote | Chargennummer | バッチ番号 |
| 616. batch to batch - (a) | de lot à lot | da lotto a lotto | de lote a lote | schubweise | バッチからバッチへ |
| 617. bath - (n) | bain | bagno | baño | Bad | 入浴 |
| 618. battered child - (n) | enfant maltraité | bambino maltrattato | niño maltratado | mißhandeltes Kind | 被虐待児 |
| 619. battery - (n) | batterie; pile | batteria; pila | batería; serie | Serie; Batterie | バッテリー、装置 |
| 620. Bayesian statistics - (n) | statistique de Bayes | statistica di Bayes | estadística de Bayes | Bayessche Statistik | ベイズ統計 |
| 621. beaklike - (a) | en forme de bec | a becco | en forma de pico | schnabelförmig | くちばしのような |

30

| English/American | French/Français | Italian/Italiano | Spanish/Español | German/Deutsch | Japanese/日本語 |
|---|---|---|---|---|---|
| 622. beard - (n) | barbe | barba | barba | Bart | 顎ひげ |
| 623. beat - (n) | battement | battito; battimento | latido | Schlag; Herzschlag | 心臓の鼓動 |
| 624. bed - (n) | lit | letto | cama | Bett | ベッド |
| 625. bed capacity - (n) | capacité de lits | capacità letti | cantidad de camas | Bettenkapazität | ベッド収容力 |
| 626. bed occupancy - (n) | occupation des lits | livello occupazione letti | camas ocupadas | Bettenbelegung | 寝台占有 |
| 627. bed rest - (n) | repos au lit | riposa a letto | reposo en cama | Bettruhe | 寝台休養 |
| 628. bedsore - (n) | escarre de décubitus | ulcera da decubito | úlcera de decúbito | Druckbrand; Decubitus | 床ずれ |
| 629. bedtime - (n) | heure du coucher | ora di andare a letto | hora de dormir | Schlafenszeit | 就寝時刻 |
| 630. bedtime dose - (n) | dose au coucher | dose prima di andare a letto | dosis a la hora de dormir | Nachtdosis | 就寝時間時の服用 |
| 631. bedwetting - (n) | énurésie nocturne | enuresi | enuresis nocturna | Bettnässen | 夜小便 |
| 632. behavior - (n) | comportement; conduite | comportamento | comportamiento; conducta | Benehmen; Verhalten | 行動 |
| 633. behavior score - (n) | score de comportement | punteggio comportamentale | puntuación de la conducta | Verhaltenspunktzahl | 行動スコア |
| 634. behavior therapy - (n) | thérapie comportementale | terapia comportamentale | terapia de la conducta | Verhaltenstherapie | 行動療法 |
| 635. behavioral - (a) | comportemental; du comportement | comportamentale; del comportamento | de la conducta | Verhaltens- | 行動の |
| 636. behavioral disorder - (n) | désordre du comportement | disordine del comportamento | trastorno de la conducta | Verhaltensstörung | 行動障害 |
| 637. belch - (n) | éructation; renvoi | eruttazione; rutto | eructo | Aufstoßen; Rülpsen | おくび |
| 638. bend backward - (v) | se pencher en arrière | ripiegarsi; piegarsi all'indietro | doblarse hacia atrás | rückwärts beugen | 後方屈折する |
| 639. bend forward - (v) | se pencher en avant | piegarsi in avanti | doblarse hacia adelante | vorwärts beugen | 前方屈折する |
| 640. bends - (n) | mal des caissons | malattia dei cassoni | enfermedad de los buzos | Taucherkrankheit; Caissonkrankheit | 屈折 |
| 641. benefit - (n) | bénéfice; avantage | beneficio; vantaggio | beneficio | Vorteil; Nutzen | 恩恵 |

31

| English/American | French/Français | Italian/Italiano | Spanish/Español | German/Deutsch | Japanese日本語 |
|---|---|---|---|---|---|
| 642. benefit - (v) | bénéficier | beneficiare | beneficiar | nützen; Vorteil haben | 利益を得る |
| 643. benefit to risk - (n) | rapport bénéfice/risque | rapporto beneficio/rischio | relación beneficio/riesgo | Nutzen-Risiko-Verhältnis | 恩恵とリスク |
| 644. benign - (a) | bénin | benigno | benigno | gutartig | 良性の |
| 645. benzodiazepine - (n) | benzodiazépine | benzodiazepina | benzodiazepina | Benzodiazepin | ベンゾジアゼピン類 |
| 646. bereavement - (n) | perte; deuil | privazione; perdita | pérdida; duelo | Trauerfall | 死別 |
| 647. best case - (n) | le meilleur cas | caso ottimale; caso migliore | mejor caso | bester Fall | 最善症例 |
| 648. beta blocker - (n) | bêtabloquant | beta-bloccante | betabloqueante | Betablocker | ベータ遮断薬 |
| 649. beta error - (n) | erreur bêta | errore beta | error beta | Beta-Fehler | β障害 |
| 650. beta receptor - (n) | récepteur bêta | recettore beta | receptor beta | Betarezeptor | ベータレセプター |
| 651. beta stimulant - (n) | bêtastimulant | beta-stimolante | beta estimulante | Betastimulans | ベータ刺激剤 |
| 652. between-patient variability - (n) | variabilité d'un patient à l'autre | variabilità tra pazienti | variabilidad entre pacientes | Variabilität zwischen Patienten | 患者間変動性 |
| 653. between treatment test - (n) | épreuve entre traitements | test intra-trattamento | prueba entre tratamientos | Zwischenuntersuchung | 治療間の試験 |
| 654. bezoar - (n) | bézoard | bezoario | bezoar; egagrópilo | Bezoar; Magenstein | 胃石 |
| 655. bias - (n) | biais; préjugé | bias; pregiudizio | propensión; prejuicio | Neigung | バイアス、ゆがみ |
| 656. bibliographic database - (n) | banque de données bibliographique | base di dati bibliografica | base de datos bibliográfica | bibliographische Datenbank | 参考文献データベース |
| 657. bibliography - (n) | bibliographie | bibliografia | bibliografía | Bibliographie | 参考文献 |
| 658. bicarbonate - (n) | bicarbonate | bicarbonato | bicarbonato | Hydrogenkarbonat | 重炭酸塩 |
| 659. biceps - (n) | biceps | bicipite | biceps | Bizeps | 二頭筋 |
| 660. bifid - (a) | bifide | bifido | bífido | zweispaltig; gespalten | 二裂の |
| 661. bifurcate - (v) | bifurquer | biforcare | bifurcarse | gabeln | 分岐する |
| 662. bifurcation - (n) | bifurcation | biforcazione | bifurcación | Gabelung; Bifurkation | 分岐 |
| 663. bigeminy - (n) | bigéminisme; pouls | bigeminismo; polso | bigeminismo; pulso | Pulsus bigeminus | 二連脈 |
| | bigéminé | bigemino | bigeminado | | |
| 664. bilateral - (a) | bilatéral | bilaterale | bilateral | zweiseitig; bilateral | 両側性の |

32

| English/American | French/Français | Italian/Italiano | Spanish/Español | German/Deutsch | Japanese/日本語 |
|---|---|---|---|---|---|
| 665. bile - (n) | bile | bile | bilis | Galle; Bilis | 胆汁 |
| 666. bile acid - (n) | acide biliaire | acido biliare | ácido biliar | Gallensäure | 胆汁酸 |
| 667. bile duct - (n) | canal biliaire | dotto biliare | conducto biliar | Gallengang | 胆管 |
| 668. bile secretion - (n) | sécrétion biliaire | secrezione biliare | secreción biliar | Gallensekretion | 胆汁分泌 |
| 669. biliary excretion - (n) | excrétion biliaire | escrezione biliare | excreción biliar | Gallenausscheidung | 胆汁排出 |
| 670. biliary tract - (n) | voie biliaire | tratto biliare | tracto biliar | Gallenwege | 胆汁路 |
| 671. bilipid membrane - (n) | membrane bilipidique | membrana bi-lipidica | membrana de doble capa lípida | Doppellipidmembran | 脂質二重膜 |
| 672. bilirubin - (n) | bilirubine | bilirubina | bilirrubina | Bilirubin | ビリルビン |
| 673. bimanual pelvic examination - (n) | examen pelvien bimanuel | esame pelvico bimanuale | examen pélvico bimanual | zweihändige Beckenuntersuchung | 双手骨盤検査 |
| 674. binary variable - (n) | variable binaire | variabilità binaria | variable binaria | binäre Variable | 二元変数 |
| 675. binding - (n) | fixation; liaison | legame | unión | Bindung; Bindemittel | 結合 |
| 676. binding - (a) | liant; fixateur | di legame | de unión; unido | bindend; verbindlich | 結合性の |
| 677. binding capacity - (n) | capacité de liaison; capacité de fixation | capacità di legare | capacidad de unión | Bindungskapazität | 結合容量 |
| 678. binding site - (n) | site de fixation; site de liaison | sito di legame | lugar de unión | Bindungsstelle | 結合部位 |
| 679. binocular - (a) | binoculaire | binoculare | binocular | binokulär | 両眼の |
| 680. binomial distribution - (n) | distribution binomiale | distribuzione binomiale | distribución binomial | Binomialverteilung | 二項の分布 |
| 681. bioassay - (n) | essai biologique | dossagio biologico | bioensayo | Lebendversuch | 生物学的検定 [法] |
| 682. bioavailability - (n) | biodisponibilité | biodisponibilità | biodisponibilidad | Bioverfügbarkeit | 生物学的利用能 |
| 683. biochemistry - (n) | biochimie | biochimica | bioquímica | Biochemie | 生化学 |
| 684. biocompatibility - (n) | biocompatibilité | biocompatibilità | biocompatibilidad | Biokompatibilität | 生体適合性 |
| 685. biocompatible materials - (n) | substances biocompatibles | materiali biocompatibili | materiales biocompatibles | biokompatible Materialien | 生体適合材料 |

33

| English/American | French/Français | Italian/Italiano | Spanish/Español | German/Deutsch | Japanese/日本語 |
|---|---|---|---|---|---|
| 686. biodegradation - (n) | biodégradation | biodegradazione | biodegradación | biologischer Abbau | 生分解 |
| 687. bioequivalence - (n) | bioéquivalence | bioequivalenza | bioequivalencia | Bioäquivalenz | 生体における等価性 |
| 688. bioethics - (n) | bioéthique | bioetica | bioética | Bioethik | 生命倫理 |
| 689. biofeedback - (n) | rétroaction biologique | biofeedback; autocontrollo biologico | biorretroacción | Biorückkoppelung | バイオフィードバック |
| 690. biogenic monoamine - (n) | monoamine biogénique | monoamina biogenica | monoamina biogénica | biogenes Monoamin | 生物起源のモノアミン |
| 691. biogenic polyamine - (n) | polyamine biogénique | poliamina biogenica | poliamina biogénica | biogenes polyamin | 生物起源のポリアミン |
| 692. biological - (a) | biologique | biologico | biológico | biologisch | 生物学の |
| 693. biological assay - (n) | titrage biologique; essai biologique | dossagio biologico | ensayo biológico | Bioassay; Lebendversuch | 生物学的検定 [法] |
| 694. biological clock - (n) | horloge biologique | orologico biologico | reloj biológico | biologische Uhr | 体内時計 |
| 695. biology - (n) | biologie | biologia | biología | Biologie | 生物学 |
| 696. biomechanics - (n) | biomécanique | biomeccanica | biomecánica | Biomechanik | 生体力学 |
| 697. biomedical engineering - (n) | génie biomédical | ingegneria biomedica | ingeniería biomédica | Biomedizinische Technik | 生物医学工学 |
| 698. biometrics - (n) | biométrie | biometria | biometría | Biometrie | 生体測定学 |
| 699. biometry - (n) | biométrie | biometria | biometría | Biometrie | 生体測定学 |
| 700. biophysics - (n) | biophysique | biofisica | biofísica | Biophysik | 生物物理学 |
| 701. biopsy - (n) | biopsie | biopsia | biopsia | Biopsie | 生検 |
| 702. biopsy needle - (n) | aiguille à biopsie | ago da biopsia | aguja de biopsia | Biopsienadel | 生検針 |
| 703. biosensor - (n) | capteur biologique | biosensore | biosensor; sensor biológico | Biosensor; Biomeßfühler | バイオセンサー |
| 704. biostatistics - (n) | biostatistique | biostatistica | bioestadística | Biostatistik | 生物統計学 |
| 705. biosynthesis - (n) | biosynthèse | biosintesi | biosíntesis | Biosynthese | 生合成 |
| 706. biotechnology - (n) | biotechnologie | biotecnologia | biotecnología | Biotechnologie | バイオテクノロジー |

34

| English/American | French/Français | Italian/Italiano | Spanish/Español | German/Deutsch | Japanese/日本語 |
|---|---|---|---|---|---|
| 707. biotrans-formation - (n) | biotransformation | biotrasformazione | biotransformación | Biotransformation; Metabolisierung | 生体内変化 |
| 708. bipolar disorder - (n) | désordre affectif bipolaire | disordine bipolare | trastorno bipolar | bipolare Psychose | 双極性障害 |
| 709. birth - (n) | naissance | nascita | nacimiento | Geburt | 出産 |
| 710. birth canal - (n) | filière pelvienne | canale del parto | canal cel parto | Geburtswege; Geburtskanal | 産道 |
| 711. birth certificate - (n) | certificat de naissance | certificato di nascita | certificado de nacimiento | Geburtsurkunde | 出生証明書 |
| 712. birth control - (n) | contrôle des naissances | controllo delle nascite | control de la natalidad | Geburtenregelung | 産児制限 |
| 713. birth control pill - (n) | pilule anticonceptionnelle | pillola anticoncezionale | píldora anticonceptiva | Antibabypille | 産児制限ピル |
| 714. birth defect - (n) | anomalie congénitale | difetto congenito | defecto congénito | Geburtsschaden | 出産異常 |
| 715. birth intervals - (n) | intervalles de naissance | intervallo tra nascite | intervalos de nacimiento | Geburtsintervalle | 出産間隔 |
| 716. birth order - (n) | ordre de naissance | ordine di nascita | orden de nacimiento | Geburtenfolge | 出生順位 |
| 717. birth rate - (n) | taux de natalité | tasso di natalità | tasa de natalidad | Geburtenziffer | 出生率 |
| 718. birth weight - (n) | poids à la naissance | peso alla nascita | peso de nacimiento | Geburtsgewicht | 出生時体重 |
| 719. birthmark - (n) | naevus; tache de naissance | nevo | marca de nacimiento | Muttermal | 先天性の皮膚斑 |
| 720. bisexual - (n) | bisexuel; hermaphrodite | bisessuale; ermafrodita | bisexual; hermafrodita | Bisexueller | 両性体 |
| 721. bisexual - (a) | bisexuel; hermaphrodite | bisessuale; ermafrodito | bisexual; hermafrodito | bisexuell | 両性の |
| 722. bisexuality - (n) | bisexualité; hermaphrodisme | bisessualità; ermafroditismo | bisexualidad; hermafroditismo | Bisexualität | 両性愛 |
| 723. bite - (n) | morsure; occlusion | morso; puntura | mordedura; oclusión | Biß; Bißwunde | 刺傷、噛むこと |
| 724. bite - (v) | mordre | mordere; morsicare | morder | beißen | 噛む |
| 725. bitter - (n) | amer; âpre | amaro | amargo | Bitterkeit | にがみ |
| 726. bizarre - (a) | bizarre | bizzarro; eccentrico | extraño; raro | bizarr; seltsam | 異様な |
| 727. black list - (n) | liste noire | lista nera | lista regra | schwarze Liste | ブラックリスト |

35

| English/American | French/Français | Italian/Italiano | Spanish/Español | German/Deutsch | Japanese/日本語 |
|---|---|---|---|---|---|
| 728. blackout - (n) | évanouissement | obnubilamento del sensorio | desmayo | kurze Ohnmacht | 一時的意識喪失 |
| 729. bladder - (n) | vessie | vescica | vejiga | Harnblase | 膀胱 |
| 730. blanch - (v) | blanchir; pâlir | sbiancare | blanquear; palidecer | erbleichen; bleichen | 漂白する、蒼白になる |
| 731. bland - (a) | fade | blando; lieve | suave | milde; reizlos | 温和な |
| 732. blank space - (n) | blanc; vide | spazio vuoto | espacio en blanco | Lücke | 空白 |
| 733. blast - (n) | cellule immature; souffle | cellula staminale; sporozoito | célula blástica; onda explosiva | Stammzelle; Explosionsdruck | …の芽細胞 |
| 734. blast crisis - (n) | crise blastique | crisi blastica | crisis blástica | Blastenschub | 急性転化 |
| 735. bleaching - (n) | décoloration | imbianchimento; imbiancamento | blanqueamiento | Bleichen | 漂白 |
| 736. bleeding - (n) | saignement; hémorragie | sanguinamento; emorragia | sangría; hemorragia | Blutung; Hämorrhagie | 出血 |
| 737. bleeding time - (n) | temps de saignement | tempo di emorragia | tiempo de sangría | Blutungszeit | 出血時間 |
| 738. blemish - (n) | défaut; tache | macchia; difetto | mancha; tacha | Fehler; Schönheitsfehler | 傷、欠点 |
| 739. blind - (v) | aveugler | accecare | cegar | blenden | 盲目にさせる |
| 740. blind - (a) | aveugle | cieco | ciego | blind | 盲目の |
| 741. blind spot - (n) | papille optique; tache aveugle | punto cieco | punto ciego | blinder Fleck | 盲点 |
| 742. blinding system - (n) | méthode en aveugle | sistema di accecamento | sistema de ceguedad | Blindstudie | 盲検方法 |
| 743. blindness - (n) | cécité | cecità | ceguera | Blindheit | 失明 |
| 744. blinking - (n) | clignotement | ammiccamento | pestañeo | Blinzeln | まばたくこと |
| 745. blister - (n) | bulle; vésicule | bolla; vesciola | bulla; vesícula | Bläschen; Blase | 水疱 |
| 746. blister package - (n) | plaquette | pacchetto trasparente | embalaje con cubierta transparente | Klarsichtpackung | 小泡治療のパッケージ |
| 747. bloated - (a) | boursouflé; gonflé | gonfio; rigonfio | hinchado | aufgetrieben; aufgebläht | むくんだ |
| 748. block - (n) | bloc; blocage | blocco | bloqueo | Block | ブロック、遮断 |
| 749. block diagram - (n) | bloc-diagramme | diagramma a blocchi | diagrama de bloques | Blockdiagramm | ブロック線図 |

36

| English/American | French/Français | Italian/Italiano | Spanish/Español | German/Deutsch | Japanese/日本語 |
|---|---|---|---|---|---|
| 750. block randomization - (n) | randomisation en bloc | randomizzazione a blocchi | randomización en bloque | Blockrandomisierung | 乱塊法 |
| 751. block size - (n) | taille des blocs | misura del blocco | tamaño de los bloques | Blockgröße | ブロックの規模 |
| 752. blockage - (n) | blocage; obstruction | blocco; ostruzione | obstrucción | Sperre | 阻害 |
| 753. blood - (n) | sang | sangue | sangre | Blut | 血液 |
| 754. blood bank - (n) | banque de sang | banca del sangue | banco de sangre | Blutbank | 血液銀行 |
| 755. blood-brain barrier [abbr] BBB - (n) | barrière hémato-encéphalique | barriera ematoencefalica, BEE | barrera hematoencefálica | Blut-Hirn-Schranke | 血液脳関門 |
| 756. blood cell - (n) | globule sanguin | cellula ematica; globulo | glóbulo sanguíneo | Blutkörperchen | 血球 |
| 757. blood cell count - (n) | numération cellulaire du sang | conta cellule ematiche | conteo de células sanguíneas | Blutzellenzählung | 血球算定 [法] |
| 758. blood chemistry - (n) | chimie sanguine | dati chimici del sangue | análisis de sangre | Blutchemie | 血液化学 |
| 759. blood clot - (n) | caillot sanguin | embolo; coagulo ematico | coágulo sanguíneo | Blutkuchen; Blutgerinnsel | 血餅 |
| 760. blood coagulation - (n) | coagulation sanguine | coagulazione ematica | coagulación de la sangre | Blutgerinnung | 血液凝固 |
| 761. blood count - (n) | hématimétrie | conta ematica; emocitometria | hematimetría | Blutkörperchenzählung | 血球算定 |
| 762. blood culture - (n) | culture sanguine; hémoculture | emocoltura | cultivo sanguíneo | Blutkultur | 血液培養 |
| 763. blood element - (n) | élément sanguin | elemento sanguigno | elemento sanguíneo | Blutbestandteil | 血液要素 |
| 764. blood factor - (n) | facteur sanguin | fattore sanguigno | factor sanguíneo | Blutfaktor | 血液因子 |
| 765. blood gas - (n) | gaz sanguin | gas ematico | gas en la sangre | Blutgas | 血液ガス |
| 766. blood group - (n) | groupe sanguin | gruppo sanguigno; emogruppo | grupo sanguíneo | Blutgruppe | 血液型群 |
| 767. blood level - (n) | niveau sanguin | livello del sangue | nivel en la sangre | Blutspiegel | 血液レベル |
| 768. blood pigment - (n) | pigment sanguin | pigmento sanguigno | pigmento sanguíneo | Blutpigment; Blutfarbstoff | 血液色素 |

37

| English/American | French/Français | Italian/Italiano | Spanish/Español | German/Deutsch | Japanese/日本語 |
|---|---|---|---|---|---|
| 769. blood platelet - (n) | plaquette sanguine | piastrina; trombocito | plaqueta sanguínea | Blutplättchen; Thrombozyt | 血小板 |
| 770. blood poisoning - (n) | septicémie; empoisonnement du sang | setticemia | envenenamiento sanguíneo | Blutvergiftung | 敗血症 |
| 771. blood preservation - (n) | préservation du sang | preservazione del sangue | preservación de la sangre | Blutkonservierung | 血液保存 |
| 772. blood pressure - (n) | pression artérielle | pressione del sangue; pressione ematica | presión arterial; presión sanguínea | Blutdruck | 血圧 |
| 773. blood protein - (n) | protéine sanguine | proteina del sangue | proteína sanguínea | Blutprotein; Bluteiweiß | 血蛋白 |
| 774. blood smear - (n) | frottis sanguin | striscio ematico | frotis de sangre | Blutausstrich | 血液塗抹標本 |
| 775. blood specimen collection - (n) | prélèvement d'échantillons sanguins | raccolta campione ematico | colección de muestras sanguíneas | Blutentnahme; Blutprobenentnahme | 血液標本収集 |
| 776. blood transfusion - (n) | transfusion sanguine | trasfusione di sangue; trasfusione ematica | transfusión de sangre | Bluttransfusion | 輸血 |
| 777. blood type - (n) | type sanguin | tipo sanguigno | grupo sanguíneo | Blutgruppe | 血液型 |
| 778. blood urea nitrogen - (n) | azote uréique sanguin | azoto ureico ematico | nitrógeno ureico en sangre | Harnstoffstickstoff im Blut | 血液尿素窒素 |
| 779. blood vessel - (n) | vaisseau sanguin | vaso sanguigno | vaso sanguíneo | Blutgefäß; Ader | 血管 |
| 780. blood viscosity - (n) | viscosité sanguine | viscosità ematica | viscosidad sanguínea | Blutviskosität | 血性粘液 |
| 781. blood volume - (n) | volume sanguin | volume del sangue | volumen sanguíneo | Blutvolumen | 血流量 |
| 782. bloodletting - (n) | saignée | salasso | sangría; efusión de sangre | Aderlaß; Blutentnahme | 放血 |
| 783. bloodshot - (a) | injecté de sang | arrossato; inflammato | inyectado en sangre; sanguinolento | blutunterlaufen | 充血した |
| 784. bloody - (a) | sanglant | sanguinante; insanguinato | sangriento; ensangrentado | blutig | 血の |
| 785. blot - (n) | tache | macchia | borrón; mancha | Fleck | しみ |
| 786. blot - (v) | tacher | macchiare; assorbire | secar; manchar | abtupfen | 吸いとる |

38

| English/American | French/Français | Italian/Italiano | Spanish/Español | German/Deutsch | Japanese/日本語 |
|---|---|---|---|---|---|
| 787. blurred vision - (n) | vision troublée | visione offuscata | visión borrosa | verschwommenes Sehvermögen | 不明瞭な視覚 |
| 788. body - (n) | corps | corpo | cuerpo | Leib; Körper | 身体、物質 |
| 789. body cavity - (n) | cavité corporelle | cavità corporea | cavidad corporal | Leibeshöhle | 体腔 |
| 790. body composition - (n) | composition corporelle | composizione corporea | composición del cuerpo | Körperzusammensetzung | 体格 |
| 791. body constitution - (n) | constitution corporelle | costituzione corporea | constitución corporal | Konstitution | 身体構成 |
| 792. body fluid - (n) | fluide corporel; liquide corporel | liquido corporeo | fluido corporal; líquido corporal | Körperflüssigkeit | 体液 |
| 793. body hair - (n) | poils corporels | peli; peluria | vello | Körperhaare | 体毛 |
| 794. body image - (n) | image corporelle | immagine corporea | imagen corporal | Körperschema | ボディイメージ |
| 795. body mass index [abbr] BMI - (n) | indice de masse corporelle | indice di massa corporea | índice de masa corporal | Körper-Massen-Index | 身体集団指数 |
| 796. body movement - (n) | mouvement corporel | movimento corporeo | movimiento corporal | Körperbewegung | 体の運動 |
| 797. body surface area - (n) | surface corporelle | superficie corporea | superficie del cuerpo | Körperoberfläche | 体表面積 |
| 798. body temperature - (n) | température corporelle | temperatura corporea | temperatura corporal | Körpertemperatur | 体温 |
| 799. body waste - (n) | excrément | escrementi | excremento | Exkrement | 身体老廃物 |
| 800. body water - (n) | eau corporelle | acqua corporea | agua del cuerpo | Körperwasser | 体水 |
| 801. body weight - (n) | poids corporel | peso del corpo | peso del cuerpo | Körpergewicht | 体重 |
| 802. boil - (n) | furoncle | foruncolo | furúnculo | Furunkel; Beule | 腫物 |
| 803. bolus - (n) | bolus | bolo | bolo | Bolus | 丸薬 |
| 804. bolus dose - (n) | dose bolus | dose bolo | dosis en bolo | Bolusdosis | ボーラス服用 |
| 805. bonding - (n) | liaison | legante | ligazón | Bindung | 結合 |
| 806. bonding agent - (n) | agent liant | agente legante | agente de ligazón | Bindemittel | 結合薬 |
| 807. bone - (n) | os | osso | hueso | Knochen | 骨 |

39

| English/American | French/Français | Italian/Italiano | Spanish/Español | German/Deutsch | Japanese/日本語 |
|---|---|---|---|---|---|
| 808. bone conduction - (n) | conduction osseuse | conduzione ossea | conducción ósea | Knochenleitung | 骨伝導 |
| 809. bone erosion - (n) | érosion osseuse | erosione dell'osso | erosión ósea | Knochenerosion | 骨侵食 |
| 810. bone fracture - (n) | fracture osseuse | frattura ossea | fractura ósea | Knochenfraktur; Knochenbruch | 骨折 |
| 811. bone graft - (n) | greffe osseuse | innesto osseo | injerto de hueso | Knochentransplantat | 骨移植 |
| 812. bone marrow - (n) | moelle osseuse | midollo osseo | médula ósea | Knochenmark | 骨髄 |
| 813. bone plate - (n) | plaque osseuse | placca ossea | placa ósea | Knochenplatte | 骨板 |
| 814. bone remodeling - (n) | remodelage osseux | ricostruzione ossea | remodelación ósea | Knochenwiederherstellung | 骨の再形成 |
| 815. bony deposit - (n) | dépôt osseux | deposito osseo | depósito óseo | Knochenablagerung | 骨性沈着物 |
| 816. bony nodule - (n) | nodule osseux | nodulo osseo | nódulo óseo | Knochenknötchen | 骨性小[結]節 |
| 817. border - (n) | bord; marge | bordo; margine | borde; margen | Rand | 境界 |
| 818. borderline - (a) | à la limite | marginale; borderline | al borde | Grenz- | 境界線の |
| 819. borderline personality disorder - (n) | désordre de personnalité marginal | disordine della personalità borderline | trastorno de personalidad fronteriza | Borderline-Persönlichkeitsstörung | 境界性人格障害 |
| 820. botanical - (a) | botanique | botanico | botánico | botanisch | 植物学の |
| 821. bottle fed - (a) | nourri au biberon | allattato artificialmente | alimentado por botella | flaschenernährt | 人工栄養で育てられた |
| 822. bottle feeding - (n) | alimentation au biberon | allattamento artificiale | alimentación con botella | Flaschenernährung | 人工栄養で育てること |
| 823. bound fraction - (n) | fraction liée | frazione ritenuta | fracción ligada; fracción unida | gebundener Anteil | 結合した（分析試料の）画分 |
| 824. bowel - (n) | intestin | intestino | intestino | Darm; Gedärm | 腸 |
| 825. bowel movement - (n) | selles | defecazione | defecación | Stuhlgang | 排泄作用 |
| 826. bowel sounds - (n) | gargouillements intestinaux | rumori intestinali | ruidos intestinales | Darmgeräusche | 腸音 |
| 827. box plot - (n) | tracé à boîtes | grafico rettangolo | gráfica en cuadros | rechteckige Darstellungsform | ボックスプロット |

40

| English/American | French/Français | Italian/Italiano | Spanish/Español | German/Deutsch | Japanese 日本語 |
|---|---|---|---|---|---|
| 828. boy - (n) | garçon | ragazzo | niño | Junge | 少年 |
| 829. braces - (n) | armatures orthopédiques; rectificateurs dentaires | sopporti; apparecchio ortodontico | aparatos ortopédicos; aparatos odontológicos | Stützapparat; Klammer | 装具 |
| 830. bradycardia - (n) | bradycardie | bradicardia | bradicardia | Bradykardie; Oligokardie | 徐脈 |
| 831. brain - (n) | cerveau; encéphale | cervello; encefalo | cerebro | Gehirn; Encephalon | 脳 |
| 832. brain abscess - (n) | abcès cérébral | ascesso cerebrale | absceso cerebral | Hirnabszeß | 脳膿瘍 |
| 833. brain chemistry - (n) | chimie cérébrale | chimica dell'encefalo | química cerebral | Gehirnchemie | 脳化学 |
| 834. brain concussion - (n) | trauma cérébral; commotion cérébrale | concussione cerebrale | concusion cerebral | Gehirnerschütterung | 脳震盪 |
| 835. brain death - (n) | mort cérébrale | morte cerebrale | muerte cerebral | Hirntod | 脳死 |
| 836. brain scan - (n) | tomographie cérébrale | tomografia dell'encefalo | tomografía cerebral | Computertomographie des Schädels | 脳スキャン |
| 837. brain stem - (n) | tronc cérébral | tronco cerebrale | tronco cerebral | (Ge)hirnstamm | 脳幹 |
| 838. brain tumor - (n) | tumeur cérébrale | tumore al cervello | tumor cerebral | Gehirntumor | 脳腫瘍 |
| 839. brain ventricle - (n) | ventricule cérébral | ventricolo cerebrale | ventrículo cerebral | Hirnkammer; Gehirnventrikel | 脳室 |
| 840. brain wave - (n) | onde cérébrale | onda cerebrale | onda cerebral | Hirnwelle | 脳波 |
| 841. branched chain - (n) | chaîne ramifiée | catena ramificata | cadena ramificada | verzweigte Kette | ［炭素鎖の］枝分かれ鎖 |
| 842. brand name - (n) | marque de fabrication | marca | marca comercial | Markenname | ブランド名 |
| 843. break in the axis - (n) | interruption de l'axe | rottura nell'asse | rotura en el axis | Bruch in der Achse | 軸の切れ目 |
| 844. breaking the blind - (n) | interruption de la méthode en aveugle | interruzione di studio cieco | interrupción del estudio ciego | Abbruch des Blindversuches | 盲目の訓練 |
| 845. breast - (n) | sein; poitrine | mammella; petto | mama; seno | Brust; Milchdrüse | 胸 |
| 846. breast fed - (a) | allaité; nourri au sein | allattato al seno | criado al pecho; amamantado | mit Muttermilch genährt; gestillt | 母乳育ちの |

41

| English/American | French/Français | Italian/Italiano | Spanish/Español | German/Deutsch | Japanese/日本語 |
|---|---|---|---|---|---|
| 847. breast tumor - (n) | tumeur mammaire | tumore mammario | tumor de la mama; tumor del seno | Brusttumor | 乳房の腫瘤 |
| 848. breastmilk - (n) | lait maternel | latte materno | leche materna | Muttermilch | 母乳 |
| 849. breath - (n) | respiration; haleine | respiro; fiato | respiración; aliento | Atem; Hauch | 呼吸 |
| 850. breath sounds - (n) | bruits respiratoires | rumore respiratorio | sonidos respiratorios | Atemgeräusche | 呼吸音 |
| 851. breathing - (n) | respiration | respiro | respiración | Atmung; Atemorgang | 呼吸 |
| 852. breathing exercise - (n) | exercice respiratoire | esercizio di respirazione | ejercicio respiratorio | Atemübung | 呼吸練習 |
| 853. breech presentation - (n) | présentation de siège | presentazione podalica | presentación de nalgas | Steißlage | 殿位 |
| 854. breeding - (n) | grossesse; gestation | allevamento | reproducción | Zucht; Fortpflanzung | 繁殖 |
| 855. brittle - (a) | fragile; friable | fragile; friabile | frágil; quebradizo | brüchig | 堅いがもろい |
| 856. broad-spectrum - (n) | large spectre | largo spettro | amplio espectro | Breitband; breites Wirkungsspektrum | 広域スペクトル |
| 857. broad-spectrum antibiotic - (n) | antibiotique à large spectre | antibiotico a largo spettro | antibiótico de amplio espectro | Breitband-Antibiotikum | 広域スペクトル抗生物質 |
| 858. broken axis - (n) | axe rupturé; axe brisé | asse fratturato; asse rotto | axis roto | gebrochene Achse | 切れた軸 |
| 859. bronchial - (a) | bronchial | bronchiale | bronquial | bronchial; Bronchien- | 気管支の |
| 860. bronchial spasm - (n) | bronchospasme | spasmo bronchiale | broncoespasmo; espasmo bronquial | Bronchialspasmus | 気管支の痙攣 |
| 861. bronchial tree - (n) | arbre bronchique | albero bronchiale | árbol bronquial | Bronchialbaum | 気管支 |
| 862. bronchiectasis - (n) | bronchiectasie | bronchiettasia | bronquiectasia | Bronchiektasie | 気管支拡張症 |
| 863. bronchiole - (n) | bronchiole | bronchiolo | bronquiolo | Bronchiole; Bronchiolus | 細気管支 |
| 864. bronchiolitis - (n) | bronchiolite | bronchiolite | bronquiolitis | Bronchiolitis | 細気管支炎 |
| 865. bronchitis - (n) | bronchite | bronchite | bronquitis | Bronchitis | 気管支炎 |
| 866. bronchoalveolar lavage - (n) | lavage bronchoalvéolaire | lavaggio bronchioalveolare | lavado broncoalveolar | bronchoalveolare Lavage | 気管支肺胞の洗浄 |

42

| English/American | French/Français | Italian/Italiano | Spanish/Español | German/Deutsch | Japanese/日本語 |
|---|---|---|---|---|---|
| 867. bronchoconstriction - (n) | bronchoconstriction | broncocostrizione | broncoconstricción | Bronchokonstriktion | 気管支収縮 |
| 868. bronchodilator - (n) | bronchodilatateur | broncodilatatore | broncodilatador | Bronchodilatator | 気管支拡張 |
| 869. bronchopulmonary dysplasia - (n) | dysplasie bronchopulmonaire | displasia broncopolmonare | displasia broncopulmonar | bronchopulmonale Dysplasie | 気管支肺形成不全 |
| 870. bronchoscopy - (n) | bronchoscopie | broncoscopia | broncoscopia | Bronchoskopie | 気管支鏡検査 |
| 871. bronchus - (n) | bronche | bronco | bronquio | Bronchie; Bronchus | 気管支 |
| 872. brow - (n) | sourcil; front | sopracciglia; fronte | ceja | Stirn | 額 |
| 873. brown fat - (n) | graisse brune | grasso bruno | grasa parda | braunes Fettgewebe | 褐色脂肪 |
| 874. bruise - (n) | contusion | contusione | contusión | Quetschung; Kontusion | 紫斑 |
| 875. bruit - (n) | bruit | rumore; soffio | soplo; sonido | Geräusch | 雑音 |
| 876. bubo - (n) | bubon | bubbone | bubón | Bubo; Leistenbeule | よこね |
| 877. buccal - (a) | buccal; oral | buccale; orale | bucal | buccal; oral | 頬の、口の |
| 878. buccal mucosa - (n) | muqueuse buccale | mucosa buccale | mucosa bucal | Wangenschleimhaut | 頬粘膜 |
| 879. budget - (n) | budget | bilancio | presupuesto | Haushaltplan | 予算 |
| 880. buffalo hump - (n) | bosse de bison | gobba di bufalo; gibbo di bufalo | cuello de búfalo; joroba de búfalo | Stiernacken | バッファローこぶ |
| 881. buffer - (n) | tampon | tampone | buffer; tampón | Puffer | 緩衝剤 |
| 882. bulging ear drums - (n) | tympan bombé; tympan protubérant | membrana timpanica protruberante | protuberancia de la membrana del tímpano | pralle Trommelhöhle | ふくらんでいる鼓膜 |
| 883. bulimia - (n) | boulimie | bulimia | bulimia | Bulimie; Adephagie | 大食 [症] |
| 884. bulla - (n) | bulle | bolla | bulla | Blase; Wasserblase | 水疱 |
| 885. bundle of His - (n) | faisceau de His | fascio di His | haz de His | Hissches Bündel; His-Bündel | ヒス束 |
| 886. bunion - (n) | oignon au gros orteil | borsite dell'alluce | bunio | Leichdorn; Ballen | 翻趾腫 |
| 887. burn - (n) | brûlure | ustione; scottatura | quemadura | Brandwunde; Verbrennung | 火傷、熱傷 |

43

| English/American | French/Français | Italian/Italiano | Spanish/Español | German/Deutsch | Japanese/日本語 |
|---|---|---|---|---|---|
| 888. burn - (v) | brûler | bruciare | quemar | brennen; verbrennen | 火傷をする |
| 889. bursa - (n) | bourse; cavité | borsa | bursa; bolsa | Sack; Beutel | 滑液嚢 |
| 890. bursal - (a) | relatif à la bourse | borsale | bursal; relacionado con una bolsa | bursal | 嚢の |
| 891. burst - (v) | éclater; éventrer | scoppiare | reventar; explotar | aufbrechen | 破裂する |
| 892. butterfly rash - (n) | éruption en papillon | eritema a farfalla | erupción en forma de mariposa | Schmetterlingsfigur | 蝶形紅斑 |
| 893. buttocks - (n) | fesses | natiche | nalga; prominencia glútea | Gesäß | 臀部 |
| 894. bypass - (n) | pontage | bypass | bypass; anastomosis | Bypass; Umgehung | バイパス |

44

| English/American | French/Français | Italian/Italiano | Spanish/Español | German/Deutsch | Japanese/日本語 |
|---|---|---|---|---|---|
| 895. cachexia - (n) | cachexie | cachessia | caquexia | Kachexie | カヘキシー　悪液質 |
| 896. cadaver - (n) | cadavre | cadavere | cadáver | Leiche | 死体 |
| 897. caffeine intoxication - (n) | intoxication à la caféine | intossificazione da caffeina | intoxicación con cafeína | Koffeinvergiftung | カフェイン中毒 |
| 898. calcification - (n) | calcification | calcificazione | calcificación | Kalzifikation; Verkalkung | 石灰化 |
| 899. calcified - (a) | calcifié | calcificato | calcificado | verkalkt | 石灰化した |
| 900. calcinosis - (n) | calcinose | calcinosi | calcinosis | Kalzinose | 石灰 [沈着] 症 |
| 901. calcium - (n) | calcium | calcio | calcio | Kalzium; Calcium | カルシウム |
| 902. calcium antagonist - (n) | antagoniste du calcium | calcio-antagonista | antagonista del calcio | Kalziumantagonist | カルシウム拮抗剤 |
| 903. calcium channel blocker - (n) | bloqueur calcique | bloccante dei canali del calcio | bloqueador de calcio | Kalziumkanalblocker | カルシウムチャンネル遮断薬 |
| 904. calcium spurs - (n) | éperons calciques | sperone di calcio | espolónes del calcio | Knochensporn | カルシウム棘突起 |
| 905. calculus - (n) | calcul; calculus | calcolo | cálculo | Stein; Konkrement | 結石 |
| 906. calibration - (n) | étalonnage | calibrazione; calibratura | calibración | Kalibrierung; Eichung | キャリブレーション |
| 907. calibration curve - (n) | courbe d'étalonnage | curva di calibrazione | curva de calibración; curva de graduación | Eichkurve | キャリブレーション曲線 |
| 908. calisthenics - (n) | gymnastique suédoise | callistenia; esercizi ginnici | calistenia | Gymnastik | 柔軟体操 |
| 909. callus - (n) | cal; durillon | callo | callo | Kallus; Knochenkallus | 仮骨 |
| 910. caloric - (a) | calorique | calorico | calórico | kalorisch; Kalorien- | 熱の |
| 911. calorie - (n) | calorie | caloria | caloría | Kalorie | カロリー |
| 912. calorimetry - (n) | calorimétrie | calorimetria | calorimetría | Kalorimetrie | 測熱 |
| 913. camera - (n) | chambre; appareil photographique | macchina fotografica; camera | cámara; compartimiento | Fotoapparat; Kammer | カメラ |
| 914. canal - (n) | canal | canale | canal | Kanal; Gang | 管 |
| 915. cancer - (n) | cancer | cancro | cáncer | Krebs | 癌 |
| 916. cancer care facility - (n) | centre de traitement du cancer | ambulatorio cura cancro | centro para el tratamiento del cáncer | Pflegeanstalt für Krebserkrankte | 癌治療施設 |

45

| English/American | French/Français | Italian/Italiano | Spanish/Español | German/Deutsch | Japanese/日本語 |
|---|---|---|---|---|---|
| 917. canine - (n) | canine | canino | canino | Eckzahn | 犬歯 |
| 918. canker - (n) | ulcère | ulcerazione | ulceración | Geschwür | 口内潰瘍 |
| 919. canker sore - (n) | chancre; ulcération aphteuse | ulcera aftosa; stomatite ulcerosa | llaga gangrenosa | Mundgeschwür | 口内びらん |
| 920. cannula - (n) | canule | cannula | cánula | Kanüle | カニューレ |
| 921. capillary - (n) | capillaire | capillare | capilar | Kapillare; Kapillargefäß | 毛細管 |
| 922. capillary dilatation - (n) | dilatation capillaire | dilatazione capillare | dilatación capilar | Kapillardilatation | 毛管拡大 |
| 923. capillary fragility - (n) | fragilité capillaire | fragilità capillare | fragilidad capilar | Kapillarfragilität | 毛管脆弱 |
| 924. capillary permeability - (n) | perméabilité capillaire | permeabilità capillare | permeabilidad capilar | Kapillarpermeabilität | 毛管透過性 |
| 925. capitation fee - (n) | forfaitaire par patient | tassa pro capite | gastos por cabeza | Kopfbetrag; Kopfgebühr | 人頭割金 |
| 926. capsule - (n) | capsule | capsula | cápsula | Kapsel | カプセル |
| 927. carbohydrate - (n) | hydrate de carbone | carboidrato | carbohidrato; hidrato de carbono | Kohlenhydrat | 炭水化物 |
| 928. carbon - (n) | carbone | carbonio | carbono | Kohlenstoff; Kohle | 炭素 |
| 929. carbon dioxide - (n) | dioxyde de carbone; bioxyde de carbone | diossido di carbonio; biossido di carbonio | dióxido de carbono | Kohlendioxid | 二酸化炭素 |
| 930. carbon monoxide - (n) | monoxyde de carbone | monossido di carbonio | monóxido de carbono | Kohlenmonoxid | 一酸化炭素 |
| 931. carbonless paper - (n) | papier autocopiant | carta copiativa senza carbone | papel autocopiante sin carbón | kohlefreies Papier | カーボンのない紙 |
| 932. carboxyhemoglobin - (n) | carboxyhémoglobine | carbossiemoglobina | carboxihemoglobina | Kohlensäurehämoglobin | 一酸化炭素ヘモグロビン |
| 933. carbuncle - (n) | furoncle | carbonchio | carbunclo | Karbunkel | 疔 |
| 934. carcinoembryonic antigen - (n) | carcinoembryonaire | carcinoembrionale | carcinoembrionario | karzinoembryonales Antigen | 癌胎児性抗原 |

| English/American | French/Français | Italian/Italiano | Spanish/Español | German/Deutsch | Japanese/日本語 |
|---|---|---|---|---|---|
| 935. carcinogen - (n) | substance cancérigène; substance cancéroçène | cancerogeno | carcinógeno | Karzinogen | 発癌物質 |
| 936. carcino-genesis - (n) | carcinogénèse | carcinogenesi; cancerogenesi | carcinogénesis | Karzinogenese | 発癌 |
| 937. carcinogenic - (a) | cancérigène; cancérogène | carcinogeno; cancerogeno | carcinogénico | karzinogen | 発癌性の |
| 938. carcino-genicity - (n) | carcinogénécité | carcinogenicità | carcinogenicidad | Karzinogenität | 発癌 |
| 939. carcinoma - (n) | carcinome | carcinoma | carcinoma | Karzinom | 癌腫 |
| 940. cardiac - (n) | cardiaque | cardiaco | cardiaco | Herzpatient; Herzmittel | 強心薬、心臓病患者 |
| 941. cardiac - (a) | cardiaque | cardiaco | cardiaco | kardial; Herz- | 心臓の |
| 942. cardiac arrest - (n) | arrêt cardiaque | arresto cardiaco | paro cardiaco | Herzstillstand | 心拍停止 |
| 943. cardiac care unit - (n) | unité de soins cardiaques | centro cardiologia | unidad coronaria | Herzabteilung | 心臓治療部 |
| 944. cardiac catheter-ization - (n) | cathétérisme cardiaque | cateterizzazione cardiaca | cateterismo cardiaco | Herzkatheter-untersuchung | 心臓カテーテル法 |
| 945. cardiac glycoside - (n) | glycoside cardiaque | glicoside cardiaco | glucósido cardiaco | Herzglykosid | 強心配糖体 |
| 946. cardiac hypertro-phy - (n) | hypertrophie cardiaque | ipertrofia cardiaca | hipertrofia cardiaca | Herzhypertrophie | 心 [臓] 肥大 |
| 947. cardiac index [abbr] CI - (n) | index cardiaque | indice cardiaco | índice cardiaco | Herzindex | 心係数 |
| 948. cardiac output - (n) | débit cardiaque | gittata cardiaca | gasto cardiaco | Herzauswurfvolumen | 心拍出量 |
| 949. cardiac rhythm - (n) | rythme cardiaque | ritmo cardiaco | ritmo cardiaco | Herzrhythmus | 心臓リズム |
| 950. cardiac shunt - (n) | shunt cardiaque | shunt cardiaco | comunicación cardiaca | Herzshunt | 心臓シャント |
| 951. cardiac tamponade - (n) | tamponnade cardiaque | tamponamento cardiaco | taponamiento cardiaco | Herztamponade | 心臓タンポナーデ |

47

| English/American | French/Français | Italian/Italiano | Spanish/Español | German/Deutsch | Japanese/日本語 |
|---|---|---|---|---|---|
| 952. cardiac volume - (n) | volume cardiaque | volume cardiaco | volumen cardiaco | Herzvolumen | 心臓容積 |
| 953. cardinal rule - (n) | règle cardinale | punto cardinale | regla cardinal | Hauptregel | 主要規則 |
| 954. cardiogenic shock - (n) | choc cardiogénique | shock cardiogeno | choque cardiogénico | kardiogener Schock | 心臓性ショック |
| 955. cardiology - (n) | cardiologie | cardiologia | cardiología | Kardiologie | 心臓学 |
| 956. cardiopulmonary bypass - (n) | pontage cardiopulmonaire | bypass cardiopolmonare | bypass cardiopulmonar | Herz-Lungen-Maschine | 心肺バイパス |
| 957. cardiopulmonary resuscitation [abbr] CPR - (n) | réanimation cardiorespiratoire, RCR | rianimazione cardiopolmonare, RCP | resucitación cardiopulmonar | kardiopulmonale Reanimation | 心肺蘇生術 |
| 958. cardiospasm - (n) | cardiospasme | cardiospasmo | cardiospasmo; espasmo cardiaco | Kardiospasmus | 胃噴門痙攣 |
| 959. cardiotonic - (n) | cardiotonique | cardiotonico | cardiotónico | Kardiotonikum; herzstärkendes Mittel | 強心薬 |
| 960. cardiotonic - (a) | cardiotonique | cardiotonico | cardiotónico | kardiotonisch | 強心性の |
| 961. cardiotoxicity - (n) | cardiotoxicité | cardiotossicità | cardiotoxicidad | Kardiotoxizität | 心臓毒性 |
| 962. cardiovascular - (a) | cardiovasculaire | cardiovascolare | cardiovascular | kardiovaskulär; Herz-Kreislauf- | 心臓血管の |
| 963. cardiovascular disease - (n) | maladie cardiovasculaire | malattia cardiovascolare | enfermedad cardiovascular | Herz-Kreislauf-Erkrankung | 心臓血管疾病 |
| 964. cardiovascular system - (n) | système cardiovasculaire | sistema cardiovascolare | aparato cardiovascular | Herz-Kreislauf-System | 心臓血管システム |
| 965. care - (n) | soins; attention | cura; attenzione | cuidado; atención | Pflege; Betreuung | 医療、看護 |
| 966. care-giver - (n) | soignant | colui presta cura | proveedor de asistencia médica | Pfleger | 看護人 |
| 967. care team - (n) | équipe traitante | gruppo medico | equipo de atención médica | Pflegegruppe | 医療チーム |

48

| English/American | French/Français | Italian/Italiano | Spanish/Español | German/Deutsch | Japanese/日本語 |
|---|---|---|---|---|---|
| 968. caries - (n) | carie | carie | carie | Karies | う蝕、カリエス |
| 969. carnal - (a) | charnel | carnale | carnal | körperlich | 肉体の |
| 970. carotene - (n) | carotène | carotene | caroteno | Karotin | カロチン |
| 971. carotid - (n) | carotid | carotide | carótida | Karotide | 頸動脈 |
| 972. carotid artery - (n) | artère carotide | arteria carotide | arteria carótida | Karotide; Arteria carotis | 頸動脈 |
| 973. carotid sinus - (n) | sinus carotidien | seno carotideo | seno carotideo | Karotissinus | 頸動脈洞 |
| 974. carpal - (a) | carpien | carpale | carpiano | karpal | 手根の |
| 975. carpal bones - (n) | os carpiens | ossa del carpo | huesos del carpo | Handwurzelknochen | 手根骨 |
| 976. carrier - (n) | porteur | portatore; vettore | portador | Träger | 保菌者 |
| 977. carrier protein - (n) | protéine porteuse | proteina vettrice | proteína transportadora | Trägerprotein | キャリア（担体）蛋白質 |
| 978. carrier state - (n) | état porteur | stato di portatore | estado portador | Übertragungsstadium | 保菌者状態 |
| 979. carry-over - (n) | reste | rimanenza | remanente | Rest; Übertrag | もちこし |
| 980. carryover effect - (n) | effet de reste | effetto rimanenza; effetto carry-over | efecto remanente | Restwirkung | もちこし効果 |
| 981. cartilage - (n) | cartilage | cartilagine | cartílago | Knorpel | 軟骨 |
| 982. case - (n) | cas | caso | caso | Fall | 症例 |
| 983. case control study - (n) | étude de cas témoin | studio caso-controllo | estudio de control de caso | Fall-Kontroll-Untersuchung | ケースコントロール研究 |
| 984. case history - (n) | anamnèse; histoire du cas | anamnesi; storia clinica | anamnesis; historia clínica | Krankengeschichte; Anamnese | 病歴 |
| 985. case record - (n) | dossier de cas | casistica | registro clínico | Krankenfallregistrierung | 症例記録 |
| 986. case report - (n) | rapport de cas | relazione medica; descrizione di un caso | informe sobre el caso | Kasuistik; Krankheitsfallbeschreibung | 症例報告書 |
| 987. case series - (n) | série clinique | serie di casi | serie ce casos | Fallserie | 症例シリーズ |
| 988. case study - (n) | étude de cas | studio caso | estudio de caso | Fallstudie | ケーススタディ |
| 989. cast - (n) | plâtre; moule | bendaggio gessato; stampo | yeso; escayola | Gips; Abdruck | ギプス包帯、鋳造物 |
| 990. casting - (n) | coulée; moulage | gesso; stampo | enyesado; escayolado | Abformen | 鋳造、鋳造物 |

| English/American | French/Français | Italian/Italiano | Spanish/Español | German/Deutsch | Japanese/日本語 |
|---|---|---|---|---|---|
| 991. castrate - (v) | castrer | castrare | castrar | kastrieren | 去勢する |
| 992. catabolism - (n) | catabolisme | catabolismo | catabolismo | Katabolismus | 異化 [作用] |
| 993. catalepsy - (n) | catalepsie | catalessi | catalepsia | Katalepsie | カタレプシー |
| 994. catalysis - (n) | catalyse | catalisi | catálisis | Katalyse | 触媒作用 [法] |
| 995. catalyst - (n) | catalyseur | catalizzatore | catalítico | Katalysator | 触媒 |
| 996. cataplexy - (n) | cataplexie | cataplessia | cataplexia | Kataplexie | 脱力発作 |
| 997. cataract - (n) | cataracte | cataratta | catarata | Katarakt; Star | 白内障 |
| 998. cataract extraction - (n) | extraction de cataracte | estrazione di cataratta | extracción de catarata | Starextraktion | 白内障摘出 |
| 999. catarrh - (n) | catarrhe | catarro | catarro | Katarrh | カタル |
| 1000. catatonia - (n) | catatonie | catatonia | catatonía | Katatonie | 緊張病 |
| 1001. catatonic - (a) | catatonique | catatonico | catatónico | kataton | 緊張病の |
| 1002. catecholamine - (n) | catécholamine | catecolamina | catecolamina | Katecholamin | カテコールアミン |
| 1003. categorical data - (n) | données catégoriques | dati categorici | datos categóricos | zu einer Kategorie gehörende Daten | カテゴリーデータ |
| 1004. categorization - (n) | catégorisation | suddivisione in categorie | categorización | Kategorisierung | カテゴリーに分けること |
| 1005. category - (n) | catégorie | categoria | categoría | Kategorie | カテゴリー |
| 1006. catgut - (n) | catgut | catgut | catgut | Catgut | 腸線 |
| 1007. catharsis - (n) | catharsis | catarsi | catarsis | Abführen; Katharsis | 浄化 |
| 1008. cathartic - (n) | cathartique | catartico | catártico | Abführmittel; Kathartikum | 下剤 |
| 1009. catheter - (n) | cathéter | catetere | catéter | Katheter | カテーテル |
| 1010. catheterization - (n) | cathétérisme | cateterizzazione | cateterismo | Katheterisierung | カテーテル法 |
| 1011. cation - (n) | cation | catione | catión | Kation | 陽イオン |
| 1012. Caucasian - (n) | Caucasien | caucasico | caucásico | Kaukasier | 白人 |
| 1013. Caucasian - (a) | caucasien | caucasico | caucásico | kaukasisch | 白人 [種] の |
| 1014. caudal - (a) | caudal | caudale | caudal | kaudal | 尾部の |

| English/American | French/Français | Italian/Italiano | Spanish/Español | German/Deutsch | Japanese/日本語 |
|---|---|---|---|---|---|
| 1015. caudate nucleus - (n) | noyau caudé | nucleo caudato | núcleo caudado | Caudatum; Nucleus caudatus | 尾状核 |
| 1016. causality - (n) | causalité | causalità | causalidad | Kausalität | 因果律 |
| 1017. cause and effect - (n) | cause et effet | causa ed effetto | causa y efecto | Ursache und Wirkung | 原因と結果 |
| 1018. cause of death - (n) | cause de la mort | causa di decesso | causa de la muerte | Todesursache | 死亡の原因 |
| 1019. cause-specific mortality - (n) | mortalité par cause spécifique | mortalità da causa specifica | mortalidad con causa específica | ursachenspezifische Mortalität | 特定原因の死亡 |
| 1020. caustic - (n) | caustique | caustico | cáustico | Ätzmittel; Kaustikum | 腐蝕剤 |
| 1021. caustic - (a) | caustique | caustico | cáustico | ätzend; kaustisch | 腐食性の |
| 1022. cauterize - (v) | cautériser | cauterizzare | cauterizar | ausbrennen; ätzen | 焼灼する |
| 1023. cavitation - (n) | cavitation | cavitazione | cavitación | Höhlenbildung | 空洞形成 |
| 1024. cavity - (n) | cavité | cavità | cavidad | Höhle | 腔 |
| 1025. cecum - (n) | cæcum | cieco | ciego | Zäkum | 盲腸 |
| 1026. ceiling effect - (n) | effet plafond | effetto limite massimo | efecto límite máximo | Maximalwert | 最高限度の効果 |
| 1027. celiac - (a) | coeliaque | celiaco | celíaco | zöliakal | 腹腔の |
| 1028. cell - (n) | cellule | cellula | célula | Zelle | 細胞 |
| 1029. cell biology - (n) | biologie cellulaire | biologia cellulare | biología celular | Zellbiologie | 細胞生物学 |
| 1030. cell clone - (n) | clone cellulaire | clone cellulare | clon celular | Zellklon | 細胞クローン |
| 1031. cell culture - (n) | culture cellulaire | coltura cellulare | cultivo celular | Zellkultur | 細胞培養 |
| 1032. cell division - (n) | division cellulaire | divisione cellulare | división celular | Zellteilung | 細胞分裂 |
| 1033. cell line - (n) | ligne cellulaire | linea cellulare | línea celular | Zellinie | 細胞系［統］ |
| 1034. cell membrane - (n) | membrane cellulaire | membrane cellulare | membrana celular | Zellmembran | 細胞膜 |
| 1035. cell wall - (n) | paroi cellulaire | parete cellulare | pared celular | Zellwand | 細胞壁 |
| 1036. cellular - (a) | cellulaire | cellulare | celular | zellulär | 細胞性の |
| 1037. cellular inclusions - (n) | inclusions cellulaires | inclusioni cellulari | inclusiones cellulares | zelluläre Einlagerungen | 細胞封入体 |

51

| English/American | French/Français | Italian/Italiano | Spanish/Español | German/Deutsch | Japanese/日本語 |
|---|---|---|---|---|---|
| 1038. cellulitis - (n) | cellulite | cellulite | celulitis | Zellgewebsentzündung | 小織炎 |
| 1039. cellulose - (n) | cellulose | cellulosa | celulosa | Zellulose | セルロース |
| 1040. cellulose - (a) | cellulosique | di cellulosa | de celulosa | Zellulose- | セルロースの |
| 1041. cement - (n) | ciment | cemento | cemento | Zement | セメント |
| 1042. center - (n) | centre | centro | centro | Zentrum; Mittelpunkt | センター |
| 1043. centigrade - (n) | centigrade | centigrado | centigrado | Grad Celsius | 百分度 |
| 1044. central - (a) | central | centrale | central | zentral; Haupt- | 中央の |
| 1045. central compartment - (n) | compartiment central | compartimento centrale | compartimiento central | Zentralkompartiment | 中央区画 |
| 1046. central laboratory - (n) | laboratoire central | laboratorio centrale | laboratorio central | Hauptlabor | 中央研究所 |
| 1047. central nervous system - (n) | système nerveux central | sistema nervoso centrale | sistema nervioso central | Zentralnervensystem | 中枢神経系 |
| 1048. central venous pressure - (n) | pression veineuse centrale | pressione venosa centrale | presión venosa central | zentraler Venendruck | 中心静脈圧 |
| 1049. centralization - (n) | centralisation | centralizzazione | centralización | Zentralisation; Zentralisierung | 集中 |
| 1050. centralized - (a) | centralisé | centralizzato | centralizado | zentralisiert | 集中型の |
| 1051. centrifugation - (n) | centrifugation | centrifugazione | centrifugación | Zentrifugation | 遠心法 |
| 1052. centrifuge - (n) | centrifugeur | centrifuga | centrifugo | Zentrifuge | 遠心器 |
| 1053. centrifuge - (v) | centrifuger | centrifugare | centrifugar | zentrifugieren | 遠心いする |
| 1054. centromere - (n) | centromère | centromero | centrómero | Zentromer | 動原体 |
| 1055. cerebellar - (a) | cérébelleux | cerebellare | cerebeloso | Kleinhirn-; zerebellär | 小脳の |
| 1056. cerebellum - (n) | cervelet | cervelletto | cerebelo | Kleinhirn; Cerebellum | 脳 |
| 1057. cerebral - (a) | cérébral | cerebrale | cerebral | zerebral; Hirn- | 大脳の |
| 1058. cerebral blood flow - (n) | irrigation cérébrale | irrigazione cerebrale | irrigación cerebral | Hirnblutfluß | 脳血流量 |

52

| English/American | French/Français | Italian/Italiano | Spanish/Español | German/Deutsch | Japanese/日本語 |
|---|---|---|---|---|---|
| 1059. cerebral cortex - (n) | cortex cérébral | corteccia cerebrale | corteza cerebral | Großhirnrinde; Cortex cerebri | 大脳皮質 |
| 1060. cerebral dominance - (n) | dominance cérébrale | dominanza cerebrale | dominancia cerebral | Seitendominanz | 大脳優位性 |
| 1061. cerebral emboli - (n) | embolie cérébrale | emboli cerebrali | embolismo cerebral | Hirnembolie | 脳塞栓 |
| 1062. cerebral ischemia - (n) | ischémie cérébrale | ischemia cerebrale | isquemia cerebral | Gehirnischämie | 脳虚血 |
| 1063. cerebral ventricle - (n) | ventricule cérébra | ventricolo cerebrale | ventrículo cerebral | Gehirnventrikel; Hirnkammer | 脳室 |
| 1064. cerebrospinal - (a) | cérébro-spinal | cerebrospinale | cerebroespinal | zerebrospinal | 脳脊髄の |
| 1065. cerebro-vascular - (a) | cérébro-vasculaire | cerebrovascolare | cerebrovascular | zerebrovaskulär | 脳血管性の |
| 1066. cerebrum - (n) | cerveau | cervello | cerebro | Großhirn; Cerebrum | 大脳 |
| 1067. certainty - (n) | certitude | certezza; sicurezza | certeza | Sicherheit | 確実性 |
| 1068. certification - (n) | certification | certificazione | certificación | Bescheinigung | 証明 |
| 1069. cerumen - (n) | cérumen | cerume | cerumen | Zerumen | 耳垢 |
| 1070. cervical - (a) | cervical | cervicale | cervical | Zervikal-; Hals-Zervix | 頸部の |
| 1071. cervix - (n) | col | cervice; collo | cuello | | 頸部 |
| 1072. cervix uteri - (n) | col de l'utérus | cervice uterina; collo dell'utero | cuello del útero | Gebärmutterhals; Cervix uteri | 子宮頸 |
| 1073. cesarian section [abbr] CS, C section - (n) | section césarienne | taglio cesareo | sección cesárea | Kaiserschnitt | 帝王切開術 |
| 1074. challenge - (n) | stimulation; provocation | stimolazione; provocazione | estímulo; provocación | Provokation; Immunitätstest | 挑戦 |
| 1075. chamber - (n) | chambre | camera; cavità | cámara | Kammer | 小室 |

| English/American | French/Français | Italian/Italiano | Spanish/Español | German/Deutsch | Japanese/日本語 |
|---|---|---|---|---|---|
| 1076. chance - (n) | possibilité; opportunité | opportunità; possibilità | casualidad; posibilidad | Möglichkeit; Zufall | 見込、機会 |
| 1077. chancre - (n) | chancre | ulcera; sifiloma primario | chancro | Schanker | 下疳 |
| 1078. change - (n) | changement; variation | cambiamento; variazione | cambio; alteración | Wandel; Veränderung | 変化 |
| 1079. change of life - (n) | ménopause | menopausa | menopausia | Menopause | 閉経 |
| 1080. change score - (n) | score de changement | punteggio di cambio | puntaje de cambio | Wechselpunktzahl | 変換値 |
| 1081. channel - (n) | canal; conduit | canale | canal | Kanal; Rille | 経路 |
| 1082. channel blocker - (n) | bloqueur du canal | bloccante del canale | bloqueador del canal | Kanalblocker | 経路遮断薬 |
| 1083. character - (n) | caractère | carattere | carácter | Charakter; Persönlichkeit | 形質 |
| 1084. characteristic - (n) | caractéristique | caratteristica | característica | Charakteristikum; Eigenschaft | 特性 |
| 1085. cheating - (n) | tromperie | imbrogliare | trampa | Betrug | ごまかし |
| 1086. checklist - (n) | liste de contrôle | lista di controllo | hoja de comprobación | Checkliste; Prüfliste | チェックリスト |
| 1087. check-up - (n) | examen médical | visita generale di controllo | chequeo; examen | Vorsorgeuntersuchung | 検診 |
| 1088. cheek - (n) | joue | guancia | mejilla | Backe | 頬 |
| 1089. chelate - (n) | chélateur | chelato | quelato | Chelat | キレート |
| 1090. chelation therapy - (n) | thérapie de chélation | terapia chelante | terapia de quelación | Chelatbildungstherapie | キレート療法 |
| 1091. chemical - (n) | substance chimique; produit chimique | prodotto chimico; sostanza chimica | producto químico; sustancia química | Chemikalie | 化学の |
| 1092. chemical analysis - (n) | analyse chimique | analisi chimica | análisis químico | chemische Analyse | 化学分析 |
| 1093. chemical burn - (n) | brûlure chimique | ustione chimica | quemadura química | Brandwunde durch Chemikalien | 化学火傷 |
| 1094. chemical development - (n) | développement chimique | sviluppo chimico | desarrollo químico | Medikamentenentwicklung | 化学の進展 |
| 1095. chemical name - (n) | nom chimique | nome chimico | nombre químico | chemischer Name | 化学薬品名 |

| English/American | French/Français | Italian/Italiano | Spanish/Español | German/Deutsch | Japanese/日本語 |
|---|---|---|---|---|---|
| 1096. chemical reaction - (n) | réaction chimique | reazione chimica | reacción química | chemische Reaktion | 化学反応 |
| 1097. chemical structure - (n) | structure chimique | struttura chimica | estructura química | chemische Struktur | 化学構造 |
| 1098. chemical synthesis - (n) | synthèse chimique | sintesi chimica | síntesis química | chemische Synthese | 化学合成 |
| 1099. chemilumines- cence - (n) | luminescence chimique | chemiluminescenza | quimioluminiscencia | Chemolumineszenz | 化学ルミネセンス |
| 1100. chemistry - (n) | chimie | chimica | química | Chemie | 化学 |
| 1101. chemolysis - (n) | chemolyse | chemiolisi | quimiólisis | Chemolyse | 化学分解 |
| 1102. chemosis - (n) | chémosis | chemosi | quemosis | Chemosis | 結膜浮腫 |
| 1103. chemotactic - (a) | chimiotactique | chemotattico | quimiotáctico | chemotaktisch | 化学走性の |
| 1104. chemotaxis - (n) | chimiotaxie | chemiotassi | quimiotaxis | Chemotaxis | 化学走性 |
| 1105. chemotherapy - (n) | chimiothérapie | chemioterapia | quimioterapia | Chemotherapie | 化学療法 |
| 1106. chest - (n) | thorax | torace | tórax | Brustkorb; Thorax | 胸 |
| 1107. chewing - (n) | mastication | masticazione | masticación | Kauen | 噛むこと |
| 1108. chiasma - (n) | chiasma | chiasma | quiasma | Chiasma; Kreuzung | 交叉 |
| 1109. child - (n) | enfant | bambino | niño | Kind | 子供 |
| 1110. child abuse - (n) | mauvais traitement des enfants | abuso minori | abuso de menores | Kindesmißhandlung | 子供虐待 |
| 1111. child care - (n) | soins des enfants | cura dell'infanzia | cuidado de los niños | Kinderpflege | 子供看護 |
| 1112. child proof container - (n) | récipient de sécurité enfants | contenitore a prova di bambino | envase a prueba de niños | kindersicherer Behälter | 子供に開けられない容器 |
| 1113. childbearing - (n) | maternité | parto; gravidanza | natalidad | Geburt | 妊娠―分娩 |
| 1114. childbearing - (a) | d'avoir des enfants | riproduttivo; fertile | fecundo; para tener hijos | gebärfähig; gebärfreudig | 妊娠可能な |
| 1115. childbirth - (n) | délivrance; accouchement | parto | parto | Geburt | 分娩 |
| 1116. childhood - (n) | enfance | infanzia | infancia; niñez | Kindheit | 幼年時代 |

55

| English/American | French/Français | Italian/Italiano | Spanish/Español | German/Deutsch | Japanese/日本語 |
|---|---|---|---|---|---|
| 1117. chill - (n) | frisson; frissonnement | infreddatura; freddo | estremecimiento; escalofrío | Kältegefühl; Schüttelfrost | 悪寒 |
| 1118. chimera - (n) | chimère | chimera | quimera | Chimäre | キメラ |
| 1119. chimeric - (a) | chimérique | chimerico | quimérico | Chimären-; chimär | キメラの |
| 1120. chimeric protein - (n) | protéine chimérique | proteina chimerica | proteína quimérica | chimäres Protein | キメラ蛋白 |
| 1121. chin - (n) | menton | mento | mentón | Kinn | 顎 |
| 1122. chiral - (a) | possédant le pouvoir rotatoire | chirale | quiral | chiral | キラル |
| 1123. chiropractic - (n) | chiropraxie; chiropractie | chiropratica | quiropráctica; quiropraxia | Chiropraxis | [脊椎] 指圧療法 |
| 1124. chi-square distribution - (n) | distribution chi-carré | distribuzione del chi quadrato | distribución de chi-cuadrado | Chi-Quadrat-Verteilung | カイ二乗分布 |
| 1125. chi-square test - (n) | épreuve chi-carré | test del chi quadrato | prueba chi-cuadrado | Chi-Quadrat Test | カイ二乗検査 |
| 1126. chloride - (n) | chlorure | cloruro | cloruro | Chlorid | 塩化物 |
| 1127. choke - (v) | s'étrangler | soffocare | sofocarse | ersticken; erwürgen | 窒息する |
| 1128. cholangiography - (n) | cholangiographie | colangiografia | colangiografía | Cholangiographie | 胆管造影（撮影）[法] |
| 1129. cholecystectomy - (n) | cholécystectomie | colecistectomia | colecistectomía | Cholezystektomie; Gallenblasenentfernung | 胆嚢摘除術 |
| 1130. cholecystitis - (n) | cholécystite | colecistite | colecistitis | Cholezystitis; Gallenblasenentzündung | 胆嚢炎 |
| 1131. cholelithiasis - (n) | cholélithiase | colelitiasi | colelitiasis | Cholelithiasis; Gallensteinleiden | 胆石症 |
| 1132. cholesterol - (n) | cholestérol | colesterolo | colesterol | Cholesterin; Cholesterol | コレステロール |
| 1133. cholinergic - (a) | cholinergique | colinergico | colinérgico | cholinerg | コリン作動 [性] の |
| 1134. cholinergic receptor - (n) | récepteur cholinergique | recettore colinergico | receptor colinérgico | cholinergischer Rezeptor | コリン作用性のレセプター |

| English/American | French/Français | Italian/Italiano | Spanish/Español | German/Deutsch | Japanese/日本語 |
|---|---|---|---|---|---|
| 1135. chondro-calcinosis - (n) | chondrocalcinose | condrocalcinosi | condrocalcinosis | Chondrocalcinose; Pseudogicht | 軟骨石灰化 [症] |
| 1136. chorda - (n) | chorda; corde | corda | cuerda; cordón | Chorda | 腱 |
| 1137. chorda tendinea - (n) | cordes tendineuses; cordage tendineux | corda tendinea | cuerdas tendinosas | Chordae tendineae; Sehnenfaden | 腱索 |
| 1138. chorea - (n) | chorée | corea | corea | Chorea | 舞踏病 |
| 1139. choreiform movement - (n) | mouvement choré forme | movimento coreiforme | movimiento coreiforme | choreatiforme Bewegung | 舞踏病的運作 |
| 1140. chorio-carcinoma - (n) | chorio-carcinome | coriocarcinoma | coriocarcinoma | Chorionkarzinom | 絨毛癌 |
| 1141. chorionic - (a) | chorionique | corionico; coriale | coriórico | Chorion- | 絨毛膜の |
| 1142. chorionic villi - (n) | villosités choriales | villi coriali | vellosidades coriónicas | Chorionzotten | 絨毛膜絨毛 |
| 1143. choroid - (n) | choroïde | coroide | coroides | Chorioidea; Aderhaut | 脈絡膜 |
| 1144. choroid plexus - (n) | plexus choroïdien | plesso coroideo | plexo coroideo | Plexus choroideus; Adergeflecht | 脈絡叢 |
| 1145. chromatin - (n) | chromatine | cromatina | cromatina | Chromatin | 染色質 |
| 1146. chroma-tography - (n) | chromatographie | cromatografia | cromatografia | Chromatographie | クロマトグラフィ |
| 1147. chromosomal deletion - (n) | délétion chromosomique | delezione cromosomi | deleción cromosómica | Chromosomendeletion; DNS-Verlust | 染色体欠失 |
| 1148. chromosome - (n) | chromosome | cromosoma | cromosoma | Chromosom | 染色体 |
| 1149. chronic - (a) | chronique | cronico | crónico | chronisch | 慢性の |
| 1150. chronic disease - (n) | maladie chronique | malattia cronica | enfermedad crónica | chronische Krankheit | 慢性病 |
| 1151. chronic obstructive pulmonary disease [abbr] COPD - (n) | maladie pulmonaire obstructive chronique | pneumopatia ostruttiva cronica | enfermedad pulmonar obstructiva crónica | chronische obstruktive Lungenerkrankung | 慢性閉塞性肺疾患 |
| 1152. chronobiology - (n) | chronobiologie | cronobiologia | cronobiología | Chronobiologie | 時計生物学 |

57

| English/American | French/Français | Italian/Italiano | Spanish/Español | German/Deutsch | Japanese/日本語 |
|---|---|---|---|---|---|
| 1153. chronology - (n) | chronologie | cronologia | cronología | zeitliche Abfolge; Chronologie | 年代学 |
| 1154. chronotropic - (a) | chronotrope | cronotropo | cronotrópico | chronotrop | 変時性の |
| 1155. chyle - (n) | chyle | chilo | quilo | Milchsaft; Chylus | キールス |
| 1156. chylomicron - (n) | chylomicron | chilomicrone | quilomicrón | Chylomikrone | カイミクロン |
| 1157. chyme - (n) | chyme | chimo | quimo | Chymus; Speisebrei | 糜汁 |
| 1158. cigarettes - (n) | cigarettes | sigaretto | cigarrillos | Zigaretten | 巻きたばこ |
| 1159. cigars - (n) | cigares | sigari | cigarros | Zigarren | 葉巻 |
| 1160. ciliary body - (n) | corps ciliaire | corpo ciliare | cuerpo ciliar | Ziliarkörper | 毛様体 |
| 1161. cilium - (n) | cil | ciglio | cilio; cilium | Flimmerhaar; Zilie | まつげ |
| 1162. cineangiography - (n) | cinéangiographie | cineangiografia | cineangiografía | Kineangiographie | 血管映画撮影 [法] |
| 1163. cineradiography - (n) | cinéradiographie | cineradiografia | cinerradiografía | Kineradiographie | シネラジオグラフィ |
| 1164. circadian rhythm - (n) | rythme circadien | ritmo circadiano | ritmo circadiano | Zirkadianrhythmus; Tagesrhythmus | 日周期リズム |
| 1165. circle - (n) | cercle | circolo | círculo | Kreis | 円 |
| 1166. circulation - (n) | circulation | circolazione | circulación | Kreislauf | 循環 |
| 1167. circulation time - (n) | temps de circulation | tempo di circolazione | tiempo de circulación | Kreislaufzeit | 循環時間 |
| 1168. circumcision - (n) | circoncision | circoncisione | circuncisión | Zirkumzision; Beschneidung | 環状切除 [術] |
| 1169. cirrhosis - (n) | cirrhose | cirrosi | cirrosis | Zirrhose | 硬変 [症] |
| 1170. clammy skin - (n) | peau moite | cute umida | piel fría y húmeda | feuchtkalte Haut | 冷たく湿った皮膚 |
| 1171. clamp - (n) | serre-joint; pince hémostatique | clamp; pinza chirurgica | clamp; pinza quirúrgica | Klammer | 鉗子、クランプ |
| 1172. clamp - (v) | clamper; pincer | clampare; pinzare | sujetar | klammern; festklammern | 締める |
| 1173. class - (n) | classe | classe | clase | Klasse; Gattung | 階級 |

| English/American | French/Français | Italian/Italiano | Spanish/Español | German/Deutsch | Japanese/日本語 |
|---|---|---|---|---|---|
| 1174. classical conditioning - (n) | conditionnement classique | condizionamento classico | condicionamiento clásico | klassische Konditionierung | 古典的条件付け |
| 1175. classification - (n) | classification | classificazione | clasificación | Klassifikation | 分類 |
| 1176. claudication - (n) | claudication | claudicazione | claudicación | Hinken | 跛行 |
| 1177. claustrophobia - (n) | claustrophobie | claustrofobia | claustrofobia | Klaustrophobie | 閉所恐怖 |
| 1178. clavicle - (n) | clavicule | clavicola | clavícula | Schlüsselbein | 鎖骨 |
| 1179. clean database - (n) | base de données nettoyée | base di dati puliti | base de datos limpia | saubere Datenbank | クリーンデータベース |
| 1180. clean file - (n) | fichier nettoyé | archivio pulito | archivo limpio | saubere Datei | クリーンファイル |
| 1181. cleaning data - (n) | données de nettoyage | dati di pulitura | datos de limpieza | Reinigungsdaten | データの整理 |
| 1182. clearance - (n) | épuration; autorisation | depurazione; autorizzazione | depuración;autorización | Klärung; Genehmigung | 浄化値、クリアランス |
| 1183. cleft - (n) | fissure | fessura | fisura | Spalte | 裂溝 |
| 1184. cleft lip - (n) | lèvre fissuré; bec-de-lièvre | cheiloschisi; labbro leporino | labio fisurado | Lippenspalte | 兎唇 |
| 1185. cleft palate - (n) | fissure palatine | palatoschisi; palato leporino | paladar fisurado | Gaumenspalte | 口蓋裂 |
| 1186. clerkship - (n) | stage hospitalier | pratica d'ospedale; internato | internado | Famulatur | 書記 |
| 1187. climacteric - (n) | climatérique | climaterio | climaterio | Klimakterium | 更年期 |
| 1188. climate - (n) | climat | clima | clima | Klima | 気候 |
| 1189. clinic - (n) | clinique | clinica; reparto ospedaliero | clínica | Klinik | 診療所 |
| 1190. clinic monitor - (n) | moniteur de clinique | monitor clinico | monitor de clínica | Überwacher der klinischen Durchführung | 診療モニター |
| 1191. clinic visit - (n) | visite à la clinique | visita clinica | visita a la clínica | Klinikbesuch | 診療のための来院 |
| 1192. clinical - (a) | clinique | clinico | clínico | klinisch | 臨床の |

| English/American | French/Français | Italian/Italiano | Spanish/Español | German/Deutsch | Japanese/日本語 |
|---|---|---|---|---|---|
| 1193. clinical assumption - (n) | hypothèse clinique | assunzione clinica | impresión clínica | klinische Annahme | 臨床的仮定 |
| 1194. clinical center - (n) | clinique | centro clinico | clínica | Klinikum | 臨床センター |
| 1195. clinical chemistry - (n) | chimie clinique | chimica clinica | química clínica | klinische Chemie | 臨床化学 |
| 1196. clinical course - (n) | cours clinique | corso clinico | curso clínico | klinischer Verlauf | 臨床コース |
| 1197. clinical deterioration - (n) | détérioration clinique | deterioramento clinico | deterioro clínico | klinische Verschlechterung | 臨床的劣化 |
| 1198. clinical development - (n) | développement clinique | sviluppo clinico | desarrollo clínico | klinische Entwicklung | 臨床開発 |
| 1199. clinical efficacy - (n) | efficacité clinique | efficacia clinica | eficacia clínica | klinische Wirksamkeit | 臨床的効能 |
| 1200. clinical endpoint - (n) | objectif clinique | obiettivo clinico | objetivo clínico | klinischer Zielpunkt | 臨床目的 |
| 1201. clinical event - (n) | événement clinique | evento clinico | evento clínico | klinisches Ereignis | 臨床上のできごと |
| 1202. clinical experience - (n) | expérience clinique | esperienza clinica | experiencia clínica | klinische Erfahrung | 臨床経験 |
| 1203. clinical importance - (n) | importance clinique | importanza clinica | importancia clínica | klinische Bedeutsamkeit | 臨床上の重要性 |
| 1204. clinical improvement - (n) | amélioration clinique | miglioramento clinico | mejoría clínica | klinische Besserung | 臨床上の改良 |
| 1205. clinical investigator - (n) | investigateur clinique | ricercatore clinico | investigador clínico | klinischer Forscher | 臨床研究者 |
| 1206. clinical investigator's brochure - (n) | brochure de l'investigateur clinique | libretto ricercatore clinico | folleto del investigador clínico | Broschüre für alle teilnehmenden Untersucher | 臨床研究者の手引き |
| 1207. clinical judgement - (n) | jugement clinique | giudizio clinico | juicio clínico | klinisches Urteil | 臨床状の判断 |

| English/American | French/Français | Italian/Italiano | Spanish/Español | German/Deutsch | Japanese/日本語 |
|---|---|---|---|---|---|
| 1208. clinical monitor - (n) | moniteur clinique | monitor clinico | monitor clínico | klinischer Überwacher | 臨床モニター |
| 1209. clinical pharmacology - (n) | pharmacologie clinique | farmacologia clinica | farmacología clínica | klinische Pharmakologie | 臨床薬理学 |
| 1210. clinical rationale - (n) | raisonnement clinicue | razionale clinico | razón clínica | klinische Gründe | 臨床原理 |
| 1211. clinical research - (n) | recherche clinique | ricerca clinica | investigación clínica | klinische Forschung | 臨床研究 |
| 1212. clinical research associate - (n) | associé de recherche clinique | associato ricerca clinica | investigador clínico adjunto | Mitarbeiter in der klinischen Forschung | 臨床研究補佐 |
| 1213. clinical response - (n) | réponse clinique | risposta clinica | respuesta clínica | klinische Reaktion | 臨床反応 |
| 1214. clinical significance - (n) | signification clinique | significato clinico | importancia clínica | klinische Bedeutung | 臨床重要性 |
| 1215. clinical signs - (n) | signes cliniques | segni clinici | signos clínicos | klinische Anzeichen | 臨床兆候 |
| 1216. clinical stage - (n) | étape clinique | stadio clinico | etapa clínica | klinische Phase | 臨床段階 |
| 1217. clinical state - (n) | état clinique | stato clinico | estado clínico | klinischer Zustand | 臨床状態 |
| 1218. clinical strategy - (n) | stratégie clinique | strategia clinica | estrategia clínica | klinische Strategie | 臨床戦略（計画） |
| 1219. clinical study - (n) | étude clinique | studio clinico | estudio clínico | klinische Studie | 臨床研究 |
| 1220. clinical symptom - (n) | symptôme clinique | sintomo clinico | síntoma clínico | klinisches Symptom | 臨床症状 |
| 1221. clinical tool - (n) | outil clinique | strumento clinico | herramienta clínica | klinisches Werkzeug | 臨床器具 |
| 1222. clinical trial - (n) | essai clinique | esperimento clinico | experimento clínico | klinischer Versuch | 臨床試験 |
| 1223. clinically significant - (a) | cliniquement significatif | clinicamente importante | de importancia clínica | klinisch von Bedeutung | 臨床的に顕著である |
| 1224. clinician - (n) | clinicien | clinico | clínico | Kliniker | 臨床家 |
| 1225. clitoris - (n) | clitoris | clitoride | clítoris | Klitoris; Kitzler | 陰核 |

61

| English/American | French/Français | Italian/Italiano | Spanish/Español | German/Deutsch | Japanese/日本語 |
|---|---|---|---|---|---|
| 1226. clockwise - (adv) | dans le sens des aiguilles d'une montre | in senso orario | en la dirección de las agujas del reloj | im Uhrzeigersinn | 右回りの |
| 1227. clone - (n) | clone | clone | clon | Klon | クローン |
| 1228. clone - (v) | cloner | clonare | clonar | klonen | クローン化する |
| 1229. clonic - (a) | clonique | clonale | clónico | klonisch | 間代性 |
| 1230. clonic movements - (n) | mouvements cloniques | movimenti clonici | movimientos clónicos | klonische Bewegungen | 間代性動作 |
| 1231. close down - (n) | fermeture | chiusura | cerrar; clausurar | Schließung | 停止 |
| 1232. close of trial - (n) | fin d'essai; fin de l'étude | fine esperimento | fin del experimento | Versuchsende | 試験の終結 |
| 1233. closed circuit anesthesia - (n) | anesthésie en circuit fermé | anestesia a circuito chiuso | anestesia a circuito cerrado | geschlossenes Narkosesystem | 閉鎖循環式麻酔 [法] |
| 1234. close-out - (n) | liquidation; termination | liquidazione | liquidación; terminación | Schließung; Räumung | 終結 |
| 1235. closure - (n) | fermeture; fin | chiusura; termine | cierre; fin | Schluß; Verschluß | 閉鎖 |
| 1236. clot - (n) | caillot | coagulo | coágulo | Klumpen; Blutgerinnsel | 凝血 |
| 1237. clot - (v) | coaguler | coagulare | coagular | koagulieren | 凝固する |
| 1238. clothes - (n) | vêtements | abiti; vestiti | vestimenta; ropa | Kleider; Kleidung | 衣服 |
| 1239. clothing - (n) | vêtements | abbigliamento; vestiario | ropa | Kleidung | 衣類 |
| 1240. clotting disorder - (n) | désordre de coagulation | disordine della coagulazione | trastorno de coagulación | Blutgerinnungsstörung | 凝固障害 |
| 1241. clotting time - (n) | temps de coagulation | tempo di coagulazione | tiempo de coagulación | Gerinnungszeit | 凝固時間 |
| 1242. cloudy - (a) | trouble; turbide | torbido; appannato | turbio | trübe | 濁っている |
| 1243. clubbing - (n) | hippocratisme | ipocratismo digitale | dedo hipocrático | keulenförmige Bindegewebsproliferation | [太鼓] ばち指形成 |
| 1244. cluster - (n) | grappe; amas | raggruppamento | agrupamiento | Anhäufung | クラスター |
| 1245. cluster analysis - (n) | analyse de grappe | analisi di raggruppamento | análisis de agrupamiento | Anhäufungsaralyse | クラスター分析 |
| 1246. coagulant - (n) | coagulant | coagulante | coagulante | Koagulans | 凝固剤 |
| 1247. coagulate - (v) | coaguler | coagulare | coagular | koagulieren | 凝固する |

62

| English/American | French/Français | Italian/Italiano | Spanish/Español | German/Deutsch | Japanese/日本語 |
|---|---|---|---|---|---|
| 1248. coagulation - (n) | coagulation | coagulazione | coagulación | Gerinnung; Koagulation | 凝固 |
| 1249. coagulation time - (n) | temps de coagulation | tempo di coagulazione | tiempo de coagulación | Gerinnungszeit | 凝固時間 |
| 1250. coarse rales - (n) | râles grossiers | rantoli grossi | estertores gruesos | grobe Rasselgeräusche | 荒い ラ音 |
| 1251. coarse rhonchi - (n) | rhonchi grossiers | ronchi grossi | roncus gruesos | grobes Röcheln | 荒い ラ音 |
| 1252. coated tablet - (n) | comprimé enrobé; tablette enrobée | pillola ricoperta | comprimido bañado; tableta bañada | Tablette mit Schutzschicht | コーチングされた錠剤 |
| 1253. cocaine addiction - (n) | cocaïnomanie | cocainomania | cocaínamanía | Kokainsucht | コカイン中毒 |
| 1254. coccyx - (n) | coccyx | coccige | cóccix | Steißbein | 尾骨 |
| 1255. cochlea - (n) | cochlée | coclea | cóclea | Kochlea; Schnecke | 蝸牛殻 |
| 1256. cochlear - (a) | cochléaire | cocleare | coclear | kochleär | 蝸牛の |
| 1257. code - (n) | code | codice | código | Kode; Vorschrift | コード |
| 1258. code - (v) | coder | codificare | codificar | kodieren | コードにする |
| 1259. code of practice - (n) | déontologie médicale | codice professionale | código de práctica | Verfahrensregeln | 開業規則 |
| 1260. coding - (n) | codage; mise en code | codice | codificación | Kodierung | コード化 |
| 1261. coding symbol - (n) | symbole de codage | simbolo di codificazione | símbolo de codificación | Kodierungszeichen | コード化シンボル |
| 1262. codon - (n) | codon | codone | codón | Kodon | コドン |
| 1263. coefficient of variation - (n) | coefficient de la variation | coefficiente di variazione | coeficiente de la variación | Variationskoeffizient | 変動係数 |
| 1264. coexisting disease - (n) | maladie coexistante | malattia coesistente | enfermedad coexistente | gleichzeitige Erkrankung | 共存する病気 |
| 1265. cognition - (n) | cognition | conoscenza | cognición | Kognition | 認識 |
| 1266. cognitive function - (n) | fonction cognitive | funzione cognitiva | funcion cognitiva | kognitive Funktion | 認識機能 |
| 1267. cognitive impairment - (n) | détérioration cognitive | alterazione cognitiva | deterioro cognitivo | kognitive Schädigung | 認識不全 |

| English/American | French/Français | Italian/Italiano | Spanish/Español | German/Deutsch | Japanese/日本語 |
|---|---|---|---|---|---|
| 1268. cogwheel rigidity - (n) | phénomène de la roue dentée | fenomeno della troclea dentata | rigidez de rueda dentada | Steifheit mit Zahnradphänomen | 歯車様強剛直 |
| 1269. cohesion - (n) | cohésion | coesione | cohesión | Kohäsion | 凝集 |
| 1270. cohort - (n) | cohorte | coorte | cohorte | Kohorte; Gruppe | コーホート |
| 1271. cohort effect - (n) | effet de cohorte | effetto coorte | efecto de grupo | Gruppeneffekt | コーホート効果 |
| 1272. cohort study - (n) | étude de cohorte | studio coorte | estudio de cohorte | Kohortenstudie | コーホート研究 |
| 1273. co-investigator - (n) | co-investigateur | coinvestigatore | coinvestigador | Mituntersucher | 共同研究者 |
| 1274. coitus - (n) | coït | coito | coito | Koitus; Beischlaf | 性交 |
| 1275. cold - (n) | rhume; froid | raffreddore; freddo | catarro; frío | Erkältung; Kälte | 感冒、寒冷 |
| 1276. cold - (a) | froid | freddo | frío | kalt | 冷たい |
| 1277. cold intolerance - (n) | intolérance au froid | intoleranza al freddo | intolerancia al frío | Überempfindlichkeit gegen Kälte | 寒冷不耐（性） |
| 1278. cold sore - (n) | herpès labial | herpes labiale | herpes labial | Herpes labialis | 口辺ヘルペス |
| 1279. cold storage - (n) | conservation par le froid | conservazione al freddo | conservación por frío | Kühllagerung | 冷蔵 |
| 1280. cold symptoms - (n) | symptômes de rhume | sintomi di raffreddamento | síntomas de catarro | Erkältungssymptome | 感冒症状 |
| 1281. colic - (n) | colique | colica | cólico | Kolik | 疝痛 |
| 1282. collaboration - (n) | collaboration | collaborazione | colaboración | Zusammenarbeit; Mitarbeit | 共同 |
| 1283. collagen - (n) | collagène | collageno | colágeno | Kollagen | コラーゲン |
| 1284. collapse - (n) | collapsus; effondrement | collasso | colapso | Kollaps | 虚脱 |
| 1285. collapse - (v) | s'effondrer; s'affaisser | avere un collasso; collassare | sufrir un colapso | kollabieren | 衰え |
| 1286. collateral - (a) | collatéral | collaterale | colateral | kollateral | 側副の |
| 1287. collateral circulation - (n) | circulation collatérale | circolazione collaterale | circulación colateral | Kollateralkreislauf; Umgehungskreislauf | 側副循環 |
| 1288. colleague - (n) | collègue | collega | colega | Kollege | 同僚 |

64

| English/American | French/Français | Italian/Italiano | Spanish/Español | German/Deutsch | Japanese/日本語 |
|---|---|---|---|---|---|
| 1289. colon - (n) | colon | colon | color | Kolon; Dickdarm | 結腸 |
| 1290. colonic - (a) | du côlon | del colon | colónico | kolisch; Dickdarm- | 結腸の |
| 1291. colonic diverticulosis - (n) | diverticulosedu côlon | diverticolosi del colon | diverticulosis colónica | Kolondivertikulose | 結腸憩室症 |
| 1292. colonoscope - (n) | colonoscope; coloscope | colonoscopio | colonoscopio | Koloskop | 結腸鏡検査 |
| 1293. colonoscopy - (n) | colonoscopie; coloscopie | colonoscopia | colonoscopia | Koloskopie; Dickdarmspiegelung | 結腸鏡検査 [法] |
| 1294. colony - (n) | colonie | colonia | colonia | Kolonie | コロニー |
| 1295. colony forming units assay - (n) | formantes colonies | test unità formanti colonie | prueba de unidades formadoras de colonias | Koloniebildungs-einheitsprobe | コロニー形成ユニットアッセイ |
| 1296. color - (n) | couleur | colore | color | Farbe | 色 |
| 1297. color blind - (a) | daltonien | daltonico | daltoniano | farbenblind | 色盲の |
| 1298. color vision - (n) | vision des couleurs | visione del colore | visión en colores | Farbensehen | 色覚視覚 |
| 1299. colorectal - (a) | colorectal | colorettale | colorectal | kolorektal | 結腸直腸の |
| 1300. colorimetry - (n) | colorimétrie | colorimetria | colorimetría | Kolorimetrie | 比色定量 |
| 1301. column - (n) | colonne | colonna | columna | Säule | カラム |
| 1302. column chart - (n) | graphique à colonnes | tabella a colonne | gráfico de columnas | Säulendiagramm | 棒グラフ |
| 1303. coma - (n) | coma | coma | coma | Koma | 昏睡 |
| 1304. combat disorder - (n) | désordre post-combat | disturbi da combattimento | trastorno post-combate | Durch Krieg hervorgerufene Störung | 闘争障害 |
| 1305. combination - (n) | combinaison | combinazione | combinación | Kombination | 組み合わせ |
| 1306. combination drug - (n) | médication combinée | farmaco composto | droga combinada | Kombinationsarzneimittel | 複合薬 |
| 1307. combined - (a) | combiné | combinato | combinado | verbunden | 結合した |
| 1308. combined centers - (n) | centres combinés | centri combinati | centros combinados | verbundene Zentren | 合同センター |
| 1309. combined data - (n) | données combinées | dati combinati | datos combinados | verbundene Daten; zusammengehörige Daten | 統合データ |

| English/American | French/Français | Italian/Italiano | Spanish/Español | German/Deutsch | Japanese 日本語 |
|---|---|---|---|---|---|
| 1310. commercial grade - (n) | classe commerciale | qualità commerciale | de grado comercial | Handelsklasse | 商業用等級 |
| 1311. commercial success - (n) | réussite commerciale | successo commerciale | éxito comercial | Erfolg auf dem Markt | 商業的成功 |
| 1312. commission - (n) | commission | commissione | comisión | Provision; Kommission | 任務 |
| 1313. committee - (n) | comité | comitato | comité | Ausschuß | 委員会 |
| 1314. common - (a) | commun | comune | común | üblich; gemeinsam | 普通の |
| 1315. common cold - (n) | rhume | raffreddore comune | catarro | Schnupfen | 感冒 |
| 1316. common protocol - (n) | protocole commun | protocollo comune | protocolo común | allgemeines Protokoll | 共通プロトコル |
| 1317. common sense - (n) | sens commun | senso comune | sentido común | gesunder Menschenverstand | 常識 |
| 1318. communicable disease - (n) | maladie transmissible | malattia contagiosa | enfermedad contagiosa | übertragbare Erkrankung | 伝染病 |
| 1319. communication - (n) | communication | comunicazione | comunicación | Kommunikation | コミュニケーション |
| 1320. community - (n) | communauté | comunità | comunidad | Gemeinschaft | 地域 |
| 1321. community based trial - (n) | étude dans une communauté | prova fatta in comunità | ensayo en una comunidad | auf ambulanter Therapie bestehende Studie | 地域試験 |
| 1322. comorbidity - (n) | comorbidité | comorbidità | comorbididad | Komorbidität | 共罹患率 |
| 1323. company - (n) | compagnie; société | società; compagnia | compañía; sociedad | Firma; Gesellschaft | 会社 |
| 1324. company culture - (n) | culture de la société | ambiente della società | cultura de compañía | Firmengeist; Firmencharakter | 会社文化 |
| 1325. comparability - (n) | comparabilité | comparabilità | comparabilidad | Vergleichbarkeit | 比較性 |
| 1326. comparability study - (n) | étude de comparabilité | studio di comparabilità | estudio de comparabilidad | Vergleichbarkeitsstudie | 比較可能的研究 |
| 1327. comparative study - (n) | étude comparative | studio comparato | estudio comparativo | Vergleichsstudie | 比較研究 |

66

| English/American | French/Français | Italian/Italiano | Spanish/Español | German/Deutsch | Japanese/日本語 |
|---|---|---|---|---|---|
| 1328. comparator medicine - (n) | médecine comparative | medicina di confronto | medicina comparativa | Vergleichermedizin | 比較測定医字 |
| 1329. comparison - (n) | comparaison | comparazione | comparación | Vergleich | 比較 |
| 1330. comparison group - (n) | groupe de comparaison | gruppo di confronto | grupo de comparación | Vergleichsgruppe | 比較グループ |
| 1331. compartment - (n) | compartiment | scompartimento; compartimento | compartimiento | Kompartiment | 区画 |
| 1332. compassionate plea protocol - (n) | protocole d'utilisation par compassion | protocollo di eccezione per compassione | protocolo de utilización por compasión | Ausnahmeprotokoll aus humanitären Gründen | 特別な配慮による（薬または治療の）プロトコル |
| 1333. compassionate use - (n) | emploi par compassion | uso per compassione | uso por compasión | Medikamentverabreichung aus humanitären Gründen | 特別な配慮による使用 |
| 1334. compatibility - (n) | compatibilité | compatibilità | compatibilidad | Kompatibilität; Verträglichkeit | 適合性 |
| 1335. compatibility trial - (n) | étude de compatibilité | test di compatibilità | ensayo de compatibilidad | Kompatibilitätsprobe | 適合性試験 |
| 1336. compelling - (a) | convaincant; irresistible | convincente; avvincente | convincente; irresistible | zwingend | 強制的な |
| 1337. compendium - (n) | compendium | compendio | compendio | Handbuch; Kompendium | 要約 |
| 1338. compensation - (n) | compensation | compenso; compensazione | compensación | Kompensation; Entschädigung | 代償 |
| 1339. competence - (n) | compétence | competenza | competencia | Kompetenz | 能力 |
| 1340. competition - (n) | compétition | competizione | competición | Konkurrenz | 競争 |
| 1341. competitive antagonist - (n) | antagoniste compétitif | antagonista competitivo | antagonista competitivo | kompetitiver Hemmstoff | 競争拮抗薬 |
| 1342. competitive bidding - (n) | enchère compétitive | offerta competitiva | ofertas en competencia | freie Ausschreibung | 競争入札 |
| 1343. competitive product - (n) | produit compétitif | prodotto competitivo | producto competitivo | Konkurrenzprodukt | 競争できる製品 |

67

| English/American | French/Français | Italian/Italiano | Spanish/Español | German/Deutsch | Japanese日本語 |
|---|---|---|---|---|---|
| 1344. complaint - (n) | maladie; symptôme | sintomo soggettivo | enfermedad; síntoma | Beschwerde | 不平、病気 |
| 1345. complement - (n) | complément | complemento | complemento | Komplement | 補体 |
| 1346. complement - (v) | compléter | complementare | complementar | ergänzen | 補う |
| 1347. complement fixation test [abbr] CFT - (n) | épreuve de fixation du complément | prova di fissazione del complemento | prueba de fijación del complemento | Komplementbindungstest | 補体結合 [反応] 検査 |
| 1348. complement receptor - (n) | récepteur du complément | recettore de complemento | receptor del complemento | Komplementrezeptor | 補体レセプター |
| 1349. complementation test - (n) | épreuve de complémentation | test di complementazione | prueba de complementación | Ergänzungstest | 相補 [性] 検査 |
| 1350. complement-fixing antibodies - (n) | anticorps de fixation du complément | anticorpi che fissano il complemento | anticuerpos de fijación del complemento | komplementbindende Antikörper | 補体結合抗体 |
| 1351. complete denture - (n) | dentition complète | dentiera completa | dentadura completa | Vollprothese | 総義歯 |
| 1352. complex - (n) | complexe | complesso | complejo; complicado | Komplex | 複合体 |
| 1353. complexion - (n) | teint | carnagione | cutis; tez | Komplexion; Gesichtsfarbe | 顔色 |
| 1354. compliance - (n) | conformité; élasticité | conformità; elasticità | conformidad; elasticidad | Einhaltung; Flexibilität | コンプライアンス、伸展性 |
| 1355. complication - (n) | complication | complicazione | complicación | Komplikation | 合併症 |
| 1356. composite - (a) | composite | composito | compuesto | zusammengesetzt | 混成の |
| 1357. compound - (n) | composé | composto | compuesto | Verbindung; Masse | 合成物 |
| 1358. compound - (a) | composé; multiple | composto | compuesto | zusammengesetzt | 複合の |
| 1359. compound patent - (n) | brevet composé | brevetto composto | patente compuesta | zusammengesetztes Patent | 複合特許 |
| 1360. compounding - (n) | composition | composizione | composición; confección | Mischen | 合成すること |
| 1361. comprehensive health care - (n) | services médicaux compréhensifs | assistenza medica completa | cobertura médica general | umfassende Gesundheitsfürsorge | 包括的健康医療 |
| 1362. compress - (n) | compresse | compressa | compresa | Kompresse | 圧迫ガーゼ |
| 1363. compress - (v) | compresser | comprimere; pressare | comprimir | komprimieren | 圧縮する |

68

| English/American | French/Français | Italian/Italiano | Spanish/Español | German/Deutsch | Japanese/日本語 |
|---|---|---|---|---|---|
| 1364. compressibili-ty - (n) | compressibilité | compressibilità | compresibilidad | Kompressionsfähigkeit | 圧縮率 |
| 1365. compression fracture - (n) | fracture par compression | frattura da compressione | fractura por compresión | Kompressionsfraktur | 圧迫骨折 |
| 1366. compulsion - (n) | compulsion | compulsione | compulsión | Zwang | 強制 |
| 1367. compulsive - (a) | compulsif | compulsivo | compulsivo | zwingend; Zwangs- | 強制的 |
| 1368. compulsive behavior - (n) | conduite compulsive | comportamento compulsivo | conducta compulsiva | Kompulsivverhalten | 強迫行為 |
| 1369. computed tomography - (n) | tomographie par ordinateur | tomografia computerizzata | tomografia computadorizada | Computertomographie | 計算断層像法 |
| 1370. computer - (n) | ordinateur | elaboratore; computer | computadora; ordenador | Computer | コンピューター |
| 1371. computer assisted - (a) | assisté par ordinateur | assistito dall' elaboratore | ayudada por computadora | computergestützt | コンピューター補助の |
| 1372. computer axial tomography [abbr] CAT - (n) | tomographie axiale par ordinateur | tomografia assiale computerizzata | tomografia axial computadorizada | Computertomogramm | コンピューター連動断層撮影 |
| 1373. computer drawings - (n) | dessins par ordinateur | disegni computerizzati | dibujos ejecutados por computadora | Computerzeichnungen | コンピューター製図 |
| 1374. computer graphics - (n) | graphiques par ordinateur | grafica computerizzata | gráficos ejecutados por computadora | Computergrafik; graphische Datenverarbeitung | コンピューターグラフィック |
| 1375. computer interface - (n) | interface par ordinateur | interfaccia computerizzata | interface de computadora | Computerschnittstelle | コンピューターインターフェイス |
| 1376. computer modeling - (n) | modelage par ordinateur | modellatura computerizzata | modelación por computadora | Modellentwurf per Computer | コンピューターモデリング |
| 1377. computer simulation - (n) | simulation par ordinateur | simulazione computerizzata | simulación por computadora | Computersimulation | コンピューターシミュレーション |
| 1378. computer terminal - (n) | terminal d'ordinateur | terminale computer | terminal de computadora | Datenstation | コンピューター端末 |

69

| English/American | French/Français | Italian/Italiano | Spanish/Español | German/Deutsch | Japanese/日本語 |
|---|---|---|---|---|---|
| 1379. computerized tomography scan [abbr] Ct scan - (n) | tomographie assistée par ordinateur | tomografia computerizzata | tomografía computadorizada | Computertomogramm | コンピューター連動断層撮影 |
| 1380. concave - (a) | concave | concavo | cóncavo | konkav | 凹の |
| 1381. conceive - (v) | concevoir | rimanere incinta | concebir | schwanger werden | 妊娠する |
| 1382. concentrating - (a) | concentrant | concentrante | concentrador | konzentrierend | 濃縮の |
| 1383. concentration - (n) | concentration | concentrazione | concentración | Konzentration | 濃度 |
| 1384. concept - (n) | concept | concetto | concepto | Konzept | 概念 |
| 1385. concept document - (n) | document conceptuel | documento di concetto | documento conceptual | Planungsdokument | 概念文書 |
| 1386. concept formation - (n) | formation conceptuelle | formazione di concetto | formación del concepto | Konzeptbildung | 概念形成 |
| 1387. conception - (n) | conception | concezione; concepimento | concepción | Konzeption; Empfängnis | 受精 |
| 1388. conclusion - (n) | conclusion; fin | conclusione | conclusión; terminación | Folgerung | 結論 |
| 1389. concomitant - (a) | concomitant | concomitante | concomitante | begleitend; gleichzeitig | 同時に生ずる |
| 1390. concomitant treatment - (n) | traitement concomitant | trattamento concomitante | tratamiento concomitante | gleichzeitige Behandlung | 付随治療 |
| 1391. concurrent - (a) | coexistant | concomitante | concurrente | parallel; gleichzeitig | 同時の |
| 1392. concurrent illness - (n) | maladie concomitante | malattia concomitante | enfermedad concurrente | gleichzeitige Krankheit | 併発病 |
| 1393. concussion - (n) | commotion cérébrale | commozione cerebrale | concusión; contusión violenta | Erschütterung | 震盪 |
| 1394. condensation - (n) | condensation | condensazione | condensación | Verdichtung; Kondensation | 濃縮 |
| 1395. condition - (n) | condition; état | condizione; patologia | condición | Zustand; Erkrankung | 状態、条件 |
| 1396. condition - (v) | conditionner | condizionare | condicionar | bedingen | 条件を設ける |
| 1397. conditioned - (a) | conditionné | condizionato | condicionado | bedingt; konditioniert | 条件付きの |

| English/American | French/Français | Italian/Italiano | Spanish/Español | German/Deutsch | Japanese/日本語 |
|---|---|---|---|---|---|
| 1398. conditioned reflex - (n) | réflexe conditionné | riflesso condizionato | reflejo condicionado | bedingter Reflex | 条件反射 |
| 1399. conditioning - (n) | conditionnement | condizionamento | condicionamiento | Konditionierung | 条件付け |
| 1400. conditioning psychology - (n) | psychologie de conditionnement | psicologia di condizionamento | psicología de condicionamiento | Konditionierungs-psychologie | 条件付け心理学 |
| 1401. condom - (n) | condom | condom | condón | Kondom | コンドーム |
| 1402. conduction - (n) | conduction | conduzione | conducción | Leitung | 伝導性 |
| 1403. conductivity - (n) | conductivité | conducibilità | conductibilidad | Leitfähigkeit | 伝導 |
| 1404. confer - (v) | conférer | conferire | conferenciar | verleihen | 相談する |
| 1405. conference - (n) | conférence | conferenza | conferencia ; congreso | Konferenz | 会議 |
| 1406. confidence interval - (n) | intervalle de confiance | intervallo di sicurezza | intervalo de confidencia | Vertrauensintervall | 信頼区間 |
| 1407. confidence limits - (n) | limites de confiance | limiti di sicurezza | límites de confidencia | Vertrauensgrenzen | 信頼限界 |
| 1408. confidentiality - (n) | confidentialité | confidenzialità | confidencialidad | Schweigepflicht; Vertraulichkeit | 秘密性 |
| 1409. confine - (n) | limite | confine; limite | límite | Grenze; Rand | 範囲、分界 |
| 1410. confinement - (n) | couches | puerperio; parto | parto; sobreparto | Bettlägrigkeit; Niederkunft | 出産、分娩 |
| 1411. confirmatory trial - (n) | essai de confirmation | test di conferma | prueba para confirmar resultados | Bestätigungsprobe | 確認試験 |
| 1412. conflict - (n) | conflit | conflitto | conflicto | Konflikt | 衝突 |
| 1413. conflict of interest - (n) | conflit d'intérêts | conflitto d'interessi | conflicto de intereses | Interessenkonflikt | 利害の衝突 |
| 1414. conformation - (n) | conformation | conformazione | conformación | Konformation; Anpassung | 立体配座 |
| 1415. confounding - (a) | confondant; confus | confondente | confundido | verwirrend | 混乱させる |
| 1416. confounding factor - (n) | facteur de confusien | fattore confondente | factor de confusión | Störfaktor | 混乱 (困惑) 因子 |

71

| English/American | French/Français | Italian/Italiano | Spanish/Español | German/Deutsch | Japanese/日本語 |
|---|---|---|---|---|---|
| 1417. confounding variable -(n) | variable de confusion | variabile confondente | variable de confusión | Störvariable | 交絡変数 |
| 1418. confusion - (n) | confusion | confusione | confusión | Verwirrung; Verwirrtheit | 錯乱（状態） |
| 1419. congener - (n) | congénère | congenere | congénere | Verwandter | 同類 |
| 1420. congenital - (a) | congénital | congenito | congénito | kongenital; ererbt | 先天性の |
| 1421. congestion - (n) | congestion | congestione | congestión | Kongestion; Anschoppung | 充血 |
| 1422. congestive - (a) | congestif | congestizio | congestivo | kongestiv | 鬱血性の |
| 1423. congestive heart failure - (n) | insuffisance cardiaque | insuffizienza cardiaca | insuficiencia cardiaca | Herzinsuffizierz | 鬱血性心不全 |
| 1424. congress - (n) | coït | coito | coito | Koitus; Geschlechtsverkehr | 性交、交合 |
| 1425. conjugate - (n) | conjugué | coniugato | conjugado | Beckendurchmesser; Conjugata | 共役 |
| 1426. conjugated - (a) | conjugué | coniugato | conjugado | gekoppelt | 共役の |
| 1427. conjugation - (n) | conjugaison | coniugazione | conjugación | Konjugation | 接合 |
| 1428. conjunctiva - (n) | conjonctive | congiuntiva | conjuntiva | Konjunktiva; Bindehaut | 結膜 |
| 1429. connection - (n) | jonction; liaison | connessione; rapporto | conexión | Verbindung | 接続 |
| 1430. connective tissue - (n) | tissu conjonctif | tessuto connettivo | tejido conectivo | Bindegewebe | 結合組織 |
| 1431. consanguinity - (n) | consanguinité | consanguineo | consanguinidad | Blutverwandschaft | 血族 |
| 1432. conscience - (n) | conscience | coscienza | conciencia | Gewissen | 良心 |
| 1433. conscious - (a) | conscient | cosciente | consciente | bewußt | 意識のある |
| 1434. conscious-ness - (n) | conscience | coscienza | consciencia | Bewußtsein | 意識 |
| 1435. consecutive - (a) | consécutif | consecutivo | consecutivo | aufeinanderfolgend | 連続的な |
| 1436. consensus - (n) | consensus | consenso | consenso | Übereinstimmung | 世論 |
| 1437. consent - (n) | consentement | consenso | consentimiento | Zustimmung | 同意 |
| 1438. consent - (v) | consentir | consentire | consentir | zustimmen | 同意する |

72

| English/American | French/Français | Italian/Italiano | Spanish/Español | German/Deutsch | Japanese/日本語 |
|---|---|---|---|---|---|
| 1439. conservation - (n) | conservation | conservazione | conservación | Konservierung; Erhaltung | 保存 |
| 1440. consolidation - (n) | consolidation | consolidamento | consolidación | Konsolidierung | 硬化 |
| 1441. constant infusion - (n) | infusion constante | infusione costante | infusión constante | Dauerinfusion | 連続注入 |
| 1442. constipation - (n) | constipation | costipazione | constipación | Verstopfung; Obstipation | 便秘 |
| 1443. constriction - (n) | constriction; étranglement | costrizione; contrazione | constricción; estrechamiento | Konstriktion; Einschnürung | 絞扼 |
| 1444. construction - (n) | construction | costruzione | construcción | Bau; Konstruktion | 構造 |
| 1445. consultant - (n) | consultant | consultatore; consulente | consultor | Berater; Konsiliararzt | 顧問医師 |
| 1446. consultation - (n) | consultation | consulto | consulta | Konsultation; Beratung | 診察をうけること |
| 1447. consume - (v) | consommer | consumare | consumir | verbrauchen; konsumieren | 消費する |
| 1448. consumer - (n) | consommateur | consumatore | consumidor | Verbraucher | 消費者 |
| 1449. consumer group - (n) | groupe de consommateurs | gruppo consumatori | grupo de consumidores | Verbrauchergruppe | 消費者グループ |
| 1450. contact - (n) | contact | contatto | contacto | Kontakt | 接触 |
| 1451. contact - (v) | se mettre en contact | mettersi in contatto | comunicar con | berühren; sich in Verbindung setzen | 接触する |
| 1452. contact dermatitis - (n) | dermatite de contact | dermatite da contatto | dermatitis de contacto | Kontaktdermatitis | 接触性皮膚炎 |
| 1453. contact lens - (n) | verre de contact | lente a contatto | lente de contacto | Kontaktlinse | コンタクトレンズ |
| 1454. contagious - (a) | contagieux | contagioso | contagioso | kontagiös; ansteckend | 伝染性の |
| 1455. container - (n) | récipient; réservoir | contenitore; recipiente | recipiente; receptáculo | Behälter; Gefäß | 容器 |
| 1456. containment - (n) | contention | ritegno | contención | Eindämmung | 封じ込め収束 |
| 1457. contaminate - (v) | contaminer | contaminare | contaminar | kontaminieren; verunreinigen | 汚染する |
| 1458. contamination - (n) | contamination | contaminazione | contaminación | Kontamination; Verunreinigung | 汚染 |

73

| English/American | French/Français | Italian/Italiano | Spanish/Español | German/Deutsch | Japanese/日本語 |
|---|---|---|---|---|---|
| 1459. content uniformity - (n) | uniformité du contenu | uniformità contenuto | uniformidad del contenido | Gleichheit des Inhalts | 内容の一様性 |
| 1460. content validity - (n) | validité du contenu | validità contenuto | validez del contenido | Validität des Inhalts | 内容の正当性 |
| 1461. contingency plan - (n) | plan d'urgence | piano contingente | medida de prevención | Ausweichplan | 万一の場合の計画 |
| 1462. contingency table - (n) | tableau de contingence | tabella di contingenza | tabla de contingencia | Kontigenztafel | 分割表 |
| 1463. continuation protocol - (n) | protocole de continuité | protocollo di continuità | protocolo de continuación | Fortsetzungsprotokoll | 継続プロトロル |
| 1464. continued - (a) | continué | continuo | continuado | weiterführend | 引き続きの |
| 1465. continuing education - (n) | formation continue | educazione continua | cursos avanzados | Weiterbildung | 継続教育 |
| 1466. continuity of patient care - (n) | soins continus du patient | cura continua dei pazienti | cuidado continuo del paciente | ununterbrochene Patientenpflege | 患者治療の継続 |
| 1467. continuous - (a) | continu | continuo | continuo | ununterbrochen, Dauer- | 連続した |
| 1468. continuous IV line - (n) | injection intraveineuse continue | infusione intravenosa continua | infusión intravenosa continua | intravenöser Dauerkatheter | 連続IVライン |
| 1469. continuum - (n) | continuum | continuo | continuo | Kontinuum | 連続体 |
| 1470. contraception - (n) | contraception | contraccezione | contracepción | Kontrazeption | 避妊 |
| 1471. contraceptive - (n) | contraceptif | contraccettivo; anticoncezionale | contraceptivo ; anticonceptivo | Verhütungsmittel; Kontrazeptivum | 避妊薬 |
| 1472. contraceptive - (a) | contraceptif; anticonceptionnel | contraccettivo; antifecondativo | contraceptivo; anticonceptivo | kontrazeptiv | 避妊の |
| 1473. contract - (n) | contrat | contratto | contrato | Vertrag | 契約 |
| 1474. contract - (v) | contracter | contrarre; contrarsi | contratar | zusammenziehen; sich zuziehen | 収縮する、病気にかかる |
| 1475. contract house - (n) | firme à contrat | azienda a contratto | firma contratada | Vertragsfirma | 契約建物 |

| English/American | French/Français | Italian/Italiano | Spanish/Español | German/Deutsch | Japanese/日本語 |
|---|---|---|---|---|---|
| 1476. contract laboratory - (n) | laboratoire à contrat;; laboratoire forfaitaire | laboratorio a contratto | laboratorio bajo contrato | Vertragslabor | 契約研究所 |
| 1477. contract manufacturer - (n) | fabricant à contrat; fabricant forfaitaire | manifattura a contratto | fabricante contratado | Vertragshersteller | 契約製造者 |
| 1478. contract office - (n) | service à contrat; service forfaitaire | ufficio a contratto | oficina contratada | Vertragsbüro | 契約事務所 |
| 1479. contract organization - (n) | organisation à contrat; organisation forfaitaire | organizzazione a contratto | organización contratada | Vertragsorganisation | 契約団体 |
| 1480. contract research - (n) | recherche à contrat; recherche forfaitaire | ricerca contratto | investigación por contrato | Vertragsforschung | 契約研究 |
| 1481. contract research organization - (n) | organisation de recherches à contrat; organisation de recherches forfaitaires | organizzazione di ricerca a contratto | organización investigadora contratada | Vertragsforschungs-organisation | 契約研究団体 |
| 1482. contract services - (n) | services à contrat; services forfaitaires | servizi a contratto | servicios contratados | vertraglich festgelegte Kundendienstleistungen | 契約サービス |
| 1483. contraction - (n) | contraction | contrazione | contracción | Kontraktion | 収縮 |
| 1484. contractor - (n) | muscle contractant | contraente; muscolo contrattile | contratista; músculo contráctil | beauftragte Firma; Schließsmuskel | 契約者、収縮筋 |
| 1485. contracture - (n) | contracture | contrattura | contractura | Kontraktur | 拘縮 |
| 1486. contra-indication - (n) | contre-indication | controindicazione | contraindicación | Kontraindikation | 禁忌 |
| 1487. contralateral - (a) | contralatéral | controlaterale | contralateral | kontralateral | （反）対側性の |
| 1488. contrast - (n) | contraste | contrasto | contraste | Kontrast | 対比 |
| 1489. contrast medium - (n) | agent de contraste | mezzo di contrasto | medio de contraste | Kontrastmedium | 造影剤 |
| 1490. contrecoup - (n) | contrecoup | contraccolpo | contragolpe | Gegenstoß; Gegenschlag | 対側衝撃 |
| 1491. control - (n) | contrôle | controllo | control | Kontrolle; Steuerung | 調節、制御 |

| English/American | French/Français | Italian/Italiano | Spanish/Español | German/Deutsch | Japanese/日本語 |
|---|---|---|---|---|---|
| 1492. control - (v) | contrôler | controllare | controlar | kontrollieren; steuern | 調節 [制御] する |
| 1493. control group - (n) | groupe de contrôle; groupe témoin | gruppo di controllo | grupo de control | Kontrollgruppe | 対照群 |
| 1494. control patient - (n) | patient de contrôle; patient témoin | paziente di controllo | paciente de control | Kontrollpatient | 対照群の患者 |
| 1495. control treatment - (n) | traitement de contrôle; traitement témoin | trattamento di controllo | tratamiento de control | Kontrollbehandlung | 対照群のための治療 |
| 1496. control value - (n) | valeur de contrôle; valeur témoin | valore di controllo | valor de control | Kontrollwert | 対照群の値 |
| 1497. controlled release technology - (n) | technologie de libération contrôlée | tecnica di rilascio controllato | tecnología de liberación controlada | Technik mit kontrollierter Freisetzung | 制御解除技術 |
| 1498. controlled trial - (n) | essai contrôlé; étude contrôlée | sperimentazione controllata | estudio controlado | kontrollierte Studie; kontrollierter Versuch | 制御された試験 |
| 1499. controversy - (n) | controverse | controversia | controversia | Kontroverse | 議論 |
| 1500. contusion - (n) | contusion | contusione | contusión | Kontusion; Quetschung | 挫傷 |
| 1501. convalescence - (n) | convalescence | convalescenza | convalescencia | Rekonvaleszenz; Genesung | 回復期 |
| 1502. convention - (n) | convention | convegno | convenio; convención | Tagung | 協議会 |
| 1503. converting - (n) | conversion | conversione | conversión | Umwandlung | 変換 |
| 1504. convex - (a) | convexe | convesso | convexo | konvex | 凸の |
| 1505. convulsion - (n) | convulsion | convulsione | convulsión | Konvulsion | 痙攣 |
| 1506. convulsive disorder - (n) | désordre convulsif | disordine convulsivo | trastorno convulsivo | Konvulsionsstörung | 痙攣性障害 |
| 1507. coordinate - (n) | coordonnée | coordinata | coordenada | Koordinate | 座標 |
| 1508. coordinating center - (n) | centre de coordination | centro coordinatore | centro coordinador | Koordinationszentrum | コーディネートセンター |
| 1509. coordination - (n) | coordination | coordinazione | coordinación | Koordination | 整合 |
| 1510. copulation - (n) | copulation | copulazione | cópula | Kopulation; Beischlaf | 性交 |
| 1511. cord - (n) | cordon | corda | cordón | Schnur | 帯 |

76

| English/American | French/Français | Italian/Italiano | Spanish/Español | German/Deutsch | Japanese/日本語 |
|---|---|---|---|---|---|
| 1512. corn - (n) | cor; durillon | callo | cuerno; callo | Hühnerauge; Klavus | うおのめ |
| 1513. cornea - (n) | cornée | cornea | córnea | Hornhaut des Auges | 角膜 |
| 1514. corneal - (a) | cornéen | corneale; corneo | corneal; de la córnea | korneal | 角膜の |
| 1515. corneal reflex - (n) | réflexe cornéen | riflesso corneale | reflejo corneal | Kornealreflex; Hornhautreflex | 角膜反射 |
| 1516. coronary - (a) | coronaire | coronario | coronaria | Koronar- | 冠状の |
| 1517. coronary artery - (n) | artère coronaire | arteria coronaria | arteria coronaria | Koronararterie | 冠状動脈 |
| 1518. coronary by-pass - (n) | pontage coronaire; pontage coronarien | bypass coronarico | bypass coronaria; puente coronario | Koronararterien-Bypass | 冠状バイパス |
| 1519. coronary care unit - (n) | unité de soins coronariens | unità di cura coronaria | unidad de cuidados coronaria | Pflegestation für Koronarpatienten | 冠状病治療部 |
| 1520. corporate mission - (n) | objectif social | oggetto sociale | objetivo social | Firmenziel | 団体任務 |
| 1521. corrected value - (n) | valeur ajustée | valore rettificato | valor corregido | korrigierter Wert | 補正数値 |
| 1522. corrective orthodontics - (n) | orthodontiques rectificatives | ortodonzia correttiva | ortodoncia correctiva | korrigierende Zahn-\Kieferbehandlung | 歯科矯正学 |
| 1523. correlation - (n) | corrélation | correlazione | correlación | Korrelation | 相互関係 |
| 1524. correlation coefficient - (n) | coefficient de corrélation | coefficiente di correlazione | coeficiente de correlación | Korrelationskoeffizient | 相関係数 |
| 1525. corrosion - (n) | corrosion | corrosione | corrosión | Korrosion | 腐食 |
| 1526. cortex - (n) | cortex | corteccia | corteza | Kortex; Rinde | 皮質 |
| 1527. corticosteroid - (n) | corticosteroïde | corticosteroide | corticosteroide | Kortikosteroid | コルチコステロイド |
| 1528. cosmetic - (n) | cosmétique | cosmetico | cosmético | Kosmetikum | 美容 |
| 1529. cosmetic - (a) | cosmétique | cosmetico | cosmético | kosmetisch | 美容術の |
| 1530. cosmetic surgery - (n) | chirurgie plastique; chirurgie cosmétique | chirurgia cosmetica; chirurgia estetica | cirugía estética | kosmetische Chirurgie | 整形外科 |
| 1531. cost - (n) | coût | costo | costo | Kosten | 費用 |

| English/American | French/Français | Italian/Italiano | Spanish/Español | German/Deutsch | Japanese/日本語 |
|---|---|---|---|---|---|
| 1532. cost-benefit analysis - (n) | analyse coûts-bénéfices | analisi costo-beneficio | análisis costes-ventajas | Kosten-Nutzen-Analyse | 原価［損失］便益分析 |
| 1533. cost-effective-ness - (n) | rentabilité; efficacité-coût | costo reale | coste eficacia; rentabilidad | Effizienz des Mitteleinsatzes | 費用効果 |
| 1534. cost-utility - (n) | coût-utilité | costo-utilità | costo-utilidad | höchste Kostenrentabilität | 原価実利 |
| 1535. cost allocation - (n) | allocation des coûts | distribuzione dei costi | distribución de costos | Kostenaufteilung; Kostenumlage | 費用の割当 |
| 1536. cost containment - (n) | contrôle des coûts | contenimento costi | contención de costos | Zurückhalten von Kosten | 費用抑制 |
| 1537. cost to benefit ratio - (n) | ratio coût-bénéfice | rapporto costo-beneficio | relación costo-beneficio | Kosten/Nutzenverhältnis | 原価と利益の割合 |
| 1538. costovertebral - (a) | costovertébral | costovertebrale | costovertebral | kostovertebral | 肋椎の |
| 1539. costovertebral angle tender-ness - (n) | douleur de l'angle costovertébral | dolorabilità angolo costovertebrale | sensibilidad del ángulo costovertebral | Druckschmerz im Kostovertebralwinkel | 肋椎角圧痛 |
| 1540. cot death - (n) | mort subite du nourrisson | morte improvvisa del neonatale | muerte infantil súbita | Krippentod; plötzlicher Kindstod | 突然死 |
| 1541. cough - (n) | toux | tosse | tos | Husten | 咳 |
| 1542. cough - (v) | tousser | tossire | toser | husten | 咳をする |
| 1543. counseling - (n) | assistance socio-psychologique | assistenza socio-psicologica | asistencia sociopsicológica | psychosoziale Beratung | カウンセリング |
| 1544. count - (n) | compte | conteggio; conto | conteo | Zählung; Zahl | 計算 |
| 1545. count - (v) | compter | contare | contar | zählen | 数える |
| 1546. counteract - (v) | contrebalancer; neutraliser | agire contro; neutralizzare | contrarrestar; neutralizar | entgegenwirken; neutralisieren | 中和する |
| 1547. counterclock-wise - (adv) | en sens inverse des aiguilles de montre | in senso antiorario | en sentido contrario a las agujas de reloj | entgegen den Uhrzeigersinn | 左回りの |

| English/American | French/Français | Italian/Italiano | Spanish/Español | German/Deutsch | Japanese/日本語 |
|---|---|---|---|---|---|
| 1548. counterfeiting - (n) | contrefaçon; falsification | contraffazione; falsificazione | falsificación | Nachahmung; Fälschung | 仮病 |
| 1549. counterirritant - (n) | révulsif | controirritante | contrairritante | Gegenreizmittel | 反対刺激剤 |
| 1550. countershock - (n) | contre-choc | defibrillazione | contrachoque | Gegenschock | カウンターショック |
| 1551. country - (n) | pays | paese | país | Staat; Land | 国 |
| 1552. course - (n) | cours | corso | curso; desarrollo | (Krankheits)verlauf | 経過 |
| 1553. covalent - (a) | covalent | covalente | covalente | kovalent | 電子対を共有する |
| 1554. covariance - (n) | covariance | covarianza | covarianza | Kovarianz | 共炎 |
| 1555. cover sheet - (n) | couverture | copertina | cubierta | Deckblatt | カバーシート |
| 1556. crack - (n) | fente; fissure | incrinatura; rottura | grieta  fisura | Hautschrunde; Riß | 割れ目 |
| 1557. crack - (v) | craquer; féler | scindere; rompere | agrietar; fisurar | anbrechen; reißen | 割れる |
| 1558. cramp - (n) | crampe | crampo | calambre | Krampf; Krampus | 痙攣 |
| 1559. cranial - (a) | crânien | cranico; craniale | craneal | kranial | 頭蓋の |
| 1560. cranial nerve - (n) | nerf crânien | nervo cranico | nervio craneal | Kranialnerv; Gehirnnerv | 脳神経 |
| 1561. cranium - (n) | crâne; boîte crânienne | cranio | cráneo | Schädel | 頭蓋 |
| 1562. craving - (n) | grand besoin | desiderio ardente | deseo vehemente | Begierde; Verlangen | 熱望 |
| 1563. creatinine - (n) | créatinine | creatinina | creatinina | Kreatinin | クレアチン |
| 1564. creatinine clearance - (n) | épuration de la créatinine | clearance della creatinina | depuración de la creatinina | Kreatinin-Clearance | クレアチニンクリアランス |
| 1565. crepitus - (n) | crépitation | crepitazione; crepito | crepitación | Krepitation | 捻髪性肺水泡音 |
| 1566. cretinism - (n) | crétinisme | cretinismo | cretinismo | Kretinismus | クレチン病 |
| 1567. crevice - (n) | crevasse; fissure | fessura | fisura | kleiner Riß; Spalte | 割れ目 |
| 1568. crib death - (n) | mort subite du nourrisson | morte improvvisa in culla | muerte en la cuna | Krippentod; plötzlicher Kindstod | 突然死 |
| 1569. crime - (n) | crime | crimine; delitto | crimen; delito | Verbrechen | 犯罪 |
| 1570. criminal psychology - (n) | psychologie criminale | psicologia criminale | psicología criminal | Kriminalpsychologie | 犯罪心理学 |
| 1571. crisis - (n) | crise | crisi | crisis | Krise | 危機 |

79

| English/American | French/Français | Italian/Italiano | Spanish/Español | German/Deutsch | Japanese/日本語 |
|---|---|---|---|---|---|
| 1572. crisis intervention - (n) | intervention de crise | intervento di crisi | intervención de crisis | Krisenintervention | 危機調停 |
| 1573. criterion - (n) | critère | criterio | criterio | Kriterium | 標準 |
| 1574. critical care - (n) | soins intensifs | cure intensive | asistencia intensiva | Intensivpflege | 臨界治療 |
| 1575. critical mass - (n) | masse critique | massa critica | masa crítica | kritische Masse | 臨界質量 |
| 1576. critical path - (n) | chemin critique; voie critique | cammino critico | camino crítico | kritscher Weg | クリティカルパス |
| 1577. critical value - (n) | valeur critique | valore critico | valor crítico | kritischer Wert | 臨界値 |
| 1578. cross-cultural - (a) | interculturel | interculturale | transcultural | interkulturell | 異文化の |
| 1579. cross-cultural comparison - (n) | comparaison interculturelle | paragone interculturale | comparación transcultural | interkultureller Vergleich | 異文化の比較 |
| 1580. cross breeding - (n) | croisement; hybridation | ibridizzazione | cruza; hibridación | Kreuzungszüchtung; Hybridisierung | 交雑 |
| 1581. cross infection - (n) | infection croisée; surinfection | infezione crociata | infección cruzada | Kreuzinfektion; gegenseitige Infizierung | 交差感染 |
| 1582. cross react - (v) | interréagir | cross-reagire | tener reacción cruzada | kreuzreagieren | 交叉反応をする |
| 1583. cross reaction - (n) | réaction croisée; interréaction | reazione crociata | reacción cruzada | Kreuzreaktion | 交差反応 |
| 1584. cross reactivity - (n) | interréactivité | reattività crociata | reactividad cruzada | Kreuzreaktivität | 交差反応性 |
| 1585. cross section - (n) | section transversale; échantillon | sezione trasversale | sección transversal; sección representativa | Querschnitt | 断面図 |
| 1586. cross sectional trial - (n) | essai transversal | test campione | prueba de corte transversal | Querschnittsprobe | 断面試験 |
| 1587. cross section study - (n) | étude transversale | studio campione | estudio de corte transversal | Querschnittstudie | 断面研究 |
| 1588. cross sensitization - (n) | sensibilisation croisée | sensibilizzazione crociata | sensibilización cruzada | Kreuzsensibilisierung | 交差感作 |

| English/American | French/Français | Italian/Italiano | Spanish/Español | German/Deutsch | Japanese/日本語 |
|---|---|---|---|---|---|
| 1589. cross tolerance - (n) | intertolérance | tolleranza crociata | tolerancia cruzada | Kreuztoleranz | 交差耐性 |
| 1590. crosshatching - (n) | contre-hachure | trateggiatura | rayados cruzados | Kreuzschraffierung | 網状の陰影をつけること |
| 1591. crossover - (n) | entrecroisement | interscambio genetico; cross-over | intercambio de genes | Cross-over; Genaustausch | 交差 |
| 1592. crossover design - (n) | dessin d'entrecroisement | disegno di cross-over | diseño de intercambio de genes | Überkreuzentwurf | 交差設計 |
| 1593. crossover trial - (n) | expérience d'entrecroisement | prova in cross-over | prueba de intercambio de genes | Überkreuzversuch | 交差試験 |
| 1594. croup - (n) | croupe; croupion | laringite difterica; croup | crup; garrotillo | Krupp | クルップ |
| 1595. crowding - (n) | entassement dentaire | affollamento dentale | amontonamiento dentario | Crowding der Zähne | 叢生 |
| 1596. crown - (n) | couronne | corona | corona | Krone; Zahnkrone | 冠 |
| 1597. crush injury - (n) | blessure par écrasement | lesione da schiacciamento | traumatismo por aplastamiento | Quetschverletzung | 圧迫傷害 |
| 1598. crust - (n) | croûte | crosta | costra; corteza | Kruste; Borke | 痂皮 |
| 1599. crutches - (n) | béquilles | grucce; stampelle | muletas | Krücken; Stützen | 松葉杖 |
| 1600. crying - (n) | pleur | pianto | lloro; llanto | Weinen | 泣き叫ぶこと |
| 1601. cryopreservation - (n) | cryopréservation | crioconservazione | criopreservación | Kryokonservierung; Kältekonservierung | 低温保存法 |
| 1602. cryoprotective agent - (n) | cryoprotecteur | agente crioprotettivo | agente crioprotector | kryoprotektive Substanz | 凍結防止剤 |
| 1603. cryosurgery - (n) | cryochirurgie | criochirurgia | criocirugía | Kryochirurgie; Kältechirurgie | 冷凍外科 |
| 1604. crystal - (n) | cristal | cristallo | cristal | Kristall | 結晶 |
| 1605. crystallin - (n) | cristallin | cristallina | cristalina | Kristallin | クリスタリン |
| 1606. crystalline - (a) | cristallin | cristallino | cristalino | kristallartig | 結晶質の |
| 1607. crystallization - (n) | cristallisation | cristallizzazione | cristalización | Kristallbildung; Kristallisierung | 結晶化 |
| 1608. cue - (n) | signal | segnale | indicación | Hinweis; Zeichen | キュー |

| English/American | French/Français | Italian/Italiano | Spanish/Español | German/Deutsch | Japanese/日本語 |
|---|---|---|---|---|---|
| 1609. cultural - (a) | culturel | cultura; ottenuto per mezzo di coltura | cultural | kulturell; Kultur- | 培養の |
| 1610. culture - (n) | culture | coltura | cultivo; cultura | Kultur | 培養 |
| 1611. culture - (v) | cultiver | coltivare | cultivar | kultivieren | 培養する |
| 1612. culture and sensitivity - (n) | culture et sensibilité | cultura e sensibilità | cultivo y sensibilidad | Kultur und Empfindlichkeit | 培養及び感受性 |
| 1613. culture medium - (n) | milieu de culture | mezzo di coltura | medio de cultivo | Kultursubstrat; Nährmedium | 培地 |
| 1614. cumulation - (n) | accumulation | accumulazione; accumulo | acumulación; amontonamiento | Kumulation | 蓄積 |
| 1615. cumulative - (a) | cumulatif | cumulativo | cumulativo | kumulativ | 蓄積の |
| 1616. cumulative dose - (n) | dose cumulative | dose accumulata | dosis cumulativa | Kumulationsdosis | 蓄積線量 |
| 1617. cumulative percent - (n) | pourcentage cumulatif | percentuale accumulata | porcentaje cumulativo | kumulative Prozent | 蓄積パーセント |
| 1618. cumulative response - (n) | réponse cumulative | risposta accumulata | respuesta cumulativa | kumulative Reaction | 蓄積反応 |
| 1619. curative treatment - (n) | traitement curatif | trattamento di cura | tratamiento curativo | Heilbehandlung | 病気に効く治療 |
| 1620. cure - (n) | cure; remède | cura; trattamento | cura | Heilung; Behandlung | 治癒 |
| 1621. cure - (v) | guérir | curare; guarire | curar | heilen | 治療する |
| 1622. cure-all - (n) | panacée | panacea | panacea; sanalotodo | Allheilmittel | 万能薬 |
| 1623. curette - (n) | curette | raschiatoio; curette | cucharilla | Kürette | キューレット |
| 1624. curriculum - (n) | programme d'études | programma di studi; curriculum di studi | currículo; plan de estudios | Lehrplan | カリキュラム |
| 1625. curriculum vitae - (n) | curriculum vitae | curriculum vitae | curriculum vitae; historial profesional | Lebenslauf | 履歴書 |
| 1626. curvature - (n) | courbure | curvatura | curvatura | Kurvatur; Krümmung | 彎曲 |

| English/American | French/Français | Italian/Italiano | Spanish/Español | German/Deutsch | Japanese/日本語 |
|---|---|---|---|---|---|
| 1627. curvilinear graph - (n) | graphique curvilinéaire | diagramma curvilineo | gráfico curvilíneo | krummlinige Darstellung | 曲線グラフ |
| 1628. cusp - (n) | cuspide | cuspide | cúspide | Spitze | 心臓弁膜尖 |
| 1629. custom - (n) | coutume; habitude | costume; abitudine | costumbre | Brauch; Sitte | 習慣 |
| 1630. cutaneous - (a) | cutané | cutaneo | cutáneo | kutan; Haut- | 皮膚の |
| 1631. cutaneous disorder - (n) | désordre cutané | disordine cutaneo | trastorno cutáneo | Hauterkrankung | 皮膚障害 |
| 1632. cutaneous nerve - (n) | nerf cutané | nervo cutaneo | nervio cutáneo | Hautnerv | 皮神経 |
| 1633. cut-off value - (n) | limite de valeur; valeur limitée | limite di valore | valor límite | Trennwert; Grenzwert | 区切りの値 |
| 1634. cyanosis - (n) | cyanose | cianosi | cianosis | Zyanose; Blausucht | チアノーゼ |
| 1635. cybernetics - (n) | cybernétique | cibernetica | cibernética | Kybernetik | サイバネティックス |
| 1636. cycle - (n) | cycle | ciclo | ciclo | Zyklus; Kreislauf | 周期 |
| 1637. cycles per second [abbr] cps - (n) | cycles par seconde; hertz | cicli al secondo; hertz | ciclos por segundo; hertz | Hertz | サイクル毎秒 |
| 1638. cyclical disease - (n) | maladie cyclique | malattia ciclica | enfermedad cíclica | zyklische Erkrankung | 周期性疾病 |
| 1639. cyst - (n) | kyste | cisti | quiste | Zyste; Blase | 嚢胞 |
| 1640. cystadeno-carcinoma - (n) | cystadénocarcinome | adenocarcinoma cistico | cistoadenocarcinoma | Zystadenokarzinom | 嚢胞腺癌 |
| 1641. cystectomy - (n) | cystectomie; kystectomie | cistectomia | cistectomía | Zystektomie | 膀胱切断術 |
| 1642. cystic - (a) | kystique | cistico | cístico | zystisch | 嚢胞性の |
| 1643. cystitis - (n) | cystite | cistite | cistitis | Zystitis | 膀胱炎 |
| 1644. cystoscopy - (n) | cystoscopie | cistoscopia | cistoscopia | Zystoskopie | 膀胱鏡検査 |
| 1645. cytogenetics - (n) | cytogénétique | citogenetica | citogenética | Zytogenetik | 細胞遺伝学 |
| 1646. cytological technique - (n) | technique cytologique | tecnica citologica | técnica citológica | Zytologieverfahren | 細胞学的技術 |
| 1647. cytology - (n) | cytologie | citologia | citología | Zytologie | 細胞学 |

| English/American | French/Français | Italian/Italiano | Spanish/Español | German/Deutsch | Japanese/日本語 |
|---|---|---|---|---|---|
| 1648. cytoplasm - (n) | cytoplasme | citoplasma | citoplasma | Zytoplasma | 原形質 |
| 1649. cytoprotective - (a) | cytoprotecteur | citoprotettivo | citoprotector | zellschützend | 細胞保護的 |
| 1650. cytoskeleton - (n) | cytosquelette | citoscheletro | citoesqueleto | Zytoskelett | 細胞骨格 |
| 1651. cytosol - (n) | cytosol | citosol | citosol | Zystol | 細胞質ゾル |
| 1652. cytotoxicity - (n) | cytotoxicité | citotossicità | citotoxicidad | Zytotoxizität | 細胞毒性 |
| 1653. cytotoxin - (n) | cytotoxine | citotossina | citotoxina | Zellgift | 細胞毒 |

84

| English/American | French/Français | Italian/Italiano | Spanish/Español | German/Deutsch | Japanese/日本語 |
|---|---|---|---|---|---|
| 1654. daily - (a) | quotidien; journalier | quotidiano; giornaliero | diario; cotidiano | täglich | 日々の |
| 1655. daily dose - (n) | dose journalière; dose quotidienne | dose giornaliera | dosis diaria; dosis por día | Tagesdosis | 日々の服用量 |
| 1656. daily living - (n) | vie quotidienne | vita quotidiana | vida diaria | tägliches Leben | 日常生活 |
| 1657. dairy product - (n) | produit laitier | prodotto caseario | producto lácteo | Milchprodukt; Molkereiprodukt | 乳製品 |
| 1658. dandruff - (n) | pellicule | forfora | caspa | (Kopf-, Haar-)schuppen | ふけ |
| 1659. dark adaptation - (n) | adaptation à l'obscurité | adattamento all'oscurità | adaptación a la oscuridad | Dunkeladaptation | 暗順応 |
| 1660. data - (n) | données | dati | datos; información | Daten | データ |
| 1661. data analysis - (n) | analyse de données | analisi dei dati | análisis de datos | Datenanalyse | データ解析 |
| 1662. data archiving - (n) | archivage de données | archiviazione dei dati | archivamiento de datos | Datenarchivierung | データ記録 |
| 1663. data audit - (n) | vérification de données | revisione dei dati | revisión de datos | Datenprüfung | データ監査 |
| 1664. data bank - (n) | banque de données | banca di dati | banco de datos | Datenbank | データバンク |
| 1665. data base - (n) | base de données | base di dati; database | base de catos | Datenbank | データベース |
| 1666. data center - (n) | centre de traitement des données | centro dati | centro de datos | Datenzentrum | データセンター |
| 1667. data clumping - (n) | regroupement de données | raggruppamento di dati | agrupación de datos | Datengruppierung | データの塊り |
| 1668. data coding - (n) | codage de données | codificazione di dati | codificación de datos | Datenkodierung | データ符号化 |
| 1669. data collection - (n) | acquisition de données | raccolta di dati | recopilación de datos | Datenerfassung; Datensammlung | データ収集 |
| 1670. data coordinating center - (n) | centre de coordination de données | centro coordinamento dati | centro de coordinador de datos | Datenkoordinierungszentrum | データコーディネートセンター |
| 1671. data display - (n) | affichage de données | visualizzatore di dati | visualización de datos | Datenanzeige | データ表示 |
| 1672. data dredging - (n) | dragage de données | spargimento dati | rastreo de datos | Datenveränderung (durch statistische Methoden) | データ整理 |

85

| English/American | French/Français | Italian/Italiano | Spanish/Español | German/Deutsch | Japanese/日本語 |
|---|---|---|---|---|---|
| 1673. data editing - (n) | préparation de données | redazione dati | edición de datos | Datenaufbereitung | データ編集 |
| 1674. data entry - (n) | entrée de données | entrata dati; immissione dati | entrada de datos | Datenerfassung | データ入力 |
| 1675. data extrapolation - (n) | extrapolation de données | estrapolazione dati | extrapolación de datos | Datenhochrechnung | データ推定 |
| 1676. data field - (n) | champ de données | campo dati | campo de datos | Datenfeld | データフィールド |
| 1677. data file - (n) | fichier de données | archivio; flusso | archivo de datos | Datei | データファイル |
| 1678. data flow - (n) | flux de données | flusso dati | flujo de datos | Datenstrom | データフロー |
| 1679. data form - (n) | fiche de données | modulo dati | formulario de datos | Datenformular | データ書式 |
| 1680. data interpretation - (n) | interprétation de données | interpretazione di dati | interpretación de datos | Datenauswertung | データ解読 |
| 1681. data item - (n) | donnée; élément de données | dato; elemento di dati | partida de datos | Datenelement; Datenwort | データ項目 |
| 1682. data misinterpretation - (n) | interprétation erronée de données | misinterpretazione di dati | interpretación falsa de datos | Datenfehlinterpretation | データ誤解読 |
| 1683. data mispresentation - (n) | présentation erronée de données | errore nella presentazione di dati | falsificación de datos | Datenverfälschung | データ誤表示 |
| 1684. data monitor - (n) | moniteur de données | monitor di dati | monitor de datos | Überwacher der Daten (einer Studie) | データ監視 |
| 1685. data point - (n) | coordonnée; point de repère | punto dati | punto de datos | einzelner Datenwert | データポイント |
| 1686. data pooling - (n) | mise en commun de données | raccolta di dati | agrupamiento de datos | Datensammlung | データプール |
| 1687. data presentation - (n) | présentation de données | presentazione di dati | presentación de datos | Datendarstellung | データ提示 |
| 1688. data processing - (n) | traitement de données | elaborazione di dati | procesamiento de datos | Datenverarbeitung | データ処理 |
| 1689. data reduction - (n) | réduction de données | riduzione di dati | reducción de datos | Datenverdichtung; Datenreduktion | データ削減 |

86

| English/American | French/Français | Italian/Italiano | Spanish/Español | German/Deutsch | Japanese/日本語 |
|---|---|---|---|---|---|
| 1690. data sheet - (n) | bordereau de données | foglio dati; documento | hoja de datos | Datenblatt; Datenbogen | データ用紙 |
| 1691. data source - (n) | source de données | fonte di dati | fuente de datos | Datenquelle | データ源 |
| 1692. data storage - (n) | mise en mémoire de données | memorizzazione di dati | memorización de datos | Datenspeicherung | データ保管 |
| 1693. data transformation - (n) | transformation de données | trasformazione di dati | transformación de datos | Datentransformation | データ変換 |
| 1694. data validation - (n) | validation des données | validazione dati | validación de datos | Datenüberprüfung | データ確認 |
| 1695. data verification - (n) | vérification des données | verifica di dati | verificación de datos | Datenprüfung | データ検査 |
| 1696. date - (n) | date | data | fecha | Datum; Tag | 日付 |
| 1697. date of admission - (n) | date d'admission | data di ammissione | fecha de admisión | Aufnahmedatum | 入院日 |
| 1698. date of expiration - (n) | date d'expiration | data di scadenza | fecha de vencimiento | Ablauftermin | 満期日 |
| 1699. datum - (n) | donnée | dato | dato; referencia | einzelner Datenpunkt; Datum | 資料 |
| 1700. day - (n) | jour; journée | giorno; giornata | día; jornada | Tag | 日 |
| 1701. day care - (n) | soins de jour | asilo; asilo nido | guardería | Tagespflege | 幼児の世話 |
| 1702. day care center - (n) | garderie; centre de soins de jour | asilo nido | guardería | Tagesstätte | 託児所 |
| 1703. daydreaming - (n) | rêverie | sognare a occhi aperti; fantasticare | ensueño; soñar despierto | Wachträumerei; Träumerei | 空想 |
| 1704. dead - (a) | mort | morto | muerto | tot | 死んでいる |
| 1705. deaf - (a) | sourd | sordo | sordo | taub; schwerhörig | 聾の |
| 1706. deaf-mute - (n) | sourd-muet | sordomuto | sordomudo | Taubstummer | 聾唖者 |
| 1707. deafness - (n) | surdité | sordità | sordera | Taubheit; Schwerhörigkeit | 聾 |
| 1708. death - (n) | décès; mort | morte | muerte | Tod | 死 |

| English/American | French/Français | Italian/Italiano | Spanish/Español | German/Deutsch | Japanese/日本語 |
|---|---|---|---|---|---|
| 1709. death certificate - (n) | acte de décès; certificat de décès | certificato di morte | partida de defunción | Totenschein; Sterbeurkunde | 死亡証明書 |
| 1710. death rate - (n) | taux de mortalité | tasso di mortalità | tasa de mortalidad | Sterbeziffer | 死亡率 |
| 1711. debilitated - (a) | débilité | debilitato | débil; con pocas fuerzas | entkräftet | 衰弱した |
| 1712. debility - (n) | débilité; faiblesse | debolezza | debilidad; falta de fuerzas | Schwäche | 弱さ、衰弱 |
| 1713. débridement - (n) | débridement | sbrigliamento | desbridamiento | Débridement | 創面切除 |
| 1714. decant - (v) | décanter | decantare | decantar | abfüllen; umfüllen | 注ぐ |
| 1715. decarboxy-lation - (n) | décarboxylation | decarbossilazione | descarboxilación | Dekarboxylation | 脱炭酸酸 |
| 1716. decay - (n) | désintégration; carie | deperimento; carie | degeneración; caries | Fäulnis; Karies | 崩壊 |
| 1717. decay - (v) | pourrir; carier | deperire; cariarsi | degenerar; cariarse | zerfallen; verfaulen | 衰退する |
| 1718. decentral-ization - (n) | décentralisation | decentralizzazione | descentralización | Dezentralisierung | 神経中枢中枢隔離 |
| 1719. deception - (n) | duperie; tromperie | inganno; frode | engaño; fraude | Täuschung; Betrug | ごまかし、幻想 |
| 1720. decerebrate state - (n) | état de décérébration | stato decerebrato | estado de decerebración | dezerebrierter Zustand | 除脳状態 |
| 1721. dechallenge - (n) | contre-stimulation; contre-provocation | disprovocazione | desestímulo; desprovocación | Rückgängigmachen der Provokation | あきらめ |
| 1722. decibel - (n) | décibel | decibel | decibel | Dezibel | デシベル |
| 1723. decidua - (n) | caduque | decidua | decidua | Dezidua | 脱落膜 |
| 1724. deciduous tooth - (n) | dent de lait | dente deciduo | diente de leche | verfallender Zahn | 第一生歯 |
| 1725. decimal - (n) | décimale | decimale | decimal | Dezimalzahl | 小数 |
| 1726. decimeter - (n) | décimètre | decimetro | decímetro | Dezimeter | デシメートル |
| 1727. decision making - (n) | prise de décision | processo decisionale | toma de decisión | Entscheidungsfindung | 意志決定 |
| 1728. decision point - (n) | point de décision | punto decisivo | punto de decisión | Entscheidungszeitpunkt | 決定時点 |

| English/American | French/Français | Italian/Italiano | Spanish/Español | German/Deutsch | Japanese/日本語 |
|---|---|---|---|---|---|
| 1729. decision theory - (n) | théorie décisionnelle | teoria delle decisioni | teoría de la decisión | Entscheidungstheorie | 決定理論 |
| 1730. decision tree (n) | arbre décisionnel | albero di decisioni | árbol de decisiones | Entscheidungsbaum | 意志決定のための枝分かれ図 |
| 1731. decline - (n) | déclin | declivio; deperimento | declinación | Verfall; Verminderung | 衰弱 |
| 1732. decline - (v) | décliner; baisser | declinare; rifiutare | declinar; disminuir | ablehnen; schwächer werden | 衰える |
| 1733. decompensation - (n) | décompensation | scompenso | descompensación | Dekompensation | 代償不全 |
| 1734. decomposition - (n) | décomposition | decomposizione | descomposición | Aufspaltung; Zersetzung | 分解 |
| 1735. decompression - (n) | décompression | decompressione | descompresión | Dekompression; Entlastung | 減圧 |
| 1736. decompression tank - (n) | caisson de décompression | camera di decompressione | tanque de descompresión | Dekompressionskammer | 減圧槽 |
| 1737. decongestant - (n) | décongestionnant | decongestionante | descongestionante | kongestionsverminderndes Mittel | 鬱血除去薬 |
| 1738. decontamination - (n) | décontamination | decontaminazione | descontaminación | Dekontamination | 除染 |
| 1739. decubitus - (n) | décubitus | decubito | decúbito | Dekubitus | 褥瘡 |
| 1740. decubitus ulcer - (n) | escarre de décubitus; ulcère de décubitus | piaga da decubito | úlcera de decúbito | Dekubitalgeschwür | 褥瘡潰瘍 |
| 1741. dedicated computer - (n) | ordinateur spécialisé | calcolatore specializzato | computadora especializada | dedizierter Computer | 専用コンピューター |
| 1742. deductive logic - (n) | déduction logique | logica deduttiva | lógica deductiva | deduktive Logik | 演繹論理 |
| 1743. deep tendon reflexes - (n) | réflexes ostéo-tend neux | riflessi tendinei profondi | reflejos tendinosos profundos | tiefe Sehnenreflexe | 深部腱反射 |

89

| English/American | French/Français | Italian/Italiano | Spanish/Español | German/Deutsch | Japanese/日本語 |
|---|---|---|---|---|---|
| 1744. deep vein thrombosis - (n) | thrombose veineuse profonde | trombosi venosa profonda | trombosis de vena profunda | tiefe Venenthrombose | 深静脈血栓症 |
| 1745. defecate - (v) | déféquer | defecare | defecar | Stuhlgang haben | 排便する |
| 1746. defecation - (n) | défécation | defecazione | defecación | Defäkation | 排便 |
| 1747. defect - (n) | défaut | difetto | defecto | Defekt; Gebrecher | 欠陥 |
| 1748. defective - (a) | défectueux | difettoso | defectuoso | Defekt - | 欠陥のある |
| 1749. defense - (n) | défense | difesa | defensa | Abwehr | 防御 |
| 1750. defense mechanism - (n) | mécanisme de défense | meccanismo di difesa | mecanismo de defensa | Abwehrmechanismus | 防御のメカニズム |
| 1751. defensive medicine - (n) | médecine défensive | medicina di difesa | medicina defensiva | defensive Medizin | 防御医学 |
| 1752. defibrillation - (n) | défibrillation | defibrillazione | desfibrilación | Defibrillation | 除細動 |
| 1753. deficiency - (n) | déficience | deficienza | deficiencia | Defizienz; Mangel | 欠乏症 |
| 1754. definition - (n) | définition | definizione | definición | Definition; Zeichenschärfe | 解像力、定義 |
| 1755. deformability - (n) | déformabilité | deformabilità | deformabilidad | Verformbarkeit | 奇形 |
| 1756. deformity - (n) | difformité | deformità | deformidad; deformación | Verformung; Deformität | 奇形 |
| 1757. degenerate - (n) | dégénéré | degenerato | degenerado | degenerierter Mensch | 変質者 |
| 1758. degenerate - (v) | dégénérer | degenerare | degenerar | degenerieren | 変質する |
| 1759. degenerate - (a) | dégénéré | degenere | degenerado | degeneriert | 変質した |
| 1760. degeneration - (n) | dégénérescence | degenerazione | degeneración | Degeneration | 変質 |
| 1761. degenerative disease - (n) | maladie dégénérative | malattia degenerativa | enfermedad degenerativa | Abbaukrankheit; degenerative Errankung | 退行性の病気 |
| 1762. degradation - (n) | dégradation | degradazione | degradación | Abbau | 分解 |
| 1763. degranulation - (n) | dégranulation | degranulazione | desgranulación | Degranulation | 脱顆粒 |
| 1764. degrees of freedom - (n) | degrés de liberté | gradi di libertà | grados de libertad | Freiheitsgrade | 自由度 |
| 1765. dehiscence - (n) | déhiscence | deiscenza | dehisencia | Dehiszenz | 裂開 |

90

| English/American | French/Français | Italian/Italiano | Spanish/Español | German/Deutsch | Japanese/日本語 |
|---|---|---|---|---|---|
| 1766. dehydrate - (v) | déshydrater | disidratare | deshidratar | dehydratisieren; dehydrieren | 脱水する |
| 1767. dehydration - (n) | déshydratation | disidratazione | deshidratación | Dehydration; Dehydrierung | 脱水 |
| 1768. déjà vu - (n) | déjà vu | già visto; déjà-vu | fenómeno de "déjà vu" | Déjà-vu-Erlebnis | 既視体験 |
| 1769. delayed - (a) | retardé; à retardement | ritardato | retrasado; retardado | verzögert | 遅延性 |
| 1770. delayed response - (n) | réponse à retardement | risposta ritardata | respuesta retardada | verzögerte Reaktion | 遅延性反応 |
| 1771. delayed type hypersensi-tivity (n) | hypersensibilité de type retardé | ipersensibilità ritardata | hipersensibilidad tipo retardada | Hypersensibilitätsreaktion vom verzögerten Typ | 遅延型過敏症 |
| 1772. deleterious - (a) | délétère; nuisible | deleterio; nocivo | deletéreo; nocivo | schädlich; nachteilig | 有害性の |
| 1773. deletion - (n) | délétion | delezione | deleción | Streichung; Löschung | 欠失 |
| 1774. delirium - (n) | délire | delirio | delirio | Delirium | せん妄 |
| 1775. delirium tremens - (n) | delirium tremens | delirium tremens | delirium tremens | Delirium tremens; Alkoholentzugsdelir | 振せんせん妄 |
| 1776. delivery - (n) | distribution; accouchement | distribuzione; parto | distribución; parto | Entbindung; Verabreichung | 分娩、配送 |
| 1777. delivery system - (n) | système de distribution | modo di distribuzione | sistema de distribución | Verabreichungssystem | 分娩系 |
| 1778. Delphi technique - (n) | technique Delphi | tecnica Delphi | técnica Delphi | Delphi Verfahren | デルフィー技術 |
| 1779. delta infection - (n) | infection delta | infezione delta | infección delta | Deltainfektion | デルタ型肝炎ウイルスの感染 |
| 1780. delta receptor - (n) | récepteur delta | recettore delta | receptor delta | Deltarezeptor | デルタレセプター |
| 1781. delusion - (n) | illusion; fantasme | delusione | delusión; ilusión | Wahn; Wahnvorstellung | 妄想 |
| 1782. dementia - (n) | démence | demenza | demencia | Demenz | 痴呆症 |
| 1783. demographic data - (n) | données démographiques | dati demografici | datos demográficos | demographische Daten | 人口統計データ |

| English/American | French/Français | Italian/Italiano | Spanish/Español | German/Deutsch | Japanese/日本語 |
|---|---|---|---|---|---|
| 1784. demographics - (n) | démographie | demografia | demografía | Demographie | 人口統計 |
| 1785. demography - (n) | démographie | demografia | demografía | Demographie | 人口統計学 |
| 1786. demyelinization, demyelination - (n) | démyélinisation | demielinizzazione | desmielinización; desmielinación | Demyelinisierung; Entmarkung | 髄鞘脱落 |
| 1787. denaturation - (n) | dénaturation | denaturazione | desnaturalización | Denaturierung | 変性 |
| 1788. dendrite - (n) | dendrite | dendrite | dendrita | Dendrit | 樹枝突起 |
| 1789. dendritic cell - (n) | cellule dendritique | cellula dendritica | célula dendrítica | dendritische Zelle | 樹枝状細胞 |
| 1790. denervation - (n) | dénervation | denervazione | desnervación | Denervation | 脱神経 |
| 1791. densitometry - (n) | densitométrie | densitometria | densitometría | Densitometrie | デンシトメトリー |
| 1792. density - (n) | densité | densità | densidad | Dichte | 密度 |
| 1793. density gradient - (n) | gradient de densité | gradiente di densità | gradiente de densidad | Dichtegradient | 密度勾配 |
| 1794. dental - (a) | dentaire | dentale; dentario | dental | dental; zahnärztlich | 歯の |
| 1795. dental calculus - (n) | calcul dentaire | calcolo dentale | cálculo dental | Zahnstein | 歯石 |
| 1796. dental care - (n) | soins dentaires | cure dentistica | cuidado dental | Zahnpflege | 歯科治療 |
| 1797. dental hygienist - (n) | hygiéniste dentaire | igienista dentale | higienista dental | Spezialist für Zahnhygiene | 歯科衛生士 |
| 1798. dental practice - (n) | pratique dentaire | trattamento dentale | práctica dental | zahnärztliche Praxis | 歯科医療 |
| 1799. dentifrice - (n) | dentifrice | dentifricio | dentífrico | Zahnputzmittel | 歯みがき剤 |
| 1800. dentin - (n) | dentine | dentina | dentina | Dentin | 象牙質 |
| 1801. dentist - (n) | dentiste | dentista; odontoiatra | dentista | Zahnarzt | 歯科医 |
| 1802. dentistry - (n) | dentisterie | odontoiatria | dentistería | Zahnheilkunde | 歯科学 |
| 1803. dentition - (n) | dentition | denti; dentatura | dentición | Zahnen; Zahnformel | 歯列 |
| 1804. denture retention - (n) | adhésion du dentier | ritenzione denti | retención de dentadura | Gebißretention | 義歯維持 |
| 1805. dentures - (n) | dentier | dentiera | dentaduras | Zahnprothese; Gebiß | 義歯 |

| English/American | French/Français | Italian/Italiano | Spanish/Español | German/Deutsch | Japanese/日本語 |
|---|---|---|---|---|---|
| 1806. deodorant - (n) | déodorant | deodorante | desodorante | Deodorant | 脱臭剤 |
| 1807. department - (n) | département; service | dipartimento; ufficio; ministero | departamento; sección | Abteilung; Station | 部門 |
| 1808. dependence liability (n) | risque de dépendance | propensione di dipendenza | riesgo de dependencia | Suchtpotential | 依存責任 |
| 1809. dependent - (a) | dépendant | dipendente | dependiente | abhängig | 依存の |
| 1810. dependent variable - (n) | variable dépendante | variabile dipendente | variable dependiente | abhängige Variable | 依存変数 |
| 1811. depilate - (v) | épiler | depilare | depilar | enthaaren; epilieren | 抜毛する |
| 1812. depilate - (v) | épuiser; réduire | vuotare; diminuire | agotar, reducir | entleeren; verbrauchen | 消耗させる |
| 1813. depletion - (n) | épuisement; réduction | deplezione; svuotamento | depleción; agotamiento | Entleerung | 消耗、除去 |
| 1814. depolarization - (n) | dépolarisation | depolarizzazione | despolarización | Depolarisation | 脱分極 |
| 1815. deposit - (n) | dépôt | deposito | depósito | Ablagerung | 沈殿物 |
| 1816. deposit - (v) | déposer | depositare | depositar | ablagern | 沈殿させる |
| 1817. depot - (n) | dépôt | deposito | depósito | Depot; Speicher | 貯蔵所 |
| 1818. depressant - (n) | déprimant | depressivo; deprimente | depresor | dämpfendes Mittel | 抑制剤 |
| 1819. depression - (n) | dépression | depressione; crisi depressiva | depresión | Depression; Schwäche | うつ病、低下 |
| 1820. deprivation - (n) | carence; privation | carenza | deprivación; privación | Deprivation | 剥奪 |
| 1821. depth perception - (n) | perception des profondeurs | percezione in profondità | percepción de profundidad | Tiefenwahrnehmung | 奥行覚 |
| 1822. derivative - (n) | dérivé | derivato | derivativo | Derivat | 誘導体 |
| 1823. derived data - (n) | données dérivées | dati derivati | datos derivados | abgeleitete Daten | 派生データ |
| 1824. dermal - (a) | cutané | dermico; cutaneo | dérmico | dermal; Haut- | 皮膚の |
| 1825. dermatitis - (n) | dermatite; dermite | dermatite | dermatitis | Dermatitis | 皮膚炎 |
| 1826. dermatology - (n) | dermatologie | dermatologia | dermatología | Dermatologie | 皮膚科学 |
| 1827. dermatosis - (n) | dermatose | dermatosi | dermatosis | Dermatose | 皮膚病 |

| English/American | French/Français | Italian/Italiano | Spanish/Español | German/Deutsch | Japanese/日本語 |
|---|---|---|---|---|---|
| 1828. descending - (a) | descendant | discendente | descendiendo; descendente | abstammend; absteigend | 下降する |
| 1829. descending colon - (n) | côlon descendant | colon discendente | colon descendente | absteigendes Kolon | 下行結腸 |
| 1830. description - (n) | description | descrizione | descripción | Beschreibung | 記述 |
| 1831. descriptive statistics - (n) | statistiques descriptives | statistica descrittiva | estadística descriptiva | beschreibende Statistik | 記述統計 |
| 1832. desensitization - (n) | désensibilisation | desensibilizzazione | desensibilización | Desensibilisierung | 脱感作 |
| 1833. desiccant - (n) | dessiccatif | disseccante | desecante | austrockendes Mittel; Trockenmittel | 乾燥剤 |
| 1834. desiccant - (a) | desséchant; siccatif | disseccante; essiccativo | desecante | austrocknend | 乾燥させる |
| 1835. desiccate - (v) | dessécher | disseccare; essiccare | desecar | austrocknen | 乾燥させる |
| 1836. desiccation - (n) | dessiccation | disseccazione | desecación | Exsikkation; Austrocknung | 乾燥 |
| 1837. design - (n) | dessin; plan | disegno; progetto | diseño; propósito | Entwurf | 設計 |
| 1838. desmosome - (n) | desmosome | desmosoma | desmosoma | Desmosom | デスモソーム |
| 1839. destructive lesion - (n) | lésion destructive | lesione distruttiva | lesión destructiva | Entartungsläsion | 破壊性病巣 |
| 1840. detachment - (n) | décollement; séparation | distacco; separazione | desprendimiento | Ablösung; Lösung | 分離 |
| 1841. detection - (n) | détection; dépistage | scoperta | descubrimiento; detección | Nachweis; Entdeckung | 検出 |
| 1842. detection limit - (n) | limite de détection | limite di scoperta | limite de detección | Nachweisgrenze | 検出限界 |
| 1843. detergent - (n) | détergent | detergente; detersivo | detergente | Reinigungsmittel | 洗剤 |
| 1844. deteriorate - (v) | détériorer | deteriorare; peggiorare | deteriorar; empeorar | verschlechtern | 劣化する |
| 1845. deterioration - (n) | détérioration | deterioramento | empeoramiento | Verschlechterung | 劣化 |
| 1846. deterrent - (n) | agent préventif | deterrente; impedimento | impedimento | Abschreckungsrmittel | 抑止物 |
| 1847. detoxication drug - (n) | médicament de détoxication | disintossicante | droga de desintoxicación | Entgiftungsmittel | 解毒剤 |

94

| English/American | French/Français | Italian/Italiano | Spanish/Español | German/Deutsch | Japanese/日本語 |
|---|---|---|---|---|---|
| 1848. deuterium - (n) | deutérium; hydrogène lourd | deuterio; idrogeno pesante | deuterio; hidrógeno pesado | Deuterium; schwerer Wasserstoff | 重水素 |
| 1849. developing country - (n) | pays en voie de développement | paese in via di sviluppo | país en vías de desarrollo | Entwicklungsland | 発展途上国 |
| 1850. development - (n) | développement | sviluppo | desarrollo | Entwicklung | 発達 |
| 1851. develop- mental - (a) | de croissance | dello sviluppo | de desarrollo | Entwicklungs- | 発達の |
| 1852. deviant - (a) | déviant; anormal | deviante; anormale | desviado | abweichend | 逸脱した |
| 1853. deviation - (n) | déviation | deviazione | desviación | Deviation; Abweichung | 偏向、逸脱 |
| 1854. device - (n) | appareil; mécanisme | strumento | dispositivo; aparato | Vorrichtung; Apparatur | 装置 |
| 1855. dextro-isomer (n) | dextro-isomère | isomero destrogiro | isómero dextrogiro | Dextroisomer | 右旋性異性体 |
| 1856. diabetes - (n) | diabète | diabete | diabetes | Diabetes; Zuckerkrankheit | 糖尿病 |
| 1857. diabetes mellitus - (n) | diabète mellitus; diabète sucré | diabete mellito | diabetes mellitus | Diabetes mellitus | 真性糖尿病 |
| 1858. diabetic - (n) | diabétique | diabetico | diabético | Diabetiker | 糖尿病患者 |
| 1859. diabetic - (a) | diabétique | diabetico | diabético | diabetisch | 糖尿病の |
| 1860. diabetic ketoacidosis - (n) | acido-cétose diabétique | cheto-acidosi diabetica | cetoacidosis diabética | Ketonkörperazidose | 糖尿病ケトアシドーシス |
| 1861. diagnosis - (n) | diagnostic | diagnosi | diagnóstico; diagnosis | Diagnose | 診断 |
| 1862. diagnostic - (n) | diagnostic | diagnostica | diagnóstico | Diagnostik | 診断学 |
| 1863. diagnostic - (a) | diagnostique | diagnostico | diagnóstico | diagnostisch | 診断の |
| 1864. diagnostic impression - (n) | impression diagnostique | impressione diagnostica | impresión diagnóstica | Verdachtsdiagnose | 診断における印象 |
| 1865. diagnostic reagent kit - (n) | ensemble de réactifs diagnostiques | cassetta reagente diagnostico | juego reactivo para diagnosticar | diagnostischer Reagenzsatz | 診断試薬セット |
| 1866. diagnostic study - (n) | étude diagnostique | studio diagnostico | estudio diagnóstico | diagnostische Untersuchung | 診断研究 |

95

| English/American | French/Français | Italian/Italiano | Spanish/Español | German/Deutsch | Japanese/日本語 |
|---|---|---|---|---|---|
| 1867. diagnostic test - (n) | épreuve diagnostique | esame diagnostico | prueba diagnóstica | diagnostische Probe | 診断検査 |
| 1868. diagnostic work-up (n) | élaboration diagnostique | elaborazione diagnostica | elaboración diagnóstica | diagnostische Aufarbeitung | 総合診断的検査 |
| 1869. diagram - (n) | diagramme | diagramma | diagrama | Diagramm | 図表 |
| 1870. dialysis - (n) | dialyse | dialisi | diálisis | Dialyse | 透析 |
| 1871. diaper - (n) | couche | pannolino | pañal | Windel; Monatsbinde | おむつ |
| 1872. diaphoresis - (n) | diaphorèse | diaforesi | diaforesis | Diaphorese | 発汗多量 |
| 1873. diaphragm - (n) | diaphragme | diaframma | diafragma | Diaphragma; Zwerchfell | 横隔膜、避妊ペッサリー |
| 1874. diarrhea - (n) | diarrhée | diarrea | diarrea | Diarrhö; Durchfall | 下痢 |
| 1875. diary - (n) | journal | diario | diario | Tagebuch | 日誌 |
| 1876. diastereo-isomer - (n) | diastéréo-isomère | diastereoisomero | diastereoisómero | Diastereoisomer | ジアステレオマー |
| 1877. diastole - (n) | diastole | diastole | diástole | Diastole | 拡張期 |
| 1878. diastolic blood pressure - (n) | pression diastolique | pressione diastolica | presión diastólica | diastolischer Blutdruck | 弛緩期 [血] 圧 |
| 1879. diastolic murmur - (n) | souffle diastolique | soffio diastolico | soplo diastólico | Diastolengeräusch | 拡張期雑音 |
| 1880. diathesis - (n) | diathèse | diatesi | diátesis | Diathese | 素質 |
| 1881. diencephalon - (n) | diencéphale | diencefalo | diencéfalo | Dienzephalon; Zwischenhirn | 間脳 |
| 1882. diet - (n) | diète; alimentation | dieta; alimentazione | dieta; alimentación | Diät; Ernährung | 食事 |
| 1883. diet - (v) | suivre un régime | stare a dieta | estar a dieta; ponerse a dieta | Diät halten | 食事療法をする |
| 1884. dietary - (a) | diététique | dietetico; di dieta | dietético | diätetisch; Nahrungs- diätetisch | 食事の |
| 1885. dietetic - (a) | diététique | dietetico; di dieta | dietético | diätetisch | 食事性の |
| 1886. dietician - (n) | diététicien | dietista; dietologo | dietista | Diätist | 栄養士 |
| 1887. differential blood count - (n) | formule leucocytaire | conta leucocitaria | recuento leucocitario | Differentialblutbild | 血球百分比 |

96

| English/American | French/Français | Italian/Italiano | Spanish/Español | German/Deutsch | Japanese/日本語 |
|---|---|---|---|---|---|
| 1888. differential count - (n) | numération différentielle | conta differenziale | recuento diferencial | Differentialbild | 白血球百分比 |
| 1889. differential diagnosis - (n) | diagnostic différentiel | diagnosi differenziale | diagnóstico diferencial | Differentialdiagnostik | 鑑別診断 |
| 1890. differentiation - (n) | différenciation | derivazione | diferenciación | Differenzierung; Unterscheidung | 分化 |
| 1891. diffuse - (v) | diffuser | diffondere | difundir | diffundieren | 放散する |
| 1892. diffuse - (a) | diffus | diffuso | difuso | diffus | 散在性の |
| 1893. diffusion - (n) | diffusion | diffusione | difusión | Diffusion | 拡散 |
| 1894. diffusion of innovation - (n) | diffusion de l'innovation | diffusione dell'innovazione | difusión de la innovación | Verbreitung von Erneuerungen | 新技術（製品）の普及 |
| 1895. diffusion study - (n) | étude de diffusion | studio della diffusione | estudio de difusión | Diffusionsstudie | 拡散研究 |
| 1896. digest - (v) | digérer | digerire | digerir | digerieren; verdauen | 消化する |
| 1897. digestion - (n) | digestion | digestione | digestión | Digestion; Verdauung | 消化［作用］ |
| 1898. digestive system - (n) | système digestif | apparato digerente | aparato digestivo | Verdauungssystem | 消化系 |
| 1899. digestive tract - (n) | appareil digestif | canale alimentare | tracto digestivo | Verdauungstrakt | 消化管 |
| 1900. digit - (n) | doigt; chiffre | dito; cifra | dedo; dígito | Finger; Zahl | 指、アラビア数字（0から9まで） |
| 1901. digital subtraction - (n) | soustraction digitale | sottrazione digitale | sustracción digital | digitale Subtraktion | デジタル減算 |
| 1902. digitalis glycosides - (n) | glucosides digitaliicues | glicosidi digitalici | glicósidos digitálicos | Digitalisglykoside | ジギタリスグリコシド |
| 1903. dilatation - (n) | dilatation | dilatazione | dilatación | Dilation | 拡張 |
| 1904. dilated pupils - (n) | pupilles dilatées | pupille dilatate | pupilas dilatadas | dilatierte Pupillen; erweiterte Pupillen | 瞳孔の拡大 |
| 1905. dilation - (n) | dilatation | dilatazione | dilatación | Dilation | 拡大 |

| English/American | French/Français | Italian/Italiano | Spanish/Español | German/Deutsch | Japanese/日本語 |
|---|---|---|---|---|---|
| 1906. dilute - (v) | diluer | diluire; allungare | diluir | verdünnen | 希釈する |
| 1907. dimensions - (n) | dimensions | dimensioni | dimensiones | Dimensionen; Größen | 寸法 |
| 1908. diminution - (n) | diminution; baisse | diminuzione; riduzione | disminución; reducción | Verminderung | 減少 |
| 1909. diopter - (n) | dioptrie | diottria | dioptría | Dioptrie | ジオプトリー |
| 1910. dipeptide - (n) | dipeptide | dipeptide | dipéptido | Dipeptid | ジペプチド |
| 1911. diplococcus - (n) | diplocoque | diplococco | diplococo | Diplococcus; Diplokokke | 双球菌 |
| 1912. diploidy - (n) | diploïdie | diploidia | diploidia | Diploidie | 二倍体 |
| 1913. diplopia - (n) | diplopie | diplopia | diplopia | Diplopie | 複視 |
| 1914. direct service cost - (n) | coût de service direct | costo servizio diretto | costo del servicio directo | direkte Dienstleistungskosten | 直接サービス費用 |
| 1915. direct to consumer advertising - (n) | publicité directe au consommateur | pubblicità diretta al consumatore | publicidad orientada directamente al consumidor | Werbung direkt zum Verbraucher | 消費者広告に直接的 |
| 1916. director - (n) | directeur | direttore | director | Direktor; Leiter | 導子 |
| 1917. dirty data (n) | données incomplètes ou non-conformes | dati non validati | datos incompletos; datos no validados | unreine Daten; schlechte Daten | 不完全データ |
| 1918. disability - (n) | invalidité; incapacité | invalidità; svantaggio | incapacidad | Behinderung Invalidität | 身体障害 |
| 1919. disability evaluation - (n) | évaluation d'invalidité | valutazione della disabilità | evaluación de la incapacidad | Beurteilung der Invalidität | 障害評価 |
| 1920. disabled - (a) | infirme; handicapé | disabile; invalido | discapaz; minusválido | behindert; arbeitsunfähig | 身体に障害のある |
| 1921. discharge - (n) | renvoi; sécrétion | secrezione; dimissione | secreción; evacuado | Ausfluß; Entlassung | 排出物、退院 |
| 1922. discharge summary (n) | résumé de renvoi | certificato di dimissione | resumen del curso hospitalario | Entlassungsbericht | 退院時の病歴と治療の要約 |
| 1923. disclosure - (n) | révélation | rivelazione | revelación | Bekanntgabe; Mitteilung | 発覚 |
| 1924. discoloration - (n) | décoloration | scoloramento | descoloramiento; descoloramiento | Verfärbung; Entfärbung | 変色 |
| 1925. discomfort - (n) | malaise; inconfort | incomodo; scomodità | incomodidad | Unwohlsein | 不快 |
| 1926. discontinuation - (n) | interruption | sospensione; interruzione | interrupción | Unterbrechung | 中絶 |

| English/American | French/Français | Italian/Italiano | Spanish/Español | German/Deutsch | Japanese日本語 |
|---|---|---|---|---|---|
| 1927. discontinued - (a) | cessé; interrompu | cessato; rotto; sospeso | interrumpido; terminado | unterbrochen | 中絶した |
| 1928. discounted rate of return - (n) | taux de rendement réduit | tasso di remunerazione scontato | tasa de rendimiento descuentado | diskontierte Rendite | 返却の割引率 |
| 1929. discovery - (n) | découverte | scoperta | descubrimiento | Entdeckung | 発見 |
| 1930. discriminant analysis - (n) | analyse discriminante | analisi discriminante | análisis discriminante | Diskriminanzanalyse | 識別分析 |
| 1931. discrimination learning - (n) | apprentissage de discrimination | imparare a discriminare | aprendizaje de discriminación | Unterscheidenslernen | 識別学習 |
| 1932. disease - (n) | maladie; affection | malattia | enfermedad | Erkrankung; Krankheit | 疾病 |
| 1933. disease of unknown origin (n) | maladie d'origine inconnue | malattia di origine ignota | enfermedad de origen desconocido | Krankheit mit unbekannter Ursache | 原因不明の病気 |
| 1934. disease specialty - (n) | maladie de spécialité | specializzazione malattia | enfermedad de especialidad | Spezialgebiet | 専門疾病 |
| 1935. disequi-librium - (n) | déséquilibre | squilibrio | desequilibrio | Ungleichgewicht | 不均衡 |
| 1936. disinfect - (v) | désinfecter | disinfettare | desinfectar | desinfizieren | 消毒する |
| 1937. disintegration - (n) | désintégration | disintegrazione | desintegración | Desintegration | 壊変 |
| 1938. disk - (n) | disque | disco | disco | Scheibe; Bandscheibe | 円板、ディスク |
| 1939. dislocate - (v) | disloquer | lussare | dislocar; descoyuntar | deslozieren | 脱臼させる |
| 1940. dislocation - (n) | dislocation; luxation | lussazione | dislocación | Dislokation; Luxation | 脱臼 |
| 1941. disorder - (n) | désordre; trouble | disturbo; turba | desarreglo; trastorno | Störung; Krankheit | 障害 |
| 1942. disorganized - (a) | désorganisé | disorganizzato | desoganizado | desorganisiert | 組織崩壊した |
| 1943. disorientation - (n) | désorientation | disorientamento | desorientación | Desorientation; Desorientierung | 失見当 |
| 1944. dispensary - (n) | dispensaire | dispensario | dispensario | Krankenhausapotheke | 診療所 |
| 1945. dispensing - (a) | distribué | distributore | distribuido | verabreichend | 調剤する |
| 1946. displacement - (n) | déplacement | spostamento; dislocazione | desplazamiento | Verlagerung; Verdrängung | 運搬 |

| English/American | French/Français | Italian/Italiano | Spanish/Español | German/Deutsch | Japanese/日本語 |
|---|---|---|---|---|---|
| 1947. display - (n) | manifestation; visualisation | manifestazione; visualizzatore | manifestación; visualización | Darstellung; Anzeige | 表示 |
| 1948. display - (v) | montrer; manifester | manifestare; visualizzare | exponer; manifestar | darstellen; anzeigen | 表示する |
| 1949. disposable - (a) | à usage unique; à jeter | monouso; da gettare | desechable | Einweg- | 使い捨ての |
| 1950. disposal of waste - (n) | enlèvement des déchets | smaltimento dei rifiuti | eliminación de desperdicios | Abfallentsorgung | 廃物処理 |
| 1951. disposition - (n) | disposition | carattere; temperamento | disposición | Bereitschaft; Anfälligkeit | 気質 |
| 1952. disqualifier - (n) | disqualificateur | squalificante | descalificador | Disqualifizierter; Ungeeigneter | 失格者 |
| 1953. dissect - (v) | disséquer | sezionare | disecar; separar | sezieren | 解剖する |
| 1954. disseminate - (v) | disséminer | disseminare | diseminar | ausbreiten | 散布する |
| 1955. disseminated disease - (n) | maladie disséminée | malattia disseminata | enfermedad diseminada | ausgebreitete Erkrankung | 播種性疾病 |
| 1956. dissemination - (n) | dissémination | disseminazione | diseminación | Dissemination; Verbreitung | 流布播種 |
| 1957. dissertation - (n) | dissertation | dissertazione di laurea; tesi | disertación; tesis | wissenschaftliche Arbeit; Doktorarbeit | 研究報告 |
| 1958. dissociation - (n) | dissociation | dissociazione | disociación | Dissoziation | 解離 |
| 1959. dissolution - (n) | dissolution | dissoluzione | disolución | Zersetzung; Auflösung | 溶解 |
| 1960. dissolve - (v) | dissoudre | sciogliere | disolver | auflösen | 溶解する |
| 1961. distal - (a) | distal | distale | distal | distal | 遠位の |
| 1962. distance - (n) | distance | distanza | distancia | Entfernung; Abstand | 距離 |
| 1963. distend - (v) | distendre | gonfiare; distendersi | dilatar; hinchar | dehnen; auftreiben | ふくらませる |
| 1964. distill - (v) | distiller | distillare | destilar | destillieren | 蒸留する |
| 1965. distilled water - (n) | eau distillée | acqua distillata | agua destilada | destilliertes Wasser | 蒸留水 |
| 1966. distinguish - (v) | distinguer | distinguere | distinguir | unterscheiden | 識別する |
| 1967. distortion - (n) | distorsion | distorsione | distorsión | Verzerrung; Distorsion | 捻挫 |
| 1968. distress - (n) | douleur; affliction | dolore; sofferenza | dolor; agotamiento | Leiden; Not | 悩み |
| 1969. distress - (v) | affliger | affliggere | doler; agotar | peinigen; beunruhigen | 悩ます |

| English/American | French/Français | Italian/Italiano | Spanish/Español | German/Deutsch | Japanese/日本語 |
|---|---|---|---|---|---|
| 1970. distributed data entry - (n) | entrée de données distribuée | entrata dati distribuzione | entrada de datos distribuida | verteilte Datenerfassung | 分散型データ入力 |
| 1971. distributed database - (n) | base de données distribuée | base di dati distribuiti | base de datos distribuida | verteilte Datenbank | 分散型データベース |
| 1972. distribution - (n) | distribution | distribuzione | distribución | Verteilung | 分布 |
| 1973. diuresis - (n) | diurèse | diuresi | diuresis | Diurese | 利尿 |
| 1974. diuretic - (n) | diurétique | diuretico | diurético | Diuretikum | 利尿剤 |
| 1975. divalent cation - (n) | cation divalent | catione divalente | catión divalente | zweiwertiges Kation | 二価陽イオン |
| 1976. divergent - (a) | divergent | divergente | divergente | divergent | 分岐する |
| 1977. diversity - (n) | diversité | diversità | diversidad | Verschiedenheit | 多様性 |
| 1978. diverticulum - (n) | diverticule | diverticolo | divertículo | Divertikel | 盲状袋 |
| 1979. divide - (v) | diviser; séparer | dividere; spartire | dividir | teilen | 分ける |
| 1980. division - (n) | division | divisione | división | Teilung | 分裂 |
| 1981. dizygotic - (a) | dizygote; bi-ovulaire | dizigotico | dicigótico | dizygot; zweieiig | 二卵性の |
| 1982. dizziness - (n) | vertige | vertigine | mareo | Benommenheit; Schwindel | 眩暈 |
| 1983. DNA [abbr. of ] deoxyribonucleic acid- (n) | acide désoxyribonucléique, ADN | acido desossiribonucleico, ADN | ácido desoxirribonucleico, ADN | Desoxyribonukleinsäure, DNS | デオキシンリボ核酸 |
| 1984. DNA fingerprinting - (n) | empreinte d'ADN | inpronta digitale ADN | identificación genética de ADN | DNS-Fingerabdruck | DNAフィンガープリンティング |
| 1985. DNA mutational analysis - (n) | analyse de mutation d'ADN | analisi di mutazione ADN | análisis de mutaciones de ADN | DNS-Mutationsanalyse | DNA突然変異分析 |
| 1986. DNA probe - (n) | sonde à ADN | sonda ADN | sonda de ADN | DNS-Sonde | DNAプローブ |
| 1987. doctor - (n) | docteur; médecin | dottore; medico | doctor médico | Arzt; Ärztin | 医師 |
| 1988. document - (n) | document | documento | documento | Dokument | 文書 |
| 1989. documentation - (n) | documentation | documentazione | documentación | Dokumentation | 文書化 |

101

| English/American | French/Français | Italian/Italiano | Spanish/Español | German/Deutsch | Japanese/日本語 |
|---|---|---|---|---|---|
| 1990. dolor - (n) | douleur | dolore; pena | dolor | Schmerz | 疼痛 |
| 1991. domestic - (a) | domestique | domestico | doméstico | häuslich; einheimisch | 家庭の |
| 1992. domestic environment - (n) | environnement domestique | ambiente domestico | ambiente doméstico | häusliche Umgebung | 家庭環境 |
| 1993. dominance - (n) | dominance | dominanza | dominancia | Dominanz | 優性 |
| 1994. dominant - (a) | dominant | dominante | dominante | dominant | 優性の |
| 1995. dominant gene - (n) | gène dominant | gene dominante | gene dominante | dominantes Gen | 優性遺伝子 |
| 1996. donor - (n) | donneur | donatore | donante | Spender | 供給者 |
| 1997. dopaminergic - (a) | dopaminergique | dopaminergico | dopaminérgico | dopaminerg | ドパミン作用性の |
| 1998. Doppler echocardi-ography - (n) | echocardiographie Doppler | ecocardiografia Doppler | ecocardiografía Doppler | Doppler-Echokardiographie | ドップラー超音波心臓検査法 |
| 1999. dormant - (a) | dormant | dormiente; in letargo | inactivo; quiescente | ruhend | 休止状態の |
| 2000. dorsal - (a) | dorsal | dorsale | dorsal | dorsal | 背面の |
| 2001. dorsiflexion - (n) | dorsiflexion; flexion dorsale | flessione dorsale | dorsiflexión | Dorsalflexion | 背屈 |
| 2002. dorsolateral - (a) | dorsolatéral | dorsolaterale | dorsolateral | dorsolateral | 外背側の |
| 2003. dosage - (n) | dosage; dose | dosaggio | dosificación | Dosierung; Dosis | 服用量 |
| 2004. dosage assign-ment - (n) | allocation de dosage | assegnazione dosaggio | asignación de la dosis | Dosierungsbestimmung | 服用量の割り当て |
| 2005. dosage form - (n) | présentation d'un médicament | presentazione del medicamento | presentación de medicamento | Darreichungsform | 投薬形式 |
| 2006. dosage regimen - (n) | régime de dosage | regime di dosaggio | régimen de dosis | Dosierungsschema | 投薬養生法 |
| 2007. dosage schedule - (n) | horaire de dosage | orario di dosaggio | horario de dosis | Dosierungsschema | 投薬予定 |
| 2008. dose - (n) | dose | dose | dosis | Dosis | 服用量 |

102

| English/American | French/Français | Italian/Italiano | Spanish/Español | German/Deutsch | Japanese/日本語 |
|---|---|---|---|---|---|
| 2009. dose - (v) | doser | dosare; somministrare una dose | administrar una dosis; medicar | dosieren | 投薬する |
| 2010. dose ascension - (n) | augmentation de dose | aumento del dosaggio | aumento de dosis | Dosiserhöhung | 服用量の上昇 |
| 2011. dose escalation - (n) | intensification de dose | incremento della dose | intensificación de dosis | Dosiseskalation | 服用量の拡大 |
| 2012. dose-interval - (n) | intervalle de dose | intervalle tra dosi | intervalo entre dosis | Intervall zwischen Dosen | 服用量の間隔 |
| 2013. dose limiting toxicity (n) | toxicité limitant la dose | dose-limite per la tossicità | toxicidad que limita la dosis | dosiseinschränkende Toxizität | 服用量制限毒性 |
| 2014. dose range - (n) | étendue des doses | limiti della posologia | margen posológico | Dosierungsbereich | 服用量範囲 |
| 2015. dose ranging (n) | détermination de l'étendue des doses | determinazione del limite del dosaggio | determinación del rango de la dosis | Dosierungsbereichs-untersuchung | 服用量範囲 |
| 2016. dose-response - (n) | dose-réponse | dose-effetto | respuesta a la dosis | Dosis-Wirkung | 服用量反応 |
| 2017. dose-response curve - (n) | courbe dose-réponse | curva dose-effetto | curva de dosis-respuesta | Dosis-Wirkungs-Kurve | 用量作用曲線 |
| 2018. dose-response relationship - (n) | relation dose-réponse; rapport dose-réponse | relazione dose-risposta; rapporto dose-risposta | relación dosis-respuesta | Dosis-Wirkungs-Beziehung | 用量作用関係 |
| 2019. dose taper (n) | diminution progressive de la dose | diminuzione graduale dose | disminución progresiva de la dosis | ausschleichende Dosierung | 服用量漸減 |
| 2020. dosimetry - (n) | dosimétrie | dosimetro | dosimetría | Dosimetrie | 線量計測 |
| 2021. dosing cycle - (n) | cycle de dosage | ciclo dosaggio | ciclo de dosis | Dosierungszyklus | 服用周期 |
| 2022. dosing paradigm (n) | paradigme de dosage | esempio dosaggio | paradigma de la dosis | Dosierungsparadigma | 服用凡例 |
| 2023. dosing record - (n) | registre de dosage | registrazione dosaggio | registro de dosis | Dosierungsverzeichnis | 服用記録 |
| 2024. dosing schedule - (n) | horaire de dosage | orario di dosaggio | horario de dosis | Dosierungsschema | 服用予定 |
| 2025. dossier - (n) | dossier | dossier | dossier | Dossier | 一件書類 |
| 2026. dot - (n) | point | punto; macchiolina | punto | Fleck; Punkt | 点 |

| English/American | French/Français | Italian/Italiano | Spanish/Español | German/Deutsch | Japanese/日本語 |
|---|---|---|---|---|---|
| 2027. double blind - (a) | à double aveugle; à double insu | a doppio cieco | doble ciego | doppelblind | 二重盲検 |
| 2028. double blind trial - (n) | essai à double aveugle; épreuve à double insu | studio a doppio cieco | ensayo doble ciego | Doppelblindversuch | 二重盲検試験 |
| 2029. double data entry - (n) | entrée de données doubles | entrata di dati doppi | entrada de datos dobles | doppelte Datenerfassung | 二重データ入力 |
| 2030. double dummy - (n) | double placebo | doppio placebo | placebo doble | Doppelplacebo | 二重偽薬 |
| 2031. double masked - (a) | doublement masqué | doppiamente mascherato | doblemente enmascarado | doppelblind | 二重盲検の |
| 2032. double placebo - (n) | double placebo | doppio placebo | placebo doble | Doppelplacebo | 二重偽薬 |
| 2033. double stranded RNA - (n) | ARN bicaténaire | ARN a doppia elica | ARN de doble cadena | doppelsträngige RNS | 二本鎖RNA |
| 2034. double vision - (n) | vision double | diplopia; vedere doppio | diplopía; visión doble | Doppelsichtigkeit | 複視 |
| 2035. douche - (n) | douche; lavage interne | doccia; irrigazione | ducha | Spülung; Dusche | 灌注 |
| 2036. douche - (v) | doucher; irriguer | fare una doccia; irrigare | duchar; irrigar | spülen | 灌注する |
| 2037. down-regu-lation - (n) | régulation à la baisse | regolazione abbassa | regulación hacia abajo | Downregulation; Herunterregulation | ダウンレギュレーション |
| 2038. Down's syndrome - (n) | syndrome de Down | sindrome di Down | síndrome de Down | Down-Syndrom | 蒙古症 |
| 2039. draft (also draught) - (n) | avant-projet; courant d'air | abbozzo; corrente d'aria | borrador; corriente de aire | Entwurf; Luftzug | 草案, 通風 |
| 2040. draft - (v) | préparer | abbozzare | preparar | entwerfen | 書く |
| 2041. drainage - (n) | drainage | drenaggio | drenaje | Drainage; Ableitung | ドレナージ |
| 2042. drawing - (n) | dessin | disegno | dibujo | Zeichnung | 製図 |
| 2043. dream - (n) | rêve | sogno | sueño | Traum | 夢 |
| 2044. dressing - (n) | pansement | fasce; bende | vendaje | Verband | 包帯 |

| English/American | French/Français | Italian/Italiano | Spanish/Español | German/Deutsch | Japanese/日本語 |
|---|---|---|---|---|---|
| 2045. drinking - (n) | boire (de l'alcool) | il bere; bevuta; alcolismo | el beber; bebida | Trinken; Alkoholkonsum | 飲酒 |
| 2046. drinking history - (n) | histoire de consommation d'alcool | storia ubriachezza | historia alcohólica | Vorgeschichte als Alkoholiker | 飲酒歴 |
| 2047. drip - (n) | perfusion; goutte-à-goutte | goccia; goccialamento | gota a gota | Tropf; Tropfen | 滴注点滴 |
| 2048. drip - (v) | laisser tomber go-utte-à-goutte | gocciolare | gotear | tröpfeln | 点滴する |
| 2049. drive - (n) | besoin; instinct | impulso | instinto; impulso | Trieb | 衝動 |
| 2050. drooling - (n) | baver; bave | scialorrea | babear | Sabbern | よだれ |
| 2051. drop-in - (n) | lecture de parasite | introduzione di bit parassiti | información parásita | Störsignal | ドロップイン |
| 2052. dropout - (n) | perte d'information | perdite di bit; ritiro | pérdida de información; pérdida accidental | Ausfall; Signalausfall | ドロップアウト |
| 2053. dropped beat - (n) | coup manquant | battito non condotto | latido fallido | ausgefallene Systole; Mobitz-Block | 心泊のぬけること |
| 2054. dropsy - (n) | hydropisie | idrope | hidropesía | Wassersucht; Hydropsia | 水腫 |
| 2055. drowsiness - (n) | somnolence | sonnolenza; torpore | somnolencia; modorra | Schläfrigkeit | 嗜眠状態 |
| 2056. drug - (n) | drogue; médicament | droga; medicamento | droga; fármaco | Medikament; Arzneimittel | 薬 |
| 2057. drug abuse - (n) | abus de drogue; abus de médicament | abuso droga | abuso de drogas | Drogenmißbrauch; Arzneimittelmißbrauch | 薬物乱用 |
| 2058. drug accountability (n) | implication d'une drogue | responsabilità dose farmaco | implicancia de una droga | Drogenverantwortlichkeit | 薬物責務 |
| 2059. drug addiction - (n) | toxicomanie | tossicomania; farmacodipendenza | drogadicción; toxicomanía | Drogenabhängigkeit; Medikamentenabhängigkeit | 薬物嗜癖 |
| 2060. drug claims (n) | prétentions d'une drogue | pretese farmaco | pretensión de una droga | Medikamenteigenschaften | 薬の効用 |
| 2061. drug delivery system - (n) | mode d'administration de drogue | modalità di somministrazione del farmaco | sistema de administración de droga | Medikamentenverabreichungssystem | 投薬システム |
| 2062. drug design - (n) | dessin médicamenteux | disegno del farmaco | diseño de la droga | Wirkstoffdesign | 薬物設計 |

| English/American | French/Français | Italian/Italiano | Spanish/Español | German/Deutsch | Japanese/日本語 |
|---|---|---|---|---|---|
| 2063. drug development - (n) | développement de médicament | sviluppo farmacologico | desarrollo de drogas | Medikamentenentwicklung | 薬物開発 |
| 2064. drug disposition - (n) | caractère de la drogue | carattere di un farmaco | carácter de la droga | Arzneimittelanordnung | 薬物性質 |
| 2065. drug holiday (n) | période sans drogue | giornate senza farmaco | período sin drogas | Medikamentenpause | 薬物休止日 |
| 2066. drug industry - (n) | industrie pharmaceutique | industria farmaceutica | industria farmacéutica | pharmazeutische Industrie | 薬物産業 |
| 2067. drug interaction - (n) | interaction médicamenteuse | interazione farmaci | interacción de drogas | Arzneimittelinteraction | 薬物相互作用 |
| 2068. drug lag - (n) | délai d'une drogue | ritardo di un farmaco | demora farmacológica | Arzneimittelverzögerung | 薬物遅延 |
| 2069. drug master file - (n) | dossier principal des drogues | schedario principale farmaco | archivo maestro de drogas | Medikamentenhaupt-verzeichnis | 薬物主要ファイル |
| 2070. drug profile (n) | profil médicamenteux | profilo farmaco | descripción de la droga | Wirkungsprofil eines Medikaments | 薬物プロファイル |
| 2071. drug receptor - (n) | récepteur médicamenteux | recettore farmaco | receptor de la droga | Medikamentrezeptor | 薬物受容体 |
| 2072. drug residue - (n) | résidu médicamenteux | residuo farmaco | residuo de la droga | Medikamentrückstand | 薬物残留 |
| 2073. drug surveillance - (n) | surveillance médicamenteuse | sorveglianza farmacologica | supervisión de la droga | Drogenüberwachung; Medikamenten-überwachung | 薬物監視 |
| 2074. drug synergism - (n) | synergie médicamenteuse | sinergismo tra farmaci | sinergismo de la droga | Medikamenten-synergismus | 薬物共力作用 |
| 2075. druggist - (n) | pharmacien | farmacista | farmacéutico | Apotheker | 薬剤師 |
| 2076. drugstore - (n) | pharmacie | farmacia | farmacia | Apotheke | ドラッグストア |
| 2077. drum - (n) | tympan | timpano; membrana timpanica | membrana timpánica | Trommelfell; Mittelohr | 鼓膜 |
| 2078. drunk - (a) | ivre; soûl | ubriaco; ebbro | borracho | betrunken | 酔っている |
| 2079. dry eyes - (n) | yeux secs; xérophtalmie | occhi asciutti | ojos secos | trockene Augen | 乾燥した目 |

| English/American | French/Français | Italian/Italiano | Spanish/Español | German/Deutsch | Japanese/日本語 |
|---|---|---|---|---|---|
| 2080. dry mouth - (n) | bouche sèche; xérostomie | bocca secca | boca seca | trockener Mund | 乾燥した口 |
| 2081. dry skin - (n) | peau sèche | cute secca; cute disidratata | piel seca | trockene Haut | 乾皮症 |
| 2082. duct - (n) | canal; conduit | dotto; condotto | conducto | Gang | 管 |
| 2083. duct gland - (n) | glande à canal; glande exocrine | dotto ghiandolare | glándula exocrina | Drüsengang | 管腺 |
| 2084. ductless gland - (n) | glande endocrine | ghiandola endocrina | glándula endocrina | Drüse ohne Ausführungsgang | 内分泌腺 |
| 2085. dull - (a) | faible; terne | sordo; insensibile; ottuso | sordo embotado | stumpf; dumpf | 鈍い |
| 2086. dullness - (n) | affaiblissement; matité | ottusità; l'essere smussato | matidez | Trübung; Dämpfung | 濁音 |
| 2087. dumb - (a) | muet | muto | mudo | stumm | 唖の |
| 2088. dumb terminal (n) | terminal muet | terminale muto | terminal simple | nichtprogrammierbare Datenstation | ダム端末 |
| 2089. dumping syndrome - (n) | syndrome de chasse | sindrome postgastrectomia | síndrome de la evacuación gástrica en torrente | Dumping-Syndrom | ダンピング症候群 |
| 2090. duodenal - (a) | duodénal | duodenale | duodenal | duodenal | 十二指腸の |
| 2091. duodenal ulcer - (n) | ulcère du duodénum | ulcera duodenale | úlcera duodenal | Duodenalulkus; Zwölffingerdarmgeschwür | 十二指腸潰瘍 |
| 2092. duodenum - (n) | duodénum | duodeno | duodeno | Zwölffingerdarm | 十二指腸 |
| 2093. dura mater - (n) | dure-mère | dura madre | dura madre | Dura mater; harte Hirnhaut | 硬脳膜 |
| 2094. duration - (n) | durée | durata | duración | Dauer | 持続期間 |
| 2095. dust - (n) | poussière | polvere | polvo | Staub | ほこり |
| 2096. dwarf - (n) | nain | nano | enano | Zwerg | 小人 |
| 2097. dwarfism - (n) | nanisme | nanismo | enanismo | Minderwuchs; Nanosomie | 小人症 |

| English/American | French/Français | Italian/Italiano | Spanish/Español | German/Deutsch | Japanese/日本語 |
|---|---|---|---|---|---|
| 2098. dye - (n) | teinture; colorant | tintura; colorante | color; tinte | Farbstoff | 色素 |
| 2099. dye - (v) | teindre; colorer | tingere; colorare | teñir | färben | 染色する |
| 2100. dying - (n) | mort | morte | muerte | Sterben | 死 |
| 2101. dynamic comparison - (n) | comparaison dynamique | paragone dinamico | comparación dinámica | dynamischer Vergleich | 動的比較 |
| 2102. dysarthria - (n) | dysarthrie | disartria | disartria | Dysarthrie | 構音障害 |
| 2103. dyscrasia - (n) | dyscrasie | discrasia | discrasia | Dyskrasie | 悪液質 |
| 2104. dysentery - (n) | dysenterie | dissenteria | disenteria | Dysenterie | 赤痢 |
| 2105. dysfunction - (n) | dysfonction | disfunzione | disfunción | Dysfunktion; Funktionsstörung | 機能障害 |
| 2106. dyskinesia - (n) | dyscinésie; dyskinésie | discinesia | disquinesia; discinesia | Dyskinesie; Bewegungsstörung | 運動障害 |
| 2107. dyslexia - (n) | dyslexie | dislessia | dislexia | Dyslexie; Legasthenie | 失読症 |
| 2108. dyslexic - (n) | dyslexique | dislessico | disléxico | Legastheniker | 失読症の人 |
| 2109. dyslexic - (a) | dyslexique | dislessico | disléxico | legasthenisch | 失読 [症] の |
| 2110. dysmenorrhea - (n) | dysménorrhée | dismenorrea | dismenorrea | Dysmenorrhö | 月経困難 [症] |
| 2111. dyspepsia - (n) | dyspepsie | dispepsia | dispepsia | Dyspepsie | 消化不良 |
| 2112. dysphagia - (n) | dysphagie | disfagia | disfagia | Dysphagie; Schluckstörung | 嚥下困難 |
| 2113. dysphasia - (n) | dysphasie | disfasia | disfasia | Dysphasie | 失語 [症] |
| 2114. dysphoria - (n) | dysphorie | disforia | disforia | Dysphorie | 不快 [気分] |
| 2115. dysplasia - (n) | dysplasie | displasia | displasia | Dysplasie | 形質異常 [症] |
| 2116. dyspnea - (n) | dyspnée | dispnea | disnea | Dyspnoea | 呼吸困難 |
| 2117. dysrhythmia - (n) | dysrhythmie | disritmia; aritmia | disritmia | Dysrhythmie | 律動異常 |
| 2118. dystonia - (n) | dystonie | distonia | distonia | Dystonie | 失調 [症] |
| 2119. dystrophy - (n) | dystrophie | distrofia | distrofia | Dystrophie | 栄養失調症. ジストロフィー |
| 2120. dysuria - (n) | dysurie | disuria | disuria | Dysurie | 排尿障害 |

| English/American | French/Français | Italian/Italiano | Spanish/Español | German/Deutsch | Japanese/日本語 |
|---|---|---|---|---|---|
| 2121. ear - (n) | oreille | orecchio | oído; oreja | Ohr | 耳 |
| 2122. ear ossicle - (n) | osselet de l'oreille | ossicino dell'orecchio | osículo del oído | Gehörknöchelchen | 耳小骨 |
| 2123. eardrum - (n) | tympan | timpano | tímpano | Trommelfell | 鼓膜 |
| 2124. early stopping rule - (n) | règle d'interruption précoce | regola dell' interruzione anticipata | regla de interrupción precoz | frühe Unterbrechungsregel | 早期停止規則 |
| 2125. eating - (n) | manger | il mangiare | el comer | Essen; Nahrungsaufnahme | 食事 |
| 2126. eating disorder - (n) | désordre de l'appétit | disordine dell'alimentazione | trastorno de la alimentación | Eßstörung | 食事障害 |
| 2127. ecchymosis - (n) | ecchymose | ecchimosi | equimosis | Ekchymose | 斑状出血 |
| 2128. echo-cardiogram - (n) | échocardiogramme | ecocardiogramma | ecocardiograma | Echokardiogramm | エコーカルジオグラム |
| 2129. echo-cardiography - (n) | échocardiographie | ecocardiografia | ecocardiografía | Echokardiographie | 心エコー検査 [法] |
| 2130. echoencephalo-graphy - (n) | échoencéphalographie | ecoencefalografia | ecoencefalografía | Echoenzephalographie | 脳エコー検査 [法] |
| 2131. echolalia - (n) | écholalie | ecolalia; ecofrasia | ecolalia | Echolalie | 反響音声 |
| 2132. eclampsia - (n) | éclampsie | eclampsia | eclampsia | Eklampsie | 子癇 |
| 2133. ecology - (n) | écologie | ecologia | ecología | Ökologie | 生態学 |
| 2134. economic analysis - (n) | analyse économique | analisi economica | análisis económico | Wirtschaftsanalyse wirtschaftliche | 経済分析 |
| 2135. economic competition - (n) | compétition économique | competizione economica | competencia económica | Konkurrenz; wirtschaftlicher Wettbewerb | 経済競争 |
| 2136. economics - (n) | économique; économie | economia | economía | Ökonomie; Wirtschaft | 経済学 |
| 2137. ectoderm - (n) | ectoderme | ectoderma | ectodermo | Ektoderm | 外胚葉 |
| 2138. ectodermal dysplasia - (n) | dysplasie ectodermique | displasia ectodermica | displasia ectodérmica | ektodermale Dysplasie | 外胚葉形成成異常 |

109

| English/American | French/Français | Italian/Italiano | Spanish/Español | German/Deutsch | Japanese 日本語 |
|---|---|---|---|---|---|
| 2139. ectopic pregnancy - (n) | grossesse ectopique | gravidanza ectopica | embarazo ectópico | ektopische Schwangerschaft | 子宮外妊娠 |
| 2140. ectopy - (n) | ectopie | ectopia | ectopia | Ektopie | 転位 |
| 2141. eczema - (n) | eczéma | eczema | eccema | Ekzem | 湿疹 |
| 2142. edema - (n) | oedème | edema | edema | Ödem | 浮腫 |
| 2143. edge - (n) | bord | bordo; spigolo | borde; margen | Kante; Rand | 辺縁 |
| 2144. edible plant - (n) | plante comestible | pianta commestibile | planta comestible | eßbare Pflanze | 食用植物 |
| 2145. edit check - (n) | contrôle d'édition | verifica redazione | control de edición | Editierungskontrolle | 編集検査 |
| 2146. edit query - (n) | demande d'édition | problema di redazione testo | demanda de edición | Editierungsabfrage | 編集質問 |
| 2147. editing - (n) | édition; rédaction | editazione; redazione | edición; redacción | Herausgabe; Redaktion | 編集 |
| 2148. editor - (n) | éditeur; rédacteur | redattore; direttore | editor; redactor | Herausgeber; Redakteur | 編集者 |
| 2149. editorial - (n) | éditorial | editoriale | editorial | Leitartikel | 論説 |
| 2150. education - (n) | éducation | educazione; istruzione | educación; formación | Erziehung | 教育 |
| 2151. educational - (a) | éducatif, d'éducation | educativo; dell'educazione | educacional | Erziehungs-; pädagogisch | 教育の |
| 2152. effect - (n) | effet | effetto | efecto | Wirkung; Effekt | 効果 |
| 2153. effective - (a) | effectif, efficace | efficace | eficaz | effektiv | 効果的な |
| 2154. effectiveness - (n) | efficacité | efficacia; efficienza | eficacia; efectividad | Effektivität | 効果 |
| 2155. efferent - (a) | efférent | efferente | eferente; centrífugo | efferent; wegführend | 遠心性の |
| 2156. efferent neuron - (n) | neurone efférent | neurone efferente | neurona eferente | efferentes Neuron | 遠心性ニューロン |
| 2157. efferent pathway - (n) | voie efférente | linea efferente | vía eferente | efferente Bahn | 遠心性経路 |
| 2158. efficacy - (n) | efficacité | efficacia | eficacia | Wirksamkeit | 効能 |
| 2159. efficacy profile - (n) | profil d'efficacité | profilo efficacia | descripción de la eficacia | Wirksamkeitsprofil | 効能プロファイル |
| 2160. efficacy score - (n) | score d'efficacité | punteggio efficacia | puntaje de eficacia | Wirksamkeitspunktzahl | 効能成績 |

| English/American | French/Français | Italian/Italiano | Spanish/Español | German/Deutsch | Japanese/日本語 |
|---|---|---|---|---|---|
| 2161. efficacy variable - (n) | variable d'efficacité | variabile efficacia | variable de eficacia | Wirksamkeitsvariable | 効能変数 |
| 2162. efficiency - (n) | efficacité; compétence | efficienza; rendimento | eficiencia; eficacia | Effizienz; Wirkungsgrad | 効率 |
| 2163. effluent - (a) | effluent | effluente | efluente | ausfließend; ausströmend | 流出する |
| 2164. effusion - (n) | effusion; épanchement | effusione; versamento | efusión; derrame | Erguß; Ausschwitzen | 滲出 |
| 2165. egg - (n) | oeuf | uovo | huevo | Ei | 卵 |
| 2166. egg count - (n) | décompte d'oeufs | conto uovi | cuenta de huevos | Eizahlbestimmung | 卵の数 |
| 2167. egg yolk - (n) | jaune d'oeuf | tuorlo; rosso d'uovo | yema de huevo | Eidotter | 卵黄 |
| 2168. ejaculation - (n) | éjaculation | eiaculazione | eyaculación | Ejakulation; Samenerguß | 射精 |
| 2169. ejection click - (n) | clic d'éjection systolique | scatto di eiezione | clic de eyección | Austreibungston | 駆出性クリック |
| 2170. ejection fraction - (n) | fraction d'éjection | frazione di eiezione | fracción de eyección | Ejektionsfraktion; Auswurfsfraktion | 駆出率 |
| 2171. elastic - (a) | élastique | elastico | elástico | elastisch | 弾性のある |
| 2172. elasticity - (n) | élasticité | elasticità | elasticidad | Elastizität | 弾力性 |
| 2173. elbow - (n) | coude | gomito | codo | Ellenbogen | 肘 |
| 2174. elderly - (a) | âgé; assez âgé | anziano; attempato | de edad; mayor | ältlich; alter | 年配の |
| 2175. elective surgery - (n) | chirurgie élective | chirurgia elettiva | cirugía electiva | elektiver Eingriff; Wahloperation | 選択手術 |
| 2176. electric - (a) | électrique | elettrico | eléctrico | elektrisch | 電気の |
| 2177. electric shock - (n) | choc électrique | shock elettrico; elettroshock | electrochoque; choque eléctrico | Elektroschock | 電気ショック |
| 2178. electrocardiogram [abbr] EKG, ECG - (n) | électrocardiogramme, ECG | elettrocardiogramma, ECG | electrocardiograma | Elektrokardiogramm, EKG | 心電図 |
| 2179. electrocardiogram leads - (n) | électrodes d'électrocardiogramme | derivazione | electrodos del electrocardiograma | Elektrokardiogramm-elektroden | 心電図誘導 |
| 2180. electrocardiography - (n) | électrocardiographie | elettrocardiografica elettrocardiografia | electrocardiografía | Elektrokardiographie | 心電図検査 [法] |

111

| English/American | French/Français | Italian/Italiano | Spanish/Español | German/Deutsch | Japanese/日本語 |
|---|---|---|---|---|---|
| 2181. electro-chemistry - (n) | électrochimie | elettrochimica | electroquímica | Elektrochemie | 電気化学 |
| 2182. electro-coagulation - (n) | électrocoagulation | elettrocoagulazione | electrocoagulación | Elektrokoagulation | 電気凝固［法］ |
| 2183. electrocon-vulsive - (a) | électroconvulsif | elettroconvulsivante | electroconvulsivo | Elektroschock-; Elektrokrampf- | 電撃ショックの |
| 2184. electrode - (n) | électrode | elettrodo | electrodo | Elektrode | 電極 |
| 2185. electroencephalo-gram - (n) | électro-encéphalogramme | elettroencefalogramma | electroencefalograma | Elektroenzephalogramm | 脳波 |
| 2186. electroencephalo-graphy - (n) | électro-encéphalographie | elettroencefalografia | electroencefalografia | Elektroenzephalographie | 脳波記録［法］ |
| 2187. electrolysis - (n) | électrolyse | elettrolisi | electrólisis | Elektrolyse | 電解 |
| 2188. electrolyte - (n) | électrolyte | elettrolito | electrólito | Elektrolyt | 電解質 |
| 2189. electrolyte imbalance - (n) | désordre électrolytique | squilibrio elettrolitico | desequilibrio de electrólitos | Elektrolytgleichgewicht-störung | 電解質不均衡 |
| 2190. electromagnetic field - (n) | champ électromagnétique | campo elettromagnetico | campo electromagnético | elektromagnetisches Feld | 電磁界 |
| 2191. electromy-ography - (n) | électromyographie | elettromiografia | electromiografia | Elektromyographie | 筋電図検査［法］ |
| 2192. electron - (n) | électron | elettrone | electrón | Elektron | 電子 |
| 2193. electron micro-scope - (n) | microscope électronique | microscopio elettronico | microscopio electrónico | Elektronenmikroskop | 電子顕微鏡 |
| 2194. electron microsco-py - (n) | microscopie électronique | microscopia elettronica | microscopía electrónica | Elektronenmikroskopie | 電子顕微鏡検査法 |
| 2195. electron transport - (n) | transport d'électrons | trasporto di elettroni | transporte de electrones | Elektronentransport | 電子輸送 |
| 2196. electronic - (a) | électronique | elettronico | electrónico | elektronisch | 電子の |
| 2197. electronic record - (n) | registre électronique | registrazione elettrica | registro electrónico | elektronische Aufzeichnung | 電子記録 |

112

| English/American | French/Français | Italian/Italiano | Spanish/Español | German/Deutsch | Japanese/日本語 |
|---|---|---|---|---|---|
| 2198. electronystagmography [abbr] ENG - (n) | électronystagmographie | elettronistagmografia | electronistagmografía | Elektronystagmographie | 電気眼振記録 [法] |
| 2199. electrooculography - (n) | électro-oculographie | elettrooculografia | electrooculografía | Elektrookulographie | 電気眼球図記録 [法] |
| 2200. electrophoresis - (n) | électrophorèse | elettroforesi | electroforesis | Elektrophorese | 電気泳動 |
| 2201. electrophysiology - (n) | électrophysiologie | elettrofisiologia | electrofisiología | Elektrophysiologie | 電気生理学 |
| 2202. electroretinography - (n) | électrorétinographie | elettroretinografia | electrorretinografía | Elektroretinographie | 網膜電図記録 [法] |
| 2203. electroshock - (n) | électrochoc | elettroshock | electrochoque | Elektroschock | 電気ショック |
| 2204. electrosurgery - (n) | électrochirurgie | elettrochirurgia | electrocirugía | Elektrochirurgie | 電気外科 |
| 2205. element - (n) | élément | elemento | elemento | Element; Grundbestandteil | 元素 |
| 2206. elements of consent - (n) | éléments du consentement | elementi di consenso | elementos de consentimiento | Aufklärungsbestandteile | 同意書の内容 |
| 2207. elevated border - (n) | bord (sur)élevé | bordo rialzato | borde elevado | erhobener Rand | 上昇境界縁 |
| 2208. elevated margin - (n) | marge (sur)élevée | margine rialzato | margen elevado | erhobener Rand | 上昇マージン |
| 2209. elevation - (n) | élévation | elevazione | elevación | Erhebung | 上昇 |
| 2210. eligibility - (n) | éligibilité; admissibilité | candidabilità | elegibilidad | Berechtigung | 適格性 |
| 2211. eligibility criteria - (n) | critères d'éligibilité; critères d'admissibilité | criteri di candidabilità | criterio de elegibilidad | Berechtigungskriterien | 適格性基準 |
| 2212. eligible - (a) | éligible; admissible | candidato | elegible; admissible | teilnahmeberechtigt | 適格の |
| 2213. eligible patient - (n) | patient éligible; patient admissible | paziente candidato | paciente elegible; paciente admissible | geeigneter Patient | 適格患者 |

113

| English/American | French/Français | Italian/Italiano | Spanish/Español | German/Deutsch | Japanese/日本語 |
|---|---|---|---|---|---|
| 2214. elimination - (n) | élimination | eliminazione | eliminación | Elimination; Ausscheidung | 除去 |
| 2215. elimination half-life - (n) | demi-vie d'élimination | emivita d'eliminazione | media vida de eliminación | Halbwertszeit der Elimination | 除去半減期 |
| 2216. elixir - (n) | élixir | elisir | elixir | Elixir | エリキシル（剤） |
| 2217. emaciation - (n) | émaciation; amaigrissement | emaciamento; dimagrimento | emaciación | Abmagerung; Auszehrung | やせること |
| 2218. emasculation - (n) | émasculation; castration | evirazione; castrazione | emasculación; castración | Entmannung; Verweiblichung | 去勢 |
| 2219. embalming - (n) | embaumement | imbalsamazione | embalsamamiento | Einbalsamierung | 死体の防腐処理 |
| 2220. embedding - (n) | incorporation; inclusion | inclusione; incorporazione | incorporación; inclusión | Einbettung | 包埋 |
| 2221. embolism - (n) | embolie | embolismo | embolismo; embolia | Embolie | 塞栓症 |
| 2222. embolization - (n) | embolisation | embolizzazione | embolización | Embolisierung | 塞栓形成 [法] |
| 2223. embolus - (n) | embolus; caillot | embolo | émbolo | Embolus | 栓子 |
| 2224. embryo - (n) | embryon | embrione | embrión | Embryo | 胎芽 |
| 2225. embryology - (n) | embryologie | embriologia | embriología | Embryologie | 胎生学 |
| 2226. embryonal - (a) | embryonnaire | embrionale | embrionario | embryonal | 胚の |
| 2227. emergency - (n) | cas urgent; urgence | emergenza; urgenza | emergencia; urgencia | Notfall | 突発事故 |
| 2228. emergency medicine - (n) | médecine d'urgence | medicina d'emergenza | medicina de emergencia | Notfallmedizin | 救急治療 |
| 2229. emergency room - (n) | salle d'urgence | reparto di pronto soccorso | sala de emergencias; sala de urgencias | Unfallstation | 救急治療部 |
| 2230. emesis - (n) | vomissement | emesi; vomito | emesis; vómito | Erbrechen | 嘔吐 |
| 2231. emetic - (n) | émétique | emetico | emético | Emetikum; Brechmittel | 吐剤 |
| 2232. emigration - (n) | émigration | emigrazione; diapedesi | emigración | Auswanderung | 遊出 |
| 2233. emission - (n) | émission | emissione | emisión | Emission; Ausstrom | 射出 |
| 2234. emission computed tomography - (n) | tomographie d'émission par ordinateur | tomografia computerizzata d'emissione | tomografía computadorizada por emisión | Computeremissions-tomographie | 射出断層撮影 [法] |

| English/American | French/Français | Italian/Italiano | Spanish/Español | German/Deutsch | Japanese/日本語 |
|---|---|---|---|---|---|
| 2235. emollient - (n) | émollient | emolliente | emoliente | Emollentium; Weichmacher | 軟膏剤 |
| 2236. emotion - (n) | émotion | emozione | emoción | Emotion | 感情 |
| 2237. emotional disorder - (n) | désordre émotionnel | disordine della sfera emotiva | trastorno emocional | emotionelle Störung | 感情障害 |
| 2238. emotional lability - (n) | labilité émotionnelle | labilità emotiva | labilidad emocional | emotionelle Labilität | 感情不安定 |
| 2239. emotive - (a) | émotif | emotivo | emotivo | gefühlsmäßig; emotional | 感情的な |
| 2240. empathy - (n) | empathie | empatia | empatía | Empathie; Einfühlung | 感情移入 |
| 2241. emphysema - (n) | emphysème | enfisema | enfisema | Emphysem | 気腫 |
| 2242. empirical - (a) | empirique | empirico | empírico | empirisch | 経験の |
| 2243. employee - (n) | employé | impiegato | empleado | Angestellter | 雇用人 |
| 2244. employment - (n) | emploi; travail | impiego; occupazione | empleo; ocupación | (An)stellung; Arbeit | 雇用 |
| 2245. empyema - (n) | empyème | empiema | empiema | Empyem | 蓄膿 |
| 2246. emulsion - (n) | émulsion | emulsione | emulsión | Emulsion | 乳剤 |
| 2247. enamel - (n) | émail | smalto | esmalte | Emaille; Zahnschmelz | エナメル |
| 2248. enantiomer - (n) | énantiomère | enantiomero | enantiómero | Enantiomer | エナンチオマー |
| 2249. encephalitis - (n) | encéphalite | encefalite | encefalitis | Enzephalitis; Gehirnentzündung | 脳炎 |
| 2250. enclosed - (a) | enfermé; inclus | rinchiuso; racchiuso | cerrado; cercado | eingeschlossen; beiliegend | 同封の |
| 2251. end of trial questionnaire - (n) | questionnaire de la fin de l'essai | questionario finale di uno studio controllato | cuestionario al final del experimento | Fragebogen zum Versuchsabschluß | 試験質問事項の終了 |
| 2252. end plate - (n) | plaque terminale | placca terminale | placa terminal | Endplatte | 終板 |
| 2253. endarterectomy - (n) | endartérectomie | endarterectomia | endarterectomía | Endarteriektomie | 動脈血管内膜切除術 |
| 2254. endemic - (a) | endémique | endemica | endémico | endemisch | 風土病 |
| 2255. endocarditis - (n) | endocardite | endocardite | endocarditis | Endokarditis | 心内膜炎 |
| 2256. endocardium - (n) | endocarde | endocardio | endocardio | Endokard | 心内膜 |

| English/American | French/Français | Italian/Italiano | Spanish/Español | German/Deutsch | Japanese/日本語 |
|---|---|---|---|---|---|
| 2257. endocrine - (a) | endocrine | endocrino | endocrino | endokrin | 内分泌腺の |
| 2258. endocrine gland - (n) | glande endocrine | ghiandola endocrina | glándula endocrina | endokrine Drüse | 内分泌腺 |
| 2259. endocrin-ology - (n) | endocrinologie | endocrinologia | endocrinología | Endokrinologie | 内分泌学 |
| 2260. endocytosis - (n) | endocytose | endocitosi | endocitosis | Endozytose | エンドサイトーシス |
| 2261. endodontics - (n) | endodontie | endodontico | endodoncia | Endodontie | 歯内治療学 |
| 2262. endogenous - (a) | endogène | endogeno | endógeno | endogen | 内因性の |
| 2263. endogenous substance receptor - (n) | récepteur de substance endogène | recettore sostanza endogena | receptor de sustancia endógena | endogener Stoffrezeptor | 内因性物質レセプター |
| 2264. endolymph - (n) | endolymphe | endolinfa | endolinfa | Endolymphe | 内リンパ |
| 2265. endometrial - (a) | endométrial | endometriale | endometrial | endometrial | 子宮内膜の |
| 2266. endo-metriosis - (n) | endométriose | endometriosi | endometriosis | Endometriose | 子宮内膜［症］ |
| 2267. endometrium - (n) | endomètre | endometrio | endometrio | Endometrium | 子宮内膜 |
| 2268. endoplasmic reticulum - (n) | réticulum endoplasmique | reticolo endoplasmatico | retículo endoplasmático | endoplasmatisches Retikulum | 小胞体 |
| 2269. endorphin - (n) | endorphine | endorfina | endorfina | Endorphin | エンドルフィン類 |
| 2270. endoscope - (n) | endoscope | endoscopio | endoscopio | Endoskop | 内視鏡 |
| 2271. endoscopic - (a) | endoscopique | endoscopico | endoscópico | endoskopisch | 内視鏡の |
| 2272. endoscopy - (n) | endoscopie | endoscopia | endoscopia | Endoskopie | 内視鏡検査［法］ |
| 2273. endosseous dental implanta-tion - (n) | implantation dentaire intraosseuse | impianto dentale endosseo | implantación dental endósea | endostale Zahnprothese | 骨内歯牙移植 |
| 2274. endothelial - (a) | endothélial | endoteliale | endotelial | endothelial | 内皮の |
| 2275. endothelium - (n) | endothélium | endotelio | endotelio | Endothel | 内皮 |
| 2276. endotoxin - (n) | endotoxine | endotossina | endotoxina | Endotoxin | 内毒素 |

116

| English/American | French/Français | Italian/Italiano | Spanish/Español | German/Deutsch | Japanese/日本語 |
|---|---|---|---|---|---|
| 2277. endpoint - (n) | point final | punto finale | punto final | Endpunkt; Zielpunkt | 終点 |
| 2278. endpoint analysis - (n) | analyse du point final | analisi del punto finale | análisis del punto final | Zielpunktanalyse | 終点分析 |
| 2279. endurance - (n) | endurance | resistenza | resistencia | Ausdauer; Belastbarkeit | 忍耐 |
| 2280. enema - (n) | lavement | clistere; clisma | enema | Klistier; Einlauf | 浣腸 |
| 2281. energy - (n) | énergie | energia | energía | Energie | エネルギー |
| 2282. engineering - (n) | ingénierie | ingegneria | ingeniería | Technologie; Technik | 工学 |
| 2283. engorged - (a) | engorgé | ingurgitato; congestionato | ingurgitado | geschwollen; prall | 充血の |
| 2284. enlarged - (a) | agrandi | allargato; ingrandito | aumentado | erweitert; vergrößert | 拡大した |
| 2285. enlargement - (n) | agrandissement | allargamento; ingrandimento | alargamiento | Erweiterung; Vergrößerung | 拡大 |
| 2286. enrollment, enrolment - (n) | enrôlement; inscription | iscrizione; registrazione | inscripción; alistamiento | Aufnahme; Anmeldung | 登録 |
| 2287. enteral - (a) | entéral | enterale | enteral | enteral | 腸内の |
| 2288. enteric - (a) | entérique | enterico | entérico | enterisch; Darm- | 腸の |
| 2289. enteric coated - (a) | Kératinisé | querantinizado | querantinizado | keratinüberzogen | 腸溶のためにコーティングされた |
| 2290. enteritis - (n) | entérite | enterite | enteritis | Enteritis | 腸炎 |
| 2291. enterochromaffin cell - (n) | cellule entéro-chromaffine | cellula enterocromafina | célula enterocromafina | enterchromaffine Zelle | 腸クロム親和細胞 |
| 2292. enterotoxin - (n) | entérotoxine | enterotossina | enterotoxina | Enterotoxin | エンテロトキシン |
| 2293. entrance - (n) | entrée | entrata; ingresso | entrada | Eingang | 入り口、入ること |
| 2294. entry criteria - (n) | critères d'entrée | criteri per ingresso | criterios de aceptación | Eingangskriterien | 入力基準 |
| 2295. enucleate - (v) | énucléer | enucleare | enuclear | entkernen; ausschälen | 摘出する |
| 2296. enuresis - (n) | énurésie | enuresi | enuresis | Enurese | 遺尿症 |
| 2297. environment - (n) | environnement | ambiente | ambiente | Umgebung; Umwelt | 環境 |
| 2298. environ-mental - (a) | environnemental | ambientale | ambiental | Umwelt- | 環境の |

| English/American | French/Français | Italian/Italiano | Spanish/Español | German/Deutsch | Japanese/日本語 |
|---|---|---|---|---|---|
| 2299. environmental factor - (n) | facteur environnemental | fattore ambientale | factor ambiental | Umweltfaktor | 環境因子 |
| 2300. environmental influence - (n) | influence environnementale | influenza ambientale | influencia ambiental | Umwelteinfluß | 環境影響 |
| 2301. enzymatic defect - (n) | défaut enzymatique | difetto enzimatico | defecto enzimático | Enzymschädigung | 酵素欠乏 |
| 2302. enzyme - (n) | enzyme | enzima | enzima | Enzym | 酵素 |
| 2303. enzymology - (n) | enzymologie | enzimologia | enzimología | Enzymologie | 酵素学 |
| 2304. eosinophil - (n) | éosinophile | eosinofilo | eosinófilo | Eosinophiler | 好酸球 |
| 2305. eosinophilia - (n) | éosinophilie | eosinofilia | eosinofilia | Eosinophilie | 好酸球増多症 |
| 2306. epicardium - (n) | épicarde | epicardio | epicardio | Epikard | 心外膜 |
| 2307. epidemic - (n) | épidémie | epidemia | epidemia | Epidemie | 流行病 |
| 2308. epidemic - (a) | épidémique | epidemico | epidémico | epidemisch | 流行性の |
| 2309. epidemiologic - (a) | épidémiologique | epidemiologico | epidemiológico | epidemiologisch | 流行病学の |
| 2310. epidemiological intelligence - (n) | intelligence épidémiologique | intelligenza epidemiologica | inteligencia epidemiológica | epidemiologische Intelligenz | 疫学上の知識 |
| 2311. epidemiology - (n) | épidémiologie | epidemiologia | epidemiología | Epidemiologie | 流行病学 |
| 2312. epidermal - (a) | épidermique | epidermico | epidérmico | epidermal | 表皮の |
| 2313. epidermis - (n) | épiderme | epidermide | epidermis | Epidermis | 表皮 |
| 2314. epididymis - (n) | épididyme | epididimo | epidídimo | Epididymis; Nebenhoden | 副睾丸 |
| 2315. epidural - (a) | épidural | epidurale | epidural | epidural | 硬［脳］膜上の |
| 2316. epigastric - (a) | épigastrique | epigastrico | epigástrico | epigastrisch | 上腹部の |
| 2317. epiglottis - (n) | épiglotte | epiglottide | epiglotis | Epiglottis; Kehldeckel | 喉頭蓋 |
| 2318. epilation - (n) | épilation; dépilation | depilazione | epilación; depilación | Epilation | 脱毛 |
| 2319. epilepsy - (n) | épilepsie | epilessia | epilepsia | Epilepsie | てんかん |
| 2320. epileptic seizure - (n) | crise d'épilepsie | crisi epilettica | ataque epiléptico | epileptischer Anfall | てんかん発作 |
| 2321. epinephrine - (n) | épinéphrine; adrénaline | epinefrina; adrenalina | epinefrina; adrenalina | Epinephrin; Adrenalin | エピネフリン |

| English/American | French/Français | Italian/Italiano | Spanish/Español | German/Deutsch | Japanese/日本語 |
|---|---|---|---|---|---|
| 2322. epiphysial plate - (n) | plaque épiphysaire | disco epifisario; cartilagine epifisaria | placa epifisaria | Epiphysenplatte; Epiphysenknorpel | 骨端板 |
| 2323. epiphysis - (n) | épiphyse | epifisi | epifisis | Epiphyse | 骨端 |
| 2324. episiotomy - (n) | épisiotomie | episiotomia | episiotomia | Episiotomie | 会陰切開 [術] |
| 2325. episode - (n) | épisode | episodio | episodio | Episode | 症状の発現 |
| 2326. epistaxis - (n) | épistaxis | epistassi | epistaxis | Epistaxis; Nasenbluten | 鼻出血 |
| 2327. epithelial - (a) | épithélial | epiteliale | epitelial | epithelial | 上皮細胞の |
| 2328. epithelial cell - (n) | cellule épithéliale | cellula epiteliale | célula epitelial | Epithelzelle | 上皮細胞 |
| 2329. epithelium - (n) | épithélium | epitelio | epitelio | Epithel | 上皮 |
| 2330. equilibrium - (n) | équilibre | equilibrio | equilibrio | Gleichgewicht | 平衡状態 |
| 2331. equipment - (n) | équipement | apparecchiatura | equipo | Gerät; Ausstattung | 器具 |
| 2332. equivalence trial - (n) | essai d'équivalence | prova equivalenza | ensayo de equivalencia | Äquivalenzprobe | 等量試験 |
| 2333. equivalent - (n) | équivalent | equivalente | equivalente | Äquivalent | 等量 |
| 2334. equivalent - (a) | équivalent | equivalente | equivalente | äquivalent | 等量の |
| 2335. equivocal results - (n) | résultats équivoques | risultati equivoci | resultados equivocos | nicht eindeutige Resultate; fragwürdige Ergebnisse | 両義の結果 |
| 2336. eradication - (n) | éradication | estirpazione | extirpación | Eradikation; Ausrottung | 絶滅 |
| 2337. erect - (a) | en érection | eretto | erecto | aufrecht; erigiert | 勃起の |
| 2338. erection - (n) | érection | erezione | erección | Erektion; Aufrichtung | 勃起 |
| 2339. erosion of skin - (n) | érosion de la peau | erosione della pelle | erosión de la piel | Hauterosion | 皮膚びらん |
| 2340. error - (n) | erreur | sbarre errore | error | Fehler | 過失 |
| 2341. error bars - (n) | barres d'erreur | barrette dell'errore | barras de error | Fehlerbalken | 誤差バー |
| 2342. error measurement - (n) | mesure d'erreurs | calcolo dell'errore | medida de errores | Fehlermessung | 誤差率測定 |
| 2343. error rate - (n) | taux d'erreurs | tasso di errore | tasa de errores | Fehlerrate | 誤差率 |
| 2344. eruption - (n) | éruption | eruzione | erupción | Eruption; Ausbruch | 発疹 |

| English/American | French/Français | Italian/Italiano | Spanish/Español | German/Deutsch | Japanese/日本語 |
|---|---|---|---|---|---|
| 2345. erythema - (n) | érythème | eritema | eritema | Erythem | 紅斑症 |
| 2346. erythroblast - (n) | érythroblaste | eritroblasto | eritroblasto | Erythroblast | 赤芽球 |
| 2347. erythrocyte - (n) | érythrocyte | eritrocito | eritrocito | Erythrozyt | 赤血球 |
| 2348. erythrocyte sedimentation rate [abbr] ES - (n) | vitesse de sédimentation érytrocytaire | velocità di eritrosedimentazione, VES | índice de sedimentación de eritrocitos | Blutkörperchensenkungs-geschwindigkeit, BSG | 赤血球沈降率 |
| 2349. erythroid progenitor cell - (n) | cellule précurseur des erythrocytes | cellula progenitrice eritroide | célula progenitora eritroide | Erythrozytenvor-äuferzelle | 赤血球先祖細胞 |
| 2350. erythro-poiesis - (n) | érythropoïèse | eritropoiesi | eritropoyesis | Erythropoiese | 赤血球生成 |
| 2351. escape clause - (n) | clause d'échappement | clausola-scappatoia | cláusula de escape | Rücktrittsklausel | 逸脱条項 |
| 2352. escape medica-tion - (n) | médication d'échappement | medicamento da scappatoia | medicación de escape | Zufluchtsmedikation | 逸脱医薬 |
| 2353. esophageal - (a) | oesophagien | esofagea | esofágio | ösophageal | 食道の |
| 2354. esophago-scopy - (n) | oesophagoscopie | esofagoscopia | esofagoscopia | Ösophagoskopie | 食道鏡検査［法］ |
| 2355. esophagus (oeso-phagus) - (n) | oesophage | esofago | esófago | Ösophagus; Speiseröhre | 食道 |
| 2356. essential - (a) | essentiel | essenziale | esencial | wesentlich | 必須の |
| 2357. esterification - (n) | estérification | esterificazione | esterificación | Esterbildung | エステル化 |
| 2358. estimate - (n) | estimation | stima; valore stimato | estimación | Schätzung; Bestimmung | 見積り |
| 2359. estimate - (v) | estimer | calcolare | estimar | schätzen; bestimnen | 見積る |
| 2360. estrogen (oestrogen) - (n) | oestrogène | estrogeno | estrógeno | Östrogen | 卵胞ホルモン |
| 2361. estrus - (n) | oestrus | estro | estro | Östrus; Brunst | 発情期 |
| 2362. ether - (n) | éther | etere | éter | Äther | エーテル |

120

| English/American | French/Français | Italian/Italiano | Spanish/Español | German/Deutsch | Japanese/日本語 |
|---|---|---|---|---|---|
| 2363. ethical approval - (n) | approbation éthique | approvazione etica | aprobación ética | Genehmigung von ethischen Grundsätzen her | 倫理的認可 |
| 2364. ethical issue - (n) | question éthique | problema etico | cuestión ética | ethische Frage | 倫理的問題 |
| 2365. ethical standard - (n) | norme éthique | standard etica | norma ética | Ethikstandard | 倫理的基準 |
| 2366. ethics - (n) | éthique | etica | ética | Ethik; Verhaltensregeln | 倫理学 |
| 2367. ethics committee - (n) | comité d'éthique | comitato etico | comité de ética | Ausschuß zur Klärung ethischer Fragen | 倫理委員会 |
| 2368. ethnic background - (n) | origine ethnique | sfondo etnico | origen étnico | ethnische Abstammung | 人種的背景 |
| 2369. ethnic group - (n) | groupe ethnique | gruppo etnico | grupo étnico | ethnische Gruppe; Volksgruppe | 人種 |
| 2370. ethology - (n) | éthologie | etologia | etología | Ethologie; Verhaltensforschung | 動物行動学 |
| 2371. etiology (aetiology) - (n) | étiologie | etiologia | etiología | Ätiologie | 病因学 |
| 2372. eugenics - (n) | eugénique | eugenetica; eugenica | eugenesia | Eugenik | 優生学 |
| 2373. euphoria - (n) | euphorie | euforia | euforia | Euphorie | 陶酔 |
| 2374. Eustachian tube - (n) | trompe d'Eustache | tromba di Eustachio | trompa de Eustaquio | Eustachische Röhre | エウスタキオ才管 |
| 2375. euthanasia - (n) | euthanasie | eutanasia | eutanasia | Euthanasie; Sterbehilfe | 安楽死 |
| 2376. evacuate - (v) | évacuer | evacuare | evacuar | evakuieren; entleeren | 排出する |
| 2377. evaluable - (a) | évaluable | valutabile | evaluable | auswertbar | 評価できる |
| 2378. evaluation - (n) | évaluation | valutazione | evaluación | Bewertung; Auswertung | 評価 |
| 2379. evening dose - (n) | dose du soir | dose serale | dosis de la tarde | Abenddosis | 夜間時の服用 |
| 2380. event rate - (n) | taux d'événements | frequenza degli eventi | tasa de eventos | Ereignisrate | 症例発生率 |
| 2381. eversion - (n) | éversion | eversione | eversión | Eversion | 外転 |

121

| English/American | French/Français | Italian/Italiano | Spanish/Español | German/Deutsch | Japanese/日本語 |
|---|---|---|---|---|---|
| 2382. every day - (adv) | tous les jours | quotidiano | todos los días | jeden Tag; täglich | 毎日 |
| 2383. every other day - (adv) | tous les deux jours | ogni due giorni; a giorni alterni | cada dos días | alle zwei Tage; jeden zweiten Tag | 一日おきに |
| 2384. evidence - (n) | évidence; preuve | evidenza; prova | evidencia; prueba | Beweis; Anzeichen | 証拠 |
| 2385. evisceration - (n) | éviscération | eviscerazione | evisceración | Eviszeration; Ausweidung | 内臓除去 [術] |
| 2386. evoked potential - (n) | potentiel évoqué | potenziale evocato | potencial evocado | evoziertes Potential | 誘発電位 |
| 2387. evolution - (n) | évolution; développement | evoluzione; sviluppo | evolución; desarrollo | Evolution; Entwicklung | 進化 |
| 2388. evulsion - (n) | évulsion | evulsione | evulsión | Evulsion; Ausreißen | 摘出 |
| 2389. exacerbation - (n) | exacerbation | esacerbazione | exacerbación | Exazerbation; Verschlimmerung | 増悪 |
| 2390. exam - (n) | examen | esame | examen | Prüfung; Untersuchung | 検査 |
| 2391. examination - (n) | examen | esame | examen | Prüfung; Untersuchung | 検査 |
| 2392. exanthema - (n) | exanthème | esantema | exantema | Exanthem | 発疹 |
| 2393. exanthematous - (a) | exanthémateux | esantematico | exantematoso | exanthematisch | 発疹の |
| 2394. excellent - (a) | excellent | eccellente | excelente | ausgezeichnet | 優秀な |
| 2395. excess risk - (n) | risque excessif | rischio eccessivo | riesgo excesivo | übermäßiges Risiko | 過剰リスク |
| 2396. excessive - (a) | excessif | eccessivo | excesivo | überstark; übermäßig | 過剰の |
| 2397. exchange - (n) | échange | scambio | cambio | Austausch | 交換 |
| 2398. exchange transfusion - (n) | exsanguino-transfusion | exanguinotrasfusione | exanguinotransfusión | Austauschtransfusion | 交換輸血 |
| 2399. excipient - (n) | excipient | eccipiente | excipiente | Arzneimittelträgersubstanz | 補形剤 |
| 2400. excise - (v) | exciser | asportare | remover quirúrgicamente | herausschneiden; exzidieren | 切除する |
| 2401. excision - (n) | excision | escissione; asportazione | escisión | Exzision | 切除 [術] |
| 2402. excitability - (n) | excitabilité | eccitabilità | excitabilidad | Erregbarkeit | 興奮性 |
| 2403. excitation - (n) | excitation | eccitazione | excitación | Erregung | 刺激 |

| English/American | French/Français | Italian/Italiano | Spanish/Español | German/Deutsch | Japanese/日本語 |
|---|---|---|---|---|---|
| 2404. exclusion criteria - (n) | critères d'exclusion | criteri di esclusione | criterios de exclusión | Ausschlußkriterien | 排他基準 |
| 2405. excrement - (n) | excrément | escremento | excremento | Kot, Exkrement | 排泄物 |
| 2406. excretion - (n) | excrétion | escrezione | excreción | Exkretion | 排泄 |
| 2407. exercise - (n) | exercice | esercizio | ejercicio | körperliche Bewegung | 運動 |
| 2408. exercise - (v) | exercer | esercitare | ejercitar | üben; trainieren | 運動する |
| 2409. exercise testing - (n) | épreuve d'exercice | prova dell'esercizio | prueba de ejercicio | Belastungstest | 運動検査 |
| 2410. exercise tolerance - (n) | tolérance à l'exercice | tolleranza all'esercizio | tolerancia al ejercicio | Belastungsfähigkeit | 運動耐性 |
| 2411. exertion - (n) | effort | sforzo; esercizio | esfuerzo | Belastung; Anstrengung | 力の行使 |
| 2412. exertional dyspnea - (n) | dyspnée d'effort | dispnea da sforzo | disnea de esfuerzo | Belastungsdyspnoe | 呼吸困難 |
| 2413. exfoliation - (n) | exfoliation | esfoliazione | exfoliación | Abschuppung; Exfoliation | 剥脱 |
| 2414. exhalation - (n) | exhalation | esalamento | exhalación | Exhalation; Ausatmen | 呼気 |
| 2415. exhaustion - (n) | épuisement; échappement | esaurimento; spossatezza | escape; agotamiento | Erschöpfung; Entleerung | 疲労ばい、消耗 |
| 2416. exhibit - (v) | exhiber | mostrare | exhibir | aufweisen; ausstellen | 処方する |
| 2417. exocrine - (a) | exocrine | esocrino | exocrino | exokrin | 外分泌の |
| 2418. exocrine gland - (n) | glande exocrine | ghiandola esocrina | glándula exocrina | exokrine Drüse | 外分泌腺 |
| 2419. exocytosis - (n) | exocytose | esocitosi | exocitosis | Exozytose | エキソサイトーシス |
| 2420. exogenous - (a) | exogène | esogeno | exogénico | exogen | 外因性の |
| 2421. exon - (n) | exon | esone | exón | Exon | エキソン |
| 2422. exophthalmos - (n) | exophtalmie | esoftalmo | exoftalmos | Exophthalmus | 眼球突出[症] |
| 2423. exotoxin - (n) | exotoxine | esotossina | exotoxina | Exotoxin | 外毒素 |

| English/American | French/Français | Italian/Italiano | Spanish/Español | German/Deutsch | Japanese/日本語 |
|---|---|---|---|---|---|
| 2424. expansion - (n) | expansion | espansione | expansión | Expansion | 膨脹 |
| 2425. expectant - (a) | expectant; enceinte | d'attesa; in attesa | expectante, encinta | erwartungsvoll; schwanger | 予想される、妊娠中の |
| 2426. expected power - (n) | puissance attendue | potere previsto | valor esperado | erwartete Kraft | 予想される効力 |
| 2427. expectorant - (n) | expectorant | espettorante | expectorante | Expektorans | 去痰剤 |
| 2428. expenditure - (n) | dépense; sortie | dispendio; consumo; spesa | gasto; despliegue | Aufwand; Verbrauch | 支出 |
| 2429. expense - (n) | dépense | spesa | gasto | Kosten; Spesen | 出費 |
| 2430. experience - (n) | expérience | esperienza | experiencia | Erfahrung; Erlebnis | 経験 |
| 2431. experience - (v) | éprouver | sentire; provare | experimentar | erfahren; erleben | 経験する |
| 2432. experiment - (n) | expérience; essai | esperimento | experimento | Versuch; Experiment | 実験 |
| 2433. experiment - (v) | expérimenter | sperimentare; condurre un esperimento | experimentar | experimentieren | 実験する |
| 2434. experimental - (a) | expérimental | sperimentale | experimental | experimentell | 実験的な |
| 2435. experimental conditions - (n) | conditions expérimentales | condizioni sperimentali | condiciones experimentales | Versuchsbedingungen | 実験条件 |
| 2436. expert - (n) | expert | esperto | experto | Experte | 専門家 |
| 2437. expert report - (n) | rapport d'un expert | relazione esperta | informe de un experto | Gutachten | 専門家報告 |
| 2438. expiration - (n) | expiration | scadenza | expiración | Exspiration; Ablauf | 呼気、死 |
| 2439. expiration date - (n) | date d'expiration | scadenza; data di scadenza | fecha de vencimiento | Verfallsdatum | 有効期限 |
| 2440. expiratory - (a) | expiratoire | espiratorio | expiratorio | exspiratorisch | 呼気[性]の |
| 2441. exploration - (n) | exploration | esplorazione | exploración | Exploration; Untersuchung | 調査 |
| 2442. exposure - (n) | exposition | esposizione | exposición | Exposition; Freilegung | 表示、露程 |
| 2443. expression - (n) | expression | espressione; spremitura | expresión | Expression; Ausdruck | 表現 |
| 2444. expression cloning - (n) | clonage par expression | clonazione espressione | clonación por expresión | Klonierung einer Ausprägungsform | 発現クローニング |

| English/American | French/Français | Italian/Italiano | Spanish/Español | German/Deutsch | Japanese/日本語 |
|---|---|---|---|---|---|
| 2445. expulsion - (n) | expulsion | espulsione | expulsión | Expulsion; Austreibung | 排泄 |
| 2446. exsanguinate - (v) | exsanguiner | dissanguare | exsanguinar; desangrar | Blut entleeren | 瀉血する |
| 2447. extended baseline - (n) | ligne de base étendue | linea di riferimento aumentato | línea de base extendida | verlängerte Standardkurve | 延長基線 |
| 2448. extension - (n) | extension; prolongement | estensione; prolungamento | extensión; prolongación | Extension; Verlängerung | 延長 |
| 2449. extension protocol - (n) | protocole d'extension | protocollo aggiuntivo | protocolo de extensión | erweitertes Protokoll | 延長プロトコル |
| 2450. extensor - (n) | extenseur | estensore; muscolo estensore | extensor | Streckmuskel | 伸筋 |
| 2451. external - (a) | externe | esterno | externo | extern; äußerlich | 外部の |
| 2452. extirpation - (n) | extirpation | estirpazione | extirpación | Exstirpation | 摘除 [術] |
| 2453. extracellular - (a) | extracellulaire | extracellulare | extracelular | extrazellulär | 細胞外の |
| 2454. extra-corporeal - (a) | extra-corporel | extracorporeo | extracorporal | extrakorporal | 体外の |
| 2455. extract - (n) | extrait | estratto | extracto | Extrakt | 抽出物 |
| 2456. extract - (v) | extraire | estrarre | extraer | extrahieren; herausziehen | 抽出する |
| 2457. extraction - (n) | extraction | estrazione | extracción | Extraktion; Herausziehen | 抽出 |
| 2458. extrahepatic - (a) | extrahépatique | extraepatico | extrahepático | extrahepatisch | 肝臓外の |
| 2459. extraneous data - (n) | données superflues | dati estranei | datos extraños | unwesentliche Daten | 外来のデータ |
| 2460. extraocular movement - (n) | mouvement extra-oculaire | movimento extraoculare | movimiento extraocular | extraokuläre Bewegung | 外眼動作 |
| 2461. extrapolation - (n) | extrapolation | estrapolazione | extrapolación | Extrapolation; Hochrechnung | 補外法 |
| 2462. extrapolation of data - (n) | extrapolation des données | estrapolazione dei dati | extrapolación de los datos | Datenhochrechnung | データの推定 |

| English/American | French/Français | Italian/Italiano | Spanish/Español | German/Deutsch | Japanese/日本語 |
|---|---|---|---|---|---|
| 2463. extrapyramidal tract - (n) | voie extra-pyramidale | tratto extrapiramidale | tracto extrapiramidal | extrapyramidales System | 錐体外路 |
| 2464. extrasystole - (n) | extrasystole | extrasistole | extrasístole | Extrasystole | 期外収縮 |
| 2465. extravasate - (n) | extravasation | stravaso | extravasación | Extravasat | 腎盂外溢流 |
| 2466. extravascular - (a) | extravasculaire | extravascolare | extravascular | extravaskulär | 脈管外の |
| 2467. extravascular lung water - (n) | liquide pulmonaire extravasculaire | liquido polmonare extravascolare | fluido pulmonar extravascular | Lungenflüssigkeit | 脈管外胸水 |
| 2468. extremity - (n) | extrémité | estremità | extremidad | Extremität | 四肢 |
| 2469. extrinsic - (a) | extrinsèque | estrinseco | extrínseco | extrinsisch | 外因の |
| 2470. extrude - (v) | expulser | estrudere; espellere | expeler | ausstoßen; auspressen | 突き出す |
| 2471. extubation - (n) | extubation | estubazione | extubación | Extubierung | 抜管法 |
| 2472. exudate - (n) | exsudat | essudato | exudado | Exsudat | 浸出液 |
| 2473. eye enucleation - (n) | énucléation de l'œil | enucleazione dell'occhio | enucleación del ojo | Enukleation des Auges | 眼球摘出［術］ |
| 2474. eye - (n) | œil | occhio | ojo | Auge | 眼 |
| 2475. eyeball - (n) | globe oculaire | globo oculare; bulbo oculare | globo ocular | Augapfel | 眼球 |
| 2476. eyebrow - (n) | sourcil | sopracciglio | ceja | Augenbraue | 眉 |
| 2477. eyeglasses - (n) | lunettes | occhiali | gafas | Brille | 眼鏡 |
| 2478. eyelash - (n) | cil | ciglio | pestaña | Wimper | 睫毛 |
| 2479. eyelid - (n) | paupière | palpebra | párpado | Augenlid | 瞼 |
| 2480. eyelid disease - (n) | maladie de la paupière | malattia della palpebra | enfermedad del párpado | Augenliderkrankung | 瞼病 |

126

| English/American | French/Français | Italian/Italiano | Spanish/Español | German/Deutsch | Japanese/日本語 |
|---|---|---|---|---|---|
| 2481. face - (n) | figure | faccia | cara | Gesicht | 顔 |
| 2482. face lift - (n) | chirurgie faciale esthétique | lifting | operación de cirugía estética | Face-Lifting; Gesichtshautstraffung | 顔の皺取り |
| 2483. face mask - (n) | masque facial | maschera facciale | máscara facial | Gesichtsmaske faziai; Gesichts- | 仮面顔 |
| 2484. facial - (a) | facial | facciale | facial | Gesichtsknochen | 顔の |
| 2485. facial bones - (n) | os faciaux | ossa della faccia | huesos faciales | Gesichtsödem | 顔面骨 |
| 2486. facial edema - (n) | oedème facial | edema facciale | edema facial | Nervus facialis | 顔面浮腫 |
| 2487. facial nerve - (n) | nerf facial | nervo facciale | nervio facial | Förderung; Erleichterung | 顔面神経 |
| 2488. facilitation - (n) | facilitation | facilitazione | facilitación | Leichtigkeit; Einrichtung | 促通 |
| 2489. facility - (n) | facilité; habilité; installation | facilità; facilitazione; edificio | facilidad; habilidad; instalación | | 才能、施設 |
| 2490. facility design - (n) | plan de la facilité | disegno edificio | diseño de la facilidad | Einrichtungsgestaltung | 施設設計 |
| 2491. fact - (n) | fait | fatto | hecho | Tatsache | 事実 |
| 2492. factitious disorders - (n) | désordres factices | disordini fattizi | trastornos facticios | vorgetäuschte Störungen | 人為的障害 |
| 2493. factor - (n) | facteur | fattore | factor | Faktor | 因子 |
| 2494. factorial analysis - (n) | analyse factorielle | analisi fattoriale | análisis factorial | Faktorenanalyse | 因数分析 |
| 2495. factorial design - (n) | dessin factoriel | disegno fattoriale | diseño factorial | Faktorenentwurf | 階乗設計 |
| 2496. factual database - (n) | banque de données factuelle | base di dati reale | base de datos factual | Tatsachendatenbank | 事実に基づくデータベース |
| 2497. faculty - (n) | faculté | facoltà; professore universitario | facultad | Fakultät; Fähigkeit | 能力．正式教員 |
| 2498. faculty practice - (n) | pratique facultaire | pratica accademica | práctica de la facultad | Privatsprechstunde der Fakultät | 正式教員による治療 |
| 2499. Fahrenheit - (n) | Fahrenheit | Fahrenheit | Fahrenheit | Fahrenheit | 華氏 |
| 2500. fail safe - (a) | sans failles | fail-safe; sicuro dai guasti | libre de fallos | pannensicher; fehlersicher | 絶対安全な |

127

| English/American | French/Français | Italian/Italiano | Spanish/Español | German/Deutsch | Japanese/日本語 |
|---|---|---|---|---|---|
| 2501. failure - (n) | défaillance; insuffisance; échec | fallimento; insufficienza | falla; insuficiencia; retraso | Ausbleiben; Versagen | 不全、失敗 |
| 2502. failure to thrive - (n) | échec de bon développement | fallimento nell'espandere | retraso del crecimiento | Gedeihstörung | 発育の遅れ |
| 2503. faint - (v) | s'évanouir | svenire; perdere i sensi | desmayarse | bewußtlos werden; in Ohnmacht fallen | 失神する |
| 2504. faintness - (n) | faiblesse; malaise | debolezza; fiacchezza | debilidad; desmayo | Schwäche; Ohnmachtsgefühl | 失神 |
| 2505. fair - (a) | juste; clair | giusto; equo; chiaro | justo; rubio; blanco | gerecht; durchschnittlich | 公平な、色白の |
| 2506. Fallopian tube - (n) | trompe de Fallope | tromba di Falloppio; tuba di Falloppio | trompa de Falopio | Eileiter | 卵管 |
| 2507. false - (a) | faux | falso | falso | falsch; Pseud- | 偽の |
| 2508. false labor - (n) | faux travail | false doglie | parto falso | Vorwehen | 仮性分娩 |
| 2509. false negative - (a) | faux négatif | falso negativo | falso negativo | falsch-negativ | 偽陰性 |
| 2510. false neurotransmitter - (n) | faux neuromédiateur | falso neurotrasmettitore | neurotransmisor falso | Pseudoneurotransmitter | 偽神経伝達物質 |
| 2511. false positive - (a) | faux positif | falso positivo | falso positivo | falsch-positiv | 偽陽性 |
| 2512. false teeth - (n) | dents fausses | denti falsi; dentiera | dientes postizos | (künstliches) Gebiß | 義歯 |
| 2513. familial - (a) | familial; héréditaire | familiare; ereditario | familiar; hereditario | familiär; hereditär | 家族性の |
| 2514. family - (n) | famille | famiglia | familia | Familie | 家族 |
| 2515. family history - (n) | histoire de la famille | anamnesi familiare; storia familiare | historial familiar | Familienanamnese | 家族歴 |
| 2516. family planning - (n) | planisme familiale | pianificazione familiare | planificación familiar | Familienplanung | 家族計画 |
| 2517. farsighted - (a) | hypermétrope | ipermetrope | hiperópico | weitsichtig; hypermetrop | 遠視の |
| 2518. fascia - (a) | fascia; aponévrose | fascia; aponeurosi | fascia; aponeurosis | Faszie | 筋膜 |
| 2519. fascial plane - (n) | plan du fascia; plan aponéurotique | piano fasciale | plano de la fascia; plano muscular | aponeurotische Ebene | ナジオンポグニオン面 |

128

| English/American | French/Français | Italian/Italiano | Spanish/Español | German/Deutsch | Japanese/日本語 |
|---|---|---|---|---|---|
| 2520. fasciculation - (n) | fasciculation | fascicolazione | fasciculación | Faszikulation; faszikuläre Zuckung | 線維束形成 |
| 2521. fasting - (n) | jeûne | digiuno | ayuno | Fasten | 断食 |
| 2522. fat - (n) | graisse | grasso; adipe; lipide | grasa; tejido adiposo | Fett; Lipid | 脂肪 |
| 2523. fat - (a) | gras; gros | grasso; adiposo | graso; gordo | fett | 脂肪の |
| 2524. fat embolism - (n) | embolie graisseuse | embolia grassosa | embolismo graso | Fettembolie | 脂肪塞栓症 |
| 2525. fat pad - (n) | coussin graisseux | cuscinetto adiposo | cobertura de grasa | Fettpolster | 脂肪パッド |
| 2526. fatal - (a) | fatal; mortel | fatale; letale | fatal; letal | letal; tödlich | 致命的な、運命の |
| 2527. fatigue - (n) | fatigue | fatica; sforzo | fatiga | Ermüdung; Müdigkeit | 疲労 |
| 2528. fatty acid - (n) | acide gras | acido grasso | ácido graso | Fettsäure | 脂肪酸 |
| 2529. fatty alcohol - (n) | alcool gras | alcool di acido grasso | alcohol graso | Fettalkohol | 脂肪アルコール |
| 2530. fatty liver - (n) | foie gras | fegato grasso | hígado graso | Fettleber | 脂肪肝 |
| 2531. fatty stool - (n) | selle graisseuse | steatorrea | defecación grasosa | Fettstuhl | 脂肪便 |
| 2532. fear - (n) | peur; crainte | paura; timore | tener miedo; temer | Furcht | 恐怖 |
| 2533. fear - (v) | craindre; avoir peur de | aver paura; temere | tener miedo; temer | fürchten | 恐れる |
| 2534. feasibility - (n) | faisabilité | fattibilità | factibilidad | Ausführbarkeit | 実現可能性 |
| 2535. febrile - (a) | fébrile; fiévreux | febbrile | febril | febril; fiebrig | 熱性の |
| 2536. fecal impaction - (n) | occlusion fécale | ritenzione fecale | impacción fecal | Koteinklemmung | 宿便 |
| 2537. fecal incontinence - (n) | incontinence fécale | incontinenza fecale | incontinencia fecal | Stuhlinkontinenz | 失禁 |
| 2538. feces - (n) | fèces | feci | heces | Fäzes | 糞便 |
| 2539. federal - (a) | fédéral | federale | federal | Bundes- | 連邦の |
| 2540. federal government - (n) | gouvernement fédéral | governo federale | gobierno federal | Bundesregierung | 連邦政府 |
| 2541. feedback - (n) | rétroaction | retroazione; feedback | retroacción | Feedback; Rückkopplung | フィードバック |
| 2542. feedback loop - (n) | boucle de rétroaction | via retroattiva | bucle de retroacción | Rückkopplungsschleife; Rückführung | フィードバックループ |

| English/American | French/Français | Italian/Italiano | Spanish/Español | German/Deutsch | Japanese/日本語 |
|---|---|---|---|---|---|
| 2543. feeding - (n) | alimentation | il nutrire; alimentazione | alimentación | Füttern; Ernährung | 栄養 |
| 2544. feeling - (n) | sensation; sentiment | sensibilità; sentimento | sensación; sentimiento | Gefühl | 感情、感覚 |
| 2545. fees and charges - (n) | frais et honoraires | costi e prezzi | honorarios y gastos | Entgelte und Gebühren | 費用と料金 |
| 2546. fellowship - (n) | bourse universitaire | borsa di studio | beca universitaria | Stipendium; Forschungskredit | 交友 |
| 2547. female - (n) | femelle | femmina | hembra; mujer | Frau; Weibchen | 女性 |
| 2548. female - (a) | femelle | femminile | femenino; hembra | weiblich | 女性の |
| 2549. female sex organs - (n) | organes sexuels femelles | organi sessuali femminili | órganos sexuales femeninos | weibliche Geschlechtsorgane | 女性性器 |
| 2550. femoral - (a) | fémoral | femorale | femoral | femoral | 大腿の |
| 2551. femur - (n) | fémur | femore | fémur | Oberschenkel; Femur | 大腿 [骨] |
| 2552. fermentation - (n) | fermentation | fermentazione | fermentación | Gärung; Fermentation | 発酵 |
| 2553. fertile - (a) | fertile; fécond | fertile; fecondo | fértil; fecundo | fruchtbar | 多産の |
| 2554. fertility - (n) | fertilité; fécondité | fertilità | fertilidad; fecundidad | Fruchtbarkeit | 受精率 |
| 2555. fertility testing - (n) | épreuve de fécondité | test di fertilità | prueba de fertilidad | Fertilitätstest | 生殖能力検査 |
| 2556. fertilization - (n) | fertilisation; fécondation | fertilizzazione; fecondazione | fertilización; fecundación | Befruchtung | 受精 |
| 2557. fester - (n) | suppuration | suppurazione | supuración | Eitergeschwür | 化膿 |
| 2558. fester - (v) | suppurer | suppurare | supurar | eitern | 化膿する |
| 2559. fetal (foetal) - (a) | foetal | fetale | fetal | fetal; fötal | 胎児の |
| 2560. fetal (foetal) disorder - (n) | désordre fœtal | disordine fetale | trastorno fetal | Fetalstörung; Fetalschädigung | 胎児障害 |
| 2561. fetal (foetal) distress - (n) | souffrance fœtale | sofferenza fetale | agotamiento fetal | Fetalkrankheit; Fetaldistreß | 胎児仮死 |
| 2562. fetal (foetal) monitor - (n) | moniteur fœtal | monitor fetale | monitor fetal | Monitor zur Überwachung des Fetusses | 胎児監視 |

130

| English/American | French/Français | Italian/Italiano | Spanish/Español | German/Deutsch | Japanese/日本語 |
|---|---|---|---|---|---|
| 2563. fetal (foetal) toxicity - (n) | toxicité fœtale | tossicità fetale | toxicidad fetal | toxische Wirkung auf den Fetus | 胎児毒性 |
| 2564. fetid - (a) | fétide | fetido | fétido | fötid; übelriechend | 悪臭の |
| 2565. fetus (foetus) - (n) | fœtus | feto | feto | Fetus; Fötus | 胎児 |
| 2566. fever - (n) | fièvre | febbre | fiebre | Fieber | 熱 |
| 2567. fever blister - (n) | herpès labial | erpete labiale | herpes labial | Lippenherpes | 急性天疱瘡 |
| 2568. fever of unknown origin - (n) | fièvre d'origine inconnue | febbre di origine sconosciuta | fiebre de origen desconocido | Fieber unbekannter Ursache | 原因不明の熱 |
| 2569. fiber - (n) | fibre | fibra | fibra | Faser | 繊維質 |
| 2570. fiber optics - (n) | optique des fibres | ottica delle fibre | óptica de las fibras | Faseroptik | 光ファイバ |
| 2571. fiberglass - (n) | fibre de verre | lana di vetro | fibra de vidrio | Fiberglas | 繊維ガラス |
| 2572. fiberoptic - (a) | fibre optique | a fibre ottiche | fibróptico | Faseroptik- | 繊維光視の |
| 2573. fibrillation - (n) | fibrillation | fibrillazione | fibrilación | Fibrillation; Flimmern | 細動 |
| 2574. fibrin - (n) | fibrine | fibrina | fibrina | Fibrin | 繊維素 |
| 2575. fibrinogen - (n) | fibrinogène | fibrinogeno | fibrinógeno | Fibrinogen | 繊維素原 |
| 2576. fibrinolysis - (n) | fibrinolyse | fibrinólisi | fibrinólisis | Fibrinolyse | フィブリン溶解 |
| 2577. fibrinolytic agent - (n) | agent fibrinolytique | agente fibrinolitico | agente fibrinolítico | Fibrinolytikum | フィブリン溶解性物質 |
| 2578. fibroblast - (n) | fibroblaste | fibroblasto | fibroblasto | Fibroblast | 繊維芽細胞 |
| 2579. fibrocystic disease - (n) | maladie fibrokystique | malattia fibrocistica | enfermedad fibroquística | fibrozystische Erkrankung | 繊維[性]嚢胞の病気 |
| 2580. fibroma - (n) | fibrome | fibroma | fibroma | Fibrom | 繊維腫 |
| 2581. fibromyalgia - (n) | fibromyalgie | fibromialgia | fibromialgia | Fibromyalgie | 繊維筋肉痛 |
| 2582. fibrosarcoma - (n) | fibrosarcome | fibrosarcoma | fibrosarcoma | Fibrosarkom | 繊維肉腫 |
| 2583. fibrosis - (n) | fibrose | fibrosi | fibrosis | Fibrose | 繊維粗織増殖 |
| 2584. fibula - (n) | péroné | fibula; perone | fibula; peroné | Wadenbein | 腓骨 |
| 2585. field - (n) | champ | campo | campo | Feld; Gebiet | 領域 |
| 2586. field monitor - (n) | moniteur clinique | monitor del campo | monitor en el campo | Überwacher eines Gebietes (einer Studie) | フィールドモニター |

131

| English/American | French/Français | Italian/Italiano | Spanish/Español | German/Deutsch | Japanese/日本語 |
|---|---|---|---|---|---|
| 2587. field report - (n) | rapport clinique | rapporto di dati da campo | información del campo | Feldbericht | フィールドレポート |
| 2588. field study - (n) | étude clinique | studio di campo | estudio en el campo | Feldstudie | フィールド研究 |
| 2589. figure [abbr] fig - (n) | figure; chiffre | illustrazione; figura | figura; cifra | Abbildung; Zahl | 数字、容姿、図解 |
| 2590. file - (n) | fichier; dossier | incartamento; archivio | fichero; archivo | Kartei; Datei | ファイル |
| 2591. filling defect - (n) | défaut de remplissage | difetto di riempimento | defecto de relleno | Füllungsdefekt; Kontrastaussparung | 充填欠損 |
| 2592. filling material - (n) | matériaux de remplissage | materiale per otturazione | material de obturación | Füllungsmaterial | 充填剤 |
| 2593. film - (n) | film; pellicule | pellicola; film; strato sottile | película | Film; Schicht | フィルム、膜 |
| 2594. filter - (n) | filtre | filtro | filtro | Filter | 沪過器 |
| 2595. filter - (v) | filtrer | filtrare | filtrar | filtrieren; filtern | 沪過する |
| 2596. filtration - (n) | filtration | filtrazione | filtración | Filtration | 沪過 |
| 2597. final - (a) | final; définitif | finale; ultimo | final | endgültig | 最終の |
| 2598. final medical report - (n) | rapport médical final | rapporto medico finale | informe médico final | medizinischer Abschlußbericht | 最終医療報告 |
| 2599. final statistical report - (n) | rapport statistique final | rapporto statistico finale | informe estadístico final | statistischer Abschlußbericht | 最終統計報告 |
| 2600. financing - (n) | financement | finanziamento | financiación | Finanzierung; Kapitalbeschaffung | 金融融資 |
| 2601. fine motor skills - (n) | motricités fines | buone capacità di movimento | motricidades finas | feine motorische Fertigkeit | 微細な運動能力 |
| 2602. fine tremor - (n) | tremblement fin | tremore fino | temblor fino | feinschlägiger Tremor | 微小振せん |
| 2603. finger - (n) | doigt | dito | dedo | Finger | 指 |
| 2604. fingernail - (n) | ongle | unghia | uña | Fingernagel | 指の爪 |
| 2605. fingerprint - (n) | empreinte digitale | impronta digitale | impresión digital | Fingerabdruck | 指紋 |
| 2606. first aid - (n) | premiers soins | pronto soccorso | primeros auxilios | Erste Hilfe | 応急手当 |

132

| English/American | French/Français | Italian/Italiano | Spanish/Español | German/Deutsch | Japanese/日本語 |
|---|---|---|---|---|---|
| 2607. first line therapy - (n) | thérapie de première ligne | terapia di prima linea | terapia de primera línea | Therapie der 1. Wahl | 至急療法 |
| 2608. first order kinetics - (n) | cinétique de premier ordre | cinetica di primo ordine | cinética de primer orden | Kinetik der 1. Ordnung | 一次関数に表せる反応 |
| 2609. first-pass effect - (n) | effet de premier passage | effetto primo passo | efecto de primer paso | first-pass Effekt | ファーストパス効果 |
| 2610. fissure - (n) | fissure; fente | fessura; solco | fisura; hendidura | Fissur; Furche | 裂溝 |
| 2611. fistula - (n) | fistule | fistola | fístula | Fistel | 瘻 |
| 2612. fit - (n) | attaque; accès | attacco; accesso | ataque; acceso | Anfall | 発作 |
| 2613. fit - (v) | adapter; ajuster | adattare; montare | adaptar; ajustar | passen; sitzen | 発作を起こす |
| 2614. fitness - (n) | bonne forme physique; aptitude | salute; forma | buen estado físico; capacidad | Eignung; Gesundheit | 健康、適合性 |
| 2615. fixation - (n) | fixation | fissazione; fissaggio | fijación | Fixierung | 固定 |
| 2616. fixative - (n) | fixatif | fissatore | fijador | Fixierungsmittel; Fixateur | 固定剤 |
| 2617. fixed - (a) | fixe | fisso | fija | fest; Fest- | 固定した |
| 2618. flaccid - (a) | flasque | flaccido | fláccido | weich; schlaff | 弛緩した |
| 2619. flaccid paralysis - (n) | paralysie flasque | paralisi flaccida | parálisis fláccida | schlaffe Lähmung | 弛緩 [性] 麻痺 |
| 2620. flare - (n) | aréole cutanée congestive | eritema; rossore | zona enrojecida | Aufflackern | 発赤 |
| 2621. flare - (v) | s'enflammer | infiammare | enrojecer | aufflackern | 発赤する |
| 2622. flatulence - (n) | flatulence | flatulento | flatulencia | Flatulenz | 鼓腸 |
| 2623. flavor (flavour) - (n) | saveur; goût | sapore; gusto | sabor; gusto | Geschmack | 味 |
| 2624. flavoring (flavouring) - (n) | assaisonnement; essence | condimento; sapore | condimento | Würze | 調味料 |
| 2625. flaw - (n) | défaut; imperfection | pecca; difetto | defecto; imperfección | Fehler; Riß | 傷 |
| 2626. flesh - (n) | chair | carne | carne | Fleisch; Muskelgewebe | 肉 |
| 2627. flexibility - (n) | flexibilité | flessibilità | flexibilidad | Flexibilität | 柔軟性 |

| English/American | French/Français | Italian/Italiano | Spanish/Español | German/Deutsch | Japanese/日本語 |
|---|---|---|---|---|---|
| 2628. flexion - (n) | flexion | flessione | flexión | Flexion; Beugung | 屈曲状態 |
| 2629. flexor - (n) | fléchisseur | flessore | flexor | Flexor | 屈筋 |
| 2630. floaters - (n) | flotteurs; corps flottants | mosche volanti | flotadores; moscas volantes | Glaskörpertrübungen | 浮遊物 |
| 2631. flora - (n) | flore | flora | flora | Flora | 植物区系 |
| 2632. flow - (n) | circulation; écoulement | flusso; scorrimento | flujo; derrame | Fluß; Strömung | 流動、流量 |
| 2633. flow - (v) | circuler; couler | scorrere; fluire | fluir | fließen | 流出する |
| 2634. flow chart - (n) | organigramme | diagramma diagnostico-terapeutico | flujograma; organigrama | Flußdiagramm | フローチャート |
| 2635. flow cytometry - (n) | cytométrie de flux | citometria a flusso | citometría de flujo | Durchflußzytometrie | フローサイトメトリー |
| 2636. flow diagram - (n) | organigramme | diagramma diagnostico-terapeutico | diagrama de flujo | Flußdiagramm | フローダイアグラム |
| 2637. flow sheet - (n) | organigramme | diagramma di flusso | flujograma | Verarbeitungdiagramm | フローシート |
| 2638. fluid - (n) | fluide; liquide | fluido | fluido; líquido | Flüssigkeit | 液体 |
| 2639. fluid and electrolyte balance - (n) | équilibre hydro-électrolytique | equilibrio fluido-elettroliti | equilibrio de fluidos y electrolitos | Flüssigkeits- und Elektrolythaushalt | 液体と電解質の均衡 |
| 2640. fluid intake - (n) | prise liquidienne | ingestione di fluidi | consumo de líquidos | Flüssigkeitsaufnahme | 液体摂取量 |
| 2641. fluid loss - (n) | perte de fluides | perdita di fluidi | pérdida de líquidos | Flüssigkeitsverlust | 液体損失 |
| 2642. fluid restriction - (n) | restriction liquidienne | restrizione fluidi | restricción de líquidos | Flüssigkeitseinschränkung | 液体制限 |
| 2643. fluidity - (n) | fluidité | fluidità | fluidez | Fließfähigkeit; flüssiger Zustand | 流動率 |
| 2644. fluke - (n) | trématode; douve | platelminta; trematode | trematodos | Plattwurm; Trematode | 吸虫類 |
| 2645. fluorescence - (n) | fluorescence | fluorescenza | fluorescencia | Fluoreszenz | 蛍光 |
| 2646. fluoridation - (n) | fluoration; fluoruration | fluorizzazione; fluororazione | fluoración; fluorización | Fluorisierung | フッ素添加 |
| 2647. fluoroscopy - (n) | fluoroscopie | fluoroscopia | fluoroscopia | Fluoroskopie | 透視診断法 |

| English/American | French/Français | Italian/Italiano | Spanish/Español | German/Deutsch | Japanese/日本語 |
|---|---|---|---|---|---|
| 2648. flush - (n) | bouffée de chaleur; afflux sanguin | arrossamento; rossore | rubor; enrojecimiento | Erröten; Gesichtsröte | 発赤 |
| 2649. flush - (v) | rougir; nettoyer à grande eau | arrossire; pulire | ruborizar; limpiar con agua | erröten; spülen | 発赤する、流す |
| 2650. flushed face - (n) | visage empourpré | faccia arrossita | rubor facial | errötetes Gesicht | 紅潮顔面 |
| 2651. flushing - (n) | bouffée congestive; lavage | rossore; flusso | enrojecimiento; lavado | Erröten; Spülung | 紅潮 |
| 2652. flutter - (n) | flutter | flutter | flutter | Flattern | 振動する |
| 2653. flux - (n) | flux | flusso | flujo | Ausfluß; Fluß | 下痢 |
| 2654. focal necrosis - (n) | nécrose focale | necrosi focale | necrosis focal | Herdnekrose | 病巣壊死 |
| 2655. focal sign - (n) | signe focal | segno focale | signo focal | Herdsymptom | 病巣症状 |
| 2656. focus - (n) | foyer; centre; focale | fuoco; focolaio | foco; centro | Herd; Brennpunkt | 焦点 |
| 2657. focus - (v) | focaliser | mettere a fuoco | enfocar | fokussieren | 焦点を合わせる |
| 2658. focus group - (n) | groupe cible | gruppo bersaglio | grupo de enfoque | Zielgruppe | 対象集団 |
| 2659. fold - (n) | pli; repli | piega; plica | pliegue; repliegue | Falte | 皺 |
| 2660. fold - (v) | plier; replier | piegare | plegar; doblar | falten; umschlagen | 折りたたむ |
| 2661. folk medicine - (n) | médecine populaire | medicina popolare | medicina popular | Volksmedizin | 民間療法 |
| 2662. follicle - (n) | follicule | follicolo | folículo | Follikel | 小胞 |
| 2663. follicular - (a) | folliculaire | follicolare | folicular | follikulär | 小胞の |
| 2664. follow up - (v) | suivre de près | eseguire esami di controllo | seguir; investigar | nachuntersuchen | 再調査をする |
| 2665. follow-up - (n) | visite de contrôle | esame di controllo; follow-up | seguimiento; investigación | Nachuntersuchung; Verlaufskontrolle | 再調査 |
| 2666. follow-up data - (n) | données de suivi | dati degli esami di controllo | datos de seguimiento | Nachuntersuchungsdaten | フォローアップデータ |
| 2667. follow-up examination - (n) | examen de contrôle | esame di controllo | reconocimiento de seguimiento | Nachuntersuchung | 再調査試験 |

| English/American | French/Français | Italian/Italiano | Spanish/Español | German/Deutsch | Japanese/日本語 |
|---|---|---|---|---|---|
| 2668. follow-up period - (n) | période de suivi médical | periodo di follow-up; periodo di controllo | periodo de seguimiento | Nachbeobachtungszeit | 再調査期間 |
| 2669. follow-up study - (n) | étude de suivi | studio di follow-up; studio di controllo | estudio de seguimiento | weiterführende Studie | 再調査研究 |
| 2670. follow-up visit - (n) | visite de contrôle | visita di follow-up; visita di controllo | visita de seguimiento | Nachuntersuchung | 再調査のための来院 |
| 2671. fontanel, fontanelle - (n) | fontanelle | fontanella | fontanela | Fontanelle | 泉門 |
| 2672. food - (n) | aliment; nourriture | cibo; alimento | alimento; nutrimento | Nahrung; Lebensmittel | 食物 |
| 2673. food allergy - (n) | allergie alimentaire | allergia alimentare | alergia alimenticia | Lebensmittelallergie | 食事性アレルギー |
| 2674. food interaction - (n) | interaction alimentaire | interazione alimentare | interacción entre alimentos | Lebensmittelinteraktion | 食品相互作用 |
| 2675. food intolerance - (n) | intolérance alimentaire | intolleranza alimentare | intolerancia alimenticia | Lebensmittel-unverträglichkeit | 食品不耐容 [症] |
| 2676. food poisoning - (n) | intoxication alimentaire | intossicazione alimentare | intoxicación alimenticia; envenenamiento alimentario | Lebensmittelvergiftung | 食品中毒 |
| 2677. foot - (n) | pied | piede | pie | Fuß | 足 |
| 2678. foot drop - (n) | pied tombant | cadente piede | pie en extensión | Fallfuß | 足下垂症 |
| 2679. footnote - (n) | note en bas de la page | nota a piè di pagina | nota al pie de la página | Fußnote; Anmerkung | 脚注 |
| 2680. foramen - (n) | foramen; orifice | forame; foro | foramen; agujero | Loch | 孔 |
| 2681. foramen magnum - (n) | trou occipital | gran forame occipitale; foro magno | foramen occipital | Hinterhauptloch; Foramenmagnum | 大後頭孔 |
| 2682. forced expiratory volume - (n) | volume expiratoire forcé | volume espiratorio forzato | volumen expiratorio forzado | Sekundenausatmungs-volumen | 最大努力呼気肺活量 |
| 2683. forceps - (n) | forceps | forcipe; pinza | fórceps | Forceps; Pinzette | 鉗子 |
| 2684. forearm - (n) | avant-bras | avambraccio | antebrazo | Unterarm | 前腕 |
| 2685. forebrain - (n) | proencéphale; cerveau antérieur | prosencefalo; cervello anteriore | prosencéfalo | Prosenzephalon; Frontalhirn | 前脳部 |

136

| English/American | French/Français | Italian/Italiano | Spanish/Español | German/Deutsch | Japanese/日本語 |
|---|---|---|---|---|---|
| 2686. forehead - (n) | front | fronte | frente | Stirn | 前頭 |
| 2687. foreign - (a) | étranger; extérieur | estraneo | extraño; ajeno | fremd | 異質の |
| 2688. foreign body - (n) | corps étranger | corpo estraneo | cuerpo extraño | Fremdkörper | 異物 |
| 2689. foreign data - (n) | données extérieures | dati estranei | datos extraños | Fremddaten | 異質データ |
| 2690. forelimb - (n) | avant membre | parte distale di un arto | antebrazo; pata delantera | Vorderbein; Vorderfuß | 前肢 |
| 2691. forensic - (a) | légal | forense; legale | forense; legal | forensisch | 法廷上の |
| 2692. forensic medicine - (n) | médecine légale | medicina legale | medicina forense; medicina legal | Gerichtsmedizin | 法医学 |
| 2693. foreskin - (n) | prépuce | prepuzio | prepucio | Vorhaut | 包皮 |
| 2694. forgetfulness - (n) | étourderie; manque de mémoire | smemoratezza; deficit di rievocazione | falta de memoria; olvido | Vergessenheit; Vergeßlichkeit | 健忘症 |
| 2695. form - (n) | forme; espèce | forma; figura; specie | forma; estado | Form; Gestalt | 形、様式 |
| 2696. formal - (a) | formel; officiel | formale; ufficiale | formal; oficial | formal; offiziell | 形式的な、正式の |
| 2697. formal logic - (n) | logique formelle | logica formale | lógica formal | formale Logik | 形式的論理 |
| 2698. format - (n) | format | formato | formato | Format; Struktur | フォーマット |
| 2699. formation - (n) | formation | formazione | formación | Bildung; Formation | 形成 |
| 2700. formula - (n) | formule | formula | fórmula | Arzneiformel; Rezept | 処方書 |
| 2701. formulary - (n) | formulaire | formulario | formulario | Medikamentenver-zeichnis; Formelnbuch | 処方集 |
| 2702. formulary committee - (n) | comité formulaire | comitati per la formulazione | comité formulario | Rezepturausschuß | 処方集委員会 |
| 2703. formulated - (a) | formulé | formulato | formulado | formuliert | 公式化した |
| 2704. formulation - (n) | formulation | formulazione | formulación | Rezept; Zubereitungsform | 公式化 |
| 2705. fornication - (n) | fornication | fornicazione | fornicación | Unzucht | 姦淫 |
| 2706. fortified - (a) | fortifié | fortificato | fortificado | verstärkt; angereichert | 強化した |
| 2707. fossa - (n) | fosse | fossa | fosa | Grube; Fossa | 窩 |

137

| English/American | French/Français | Italian/Italiano | Spanish/Español | German/Deutsch | Japanese/日本語 |
|---|---|---|---|---|---|
| 2708. foul discharge - (n) | suintement infect; écoulement nauséabond | secrezione maleodorante | supuración con mal olor | überriechender Ausfluß | 不快な排出物 |
| 2709. foundation - (n) | fondation; base | base; supporto; fondazione | soporte; base | Grundlage; Stiftung | 基礎、財団 |
| 2710. fraction - (n) | fraction | frazione | fracción | Fraktion; Bruch | 分数 |
| 2711. fractionation - (n) | fractionnement | frazionamento | fraccionamiento | Fraktionierung | 分別 |
| 2712. fracture - (n) | fracture | frattura | fractura | Fraktur; Bruch | 骨折 |
| 2713. fragility - (n) | fragilité | fragilità | fragilidad | Zerbrechlichkeit; Fragilität | 脆弱な性質 |
| 2714. fragment - (n) | fragment; morceau | frammento; pezzo | fragmento | Fragment; Bruchstück | 断片 |
| 2715. fragmentation - (n) | fragmentation | frammentazione | fragmentación | Fragmentierung | 細分 |
| 2716. frail - (a) | frêle; faible | delicato; fragile | frágil; quebradizo | zerbrechlich; gebrechlich | もろい、弱い |
| 2717. frameshift mutation - (n) | mutation de déplacement de structure | mutazione frameshift | mutación por cambio de encuadre | Rasterverschiebungs-mutation | 読み枠突然変異 |
| 2718. framework - (n) | structure; cadre | stroma | soporte; soporte protésico | Stützgerüst | 骨組み |
| 2719. fraternal twins - (n) | jumeaux hétérozygotes | gemelli biovulari; gemelli dizigotici | gemelos fraternos | zweieiige Zwillinge | 二卵性双生児 |
| 2720. fraud - (n) | fraude; supercherie | frode | fraude | Betrug | 詐欺 |
| 2721. freckle - (n) | tache de rousseur | lentiggine; efelide | peca; lentigo | Sommersprosse | 雀斑 |
| 2722. free radical - (n) | radical libre | radicale libero | radical libre | freies Radikal | 遊離基 |
| 2723. freedom - (n) | liberté | libertà | libertad | Freiheit | 自由 |
| 2724. freeze drying - (n) | lyophilisation | liofilizzazione | liofilizar | Gefriertrocknung | 凍結乾燥 |
| 2725. freeze-dried - (a) | lyophilisé | liofilizzato | liofilizado | gefriergetrocknet | 凍結乾燥の |
| 2726. freezing - (n) | congélation | congelamento | congelación | Einfrieren | 冷凍 |
| 2727. fremitus - (n) | frémissement | fremito | frémito | Fremitus | 振動 |
| 2728. frenulum - (n) | frein | frenulo | frénulo | Frenulum; Bändchen | 小帯 |
| 2729. frenzy - (n) | frénésie | frenesia | frenesí | Wahnsinn | 狂暴 |

| English/American | French/Français | Italian/Italiano | Spanish/Español | German/Deutsch | Japanese/日本語 |
|---|---|---|---|---|---|
| 2730. frequency - (n) | fréquence | frequenza | frecuencia | Frequenz; Häufigkeit | 周波数、頻度 |
| 2731. frequency distribution - (n) | distribution de fréquence | distribuzione di frequenza | distribución de frecuencia | Häufigkeitsverteilung | 度数分布 |
| 2732. fresh water - (n) | eau fraîche; eau douce | acqua dolce | agua fresca; agua dulce | Süßwasser | 淡水 |
| 2733. friable - (a) | friable | friabile | friable | zerreibbar; bröcklig | 脆い |
| 2734. friable mucosa - (n) | muqueuse friable | mucosa friabile | mucosa friable | sprüngige Schleimhaut | 脆い粘膜 |
| 2735. friction - (n) | friction | frizione | fricción | Reibung; Friktion | 摩擦 |
| 2736. friction rub - (n) | frottement péricardique | rumore di sfregamento | frote pericárdico | Reibegeräusch | 摩擦音 |
| 2737. frigidity - (n) | frigidité | frigidità | frigidez | Frigidität | 冷感症 |
| 2738. fringe benefit - (n) | avantage accessoire | indennità accessoria | beneficio complementario | (Gehalts-)nebenleistung | 特別給与 |
| 2739. frontal - (a) | frontal | frontale | frontal | frontal; Stirn- | 前面の |
| 2740. frontal sinus - (n) | sinus frontal | seno frontale | seno frontal | Stirnbeinhöhle | 前頭洞 |
| 2741. frozen section - (n) | section congelée | sezione congelata | sección congelada | Gefrierschnitt | 凍結切片 |
| 2742. fruit - (n) | fruit | frutto | fruto; fruta | Frucht; Obst | 果実 |
| 2743. frustration - (n) | frustration | frustrazione | frustración | Frustration | フラストレーション |
| 2744. full scale production - (n) | production à grande échelle | produzione in grande scala | producción a capacidad máxima | groß angelegte Veranstaltung | 多量生産 |
| 2745. fulminant - (a) | fulminant | fulminante | fulminante | fulminant; foudroyant | 電撃性の |
| 2746. function - (n) | fonction | funzione | función | Funktion | 機能 |
| 2747. functional - (a) | fonctionnel | funzionale | funcional | funktionell | 機能性の |
| 2748. functional status - (n) | état fonctionnel | stato funzionale | estado funcional | Funktionsstatus | 機能性状態 |
| 2749. fund raising - (n) | levée des fonds | raccolta fondi | recolección de fondos | Geldbeschaffung | 資金収集 |
| 2750. fundamental research - (n) | recherche fondamentale | ricerca fondamentale | investigación fundamental | Grundlagenforschung | 基礎研究 |

139

| English/American | French/Français | Italian/Italiano | Spanish/Español | German/Deutsch | Japanese/日本語 |
|---|---|---|---|---|---|
| 2751. funding agency - (n) | agence de financement | agenzia sponsorizzatrice | agencia que provee fondos | Stiftung | 投資機関 |
| 2752. funding award - (n) | bourse de financement | borsa di studio | adjudicación de fondos | Geldstipendium | 投資裁定 |
| 2753. fundus - (n) | fond | fondo | fondo | Grund; Fundus | 基底 |
| 2754. funeral - (n) | funérailles | funerale | funeral | Bestattung | 葬式 |
| 2755. fungal - (a) | fongique | fungino | fúngico | pilzartig; Pilz- | 真菌の |
| 2756. fungicide - (n) | fongicide | fungicida | fungicida | Fungizid | 殺真菌薬 |
| 2757. fungus - (n) | fongus | fungo | hongo | Pilz | 菌類 |
| 2758. fusion - (n) | fusion | fusione | fusión | Fusion | 融合 |
| 2759. future trend - (n) | tendance future | direzioni future | tendencia futura | zukünftige Entwicklung; Entwicklungstendenz | 将来の傾向 |

| English/American | French/Français | Italian/Italiano | Spanish/Español | German/Deutsch | Japanese/日本語 |
|---|---|---|---|---|---|
| 2760. gag reflex - (n) | réflexe pharyngé | riflesso faringeo | reflejo faríngeo | Würgereflex; Rachenreflex | 嘔吐反射 |
| 2761. gait - (n) | démarche | passo; andatura | marcha | Gang; Gangart | 歩きぶり |
| 2762. galactorrhea - (n) | galactorrhée | galattorrea | galactorrea | Galaktorrhö; Milchfluß | 乳汁漏出[症] |
| 2763. galactosemia - (n) | galactosémie | galattosemia | galactosemia | Galaktosämie | ガラクトース血[症] |
| 2764. gallbladder - (n) | vésicule biliaire | cistifellea | vesícula biliar | Gallenblase | 胆嚢 |
| 2765. gallop - (n) | galop | galoppo | galope | Galopp | 奔馬律 |
| 2766. gallop rhythm - (n) | rythme de galop | ritmo di galoppo | ritmo de galope | Galopprhythmus | 奔馬[性]リズム |
| 2767. gallstone - (n) | calcul biliaire | calcolo biliare | cálculo biliar | Gallenstein; Gallenkonkrement | 胆石 |
| 2768. galvanic skin response - (n) | réponse cutanée galvanique | risposta galvanica cutanea | respuesta galvánica de la piel | galvanischer Hautreflex | 平流電流の皮膚反応 |
| 2769. gambling - (n) | jeu; spéculation | speculazione; scommessa | especulación; apuesta | Glücksspiel | 賭博 |
| 2770. gamma globulin - (n) | gamma-globuline | gammaglobulina | gammaglobulina | Gammaglobulin | ガンマグロブリン |
| 2771. gamma rays - (n) | rayons gamma | raggi gamma | rayos gamma | Gammastrahlen | ガンマ線 |
| 2772. gamma receptor - (n) | récepteur gamma | recettore gamma | receptor gamma | Gammarezeptor | ガンマレセプター |
| 2773. ganglioma - (n) | gangliome | ganglioma | ganglioma | Gangliom | 神経節腫瘍 |
| 2774. ganglion - (n) | ganglion | ganglio | ganglio | Ganglion | 神経節 |
| 2775. ganglionic - (a) | ganglionnaire | gangliare; ganglionare | ganglionar | Ganglien- | 神経節の |
| 2776. gangrene - (n) | gangrène | gangrena | gangrena | Gangrän | 壊疽 |
| 2777. Gantt chart - (n) | dossier de Gantt | diagramma di Gantt | diagrama de Gantt | Gantt-Diagramm | ギャントチャート |
| 2778. gargle - (n) | gargarisme | colluttorio per gargarismi | gargarismo | Mundwasser | うがい薬 |
| 2779. gargle - (v) | se gargariser | gargarizzare | gargarizar | gurgeln | うがいをする |
| 2780. gas - (n) | gaz | gas | gas | Gas | ガス |
| 2781. gas gangrene - (n) | gangrène gazeuse | gangrena gassosa | gangrena gaseosa | Gasgangrän | ガス壊疽 |

| English/American | French/Français | Italian/Italiano | Spanish/Español | German/Deutsch | Japanese/日本語 |
|---|---|---|---|---|---|
| 2782. gaseous - (a) | gazeux | gassoso | gaseoso | gasförmig | ガス状の |
| 2783. gasping - (a) | haletant; suffocant | respiro affannoso; fame d'aria | jadeante; respirando con dificultad | keuchend; schwer atmend | あえぎ呼吸 |
| 2784. gastric - (a) | gastrique | gastrico | gástrico | gastrisch; Magen- | 胃の |
| 2785. gastric aspirate - (n) | aspiration gastrique | aspirazione gastrica | aspiración gástrica | Magenaspirat | 胃の吸引（液） |
| 2786. gastric fundus - (n) | fundus gastrique | fondo gastrico | fondo gástrico | Magenfundus | 胃底 |
| 2787. gastric juice - (n) | suc gastrique | succo gastrico | jugo gástrico | Magensaft | 胃液 |
| 2788. gastric lavage - (n) | lavage gastrique | lavanda gastrica | lavado gástrico | Magenspülung | 胃洗浄 |
| 2789. gastro-enterology - (n) | gastro-entérologie | gastroenterologia | gastroenterología | Gastroenterologie | 胃腸病学 |
| 2790. gastroesophageal reflux - (n) | reflux gastro-oesophagien | riflusso gastroesofageo | reflujo gastroesofágico | gastroösophagealer Reflux | 胃食道逆流 |
| 2791. gastrointestinal [abbr] GI - (a) | gastro-intestinal | gastrointestinale | gastrointestinal | gastrointestinal | 胃腸の |
| 2792. gastrointestinal tract - (n) | tractus gastro-intestinal; tube digestif | tratto gastrointestinale | tracto gastrointestinal | Magen-Darm-Kanal; Verdauungsapparat | 胃腸管 |
| 2793. gastroscopic examination - (n) | examen gastroscopique | esame gastroscopica | examen gastroscópico | gastroskopische Untersuchung | 胃鏡検査 |
| 2794. gastroscopy - (n) | gastroscopie | gastroscopia | gastroscopia | Gastroskopie | 胃鏡検査法 |
| 2795. Gaussian distribution - (n) | distribution de Gauss | distribuzione gaussiana | distribución de Gauss | Gauss-Kurve, Gauss-Normalverteilung | ガウス分布 |
| 2796. gauze - (n) | gaze | garza | gasa | Gaze; Mull | ガーゼ |
| 2797. gavage - (n) | gavage | alimentazione mediante sonda gastrica | alimentación por sonda | Ernährung über eine Magensonde | 摂食 |
| 2798. gay - (n) | homosexuel | omosessuale | homosexual | Homosexueller | 同性愛主義者 |
| 2799. gay - (a) | homosexuel | omosessuale | homosexual | homosexuell | 同性愛の |

| English/American | French/Français | Italian/Italiano | Spanish/Español | German/Deutsch | Japanese/日本語 |
|---|---|---|---|---|---|
| 2800. gel - (n) | gel | gel | gel | Gel | ゲル |
| 2801. gel - (v) | se gélifier | gelificare | aglutinarse | gelatinieren | ゲル化する |
| 2802. gelatin capsule - (n) | capsule de gélatine | capsula di gelatina | cápsula de gelatina | Gelatinekapsel | ゼラチンカプセル |
| 2803. gender - (n) | genre; sexe | sesso; genere | género; sexo | Geschlecht; Genus | 性 |
| 2804. gender identity - (n) | identité sexuelle | identità sessuale | identidad sexual | Geschlechtsidentität | 性同一性 |
| 2805. gene - (n) | gène | gene | gene | Gen | 遺伝子 |
| 2806. gene amplification - (n) | amplification génique | amplificazione genica | amplificación de genes | Genamplifikation | 遺伝子の増幅 |
| 2807. gene mapping - (n) | cartographie génique | compilazione di mappa genetica | mapeo de genes | Genkartierung | 遺伝子地図 |
| 2808. genealogy tree - (n) | arbre généalogique | albero genealogico | árbol genealógico | Stammbaum | 系統樹 |
| 2809. general - (a) | général | generale | general | generell; allgemein | 一般の |
| 2810. general population - (n) | population générale | popolazione generale | población general | Öffentlichkeit; Allgemeinheit | 総人口 |
| 2811. general practitioner - (n) | médecin généraliste | medico generico | médico generalista | praktischer Arzt | 一般開業医 |
| 2812. general well-being - (n) | bien-être général | benessere generale | salud en general | allgemeines Wohl | 一般福祉 |
| 2813. generalization - (n) | généralisation | generalizzazione | generalización | Generalisierung | 一般化 |
| 2814. generalized - (a) | généralisé | generalizzato | generalizado | ausgebreitet; generalisiert | 一般化された |
| 2815. generalized seizure - (n) | convulsion généralisée | crisi generalizzata | convulsión generalizada | generalisierter Anfall | 汎発性てんかん発作 |
| 2816. generic - (n) | générique | genericità; generico; farmaco generico | medicamento genérico | Generikum; Freiname | 属 |

143

| English/American | French/Français | Italian/Italiano | Spanish/Español | German/Deutsch | Japanese/日本語 |
|---|---|---|---|---|---|
| 2817. generic - (a) | générique | generico | genérico | Gattung | 属の |
| 2818. genetic - (a) | génétique | genetico | genético | genetisch | 遺伝の |
| 2819. genetic code - (n) | code génétique | codice genetico | código genético | genetischer Kode | 遺伝子暗号 |
| 2820. genetic cross - (n) | croisement génétique | incrocio genetica | cruce genético | genetische Kreuzung | 遺伝子交差 |
| 2821. genetic engineering - (n) | génie génétique | ingegneria genetica | ingeniería genética | Gen-Manipulation | 遺伝子工学 |
| 2822. genetic makeup - (n) | composition génétique | composizione genetico | composición genética | Gen-Zusammensetzung | 遺伝子構成 |
| 2823. genetic polymorphism - (n) | polymorphisme génétique | polimorfismo genetico | polimorfismo genético | genetische Polymorphie | 遺伝子多形 |
| 2824. genetic recombination - (n) | recombination génétique | ricombinazione genetica | recombinación genética | genetische Rekombination | 遺伝的組換え |
| 2825. genetic suppression - (n) | suppression génétique | soppressione genetica | supresión genética | genetische Unterdrückung | 遺伝子抑圧 |
| 2826. genetic transcription - (n) | transcription génétique | trascrizione genetica | transcripción genética | genetische Transkription | 遺伝子転写 |
| 2827. genetic transduction - (n) | transduction génétique | trasduzione genetica | transducción genética | genetische Transduktion | 遺伝子形質導入 |
| 2828. geniculate body - (n) | corps géniculé | corpo genicolato | cuerpo geniculado | Corpus geniculatum | 膝状体 |
| 2829. genital - (a) | génital | genitale | genital | genital; geschlechtlich | 生殖器の |
| 2830. genital organs - (n) | organes génitaux | organi genitali | órganos genitales | Geschlechtsorgane | 性器 |
| 2831. genitalia - (n) | organes génitaux | genitali | genitales | Genitalien | 生殖器 |
| 2832. genitals - (n) | organes génitaux | genitali | genitales | Genitalien | 生殖器 |
| 2833. genitourinary - (a) | génito-urinaire | urogenitale; genitourinario | genitourinario | urogenital | 尿性器の |
| 2834. genome - (n) | génome | genoma | genoma | Genom | ゲノム |

144

| English/American | French/Français | Italian/Italiano | Spanish/Español | German/Deutsch | Japanese/日本語 |
|---|---|---|---|---|---|
| 2835. genomic library - (n) | bibliothèque du génome | biblioteca genomica | biblioteca genómica | genomische DNS-Bank | ゲノムライブラリー |
| 2836. genotype - (n) | génotype | genotipo | genotipo | Genotyp | 遺伝型 |
| 2837. genus - (n) | genre | genere | género | Gattung | 属 |
| 2838. geometric mean - (n) | moyenne géométrique | media geometrica | media geométrica | geometrisches Mittel | 相乗平均 |
| 2839. geriatric - (a) | gériatrique | geriatrico | geriátrico | geriatrisch | 老年医学の |
| 2840. germ - (n) | germe | germe | germen | Keim | 微生物 |
| 2841. germ cell - (n) | cellule germinale | cellula germinale | célula germinal | Keimzelle | 生殖細胞 |
| 2842. germinal - (a) | germinal | germinale | germinal | germinal; germinativ | 胚の |
| 2843. germinal tissue - (n) | tissu germinal | tessuto germinale | tejido germinal | Keimgewebe | 胚組織 |
| 2844. gerontology - (n) | gérontologie | gerontologia | gerontología | Gerontologie; Geratologie | 老人学 |
| 2845. gestation - (n) | gestation | gestazione | gestación | Gestation; Schwangerschaft | 妊娠 |
| 2846. gestational - (a) | gestationnel | gestazionale | gestacional | Gestations-; Schwangerschafts- | 懐妊の |
| 2847. giant cell - (n) | cellule géante | cellula piramidale gigante | célula gigante | Riesenzelle | 巨細胞 |
| 2848. giddiness - (n) | vertige | vertigini | vértigo | Schwindel | 眩暈 |
| 2849. gigantism - (n) | gigantisme | gigantismo | gigantismo | Gigantismus | 巨大症 |
| 2850. gingiva - (n) | gencive | gengiva | encía | Gingiva; Zahnfleisch | 歯肉 |
| 2851. gland - (n) | glande | ghiandola | glándula | Drüse | 腺 |
| 2852. glans - (n) | gland | glande | glande | Eichel | 亀頭 |
| 2853. glass - (n) | verre | vetro | vidrio | Glas | ガラス |
| 2854. glasses - (n) | lunettes | occhiali | anteojos | Brille | 眼鏡 |
| 2855. glaucoma - (n) | glaucome | glaucoma | glaucoma | Glaukom | 緑内障 |
| 2856. glioblastoma - (n) | glioblastome | glioblastoma | glioblastoma | Glioblastom | 神経膠芽腫 |
| 2857. glioma - (n) | gliome | glioma | glioma | Gliom | 神経膠腫 |

145

| English/American | French/Français | Italian/Italiano | Spanish/Español | German/Deutsch | Japanese/日本語 |
|---|---|---|---|---|---|
| 2858. global clinical evaluation - (n) | évaluation clinique globale | valutazione clinica globale | evaluación clínica general | globale klinische Auswertung | 世界的な臨床評価 |
| 2859. global development - (n) | développement global | sviluppo globale | desarrollo global | globale Entwicklung | 世界的な発展 |
| 2860. global evaluation - (n) | évaluation globale | valutazione globale | evaluación global | globale Auswertung | 世界的な評価 |
| 2861. global introspection - (n) | introspection globale | introspezione globale | introspección global | globale Introspektion | 世界的な内省 |
| 2862. globin - (n) | globine | globina | globina | Globin | 血色素蛋白 |
| 2863. globulin - (n) | globuline | globulina | globulina | Globulin | グロブリン |
| 2864. glomerular filtration rate [abbr] GFR - (n) | taux de filtration glomérulaire | tasso di filtrazione glomerulare | tasa de filtración glomerular | Glomerulusfiltrationsrate | 糸球体沪過値 |
| 2865. glomerulonephritis - (n) | glomérulonéphrite | glomerulonefrite | glomerulonefritis | Glomerulonephritis | 糸球体腎炎 |
| 2866. glossa - (n) | langue | lingua | lengua | Zunge | 舌 |
| 2867. glottis - (n) | glotte | glottide | glotis | Stimmapparat; Glottis | 舌炎 |
| 2868. glucocorticoid - (n) | glucocorticoïde | glucocorticoide | glucocorticoide | Glukokortikoid | グルココルチコイド |
| 2869. gluconeogenesis - (n) | gluconéogénèse | gluconeogenesi | gluconeogénesis | Glukoneogenese | 糖質新生 |
| 2870. glucose - (n) | glucose | glucosio; glucoso | glucosa | Glukose | グルコース |
| 2871. glucose tolerance test [abbr] GTT - (n) | épreuve de tolérance au glucose | test di tolleranza al glucosio | prueba de tolerancia a la glucosa | Glukosetoleranztest | グルコース耐容性検査 |
| 2872. gluteal - (a) | fessier | gluteo | glúteo | gluteal | 臀筋の |
| 2873. glycogen - (n) | glycogène | glicogeno | glucógeno | Glykogen | グリコーゲン |
| 2874. glycosuria - (n) | glycosurie | glicosuria | glucosuria | Glykosurie | 糖尿 |
| 2875. goal - (n) | but; objectif | scopo; fine | meta; objetivo | Ziel | 目標 |

| English/American | French/Français | Italian/Italiano | Spanish/Español | German/Deutsch | Japanese/日本語 |
|---|---|---|---|---|---|
| 2876. goiter - (n) | goitre | gozzo | bocio | Kropf; Struma | 甲状腺腫 |
| 2877. gold - (n) | or | oro | oro | Gold | 金 |
| 2878. gold standard - (n) | mesure étalon | standard di riferimento | patrón oro | Goldstandard | 金本位制 |
| 2879. golden rule - (n) | règle d'or | principio informatore | regla de oro | goldene Regel; goldene Sittenregel | 黄金律 |
| 2880. Golgi apparatus - (n) | appareil de Golgi | apparato del Golgi | aparato de Golgi | Golgi-Apparat | ゴルジ装置 |
| 2881. gonad - (n) | gonade | gonade | gónada | Gonade | 生殖腺 |
| 2882. good - (a) | bon | buono | bueno | gut | 良好な |
| 2883. good clinical practice - (n) | bonne pratique clinique | buona pratica clinica | buena práctica clínica | standardisierte klinische Praktiken | 良好な臨床診察 |
| 2884. good clinical trial practice - (n) | bonne pratique d'essai clinique | buona pratica di test clinichi | buena práctica de ensayo clínico | standardisierte klinische Durchführung einer Studie | 良好な試験的臨床診察 |
| 2885. good laboratory practice - (n) | bonne pratique de laboratoire | buona pratica di laboratorio | buena práctica de laboratorio | standardisierte Laborpraktiken | 良好な研究室実験実施 |
| 2886. good manufacturing practice - (n) | bonne pratique de fabrication | buona pratica industriale | buena práctica de fabricación | standardisierte Herstellungspraktiken | 良好な医薬品の製造及び品質管理に関する実施 |
| 2887. governing - (a) | gouvernant | governante; amministratore | directivo | leitend | 抑制する |
| 2888. governing board - (n) | conseil d'administration | consiglio d'amministrazione | junta directiva | Vorstand | 抑制部 |
| 2889. government - (n) | gouvernement | governo | gobierno | Regierung | 政府 |
| 2890. government agency - (n) | agence gouvernementale | agenzia governativa | agencia del gobierno | Verwaltungsbehörde | 抑制機関 |
| 2891. Graafian follicle - (n) | follicule de Graaf | follicolo di Graaf | folículos de Graaf | Graaf-Follikel | グラーフ小胞 |
| 2892. gradual onset - (n) | début graduel | insorgenza graduale | comienzo gradual | allmählicher Ausbruch | 段階的開始 |

147

| English/American | French/Français | Italian/Italiano | Spanish/Español | German/Deutsch | Japanese/日本語 |
|---|---|---|---|---|---|
| 2893. graduate education - (n) | éducation de troisième cycle | istruzione di perfezionamento dopo la laurea | educación para graduados | Studium für Studenten mit abgeschlossenem Bakkalaureat | 大学院教育 |
| 2894. graduated scale - (n) | échelle graduée | misura graduata | escala graduada | abgestufte Gradeinteilung | 段階的重量計 |
| 2895. graft - (n) | greffe; greffon | innesto; trapianto | injerto | Transplantat; Transplantation | 移植、移植片 |
| 2896. graft - (v) | greffer | innestare; trapiantare | injertar | transplantieren; verpflanzen | 移植する |
| 2897. graft versus host - (n) | greffon contre l'hôte | trapianto verso l'ospite | injerto contra huésped | Transplantat gegen Empfänger | 移植片一宿主 |
| 2898. gram - (n) | gramme | grammo | gramo | Gramm | グラム |
| 2899. Gram-negative - (a) | Gram-négatif | gram-negativo | gramnegativo | gramnegativ | グラム陰性 |
| 2900. Gram-positive - (a) | Gram-positif | gram-positivo | grampositivo | grampositiv | グラム陽性 |
| 2901. grand mal - (n) | épilepsie grand-mal | grande male | epilepsia gran mal | Grand-mal-Epilepsie | 大発作 |
| 2902. grant - (n) | subvention; allocation | concessione; borsa di studio | subvención; beca | Subvention; Stipendium | 補助金 |
| 2903. granulation - (n) | granulation | granulazione | granulación | Granulation | 肉芽 |
| 2904. granule - (n) | granule | granulo | gránulo | Körnchen | 顆粒 |
| 2905. granulocyte - (n) | granulocyte | granulocità | granulocito | Granulozyt | 顆粒球細胞 |
| 2906. granuloma - (n) | granulome | granuloma | granuloma | Granulom | 肉芽腫 |
| 2907. granulomatous - (a) | granulomateux | granulomatoso | granulomatoso | granulomatös | 肉芽腫性の |
| 2908. granulosa cell - (n) | cellule de la granulosa | cellula della granulosa | célula de la granulosa | Granulosazelle | 顆粒膜細胞 |
| 2909. graphics - (n) | graphisme | grafici | gráficos | Grafik | 図解 |
| 2910. grass - (n) | herbe | erba | pasto | Gras | 草 |

148

| English/American | French/Français | Italian/Italiano | Spanish/Español | German/Deutsch | Japanese/日本語 |
|---|---|---|---|---|---|
| 2911. gravid - (a) | gravide; enceinte | gravido; pregno | grávida; embarazada | gravid; schwanger | 妊娠の |
| 2912. gray matter - (n) | substance grise | sostanza grigia | sustancia gris | graue Substanz | 灰白質 |
| 2913. grid - (n) | grille | grata; griglia | rejilla; cuadrícula | Gitter; Raster | グリッド |
| 2914. grief - (n) | chagrin; douleur | afflizione; sofferenza | pesar; pesadumbre | Kummer; Trauer | 悲嘆 |
| 2915. grief reaction - (n) | réaction de douleur | reazione alla sofferenza | reacción de pesar | Trauerreaktion | 悲嘆反応 |
| 2916. grip strength - (n) | force de préhension | forza di prensione | fuerza de prehensión | Greifstärke | 握力の強さ |
| 2917. groin - (n) | aine | inguine | ingle | Leiste | 鼠径部 |
| 2918. groove - (n) | sillon; cannelure | solco | surco; canal | Furche; Rinne | 溝 |
| 2919. gross pathology - (n) | pathologie macroscopique | patologia macroscopica | patología macroscópica | Makropathologie | 肉眼病理学 |
| 2920. group - (n) | groupe | gruppo | grupo | Gruppe | 群 |
| 2921. group - (v) | grouper; disposer en groupes | raggruppare; disporre a gruppi | agrupar | gruppieren | 分類する |
| 2922. group data - (n) | données de groupe | dati del gruppo | datos de grupo | Gruppendaten | グループデータ |
| 2923. group sequential analysis - (n) | analyse séquentielle de groupe | analisi sequenziale a gruppi | análisis secuencial de grupo | Gruppensequentialanalyse | グループ逐続分析 |
| 2924. growth - (n) | croissance | crescita; accrescimento | crecimiento | Wachstum; Größenzunahme | 成長 |
| 2925. growth factor - (n) | facteur de croissance | fattore di accrescimento; fattore di crescita | factor de crecimiento | Wachstumsfaktor | 成長因子 |
| 2926. growth factor receptor - (n) | récepteur du facteur de croissance | recettore di fattore crescita | receptor del factor de crecimiento | Wachstumsfaktorrezeptor | 成長因子レセプター |
| 2927. growth plate - (n) | plaque de croissance | piano di crescita | placa de crecimiento | Wachstumszone | 成長板 |
| 2928. guide - (n) | guide | guida | guía | Führer; Führung | ガイド |
| 2929. guide - (v) | guider | guidare | guiar | führen; anleiten | 案内する |
| 2930. guideline - (n) | ligne directrice; ligne de conduite | linea di condotta | directriz; norma | Richtlinie; Empfehlung | ガイドライン |
| 2931. guinea pig - (n) | cobaye | porcellino d'India; cavia | cobayo | Meerschweinchen; [fig] Versuchskaninchen | モルモット |

| English/American | French/Français | Italian/Italiano | Spanish/Español | German/Deutsch | Japanese/日本語 |
| --- | --- | --- | --- | --- | --- |
| 2932. gum - (n) | gomme; gencive | gomma; gengiva | goma; encía | Gummi; Zahnfleisch | ゴム、歯肉 |
| 2933. gut - (n) | intestin; boyau | intestino | intestino | Darm | 腸 |
| 2934. gynecology (gynae-cology) - (n) | gynécologie | ginecologia | ginecología | Gynäkologie | 婦人科学 |
| 2935. gyne-comastia - (n) | gynécomastie | ginecomastia | ginecomastia | Gynäkomastie | 女性化乳房 |

| English/American | French/Français | Italian/Italiano | Spanish/Español | German/Deutsch | Japanese/日本語 |
|---|---|---|---|---|---|
| 2936. habit - (n) | habitude | abitudine | hábito | Gewohnheit; Angewohnheit | 習性 |
| 2937. habitus - (n) | habitus | habitus | hábito | Habitus; Körperbeschaffenheit | 体質 |
| 2938. hair - (n) | cheveux; poil | pelo: capello | cabello; pelo | Haar | 毛 |
| 2939. hair distribution - (n) | distribution des cheveux | distribuzioni dei peli | distribución del cabello; pelo | Haarverteilung | 毛髪の分布 |
| 2940. hair follicle - (n) | follicule pileux | follicolo pilifero | folículo capilar | Haarfollikel | 毛包 |
| 2941. hair loss - (n) | perte des cheveux | perdita dei capelli; caduta dei capelli | pérdida del cabello; caída de cabello | Haarausfall | 毛髪の損失 |
| 2942. half-life - (n) | demi-vie | emivita | vida media | Halbwertszeit | 半減期 |
| 2943. half-tone - (n) | demi-ton | semitono | medio tono | Halbton; halber Ton | 半音 |
| 2944. halitosis - (n) | mauvaise haleine | alitosi | halitosis | Mundgeruch | 口臭 |
| 2945. hallucination - (n) | hallucination | allucinazione | alucinación | Halluzination | 幻覚 |
| 2946. halogen - (n) | halogène | alogeno | halógeno | Halogen | ハロゲン |
| 2947. hand - (n) | main | mano | mano | Hand | 手 |
| 2948. hand-filled capsule - (n) | capsule remplie à la main | capsule riempite a mano | cápsula rellenada a mano | mit der Hand abgefüllte Kapsel | 手づめのカプセル |
| 2949. handling - (n) | manipulation | maneggiamento | manejo | Handhabung | 取り扱い |
| 2950. handwashing - (n) | lavage des mains | lavaggio delle mani | lavado de las manos | Händewaschen | 手を洗うこと |
| 2951. hangover - (n) | reste | postumi dell'ubriachezza | resaca | Kater | 二日酔い |
| 2952. haploid - (a) | haploïde | aploide | haploide | haploid | 半数体 |
| 2953. haplotype - (n) | haplotype | aplotipo | haplotipo | Haplotyp | ハプロタイプ |
| 2954. happiness - (n) | félicité; bonheur | felicità | felicidad | Glück | 幸福 |
| 2955. hard endpoint - (n) | objectif spécifique majeur | punto finale ben definibile | punto final definido | hartes Endziel | 最終的な目的 |
| 2956. hard outcome - (n) | issue majeure; conséquence majeure | risultato ben definibile | resultado definido | hartes (statistisch signifikantes) Ergebnis | 明解な結果 |

151

| English/American | French/Français | Italian/Italiano | Spanish/Español | German/Deutsch | Japanese/日本語 |
|---|---|---|---|---|---|
| 2957. hardware - (n) | hardware; matériel | hardware | hardware; equipos | Hardware | ハードウェア |
| 2958. hatch marks - (n) | marques d'hachures | marchi di indentatura | marcas de rayas cruzadas | schraffierte Linier | ハッチングマーク |
| 2959. hay fever - (n) | fièvre des foins | febbre da fieno; pollinosi | fiebre del heno | Heuschnupfen | 枯れ草熱 |
| 2960. hazard - (n) | risque | rischio | riesgo | Gefahr | 危険 |
| 2961. hazardous substance - (n) | substance dangereuse | sostanza pericolosa | sustancia peligrosa | gefährlicher Stoff / Gefahrstoff | 危険物質 |
| 2962. head - (n) | tête | capo; testa | cabeza | Kopf | 頭 |
| 2963. head count - (n) | comptage des têtes | conto dei soggetti | conteo de las personas | Zählung; Erhebung | 国勢調査 |
| 2964. head injury - (n) | traumatisme crânien | trauma cranico | traumatismo del cráneo | Kopfverletzung; Schädeltrauma | 頭部損傷 |
| 2965. headache - (n) | céphalée; mal de tête | cefalea; mal di testa | cefalea; dolor de cabeza | Kopfschmerz | 頭痛 |
| 2966. heal - (v) | guérir | sanare; guarire | curar; sanar | heilen | 治る |
| 2967. healing - (n) | guérison | guarigione | curativo | Heilung | 治癒 |
| 2968. health - (n) | santé | salute | salud | Gesundheit | 健康 |
| 2969. health aide - (n) | aide à la santé | aiuto sanitario | personal auxiliar de la salud | Krankenpflegehelfer | 健康援助の人 |
| 2970. health care - (n) | soins de santé | assistenza sanitaria | servicio de salud | Gesundheitsfürsorge | 健康管理 |
| 2971. health catchment area - (n) | zone de service-santé | distretto sanitario | zona de servicio de salud | Einzugsbereich einer Gesundheitseinrichtung) | 健康流域 |
| 2972. health center - (n) | centre de santé | centro sanitario | centro médico | Gesundheitszentrum; Ärztezentrum | 健康センター |
| 2973. health education - (n) | éducation de santé | educazione sanitaria | educación sanitaria | Gesundheitserziehung | 保健教育 |
| 2974. health facility - (n) | installation de santé | ambulatorio sanitario | instalación de asistencia médica | Gesundheitseinrichtung | 健康施設 |
| 2975. health insurance - (n) | assurance médicale; assurance-santé | assicurazione per la salute | seguro de enfermedad | Krankenversicherung; Krankenkasse | 健康保険 |

| English/American | French/Français | Italian/Italiano | Spanish/Español | German/Deutsch | Japanese/日本語 |
|---|---|---|---|---|---|
| 2976. health mainte- nance organiza- tion [abbr] HMO - (n) | organisation de maintien de la santé | organizzazione mantenimento sanitario | organización que presta servicios de salud | Gesundheitserhaltungs- organisation | 健康維持団体 |
| 2977. health planning - (n) | planification de santé | pianificazione sanitaria | planificación sanitaria | Gesundheitsplanung | 健康計画 |
| 2978. health service - (n) | service de santé | servizio sanitario | servicio de salud | Gesundheitswesen | 健康サービス |
| 2979. health status - (n) | état de santé | condizione di salute | estado físico | Gesundheitszustand | 健康状態 |
| 2980. healthy - (a) | sain; en bonne santé | sano; in buona salute | sano; en buen estado de salud | gesund | 健康な |
| 2981. hearing - (n) | ouïe | udito | oído | Hören | 聴力 |
| 2982. hearing aid - (n) | prothèse auditive | protesi acustica | aparato acústico | Hörgerät | 補聴器 |
| 2983. hearing loss - (n) | perte auditive | perdita uditiva | sordera | Hörverlust | 聴力損失 |
| 2984. hearing test - (n) | épreuve d'audition | test della funzione uditiva | examen de oído | Hörprüfung | 聴覚検査 |
| 2985. heart - (n) | coeur | cuore | corazón | Herz | 心臓 |
| 2986. heart arrest - (n) | arrêt cardiaque | arresto cardiaco | paro cardíaco | Herzstillstand | 心臓停止 |
| 2987. heart attack - (n) | crise cardiaque | attacco cardiaco | ataque cardíaco | Herzanfall; Herzinfarkd | 心臓発作 |
| 2988. heart block - (n) | blocage du coeur | blocco cardiaco | bloqueo cardíaco | Herzblock | 心臓ブロック |
| 2989. heart disease - (n) | maladie cardiaque | cardiopatia | enfermedad cardíaca | Herzerkrankung | 心臓病 |
| 2990. heart failure - (n) | défaillance cardiaque; insuffisance cardiaque | scompenso cardiaco; insufficienza cardiaca | fallo cardíaco; insuficiencia cardíaca | Herzversagen; Herzinsuffizienz | 心不全 |
| 2991. heart massage - (n) | massage cardiaque | massaggio cardiaco | masaje cardíaco | Herzmassage | 心臓マッサージ |
| 2992. heart murmur - (n) | souffle cardiaque | soffio cardiaco | soplo cardíaco | Herzgeräusch | 心臓雑音 |
| 2993. heart muscle - (n) | muscle cardiaque | muscolo cardiaco | músculo cardíaco | Herzmuskel | 心筋 |
| 2994. heart rate - (n) | fréquence cardiaque | frequenza cardiaca | frecuencia cardíaca | Herzfrequenz | 心度数 |
| 2995. heart sound - (n) | bruit cardiaque | rumore cardiaco; tono cardiaco | sonido cardíaco | Herzton | 心音 |

153

| English/American | French/Français | Italian/Italiano | Spanish/Español | German/Deutsch | Japanese/日本語 |
|---|---|---|---|---|---|
| 2996. heart transplant - (n) | transplantation cardiaque | trapianto cardiaco | trasplante cardiaco | Herztransplantation | 心臓移植 |
| 2997. heart valve - (n) | valve cardiaque | valvola cardiaca | válvula cardiaca | Herzklappe | 心臓弁 |
| 2998. heartbeat - (n) | battement du cœur | battito cardiaco | latido del corazón | Herzschlag | 心拍 |
| 2999. heartburn - (n) | pyrosis | pirosi | pirosis | Sodbrennen | 胸やけ |
| 3000. heart-lung machine - (n) | cœur-poumon artificiel | macchina cuore-polmoni | bomba corazón pulmón | Herz-Lungen-Maschine | 人工心肺 |
| 3001. heart-lung transplantation - (n) | transplantation cœur-poumon | trapianto cuore-polmone | trasplante cardiopulmonar | Herz-Lungen-Transplantation | 心肺移植 |
| 3002. heat - (n) | chaleur | calore; caldo | calor | Hitze; Wärme | 熱 |
| 3003. heat - (v) | chauffer | scaldare; riscaldare | calentar | erhitzen; erwärmen | 熱する |
| 3004. heat exhaustion - (n) | épuisement à la chaleur | collasso da calore | golpe por calor | Wärmestau mit allgemeiner Erschöpfung | 暑気当たり |
| 3005. heat intolerance - (n) | intolérance à la chaleur | intolleranza al caldo | intolerancia al calor | Wärmeunverträglichkeit | 熱不耐容 |
| 3006. heat loss - (n) | perte calorifique | perdita di calore | pérdida de calor | Wärmeverlust | 熱損失 |
| 3007. heat shock - (n) | coup de chaleur | shock da calore | choque por calor | Hitzeschock | 熱ショック |
| 3008. heat shrink seal - (n) | scellé thermocontractile | chiusura termocontrattile | sello termocontraible | Heißsiegel | 熱収縮密封 |
| 3009. heating - (n) | chauffage | riscaldamento | calefacción | Erwärmung; Heizung | 暖房 |
| 3010. heavy metal poisoning - (n) | intoxication aux métaux lourds | avvelemento de metallo pesante | envenenamiento por metales pesados | Schwermetallvergiftung | 重金属中毒 |
| 3011. heel - (n) | talon | calcagno; tallone | talón | Absatz; Ferse | 踵 |
| 3012. height - (n) | taille; grandeur | altezza | altura | Höhe | 高度 |
| 3013. helium - (n) | hélium | elio | helio | Helium | ヘリウム |
| 3014. helminth - (n) | helminthe | elminte | helminto | Helminthe | 寄生虫 |
| 3015. hemagglutination - (n) | hémagglutination | emoagglutinazione | hemaglutinación | Hämagglutination | 赤血球凝集反応 |

154

| English/American | French/Français | Italian/Italiano | Spanish/Español | German/Deutsch | Japanese=日本語 |
|---|---|---|---|---|---|
| 3016. hemangioma - (n) | hémangiome | emangioma | hemangioma | Hämangiom | 血管腫 |
| 3017. hemarthrosis - (n) | hémarthrose | emartrosi | hemartrosis | Hämarthros | 出血性関節症 |
| 3018. hematemesis - (n) | hématémèse | ematemesi | hematemesis | Hämatemesis; Bluterbrechen | 吐血 [症] |
| 3019. hematocrit [abbr] HCT, HT - (n) | hématocrite | ematocrito | hematócrito | Hämatokrit | ヘマトクリット |
| 3020. hematologic - (a) | hématologique | ematologico | hematológico | hämatologisch | 血液学の |
| 3021. hematology - (n) | hématologie | ematologia | hematología | Hämatologie | 血液学 |
| 3022. hematoma - (n) | hématome | ematoma | hematoma | Hämatom | 血腫 |
| 3023. hemato-poiesis - (n) | hématopoïèse | emopoiesi | hematopoyesis | Hämatopoese | 造血 |
| 3024. hematopoietic stem cell - (n) | cellule souche hématopoïétique | cellula staminale ematopoietica | célula progenitora hematopoyética | hämatopoetische Stammzelle | 造血幹細胞 |
| 3025. hematuria - (n) | hématurie | ematuria | hematuria | Hämaturie | 血尿 [症] |
| 3026. hemialgia - (n) | hémialgie; hémicrânie | emialgia | hemialgia; hemicránea | Hemialgia; Halbseitenschmerz | 片頭痛 |
| 3027. hemic system - (n) | système hémique | sistema ematico | sistema hémico | hämorrheologisches System | 血液系 |
| 3028. hemiplegia - (n) | hémiplégie | emiplegia | hemiplejía | Hemiplegie | 片麻痺 |
| 3029. hemisphere - (n) | hémisphère | emisfero | hemisferio | Hemisphäre | 半球 |
| 3030. hemodialysis (haemo-dialysis) - (n) | hémodialyse | emodialisi | hemodiálisis | Hämodialyse | 血液透析 |
| 3031. hemo-dynamics - (n) | hémodynamique | emodinamica | hemodinámica | Hämodynamik | 血行力学 |
| 3032. hemoglobin [abbr] Hb - (n) | hémoglobine | emoglobina | hemoglobina | Hämoglobin | ヘモグロビン |
| 3033. hemoglobin-opathy - (n) | hémoglobinopathie | emoglobinopatia | hemoglobinopatía | Hämoglobinopathie | 血球素病 |

| English/American | French/Français | Italian/Italiano | Spanish/Español | German/Deutsch | Japanese 日本語 |
|---|---|---|---|---|---|
| 3034. hemoglobin-uria - (n) | hémoglobinurie | emoglobinuria | hemoglobinuria | Hämoglobinurie | 血色素尿症 |
| 3035. hemolysis - (n) | hémolyse | emolisi | hemólisis | Hämolyse | 溶血 |
| 3036. hemolytic - (a) | hémolytique | emolitico | hemolítico | hämolytisch | 溶血性の |
| 3037. hemolytic anemia - (n) | anémie hémolytique | anemia emolitica | anemia hemolítica | hämolytische Anämie | 溶血性貧血 |
| 3038. hemo-perfusion - (n) | hémoperfusion | emoperfusione | hemoperfusión | Hämoperfusion | 血液灌流 |
| 3039. hemophilia - (n) | hémophilie | emofilia | hemofilia | Hämophilie | 血友病 |
| 3040. hemoptysis - (n) | hémoptysie | emottisi | hemoptisis | Hämoptyse | 喀血 |
| 3041. hemorrhage - (n) | hémorragie | emorragia | hemorragia | Hämorrhagie | 出血 |
| 3042. hemorrhagic diathesis - (n) | diathèse hémorragique | diatesi emorragica | diátesis hemorrágica | hämorrhagische Diathese | 出血性素質 |
| 3043. hemorrhagic shock - (n) | choc hémorragique | shock emorragico | choque hemorrágico | hämorrhagischer Schock | 出血性ショック |
| 3044. hemorrhoid - (n) | hémorroïde | emorroide | hemorroide | Hämorrhoide | 痔 |
| 3045. hemostasis - (n) | hémostase | emostasi | hemostasia | Hämostase | 止血 |
| 3046. hemostat - (n) | hémostatique | pinza emostatica | hemóstato | Gefäßklemme | 止血鉗子 |
| 3047. heparin lock - (n) | régulateur du débit de l'héparine | dispositivo regolatore | dispositivo regulador de heparina | Heparinflußregulator | ヘパリンロック |
| 3048. hepatic - (a) | hépatique | epatico | hepático | hepatisch | 肝の |
| 3049. hepatitis - (n) | hépatite | epatite | hepatitis | Hepatitis | 肝炎 |
| 3050. hepatojugular reflux - (n) | reflux hépato-jugulaire | riflesso epato-giugulare | reflujo hepatoyugular | hepatojugulärer Reflux | 肝-頸静脈逆流 |
| 3051. hepatolenticular degeneration - (n) | dégénération hépatolenticulaire | degenerazione epatolenticolare | degeneración hepatolenticular | hepatolentikuläre Degeneration | 肝レンズ核変性 [症] |
| 3052. hepatology - (n) | hépatologie | epatologia | hepatología | Hepatologie | 肝学 |
| 3053. hepatoma - (n) | hépatome | epatoma | hepatoma | Hepatom | 肝癌 |

156

| English/American | French/Français | Italian/Italiano | Spanish/Español | German/Deutsch | Japanese/日本語 |
|---|---|---|---|---|---|
| 3054. hepato-megaly - (n) | hépatomégalie | epatomegalia | hepatomegalia | Hepatomegalie | 肝腫［大］ |
| 3055. herb - (n) | herbe | erba | hierba | Kraut; Pflanze | 薬草 |
| 3056. herbal medicine - (n) | remède galénique | medicinale naturale | medicina herbaria | Kräutermedizin | 薬草学 |
| 3057. herbicide - (n) | herbicide | erbicida | herbicida | Herbizid | 除草剤 |
| 3058. hereditary - (a) | héréditaire | ereditario | hereditario | hereditär; erblich | 遺伝性の |
| 3059. heredity - (n) | hérédité | eredità | herencia | Vererbung; Heredität | 遺伝 |
| 3060. hermaphrodit-ism - (n) | hermaphrodisme | ermafroditismo | hermafroditismo | Hermaphroditismus | 半陰陽 |
| 3061. hernia - (n) | hernie | ernia | hernia | Hernie; Bruch | ヘルニア |
| 3062. herniated disk - (n) | hernie discale | ernia del disco | hernia de disco | Diskushernie | 脱出椎間板 |
| 3063. heroin depen-dence - (n) | héroïnomanie | eroinomania | heroinomania | Heroinabhängigkeit | ヘロイン中毒 |
| 3064. herpetic - (a) | herpétique | erpetico | herpético | herpetisch; Herpes- | ヘルペス［性］の |
| 3065. hertz [abbr] Hz - (n) | hertz | hertz | hertz | Hertz | ヘルツ |
| 3066. heterologous - (a) | hétérologue | eterologo | heterólogo | heterolog | 異種の |
| 3067. heterophil - (a) | hétérophile | eterofilo | heterófilo | heterophil | 異染［性］の |
| 3068. heterosexual - (n) | hétérosexuel | eterosessuale | heterosexual | Heterosexueller | 異性愛主義者 |
| 3069. heterosexual - (a) | hétérosexuel | eterosessuale | heterosexual | heterosexuell | 異性愛の |
| 3070. heterotopic - (a) | hétérotopique | eterotopico | heterotópico | heterotop | 異位元素の |
| 3071. heterozygote - (n) | hétérozygote | eterozigote | heterozigoto | Heterozygot | ヘテロ接合体 |
| 3072. hiatal hernia - (n) | hernie hiatale | ernia iatale | hernia hiatal | Hiatushernie | 裂孔ヘルニア |
| 3073. hiatus - (n) | hiatus; aperture | hiatus; apertura | hiato; abertura | Hiatus; Lücke | 裂孔 |
| 3074. hiccups - (n) | hoquet | singhiozzo | hipo | Schluckauf | しゃっくり |
| 3075. hierarchy - (n) | hiérarchie | gerarchia | jerarquía | Hierarchie | 分類段階 |

157

| English/American | French/Français | Italian/Italiano | Spanish/Español | German/Deutsch | Japanese/日本語 |
|---|---|---|---|---|---|
| 3076. high dose - (n) | haute dose | dose alta | dosis alta | hohe Dosis | 多量投薬 |
| 3077. high frequency - (n) | haute fréquence | alta frequenza | alta frecuencia | Hochfrequenz | 高周波 |
| 3078. high pressure - (n) | haute pression | alta pressione | alta presión | Hochdruck | 高圧 |
| 3079. high risk - (n) | haut risque | alto rischio | alto riesgo | hohes Risiko | ハイリスク |
| 3080. highly bound drug - (n) | médicament fortement lié | sostanza con alta affinità plasmatica | droga altamente ligada | Medikament mit hoher Bindungsaffinität | 高結合薬 |
| 3081. high-tech - (n) | haute-technologie | high-tech; alta tecnologia | alta tecnología | Spitzentechnologie; Hi-tech | ハイテク |
| 3082. high-tech - (a) | de haute-technologie; de pointe | high-tech; altamente tecnologico | de alta tecnología | Hi-tech-; technologisch anspruchsvoll | ハイテクの |
| 3083. hilus - (n) | hile | ilo | hilio | Pforte; Hilus | 門 |
| 3084. hindbrain - (n) | rhombencéphale | rombencefalo | rombencéfalo | Rhombenzephalon | 後頭 |
| 3085. hind limb - (n) | membre postérieur | arto posteriore | miembro posterior | Hinterbein | 後肢 |
| 3086. hip - (n) | hanche | anca | cadera | Hüfte | 臀部 |
| 3087. hip joint - (n) | articulation de la hanche | articolazione dell'anca | articulación de la cadera | Hüftgelenk | 股関節 |
| 3088. hippocampus - (n) | hippocampe | ippocampo | hipocampo | Ammonshorn; Hippocampus | 海馬 |
| 3089. hirsute - (a) | hirsute | irsuto | hirsuto | hirsutistisch; haarig | 粗毛の |
| 3090. Hispanic - (a) | hispanique | ispanico | hispánico | hispanisch | ヒスパニックの |
| 3091. histamine - (n) | histamine | istamina | histamina | Histamin | ヒスタミン |
| 3092. histaminergic - (a) | histaminergique | istaminergico | histaminérgico | histaminerg | ヒスタミン作用性の |
| 3093. histiocytosis - (n) | histiocytose | istiocitosi | histiocitosis | Histiozytose | 組織球増殖額[症] |
| 3094. histocompatibility - (n) | histocompatibilité | istocompatibilità | histocompatibilidad | Histokompatibilität | 組織適合性 |
| 3095. histocytochemistry - (n) | histocytochimie | istocitochimica | histocitoquímica | Histocytochemie | 組織化学 |
| 3096. histogram - (n) | histogramme | istogramma | histograma | Histogramm | ヒストグラム |

| English/American | French/Français | Italian/Italiano | Spanish/Español | German/Deutsch | Japanese/日本語 |
|---|---|---|---|---|---|
| 3097. histological - (a) | histologique | istologico | histológico | histologisch | 組織学の |
| 3098. histological section - (n) | coupe histologique | sezione istologica | sección histológica | histologischer Schnitt | 組織切片 |
| 3099. histologist - (n) | histologiste | istologo | histólogo | Histologe | 組織学者 |
| 3100. histology - (n) | histologie | istologia | histología | Histologie | 組織学 |
| 3101. histopathology - (n) | histopathologie | istopatologia | histopatología | Histopathologie | 組織病理学 |
| 3102. historical baseline - (n) | ligne de base historque | livello di base storico | línea de base histórica | übernommene Standardkurve | 歴史的基線 |
| 3103. historical control - (n) | témoin historique; contrôle historique | controllo storico | control histórico | übernommene Kontrolle | 歴史的コントロール |
| 3104. history - (n) | histoire; anamnèse | storia; anamnesi | historia; anamnesis | Anamnese | 既往症 |
| 3105. history taking - (n) | prise de l'histoire médicale | anamnesi | obtención de la historia clínica; anamnesis | Anamneseaufnahme | 病歴を記入すること |
| 3106. hives - (n) | uticaire | orticaria | urticaria | Urtikaria; Nesselfieber | 蕁麻疹 |
| 3107. hoarseness - (n) | enrouement | raucedine | ronquera | Heiserkeit | しわがれ声 |
| 3108. holistic health - (n) | santé holistique | salute olistica | salud holística | ganzheitliche Gesundheit | 健康全体論 |
| 3109. Holter monitor - (n) | moniteur de Holter | monitore Holter | monitor de Holter | Holter-Monitor | ホルターモニター |
| 3110. home - (n) | maison; domicile | casa; dimora | casa; domicilio | Heim; Pflegeheim | 家庭 |
| 3111. home care - (n) | soins à domicile | assistenza domiciliare | atención en la casa; atención a domicilio | Hauspflege | 家庭療養 |
| 3112. homeless - (a) | sans abris | senza casa | sin hogar | obdachlos | 家のない |
| 3113. homeopathy - (n) | homéopathie | omeopatia | homeopatía | Homöopathie | 同毒療法 |
| 3114. homeostasis - (n) | homéostasie | omeostasi | homeostasis | Homöostase | 動的平衡 |
| 3115. homicide - (n) | homicide | omicidio | homicidio | Mord | 殺人 |
| 3116. homogenate - (n) | homogénat | omogenato | homogenado | Homogenat | ホモジネート |
| 3117. homogeneity - (n) | homogénéité | omogeneità | homogeneidad | Homogenität | 同質 |

159

| English/American | French/Français | Italian/Italiano | Spanish/Español | German/Deutsch | Japanese/日本語 |
|---|---|---|---|---|---|
| 3118. homo-geneous - (a) | homogène | omogeneo | homogéneo | homogen | 同質の |
| 3119. homograft - (n) | homogreffe | innesto omologo; omotrapianto | homoinjerto | Homotransplantat | 同種移植片 |
| 3120. homologous - (a) | homologue | omologo | homólogo | homolog | 相同性の |
| 3121. homology - (n) | homologie | omologia | homología | Homologie | 相同 |
| 3122. homosexual - (n) | homosexuel | omosessuale | homosexual | Homosexueller | 同性愛主義者 |
| 3123. homosexual - (a) | homosexuel | omosessuale | homosexual | homosexuell | 同性愛の |
| 3124. homo-sexuality - (n) | homosexualité | omosessualità | homosexualidad | Homosexualität | 同性愛 |
| 3125. homozygote - (n) | homozygote | omozigote | homocigoto | Homozygot | ホモ接合体 |
| 3126. homozygous - (a) | homozygote | omozigotico | homocigótico | homozygot | ホモ接合の |
| 3127. horizontal - (a) | horizontal | orizzontale | horizontal | horizontal | 水平の |
| 3128. hormonal contraceptive - (n) | contraceptif hormonal | contracettivo ormonale | anticonceptivo hormonal | hormonales Verhütungsmittel | ホルモン性避妊薬 |
| 3129. hormone - (n) | hormone | ormone | hormona | Hormon | ホルモン |
| 3130. hormone dependent - (a) | hormono-dépendant | ormonodipendente | dependiente de hormonas | hormonabhäng g | ホルモン依存の |
| 3131. hormono-therapy - (n) | hormonothérapie | ormonoterapia; terapia ormonale | terapia con hormonas | Hormontherapie | ホルモン療法 |
| 3132. horny tissue - (n) | tissu calleux | tessuto corneo | tejido córneo | hornartiges Gewebe | 角質組織 |
| 3133. hospice - (n) | hospice | ospizio | hospicio | Hospiz; Sterbeklinik | ホスピス, 収容所 |
| 3134. hospice care - (n) | soins dans un hospice | assistenza in ospizio | atención en un hospicio | Hospizpflege | ホスピス療養 |
| 3135. hospital - (n) | hôpital | ospedale | hospital | Krankenhaus | 病院 |
| 3136. hospital admission - (n) | admission à l'hôpital | ammissione ospedaliera | admisión al hospital | Krankenhausei nlieferung | 入院 |
| 3137. hospital chart - (n) | dossier d'hôpital | dossier ospedaliero | ficha clínica | Krankenhaustabelle | 病院チャート |
| 3138. hospital stay - (n) | séjour à l'hôpital | degenza ospedaliera | estadía en el hospital | Krankenhausaufenthalt | 入院 |

| English/American | French/Français | Italian/Italiano | Spanish/Español | German/Deutsch | Japanese/日本語 |
|---|---|---|---|---|---|
| 3139. hospitalization - (n) | hospitalisation | ospedalizzazione | hospitalización | Krankenhauseinweisung | 入院 |
| 3140. host - (n) | hôte | ospite | huésped | Wirt | 宿主 |
| 3141. host resistance - (n) | résistance de l'hôte | resistenza dell'ospite | resistencia del huésped | Wirtsresistenz | 宿主抵抗 |
| 3142. hostility - (n) | hostilité | ostilità | hostilidad | Feindseligkeit | 敵意 |
| 3143. host-parasite relations - (n) | rapport hôte-parasite | relazioni ospite-parassite | relación huésped-parásito | Wirt-Parasit-Beziehungen | 宿主ー寄生体関係 |
| 3144. hot flash - (n) | bouffée de chaleur | vampata di calore | sofoco de calor | fliegende Hitze | のぼせ |
| 3145. hot line - (n) | ligne ouverte | hotline | teléfono rojo | Telefonberatung | ホットライン |
| 3146. house staff - (n) | internes | staff permanente | internos | Hauspersonal | 宿直医員 |
| 3147. housekeeping - (n) | ménage économe de maison | governo della casa | gobierno de la casa | Haushalten | 家事 |
| 3148. housing - (n) | logement | alloggio | vivienda | Wohnung | 収容 |
| 3149. human - (n) | humain | essere umano | humano | Mensch | 人間 |
| 3150. human - (a) | humain | umano | humano | menschlich | 人間の |
| 3151. human body - (n) | corps humain | corpo umano | cuerpo humano | menschlicher Körper | 人体 |
| 3152. human experimentation committee - (n) | comité d'expérimentation humaine | comitato | comité de experimentación en seres humanos | Ausschuß zur Entscheidung über Menschenversuche | 人体実験委員会 |
| 3153. human pharmacology - (n) | pharmacologie humaine | farmacologia umana | farmacología humana | Menschenpharmakologie | 人体薬理学 |
| 3154. human stem cell - (n) | cellule souche humaine | cellula staminale umana | célula progenitora humana | menschliche Stammzelle | 人体幹細胞 |
| 3155. human testing - (n) | essai sur les êtres humains | test sul corpo umano | ensayos sobre seres humanos | Menschenversuch | 人体実験 |
| 3156. humanitarian protocol - (n) | protocole humanitaire | protocollo umanitario | protocolo humanitario | humanitäres Protokoll | 人道主義プロトコル |

161

| English/American | French/Français | Italian/Italiano | Spanish/Español | German/Deutsch | Japanese/日本語 |
|---|---|---|---|---|---|
| 3157. humerus - (n) | humérus | omero | húmero | Oberarm | 上腕骨 |
| 3158. humidity - (n) | humidité | umidità | humedad | Feuchtigkeit | 湿度 |
| 3159. humoral - (a) | huméral | umorale | humoral | humoral | 体液の |
| 3160. hunchback - (n) | cyphose | cifosi | cifosis | Kyphose | 亀背 |
| 3161. hunger - (n) | faim | fame | hambre | Hunger | 飢餓 |
| 3162. hyaline cartilage - (n) | cartilage hyalin | cartilagine ialina | cartílago hialino | Hyalinknorpel | 硝子軟骨 |
| 3163. hyaline cast - (n) | cylindre hyalin | cilindro ialino | cilindro hialino | Hyalinzylinder | 硝子樣円柱 |
| 3164. hyaline membrane - (n) | membrane hyaline | membrana ialina | membrana hialina | hyaline Membran | 硝子膜 |
| 3165. hybrid - (n) | hybride | ibrido | híbrido | Hybrid | 混種 |
| 3166. hybrid - (a) | hybride | ibrido | híbrido | hybrid | 混種の |
| 3167. hybridization - (n) | hybridation | ibridazione | hibridización | Hybridisierung | 交雑 |
| 3168. hybridoma - (n) | hybridome | ibridoma | hibridoma | Hybridzelle | ハイブリドーマ |
| 3169. hydrated - (a) | hydraté | idratato | hidratado | hydriert | 水和物の |
| 3170. hydrocarbon - (n) | hydrocarbone | idrocarburo | hidrocarburo | Kohlenwasserstoff | 炭化水素 |
| 3171. hydrocele - (n) | hydrocèle | idrocele | hidrocele | Hydrozele | 水瘤 |
| 3172. hydrocephalus - (n) | hydrocéphalie | idrocefalo | hidrocéfalo | Hydrozephalus; Wasserkopf | 水頭症 |
| 3173. hydrogen - (n) | hydrogène | idrogeno | hidrógeno | Wasserstoff | 水素 |
| 3174. hydrogen bond - (n) | liaison d'hydrogène | legame idrogeno | enlace de hidrógeno | Wasserstoffbrücke | 水素結合 |
| 3175. hydrolysis - (n) | hydrolyse | idrolisi | hidrólisis | Hydrolyse | 加水分解 |
| 3176. hydrophilic - (a) | hydrophile | idrofilo | hidrofílico | hydrophil | 親水性の |
| 3177. hydrophobic - (a) | hydrophobe | idrofobo; idrofobico | hidrofóbico | hydrophobisch | 疎水性の |
| 3178. hydroxylation - (n) | hydroxylation | idrossilazione | hidroxilación | Hydroxylierung | 水酸化 |
| 3179. hygiene - (n) | hygiène | igiene | higiene | Hygiene | 衛生学 |
| 3180. hymen - (n) | hymen | imene | himen | Hymen; Jungfernhäutchen | 処女膜 |

162

| English/American | French/Français | Italian/Italiano | Spanish/Español | German/Deutsch | Japanese/日本語 |
|---|---|---|---|---|---|
| 3181. hyper- - (prefix) | hyper- | iper- | hiper- | Hyper-; Über- | 過剰の |
| 3182. hyperacidity - (n) | hyperacidité | iperacidità | hiperacidez | Hyperazidität; Übersäuerung | 過酸症 |
| 3183. hyperactive - (a) | hyperactif | iperattivo | hiperactivo | hyperaktiv | 機能亢進の |
| 3184. hyperactive reflex - (n) | hyperréflexie | riflesso iperattivo | reflejo hiperactivo | übersteigerter Reflex | 機能亢進反射 |
| 3185. hyperactivity - (n) | hyperactivité | iperattività | hiperactividad | Hyperaktivität | 機能亢進 |
| 3186. hyperalgesia - (n) | hyperalgésie | iperalgesia | hiperalgesia | Hyperalgesie | 痛覚過敏 |
| 3187. hyperbaric oxygen - (n) | oxygène hyperbare | ossigeno iperbarico | oxígeno hiperbárico | hyperbarer Sauerstoff | 高圧酸素 |
| 3188. hypercalcemia - (n) | hypercalcémie | ipercalcemia | hipercalcemia | Hyperkalzämie | 高カルシウム血 [症] |
| 3189. hypercapnia - (n) | hypercapnie | ipercapnia | hipercapnia | Hyperkapnie | 炭酸過剰 |
| 3190. hypercholesterolemia - (n) | hypercholestérolémie | ipercolesterolemia | hipercolesterolemia | Hypercholesterinämie | 高コレステロール血 [症] |
| 3191. hyperchromic - (a) | hyperchromique | ipercromico | hipercrómico | hyperchrom | 高色素性の |
| 3192. hyperemia - (n) | hyperémie | iperemia | hiperemia | Hyperämie | 充血 |
| 3193. hyperesthesia - (n) | hyperesthésie | iperestesia | hiperestesia | Hyperästhesie | 感覚過敏 [症] |
| 3194. hyperfunction - (n) | hyperfonction | iperfunzione | hiperfunción | Überfunktion | 機能亢進 |
| 3195. hyperglycemia - (n) | hyperglycémie | iperglicemia | hiperglucemia | Hyperglykämie | 血糖過多症 |
| 3196. hyperkalemia - (n) | hyperkaliémie | iperpotassiemia; iperkaliemia | hiperpotasemia | Hyperkaliämie; Hyperkaliämie | 高カリウム [症] |
| 3197. hyperkinesia - (n) | hypercinésie; hyperkinésie | ipercinesia | hipercinesia | Hyperkinesie | 過運動症 |
| 3198. hyperlipidemia - (n) | hyperlipidémie | iperlipidemia | hiperlipidemia | Hyperlipidämie; Hyperlipämie | 高脂肪血 [症] |

| English/American | French/Français | Italian/Italiano | Spanish/Español | German/Deutsch | Japanese/日本語 |
|---|---|---|---|---|---|
| 3199. hyperlipopro-teinemia - (n) | hyperlipoprotéinémie | iperlipoproteinemia | hiperlipoproteinemia | Hyperlipoproteinämie | 高リポ蛋白血［症］ |
| 3200. hyper-natremia - (n) | hypernatrémie | ipernatriemia | hipernatremia | Hypernatriämie | 高ナトリウム血［症］ |
| 3201. hyperostosis - (n) | hyperostose | iperostosi | hiperostosis | Hyperostosis | 過骨症 |
| 3202. hyperparathyroi-dism - (n) | hyperparathyroïdisme | iperparatiroidismo | hiperparatiroidismo | Hyperparathyreoidismus | 上皮小体［機能］亢進［症］ |
| 3203. hyperphagia - (n) | hyperphagie | iperfagia | hiperfagia | Hyperphagie | 暴食 |
| 3204. hyperplasia - (n) | hyperplasie | iperplasia | hiperplasia | Hyperplasie | 過形成 |
| 3205. hyper-reactivity - (n) | hyperréactivité | iperreattività | hiperreactividad | Hyperreaktivität | 過剰反応 |
| 3206. hyperreflexia - (n) | hyperréflexie | iperreflessia | hiperreflexia | Hyperreflexie | 反射異常亢進 |
| 3207. hyper-sensitive - (a) | hypersensible | ipersensibile | hipersensible | überempfindlich | 過敏の |
| 3208. hypersensi-tivity - (n) | hypersensibilité | ipersensibilità | hipersensibilidad | Überempfindlichkeit | 過敏症 |
| 3209. hypertension - (n) | hypertension | ipertensione | hipertensión | Hypertension; Hypertonie | 高血圧症 |
| 3210. hyperthermia - (n) | hyperthermie | ipertermia | hipertermia | Hyperthermie | 異常高熱 |
| 3211. hyper-thyroidism - (n) | hyperthyroïdisme | ipertiroidismo | hipertiroidismo | Hyperthyreoidismus; Hyperthyreose | 甲状腺機能亢進［症］ |
| 3212. hypertonic saline - (n) | salin hypertonique | soluzione salina ipertonica | salina hipertónica | hypertonische Salzlösung | 高張塩水 |
| 3213. hypertonic solution - (n) | solution hypertonique | soluzione ipertonica | solución hipertónica | hypertonische Lösung | 高張溶液 |
| 3214. hypertonicity - (n) | hypertonicité | ipertonia | hipertonicidad | Hypertonie | 高張性 |
| 3215. hypertriglyce-ridemia - (n) | hypertriglycéridémie | ipertrigliceridemia | hipertrigliceridemia | Hypertriglyzeridämie | 高トリグリセリド血症 |
| 3216. hypertrophic - (a) | hypertrophique | ipertrofico | hipertrófico | hypertroph | 肥大性の |

164

| English/American | French/Français | Italian/Italiano | Spanish/Español | German/Deutsch | Japanese/日本語 |
|---|---|---|---|---|---|
| 3217. hypertrophy - (n) | hypertrophie | ipertrofia | hipertrofia | Hypertrophie | 肥大 |
| 3218. hyperventilation - (n) | hyperventilation | iperventilazione | hiperventilación | Hyperventilation | 換気亢進 |
| 3219. hypnosis - (n) | hypnose | ipnosi | hipnosis | Hypnose | 催眠 |
| 3220. hypnotic - (a) | hypnotique | ipnotico | hipnótico | hypnotisch | 催眠の |
| 3221. hypo- - (prefix) | hypo- | ipo- | hipo- | Hypo-; Unter- | 不足の |
| 3222. hypochondria - (n) | hypochondrie | ipocondria | hipocondria | Hypochondrie | ヒポコンドリア症 |
| 3223. hypochondriac - (n) | hypocondriaque | ipocondriaco | hipocondríaco | Hypochonder | ヒポコンドリア症患者 |
| 3224. hypochondriasis - (n) | hypochondrie | ipocondria | hipocondria | Hypochondrie | 心気症 |
| 3225. hypochromic - (a) | hypochromique | ipocromico | hipocrómico | hypochrom | 血色減少の |
| 3226. hypodermic syringe - (n) | seringue hypodermique | siringa ipodermica | jeringa hipodérmica | Spritze zur subkutanen Injektion | 皮下注射器 |
| 3227. hypofunction - (n) | hypofonction | ipofunzione | hipofunción | Unterfunktion | 機能減退 |
| 3228. hypoglycemic - (a) | hypoglycémique | ipoglicemico | hipoglucémico | Hypoglykämie | 低血糖［症］の |
| 3229. hypolipoproteinemia - (n) | hypolipoprotéinémie | ipolipoproteinemia | hipolipoproteinemia | Hypolipoproteinämie | 低リポ蛋白血［症］ |
| 3230. hypomenorrhea - (n) | hypoménorrhée | ipomenorrea | hipomenorrea | Hypomenorrhö | 過小月経 |
| 3231. hyponatremia - (n) | hyponatrémie | iponatriemia | hiponatremia | Hyponatriämie | 低ナトリウム血［症］の |
| 3232. hypophysectomy - (n) | hypophysectomie | ipofisectomia | hipofisectomia | Hypophysektomie | 下垂体切除［術］ |
| 3233. hypophysis - (n) | hypophyse | ipofisi | hipófisis | Hypophyse | 脳下垂体 |
| 3234. hypopituitarism - (n) | hypopituitarisme | ipopituitarismo | hipopituitarismo | Hypopituitarismus | 脳下垂体機能不全 |
| 3235. hypoplasia - (n) | hypoplasie | ipoplasia | hipoplasia | Hypoplasie | 発育不全 |
| 3236. hypotension - (n) | hypotension | ipotensione | hipotensión | Hypotension; Hypotonie | 低血圧［症］ |

| English/American | French/Français | Italian/Italiano | Spanish/Español | German/Deutsch | Japanese/日本語 |
|---|---|---|---|---|---|
| 3237. hypothalamo-hypophyseal system - (n) | système hypothalamo-hypophysaire | sistema ipotalamo ipofisario | sistema hipotalamohipofisario | Hypothalamus-Hypophysen-System | 視床下部－下垂体系 |
| 3238. hypo-thalamus - (n) | hypothalamus | ipotalamo | hipotálamo | Hypothalamus | 視床下部 |
| 3239. hypothermia - (n) | hypothermie | ipotermia | hipotermia | Hypothermie | 冷却法 |
| 3240. hypothesis - (n) | hypothèse | ipotesi | hipótesis | Hypothese | 仮説 |
| 3241. hypothetical - (a) | hypothétique | ipotetico | hipotético | hypothetisch | 仮説の |
| 3242. hypothyroid - (a) | hypothyroïdien | ipotiroideo | hipotiroideo | hypothyreoid | 甲状腺機能低下の |
| 3243. hypo-thyroidism - (n) | hypothyroïdisme | ipotiroidismo | hipotiroidismo | Hypothyreoidismus; Hypothyreose | 甲状腺機能低下［症］ |
| 3244. hypotonia - (n) | hypotonie | ipotonia | hipotonía | Hypotonie | 低張 |
| 3245. hypotonic - (a) | hypotonique | ipotonico | hipotónico | hypoton | 低張性の |
| 3246. hypoxemia (hypoxaemia) - (n) | hypoxémie | ipossiemia | hipoxemia | Hypoxämie | 血中酸素減少症 |
| 3247. hypoxia - (n) | hypoxie | ipossia | hipoxia | Hypoxie | 低酸素症 |
| 3248. hysterectomy - (n) | hystérectomie | isterectomia | histerectomía | Hysterektomie | 子宮摘除術 |
| 3249. hysteria - (n) | hystérie | isteria | histeria | Hysterie | ヒステリー |
| 3250. hysterosalpingo-graphy - (n) | hystérosalpingographie | isterosalpingografia | histerosalpingografía | Hysterosalpingographie | 子宮卵管造影（撮影）［法］ |

166

| English/American | French/Français | Italian/Italiano | Spanish/Español | German/Deutsch | Japanese/日本語 |
|---|---|---|---|---|---|
| 3251. iatrogenic - (a) | iatrogénique | iatrogeno | iatrogénico | iatrogen | 医原性の |
| 3252. ichthyosis - (n) | ichtyose | ittiosi | ictiosis | Ichthyose; Schuppenkrankheit | 魚鱗癬 |
| 3253. icteric - (a) | ictère | itterico | ictérico | ikterisch | 黄疸の |
| 3254. ideation - (n) | idéation | ideazione | ideación | Ideation; Ideenbildung | 表象 |
| 3255. identical twins - (n) | jumeaux identiques; jumeaux monozygotes | gemelli monozigotici | gemelos idénticos; gemelos monocigóticos | eineiige Zwillinge | 一卵性双生児 |
| 3256. identification [abbr] ID - (n) | identification | identificazione | identificación | Identifizierung; Kennzeichnung | 同定 |
| 3257. identification code - (n) | code d'identification | codice di identificazione | código de identificación | Kenncode; Identifikationscode | 個人識別コード |
| 3258. identification number - (n) | numéro d'identification | numero di identificazione | número de identificación | Identifikationsnummer | 個人識別番号 |
| 3259. idiopathic - (a) | idiopathique | idiopatico | idiopático | idiopathisch | 特発性疾患の |
| 3260. idiosyncrasy - (n) | idiosyncrasie | idiosincrasia | idiosincrasia | Idiosynkrasie; Eigenheit | 特異体質 |
| 3261. idiot - (n) | idiot | idiota | idiota | Idiot; Schwachsinniger | 白痴者 |
| 3262. idiot savant - (n) | idiot-savant | idiota erudito | idiota sabio | Idiot-Savant | 白痴学者 |
| 3263. ileal - (a) | iléal | ileale | ileal | Ileum- | 回腸の |
| 3264. ileocecal valve - (n) | valvule iléo-cæcale | valvola ileocecale | válvula ileocecal | Ileozökalklappe | 回盲弁 |
| 3265. ileostomy - (n) | iléostomie | ileostomia | ileostomía | Ileostomie | 回盲フィステル形成 [術] |
| 3266. ileum - (n) | iléon | ileo | ileon | Ileum; Krummdarm | 回腸 |
| 3267. ileus - (n) | iléus | ileo | ileo | Ileus; Darmverschluß | 腸閉塞症 |
| 3268. iliac (ileac) crest - (n) | crête iliaque | cresta iliaca | cresta ilíaca | Darmbeinkamm | 腸骨稜 |
| 3269. ilium - (n) | ilion | ilio | ilion | Ilium; Darmbein | 腸骨 |
| 3270. ill health - (n) | mauvaise santé | cattiva salute | mala salud | Gesundheitsbeeinträchtigung | 不健康 |

167

| English/American | French/Français | Italian/Italiano | Spanish/Español | German/Deutsch | Japanese/日本語 |
|---|---|---|---|---|---|
| 3271. illicit drug history - (n) | histoire d'utilisation de drogues illicites | storia di uso di droga illecita | historia de uso de drogas ilícitas | Vorgeschichte als Drogenmißbraucher | 不正の薬歴 |
| 3272. illness - (n) | maladie | malattia | enfermedad | Krankheit | 病気 |
| 3273. illusion - (n) | illusion | illusione | ilusión | Illusion; Wahnvorstellung | 錯覚 |
| 3274. illustration - (n) | illustration | illustrazione | ilustración | Abbildung | 説明図 |
| 3275. image - (n) | image | immagine | imagen | Bild | 像 |
| 3276. imaging - (n) | imagerie | formazione di immagini | formación de imágenes | Bildgebung | イメージング |
| 3277. imbalance - (n) | déséquilibre | squilibrio | desequilibrio | Ungleichgewicht | 平衡異常 |
| 3278. imbecile - (a) | imbécile | imbecille | imbécil | imbezil | 痴愚の |
| 3279. imitative behavior - (n) | comportement d'imitation | comportamento imitativo | conducta imitativa | imitatives Verhalten; nachahmendes Benehmen | 模倣行為 |
| 3280. immature - (a) | immature | immaturo | inmaduro | unreif | 未成熟の |
| 3281. immediate - (a) | immédiat | immediato | inmediato | sofort | 即座の |
| 3282. immediately - (adv) | immédiatement | immediatamente | inmediatamente | sofort | 即座に |
| 3283. immigration - (n) | immigration | immigrazione | inmigración | Einwanderung | 移住 |
| 3284. immiscible - (a) | non miscible | immiscibile | inmiscible | unvermischbar | 混合できない |
| 3285. immobile - (a) | immobile | immobile | inmóvil | immobil; unbeweglich | 不動の |
| 3286. immobilization - (n) | immobilisation | immobilizzazione | inmovilización | Immobilisierung | 不動 [化] |
| 3287. immobilized - (a) | immobilisé | immobilizzato | inmovilizado | immobilisiert | 不動の |
| 3288. immune - (a) | immunisé | immune | inmune | immun | 免疫の |
| 3289. immune system - (n) | système immunitaire | sistema immunitario | sistema inmunológico | Immunsystem | 免疫系 |
| 3290. immunity - (n) | immunité | immunità | inmunidad | Immunität | 免疫 [性] |
| 3291. immunization - (n) | immunisation | immunizzazione | inmunización | Immunisierung | 免役すること |

168

| English/American | French/Français | Italian/Italiano | Spanish/Español | German/Deutsch | Japanese/日本語 |
|---|---|---|---|---|---|
| 3292. immunoassay - (n) | immunoessai | prova immunoenzimatica | inmunoensayo | Immunoassay; Immuntest | 免疫学的検定 [法] |
| 3293. immunochemistry - (n) | immunochimie | immunochimica | inmunoquímica | Immunchemie | 免疫化学 |
| 3294. immunocompetence - (n) | immunocompétence | immunocompetenza | inmunocompetencia | Immunkompetenz | 免疫能 |
| 3295. immunocompromised host - (n) | hôte immunocompromis | ospite immunocompromesso | huésped inmunocomprometido | immungeschwächter Wirt | 免疫力低下宿主 |
| 3296. immunodeficiency - (n) | immunodéficience | immunodeficienza | inmunodeficiencia | Immundefekt; Immundefizienz | 免疫不全 |
| 3297. immunodiffusion - (n) | immunodiffusion | immunodiffusione | inmunodifusión | Immunodiffusion | 免疫拡散 [法] |
| 3298. immunoelectrophoresis - (n) | immuno-électrophorèse | immunoelettroforesi | inmunoelectroforesis | Immunelektrophorese | 免疫電気泳動法 |
| 3299. immunogenetics - (n) | immunogénétique | immunogenetica | inmunogenética | Immungenetik | 免疫遺伝学 |
| 3300. immunoglobulin [abbr] Ig - (n) | immunoglobuline, Ig | immunoglobulina, Ig | inmunoglobulina, Ig | Immunglobulin, Ig | 免疫グロブリン |
| 3301. immunohistochemistry - (n) | immunohistochimie | immunoistochimica | inmunohistoquímica | Immunhistochemie | 免疫組織化学 |
| 3302. immunologic - (a) | immunologique | immunologica | inmunológico | immunologisch | 免疫の |
| 3303. immunology - (n) | immunologie | immunologia | inmunología | Immunologie | 免疫学 |
| 3304. immunophenotyping - (n) | typage immunologique | immunofenotipo; tipizzazione immunologica | inmunofenotipo | Immunphänotypisierung | 免疫表現型 |
| 3305. immunoproliferative disorder - (n) | syndrome immunoprolifératif | disordine immunoproliferativo | trastorno inmunoproliferativo | immunproliferative Störung | 免疫増殖性障害 |
| 3306. immunosorbent - (n) | immunoadsorbant | immunosorbente | inmunobsorbente | Immunoadsorbens | 免疫吸着剤 |

| English/American | French/Français | Italian/Italiano | Spanish/Español | German/Deutsch | Japanese/日本語 |
|---|---|---|---|---|---|
| 3307. immunosuppressant - (n) | immunosuppresseur | immunosoppressore | inmunosupresor | immunsupprimierende Substanz | 免疫抑制薬 |
| 3308. immunosuppression - (n) | immunosuppression | immunosoppressione | inmunosupresión | Immunsuppression | 免疫抑制 |
| 3309. immunosuppressive - (a) | immunosuppressif | immunosoppressivo | inmunosupresivo | immunosupprimierend | 免疫抑制性の |
| 3310. immunotherapy - (n) | immunothérapie | immunoterapia | inmunoterapia | Immuntherapie; Immunotherapie | 免疫療法 |
| 3311. immunotoxin - (n) | immunotoxine | immunotossina | inmunotoxina | Antitoxin | 免疫毒素 |
| 3312. impacted - (a) | inclus | incuneato; incastrato | impactado | impaktiert; eingeklemmt | 埋状した |
| 3313. impaired - (a) | diminué; détérioré | alterato | disminuido; deteriorado | gestört; geschwächt | 不全の |
| 3314. impairment - (n) | affaiblissement; détérioration | indebolimento; alterazione | disminución; deterioración | Beeinträchtigung; Schädigung | 悪化 |
| 3315. impedance - (n) | impédance | impedanza7 | impedancia | Impedanz | インピーダンス |
| 3316. imperforate - (a) | imperforé | imperforato | imperforado | nicht perforiert; atretisch | 閉鎖した |
| 3317. impermeable - (a) | imperméable | impermeabile | impermeable | impermeabel; undurchlässig | 不浸透性の |
| 3318. implant - (n) | greffe; implant | innesto; impianto | implante; injerto | Implantat | 移植 |
| 3319. implant - (v) | implanter | innestare; impiantare | implantar | implantieren | 移植する |
| 3320. implantable - (a) | implantable | innestabile; impiantabile | implantable | implantierbar | 移植可能の |
| 3321. implantable defibrillator - (n) | défibrillateur implantable | defibrillatore innestabile | desfibrilador implantable | implantierbarer Defibrillator | 移植可能除細動器 |
| 3322. implanted electrode - (n) | électrode implantée | elettrodo impiantato | electrodo implantado | implantierte Elektrode | 移植電極 |
| 3323. implosive - (a) | implosif | implosivo | implosivo | implosiv | 内破の |
| 3324. impotence - (n) | impotence | impotenza | impotencia | Impotenz | 陰萎 |
| 3325. impregnation - (n) | imprégnation | impregnazione; fecondazione | impregnación | Imprägnierung | 精子侵入 |
| 3326. impression - (n) | impression | impronta | impresión | Abdruck; Eindruck | 印象 |

170

| English/American | French/Français | Italian/Italiano | Spanish/Español | German/Deutsch | Japanese/日本語 |
|---|---|---|---|---|---|
| 3327. improvement - (n) | amélioration | miglioramento | mejoría; mejoramiento | Besserung | 改良 |
| 3328. impulse - (n) | impulsion | impulso | impulso | Impuls; Reiz | 衝動 |
| 3329. impulsive behavior - (n) | conduite impulsive | comportamento impulsivo | conducta impulsiva | Spontanverhalten | 衝動的行為 |
| 3330. impurity - (n) | impureté | impurezza; impurità | impureza | Verunreinigung | 不純物 |
| 3331. imputation - (n) | imputation | imputazione | imputación | Bezichtigung | 非難 |
| 3332. in extremis - (a) | in extremis | in extremis | in extremis | in extremis; im Sterben liegend | 臨終の |
| 3333. in situ - (a) | in situ | in situ; in loco | in situ | in situ | 本来の位置の |
| 3334. in vitro - (a) | in vitro | in vitro | in vitro | künstlich; In-vitro- | 試験管内の |
| 3335. in vivo - (a) | in vivo | in vivo | in vivo; en el cuerpo vivo | in vivo; im lebendigen Organismus | 生体内の |
| 3336. inactivate - (v) | inactiver; rendre inactif | inattivare; rendere inattivo | inactivar | inaktivieren | 不活性化する |
| 3337. inactivated - (a) | inactivé | inattivato | inactivado | inaktiviert | 不活性化した |
| 3338. inactive - (a) | inactif; inerte | inattivo | inactivo | untätig; passiv | 不活性の |
| 3339. inappropriate behavior - (n) | comportement inapproprié | comportamento inappropriato | conducta impropia | unangebrachtes Verhalten | 不適切行動 |
| 3340. inborn - (a) | congénital; inné | congenito; innato | innato; congénito | kongenital; angeboren | 先天 [性] の |
| 3341. inbred - (a) | consanguin | consanguineo | consanguíneo | Inzucht- | 同系の |
| 3342. incest - (n) | inceste | incesto | incesto | Inzest; Blutschande | 近親相姦 |
| 3343. incidence - (n) | incidence | incidenza | incidencia | Inzidenz; Vorkommen | 病気の起こる頻度 |
| 3344. incipient - (a) | naissant | incipiente | incipiente | beginnend; initial | 初期の |
| 3345. incise - (v) | inciser; faire une incision dans | incidere | cortar; hacer una incisión en | schneiden | 切開する |
| 3346. incision - (n) | incision | incisione | incisión | Inzision; Schnitt | 切開 [術] |
| 3347. incisor - (n) | incisive | dente incisivo | incisor; incisivo | Schneidezahn | 切歯 |
| 3348. inclusion body - (n) | corps d'inclusion | corpo incluso | cuerpo de inclusión | Einschlußkörperchen | 封入体 |

| English/American | French/Français | Italian/Italiano | Spanish/Español | German/Deutsch | Japanese/日本語 |
|---|---|---|---|---|---|
| 3349. inclusion criteria - (n) | critères d'inclusion | criteri di inclusione | criterios de inclusión | Einschlußkriterien | 包含基準 |
| 3350. incoherent - (a) | incohérent | incoerente | incoherente | inkohärent | 相反する |
| 3351. income - (n) | revenu | reddito; entrata | ingreso | Einkommen | 所得 |
| 3352. incompatible - (a) | incompatible | incompatibile | incompatible | inkompatibel; nicht verträglich | 不適合の |
| 3353. incompetence - (n) | incompétence | incompetenza | incompetencia | Unfähigkeit | 無能力 |
| 3354. incomplete block - (n) | bloc incomplet | blocco incompleto | bloqueo incompleto | unvollständiger Block | 不完全ブロック |
| 3355. incomplete penetrance of gene - (n) | pénétrance incomplète du gène | penetrazione incompleta del gene | penetrancia incompleta del gene | unvollständige Penetranz der Gene | 不完全遺伝子浸透度 |
| 3356. inconclusive results - (n) | résultats peu concluants | risultati inconclusivi | resultados poco convincentes | nicht überzeugende Ergebnisse | 決定的でない結果 |
| 3357. incontinence - (n) | incontinence | incontinenza | incontinencia | Inkontinenz | 失禁 |
| 3358. incoordination - (n) | incoordination; ataxie | incoordinazione; atassia | incoordinación; sacudida atáxica | Inkoordination; Ataxie | 不同格 |
| 3359. increase - (n) | augmentation; intensification | aumento; incremento | incremento; aumento | Zunahme; Anstieg | 増加 |
| 3360. increase - (v) | augmenter; intensifier | aumentare; incrementare | incrementar; aumentar | zunehmen; wachsen | 増加する |
| 3361. incubate - (v) | incuber; être en incubation | incubare; mantenere in incubazione | incubar | inkubieren; ausbrüten | 保温する |
| 3362. incubation - (n) | incubation | incubazione | incubación | Inkubation; Ausbrütung | 潜伏 |
| 3363. incubation period - (n) | période d'incubation | periodo di incubazione | periodo de incubación | Inkubationszeit; Ausbrütungszeit | 潜伏期 |
| 3364. incubator - (n) | incubateur; couveuse | incubatrice | incubadora | Inkubator; Brutapparat | 孵卵器 |
| 3365. incurable - (a) | incurable; inguérissable | incurabile; inguaribile | incurable | unheilbar | 不治の |

172

| English/American | French/Français | Italian/Italiano | Spanish/Español | German/Deutsch | Japanese/日本語 |
|---|---|---|---|---|---|
| 3366. indemnification - (n) | indemnisation | indennizzo | indemnización | Entschädigung | 賠償 |
| 3367. indentation - (n) | indentation; dentelure | incisura; dentellatura | indentación; muesca | Auszackung | 窩洞形成 |
| 3368. independent - (a) | indépendant | indipendente | independiente | unabhängig | 独立の |
| 3369. independent variable - (n) | variable indépendante | variabile indipendente | variable independiente | unabhängige Variable | 独立変数 |
| 3370. index - (n) | index | indice | índice | Index; Register | 指標 |
| 3371. index case - (n) | cas d'index | paziente originale | caso índice | Indexpatient | インデックスケース |
| 3372. indexing - (n) | classement | rubricazione | indexación; modificación por índice | Indizierung; Bezifferung | 表示すること |
| 3373. indication - (n) | indication | indicazione | indicación | Indikation; Anzeige | 指示 |
| 3374. indicator - (n) | indicateur | indicatore | indicador | Indikator; Anzeiger | 指示薬 |
| 3375. indicator dilution technique - (n) | technique de dilution avec indicateur | tecnica di diluizione dell'indicatore | técnica de dilución indicadora | Farbstoffverdünnungsmethode | 指示薬希釈法 |
| 3376. indigenous - (a) | indigène | indigeno | indígena | eingeboren; einheimisch | 地元の |
| 3377. indigestion - (n) | indigestion | indigestione | indigestión | Verdauungsstörung | 消化不良 |
| 3378. indirect costs - (n) | coûts indirects | costi indiretti | costos indirectos | indirekte Kosten | 間接的費用 |
| 3379. indisposition - (n) | indisposition | indisposizione | indisposición | Unwohlsein | 軽症 |
| 3380. indistinguishable - (a) | indifférenciable | indistinguibile | indistinguible | ununterscheidbar | 区別がつかない |
| 3381. individual - (n) | individu | individuo; uomo singolo | individuo | Individuum | 個人 |
| 3382. individual - (a) | individuel | individuale; singolo | individual | individuell | 個人の |
| 3383. individuality - (n) | individualité | individualità | individualidad | Individualität | 個性 |
| 3384. induced - (a) | induit; provoqué | indotto; provocato | inducido | induziert | 誘発された |
| 3385. induced labor - (n) | travail induit; travail provoqué | parto indotto | parto inducido | künstlich eingeleitete Wehen | 誘発分娩 |
| 3386. inducer - (n) | inducteur | induttore | inductor | Induktor | 誘発因子 |
| 3387. induction - (n) | induction; provocation | induzione | inducción | Induktion; Einleitung | 誘導 |

| English/American | French/Français | Italian/Italiano | Spanish/Español | German/Deutsch | Japanese/日本語 |
|---|---|---|---|---|---|
| 3388. inductive logic - (n) | logique inductive | logica induttiva | lógica inductiva | induktive Logik | 帰納論 |
| 3389. induration - (n) | induration | indurazioni | induración | Induration; Verhärtung | 硬化 |
| 3390. industry - (n) | industrie | industria | industria | Industrie | 産業 |
| 3391. indwelling catheter - (n) | sonde à demeure | catetere a permanenza | sonda permanente | Verweilkatheter; Dauersonde | 留置カテーテル |
| 3392. inebriation - (n) | enivrement | inebriamento; intossicazione | inebriación | Trunkenheit; Rauschzustand | 麻酔 |
| 3393. ineffective - (a) | inefficace | inefficace | ineficaz | unwirksam | 効果のない |
| 3394. ineligible - (a) | inéligible | non candidabile | inelegible | untauglich; ungeeignet | 不適格の |
| 3395. ineligible patient - (n) | patient inéligible | paziente non candidabile | paciente no elegible | ungeeigneter Patient | 不適格患者 |
| 3396. inert - (a) | inerte | inerte | inerte | inert | 不活性の |
| 3397. inertia - (n) | inertie | inerzia | inercia | Inertie; Trägheit | 慣性 |
| 3398. infant - (n) | nouveau-né | neonato | infante | Neugeborenes | 乳児 |
| 3399. infantile - (a) | infantile | infantile | infantil | infantil; kindlich | 乳児の |
| 3400. infarct - (n) | infarctus | infarto | infarto | Infarkt | 梗塞 |
| 3401. infarction - (n) | infarctus; infarcissement | infarcimento; infarto | infarto; infartación | Infarzierung; Infarkt | 梗塞 |
| 3402. infect - (v) | infecter | infettare | infectar | infizieren | 感染する |
| 3403. infection - (n) | infection | infezione | infección | Infektion | 感染 |
| 3404. infectious - (a) | infectieux | infettivo | infeccioso | infektiös | 感染の |
| 3405. infectious disease - (n) | maladie infectieuse | malattia infettiva | enfermedad infecciosa | ansteckende Krankheit; infektiöse Krankheit | 伝染病 |
| 3406. inferior - (a) | inférieur | inferiore | inferior | minderwertig; untergeordnet | 下位の |
| 3407. infertile - (a) | infertile; stérile | infecondo; sterile | no fértil; estéril | unfruchtbar | 生殖力のない |
| 3408. infertility - (n) | infertilité | infertilità; sterilità | infertilidad | Infertilität; Unfruchtbarkeit | 不妊症 |

174

| English/American | French/Français | Italian/Italiano | Spanish/Español | German/Deutsch | Japanese/日本語 |
|---|---|---|---|---|---|
| 3409. infestation - (n) | infestation | infestazione | infestación | Infestation; Parasitenbefall | 寄生 |
| 3410. infiltrate - (n) | infiltrat | infiltrato | infiltrado | Infiltrat | 浸潤 |
| 3411. infiltrate - (v) | infiltrer | infiltrare | infiltrar | infiltrieren | 浸潤する |
| 3412. infirm - (a) | infirme | infermo; debole | enfermizo; enfermo | unsicher; schwach | 弱い |
| 3413. infirmary - (n) | infirmerie; hôpital | infermeria; ospedale | enfermería; hospital | Pflegestation; Krankenrevier | 医務室．病院 |
| 3414. infirmity - (n) | infirmité | infermità | enfermedad | Schwäche; Gebrechlichkeit | 虚弱 |
| 3415. inflammation - (n) | inflammation | inflammazione | inflamación | Inflammation; Entzündung | 炎症 |
| 3416. inflammatory - (a) | inflammatoire | inflammatorio | inflamatorio | entzündlich | 炎症性の |
| 3417. inflammatory disorder - (n) | désordre inflammatoire | disordine inflammatorio | trastorno inflamatorio | entzündliche Störung | 炎症障害 |
| 3418. inflate - (v) | gonfler; dilater | gonfiare | inflar; hinchar | aufblähen; insufflieren | 膨張する、膨張させる |
| 3419. influenza - (n) | influenza; grippe | influenza | influenza; gripe | Grippe; Influenza | インフルエンザ |
| 3420. informatics - (n) | informatique | informatica | informática | Informatik | 情報学 |
| 3421. information - (n) | information; renseignements | informazione | información | Informationen; Auskunft | 情報 |
| 3422. information service - (n) | service d'information | servizio informazioni | servicio de información | Informationsdienst | 情報サービス |
| 3423. information technology - (n) | technologie d'information | tecnologia di informazione | tecnología de información | Informationstechnik | 情報テクノロジー |
| 3424. informed consent - (n) | consentement éclairé | consenso informato | consentimiento informado | Einwilligung nach sachkundiger Aufklärung | 通知承諾 |
| 3425. infrared - (n) | infrarouge | infrarosso | infrarrojo | Infrarot | 赤外部 |
| 3426. infrared rays - (n) | rayons infrarouges | raggi infrarossi | rayos infrarrojos | Infrarotstrahlen | 赤外線 |
| 3427. infrared spectrum - (n) | spectre infrarouge | spettro infrarosso | espectro infrarrojo | Infrarotspektrum | 赤外線スペクトル |

| English/American | French/Français | Italian/Italiano | Spanish/Español | German/Deutsch | Japanese/日本語 |
|---|---|---|---|---|---|
| 3428. infusion - (n) | infusion | infusione | infusión | Infusion; Aufguß | 浸出液 |
| 3429. infusion pump - (n) | pompe à l'infusion | pompa d'infusione | bomba de infusión | Infusionspumpe | 注入ポンプ |
| 3430. ingest - (v) | ingérer | ingerire | ingerir | aufnehmen; zu sich nehmen | 摂取する |
| 3431. ingredient - (n) | ingrédient | ingrediente | ingrediente | Bestandteil | 成分 |
| 3432. inguinal - (a) | inguinal | inguinale | inguinal | inguinal; Leisten- | 鼠径の |
| 3433. inguinal canal - (n) | canal inguinal | canale inguinale | canal inguinal | Inguinalkanal; Leistenkanal | 鼠径管 |
| 3434. inhalant - (n) | inhalant | inalente | inhalante | Inhalationsmittel | 吸入剤 |
| 3435. inhalation - (n) | inhalation | inalazione | inhalación | Inhalation | 吸入 |
| 3436. inhale - (v) | inhaler | inalare | inhalar | inhalieren; einatmen | 吸入する |
| 3437. inherent - (a) | inhérent | inerente; innato | inherente; intrínseco | inhärent; innewohnend | 生まれつきの |
| 3438. inheritance - (n) | héritage | eredità; erditarietà | herencia | Vererbung | 遺伝 |
| 3439. inherited disease - (n) | maladie héréditaire | malattia ereditaria | enfermedad hereditaria | vererbte Krankheit; Erbkrankheit | 遺伝病 |
| 3440. inhibition - (n) | inhibition | inibizione | inhibición | Inhibition; Hemmung | 抑制 |
| 3441. inhibitor - (n) | inhibiteur | inibitore | inhibidor | Inhibitor; Hemmstoff | 抑制因子 |
| 3442. in-house - (a) | interne | a casa; interno all'azienda | interno; local | intern; im Hause | 構内の |
| 3443. initial dose - (n) | dose initiale | dose iniziale | primera dosis | Anfangsdosis; Ausgangsdosis | 初期服用量 |
| 3444. initials - (n) | initiales | iniziali | iniciales | Initialen; Anfangsbuchstaben | 頭文字 |
| 3445. initiation - (n) | initiation; commencement | iniziazione | inicio | Initiation; Einführung | 発足 |
| 3446. inject - (v) | injecter | iniettare | inyectar | injizieren | 注射する |
| 3447. injected conjunctiva - (n) | conjonctive injectée | congiuntiva iniettata | conjuntiva inyectada | injizierte Konjunktiva | 結膜充血 |

176

| English/American | French/Français | Italian/Italiano | Spanish/Español | German/Deutsch | Japanese/日本語 |
|---|---|---|---|---|---|
| 3448. injection - (n) | injection | iniezione | inyección | Injektion | 注射 |
| 3449. injury - (n) | blessure; lésion | lesione; danno | herida; lesión | Verletzung | 傷害 |
| 3450. injury severity score - (n) | échelle de sévérité de la blessure | punteggio della severità della lesione | puntaje de severidad de la lesión | Schweregrad der Verletzung | 傷害重度スコア |
| 3451. inlay - (n) | obturation; greffe encastrée | intarsio; innesto endo-cavitario | obturación; injerto en "inlay" | Zahnfüllung | インレー |
| 3452. innate - (a) | inné | innato | innato | angeboren | 先天性の |
| 3453. inner ear - (n) | oreille interne | orecchio interno | oído interno | Innenohr | 内耳 |
| 3454. innervate - (v) | innerver | innervare | inervar | innervieren | 神経刺激を与える |
| 3455. innocent - (a) | innocent | innocente | inocente | harmlos; benigne | 良性の |
| 3456. innocuous - (a) | inoffensif | innocuo | inocuo; inofensivo | unschädlich | 無害の |
| 3457. innovation - (n) | innovation | innovazione | innovación | Innovation; Neuerung | 新制度 |
| 3458. inoculate - (v) | inoculer; vacciner | inoculare; vaccinare | inocular | inokulieren; impfen | 接種する |
| 3459. inoperable - (a) | inopérable | inoperabile | inoperable | inoperabel | 手術が不可能の |
| 3460. inotropic - (a) | inotrope | inotropo | inotrópico | inotrop | 変力 [性] の |
| 3461. inpatient - (n) | patient hospitalisé | degente; paziente interno | paciente interno | stationärer Patient | 入院患者 |
| 3462. inpatient clinic - (n) | clinique interne | clinica degenti | clínica residente | Klinik für stationäre Patienten | 入院患者のクリニック |
| 3463. in-process testing - (n) | essai interprocessus | prova interprocesso | ensayo interprocesal | Zwischenprüfung | 進行中の検査 |
| 3464. inquest - (n) | enquête | investigazione; indagine | indagación | Ermittlung; Leichenschau | 検屍 |
| 3465. insane - (n) | aliéné; dément | pazzo; demente | insano; lunática loco; demente | Geisteskranker | 精神病 |
| 3466. insane - (a) | aliéné; dément | pazzo; demente | loco; demente | geisteskrank | 精神病の |
| 3467. insanity - (n) | aliénation mentale; démence | pazzia; demenza; insania | locura; demencia | Geisteskrankheit | 精神錯乱 |
| 3468. insect - (n) | insecte | insetto | insecto | Insekt | 昆虫 |
| 3469. insecticide - (n) | insecticide | insetticida | insecticida | Insektizid | 殺虫剤 |

177

| English/American | French/Français | Italian/Italiano | Spanish/Español | German/Deutsch | Japanese/日本語 |
|---|---|---|---|---|---|
| 3470. insemination - (n) | insémination | inseminazione | inseminación | Insemination | 受精 |
| 3471. insensible water loss - (n) | perte d'eau insensible | perdita d'acqua | pérdida de agua | unmerklicher Wasserverlust | 不感蒸泄 |
| 3472. insensitive - (a) | insensible | insensibile | insensible | unempfindlich | 無感覚な |
| 3473. insertion - (n) | insertion | inserzione | inserción | Insertion; Einfügung durch Insertion | 挿入 [術] |
| 3474. insertional - (a) | inséré | inseribile | insertado | | 挿入性の |
| 3475. insidious - (a) | insidieux | insidioso | insidioso | schleichend; tückisch | 潜行性の |
| 3476. insoluble - (a) | insoluble | insolubile | insoluble | insolubel; unlöslich | 不溶性の |
| 3477. insomnia - (n) | insomnie | insonnia | insomnio | Insomnie; Schlaflosigkeit | 不眠症 |
| 3478. inspection - (a) | inspection | ispezione | inspección | Inspektion | 視診 |
| 3479. inspiration - (n) | inspiration | inspirazione | inspiración | Inspiration; Einatmung | 吸息、刺激 |
| 3480. inspiratory - (a) | inspiratoire | inspiratorio | inspiratorio | Inspirations-; inspiratorisch | 吸息の |
| 3481. inspire - (v) | inspirer | inspirare; inalare | inspirar | inhalieren; einatmen | 息を吸う |
| 3482. instability - (n) | instabilité | instabilità | inestabilidad | Instabilität | 不安定 |
| 3483. instillation - (n) | instillation | istillazione | instilación | Einträufelung | 点滴注入 |
| 3484. instinct - (n) | instinct | istinto | instinto | Instinkt; Trieb | 本能 |
| 3485. institute - (n) | institut | istituto | instituto | Institut; Anstalt | 研究所 |
| 3486. institution - (n) | institution | istituzione; istituto | institución | Einrichtung; Anstalt | 機関 |
| 3487. institutional - (a) | institutionnel | istituzionale | institucional | institutionsmäßig; angeordnet | 機関の |
| 3488. institutional memory - (n) | mémoire institutionnelle | memoria istituzionale | memoria institucional | Institutionserfahrung | 機関記憶 |
| 3489. institutional review board - (n) | conseil de révision institutionnel | consiglio revisione istituzionale | consejo de revisión institucional | Institutionsüberprüfungsausschuß | 機関の管理組織 |
| 3490. institutionalization - (n) | institutionnalisation | istituzionalizzazione | institucionalización | Institutionalisierung | 制度化 |
| 3491. instructions - (n) | instructions; directives | istruzioni | instrucciones | Anweisungen; Anleitungen | 教示 |

| English/American | French/Français | Italian/Italiano | Spanish/Español | German/Deutsch | Japanese/日本語 |
|---|---|---|---|---|---|
| 3492. instructions to authors - (n) | directives aux auteurs | istruzioni agli autori | instrucciones para los autores | Richtlinien für die Verfasser | 著者への指示 |
| 3493. instrument - (n) | instrument; appareil | strumento; apparecchio | instrumento | Instrument | 器具 |
| 3494. instrumentation - (n) | instrumentation | strumentazione | instrumentación | instrumentelle Ausstattung; apparative Ausstattung | 器具の使用 |
| 3495. insufficiency - (n) | insuffisance | insufficienza | insuficiencia | Insuffizienz | 不全［症］ |
| 3496. insufficient relief - (n) | soulagement insuffisant | insufficiente sollievo | alivio insuficiente | unzureichende Besserung | 不完全な治 |
| 3497. insufflate - (v) | insuffler | insufflare | insuflar | insufflieren | 吹き入れる |
| 3498. insulin - (n) | insuline | insulina | insulina | Insulin | インシュリン |
| 3499. insulin dependent - (a) | insulino-dépendant | insulino dipendente | insulino dependiente | insulinabhängig | インシュリン依存性の |
| 3500. insurance - (n) | assurance | assicurazione | seguro | Versicherung | 保険 |
| 3501. insurance claim - (n) | réclamation d'assurance | reclamo assicurazione | reclamación de seguro | Versicherungsanspruch | 保険申請 |
| 3502. intake - (n) | apport; prise | apporto; afflusso | aportación; consumo | Aufnahme | 摂取量 |
| 3503. intangible costs - (n) | coûts intangibles | costi intangibile | costos intangibles | unbestimmte Kosten | 不明瞭費用 |
| 3504. integration - (n) | intégration | integrazione | integración | Integration; Integrierung | 同化 |
| 3505. integrity - (n) | intégrité | integrità | integridad | Integrität; Einheit | 統合性 |
| 3506. integument - (n) | tégument | tegumento | integumento | Integument | 外皮 |
| 3507. intellect - (n) | intellect | intelletto | intelecto | Intellekt | 知性 |
| 3508. intelligence - (n) | intelligence | intelligenza | inteligencia | Intelligenz | 知能 |
| 3509. intelligence quotient [abbr] IQ - (n) | quotient intellectuel, QI | quoziente d'intelligenza, QI | cociente intelectual, CI | Intelligenzquotient, IQ | 知能指数 |
| 3510. intelligence test - (n) | épreuve d'intelligence | test d'intelligenza | prueba de inteligencia | Intelligenztest | 知能検査 |

179

| English/American | French/Français | Italian/Italiano | Spanish/Español | German/Deutsch | Japanese日本語 |
|---|---|---|---|---|---|
| 3511. intelligent terminal - (n) | terminal intelligent | terminale intelligente | terminal inteligente | intelligente Darstellung | インテリジェント端末 |
| 3512. intemperance - (n) | intempérance | intemperanza | intemperancia | Maßlosigkeit | 不節制 |
| 3513. intensity of reaction - (n) | intensité de la réaction | intensità della reazione | intensidad de la reacción | Reaktionsintensität | 反応の強度 |
| 3514. intensive - (a) | intensif | intensivo | intensivo | intensiv | 集中的な |
| 3515. intensive care - (n) | soins intensifs | cure intensiva | cuidados intensivos | Intensivpflege | 集中治療 |
| 3516. intensive care unit [abbr] ICU - (n) | unité de soins intensifs | reparto cure intensiva | unidad de vigilancia intensiva | Intensivbehandlungseinheit; Intensivstation | 集中治療部 |
| 3517. intensive treatment unit - (n) | unité de traitement intensif | reparto terapia intensiva | unidad de tratamiento intensivo | Intensivbehandlungseinheit; Intensivstation | 集中治療部 |
| 3518. intentional overdosage - (n) | surdose intentionnelle | sopradossaggio intenzionale | sobredosis intencional | absichtliche Überdosierung | 故意の過剰投薬 |
| 3519. interaction - (n) | interaction | interazione | interacción | Interaktion; Wechselwirkung | 相互作用 |
| 3520. intercalating agent - (n) | agent d'interaction | agente interpolante | agente de intercalación | interkalierendes Agens | 介在物質 |
| 3521. intercellular junction - (n) | jonction intercellulaire | giunzione intercellulare | unión intercelular | Zellverbindung | 細胞間結合 |
| 3522. intercostal - (a) | intercostal | intercostale | intercostal | interkostal | 肋間の |
| 3523. intercourse - (n) | relation; coït | rapporto; coito | trato; coito | Verkehr; Koitus | 性交 |
| 3524. inter-disciplinary - (a) | interdisciplinaire | interdisciplinare | interdisciplinario | interdisziplinär | 学際の |
| 3525. interferon - (n) | interféron | interferone | interferón | Interferon | インターフェロン |
| 3526. interim - (n) | intérim | interim; intervallo | interin; intermedio | Zwischenzeit; nterim | 中間期 |
| 3527. interim - (a) | intérimaire; provisoire | provvisorio; temporaneo | interino; intermedio | vorläufig; Übergangs- | 中間の |
| 3528. interim analysis - (n) | analyse provisoire | analisi temporanea | análisis interino | vorläufige Analyse | 中間分析 |

| English/American | French/Français | Italian/Italiano | Spanish/Español | German/Deutsch | Japanese/日本語 |
|---|---|---|---|---|---|
| 3529. intermittent - (a) | intermittent | intermittente | intermitente | intermittierend | 間欠性の |
| 3530. intermittent claudication - (n) | claudication intermittente | claudicazione intermittente | claudicación intermitente | intermittierendes Hinken | 間欠性跛行性 |
| 3531. intermittent positive pressure ventilation - (n) | ventilation à pression positive intermittente | ventilazione a pressione positiva intermittente | ventilación de presión positiva intermitente | intermittierende Überdruckbeatmung | 間欠性陽圧換気 |
| 3532. internal audit - (n) | vérification interne | riscontro interno | auditoría interna | innerbetriebliche Revision | 内部監査 |
| 3533. internal medicine - (n) | médecine interne | medicina interna | medicina interna | innere Medizin | 内科 |
| 3534. internal validity - (n) | validité interne | validità interna | validez interna | interne Validität | 内部有効性 |
| 3535. international - (a) | international | internazionale | internacional | international | 国際的 |
| 3536. international unit [abbr] IU - (n) | unité internationale | unità internazionale | unidad internacional | internationale Einheit | 国際単位 |
| 3537. interneuron - (n) | interneurone | interneurone | interneurona | Interneuron | 介在ニューロン |
| 3538. internist - (n) | interniste | internista | internista | Internist | 内科医 |
| 3539. internship - (n) | internat | internato | internado | Praktikum | インターン |
| 3540. interphase - (n) | interphase | interfase | interfase | Interphase | 中間期 |
| 3541. interpretation - (n) | interprétation | interpretazione | interpretación | Interpretation; Auswertung | 解釈 |
| 3542. interspace - (n) | interstice | spazio intermedio | interespacio | Zwischenraum | 間空 |
| 3543. interstitial - (a) | interstitiel | interstiziale | intersticial | intersttitiell | 間質性の |
| 3544. interval - (n) | intervalle | intervallo | intervalo | Intervall; Zwischenzeit | 中間期 |
| 3545. interval data - (n) | données d'intervalle | dati d'intervallo | datos del intervalo | Intervalldaten | 中間データ |
| 3546. intervention - (n) | intervention | intervento | intervención | Intervention | 介在 |
| 3547. interventional radiography - (n) | radiographie interventionnelle | radiografia d'intervento | radiografía intervencionista | Verlaufs-Röntgenaufnahme | インターベンショナルラジオグラフィー |

| English/American | French/Français | Italian/Italiano | Spanish/Español | German/Deutsch | Japanese/日本語 |
|---|---|---|---|---|---|
| 3548. interventricular - (a) | interventriculaire | interventricolare | interventricular | interventrikulär | 心室間の |
| 3549. intervertebral disk - (n) | disque intervertébral | disco intervertebrale | disco intervertebral | Bandscheibe | 椎間 [円] 板 |
| 3550. interview - (n) | entrevue; interview | colloquio; intervista | entrevista | Befragung; Interview | 会見 |
| 3551. interview - (v) | avoir une entrevue avec; interviewer | avere un colloquio; intervistare | entrevistar | interviewen | 会見する |
| 3552. intestinal - (a) | intestinal | intestinale | intestinal | intestinal; Darm- | 腸の |
| 3553. intestinal absorption - (n) | absorption intestinale | assorbimento intestinale | absorción intestinal | intestinale Resorption | 腸管吸収 |
| 3554. intestinal bleeding - (n) | hémorragie intestinale | emorragia intestinale | hemorragia intestinal | Darmblutung | 腸管出血 |
| 3555. intestinal pain - (n) | douleur intestinale | dolore intestinale | dolor intestinal | Darmschmerz | 腸管痛 |
| 3556. intestine - (n) | intestin | intestino | intestino | Darm; Intestinum | 腸 |
| 3557. intima - (n) | intima | intima | íntima | Intima | 動脈内膜 |
| 3558. intolerance - (n) | intolérance | intolleranza | intolerancia | Unverträglichkeit; Intoleranz | 不耐容 [症] |
| 3559. intolerant - (n) | intolérant | intollerante | intolerante | unverträglich; intolerant | 不耐容の |
| 3560. intoxication - (n) | intoxication | intossicazione | intoxicación | Intoxikation; Vergiftung | 中毒 |
| 3561. intra-arterial - (a) | intra-artériel | intrarterioso | intraarterial | intraarteriell | 動脈内の |
| 3562. intra-articular - (a) | intra-articulaire | intrarticolare | intraarticular | intraartikulär | 関節内の |
| 3563. intracellular - (a) | intracellulaire | intracellulare | intracelular | intrazellulär | 細胞内の |
| 3564. intracranial pressure - (n) | pression intracrânienne | pressione intracranica | presión intracraneal | intrakranieller Druck | 脳内圧 |
| 3565. intradermal - (a) | intradermique | intradermico | intradérmico | intradermal | 皮内の |
| 3566. intrahepatic - (a) | intrahépatique | intraepatico | intrahepático | intrahepatisch | 肝臓内の |
| 3567. intralesional - (a) | intralésionnel | intralesionale | localizado en la lesión | in einer Läsion | 病巣内の |
| 3568. intramural - (a) | intramural | intramurale | intramural | intramural | 壁内の |
| 3569. intramuscular - (a) | intramusculaire | intramuscolare | intramuscular | intramuskulär | 筋肉内の |

| English/American | French/Français | Italian/Italiano | Spanish/Español | German/Deutsch | Japanese/日本語 |
|---|---|---|---|---|---|
| 3570. intranasal - (a) | intranasal | intranasale | intranasal | intranasal | 鼻内の |
| 3571. intraocular - (a) | intra-oculaire | intraoculare | intraocular | intraokular | 眼球内の |
| 3572. intraocular lens - (n) | lentille intra-oculaire | lente intraoculare | lente intraocular | intraokulare Linse | 眼内レンズ |
| 3573. intraocular pressure - (n) | pression intra-oculaire | pressione intraoculare | presión intraocular | Intraokulardruck; Augeninnendruck | 内眼圧 |
| 3574. intraoperative - (a) | intraopératoire | intraoperatorio | intraoperatorio | intraoperativ | [外科] 手術中の |
| 3575. intra-peritoneal - (a) | intrapéritonéal | intraperitoneale | intraperitoneal | intraperitoneal | 腹腔内の |
| 3576. intrapleural - (a) | intrapleural | intrapleurico | intrapleural | intrapleural | 胸膜腔内の |
| 3577. intratracheal - (a) | intratrachéal | intratracheale | intratraqueal | intratracheal | 気管内の |
| 3578. intrauterine device [abbr] IUD - (n) | dispositif anti-conceptionel intra-uterin | contraccettivo intrauterino | dispositivo intrauterino, DIU | Intrauterinpessar; Intrauterinspange | 子宮内 [避妊] 器具 |
| 3579. intravascular - (a) | intravasculaire | intravascolare | intravascular | intravaskulär | 脈管内の |
| 3580. intravenous [abbr] IV - (a) | intraveineux | intravenoso | intravenoso | intravenös | 静脈 [内] の |
| 3581. intra-ventricular - (a) | intraventriculaire | intraventricolare | intraventricular | intraventrikulär | 心室内の |
| 3582. intravesical - (a) | intravésical | intravescicale | intravesical | intravesikal | 膀胱内の |
| 3583. intrinsic activity - (n) | activité intrinsèque | attività intrinseca | actividad intrínseca | intrinsische Aktivität | 内因性活性 |
| 3584. introduction - (n) | introduction | introduzione | introducción | Einführung | 導入 |
| 3585. intron - (n) | intron | introne | intrón | Intron | イントロン |
| 3586. introvert - (a) | introverti | introvertito | introvertido | introvertiert | 内省的な |
| 3587. intubation - (n) | intubation | intubazione | intubación | Intubation | 挿管法 |
| 3588. invalid - (n) | invalide; malade | invalido; malato | inválido; incapacitado | Invalide | 病人 |
| 3589. invalid - (a) | invalide; malade | non valido; invalido | inválido; incapacitado | ungültig; körperbehindert | 病弱の |
| 3590. invasive procedure - (n) | procédure invasive | procedura invasiva | procedimiento invasor | invasives Verfahren | 侵襲的手順 |

| English/American | French/Français | Italian/Italiano | Spanish/Español | German/Deutsch | Japanese/日本語 |
|---|---|---|---|---|---|
| 3591. inventory - (n) | inventaire | inventario | inventario | Inventar | 在庫品 |
| 3592. inventory - (v) | inventorier | inventariare | inventariar | inventarisieren | 在庫品調査をする |
| 3593. inventory turns - (n) | rotation d'inventaire | rotazioni dell'inventario | turnos de inventario | Lagerumschlag | 在庫品の回転 |
| 3594. inversion - (n) | inversion | inversione | inversión | Inversion; Wendung | 逆位、反転 |
| 3595. invertebrate - (n) | invertébré | invertebrato | invertebrado | wirbelloses Tier | 無脊椎動物 |
| 3596. invertebrate - (a) | invertébré | invertebrato | invertebrado | wirbellos | 無脊椎の |
| 3597. inverted - (a) | interverti | invertito | invertido | umgekehrt | 逆性の |
| 3598. inverted histogram - (n) | histogramme inversé | istogramma invertito | histograma invertido | umgekehrtes Histogramm | 逆ヒストグラム |
| 3599. investigate - (v) | examiner; étudier | investigare | investigar | untersuchen; erforschen | 調査する |
| 3600. investigation - (n) | investigation | investigazione | investigación | Untersuchung; Erforschung | 調査 |
| 3601. investigational drug - (n) | médicament à l'étude | farmaco investigativo | droga investigacional | zu untersuchendes Arzneimittel | 調査中薬品 |
| 3602. investigational new drug application - (n) | application dans l'étude d'un nouveau médicament | applicazione investigativa di un nuovo farmaco | solicitud de una nueva droga investigacional | Antrag zur Durchführung einer klinischen Studie | 調査中新薬願い |
| 3603. investigational site - (n) | site d'investigation | sito investigativo | sitio de la investigación | Untersuchungsstelle | 調査中（薬品投与）部位 |
| 3604. investigator - (n) | investigateur | investigatore | investigador | Ermittler; Untersucher | 調査者 |
| 3605. investigator comment - (n) | commentaire de l'investigateur | commento investigatore | comentario del investigador | Bemerkung des Untersuchers | 調査者コメント |
| 3606. investigator file - (n) | dossier de l'investigateur | incartamento investigatore | archivo del investigador | Dossier des Untersuchers | 調査者ファイル |
| 3607. investigator's brochure - (n) | brochure de l'investigateur | opuscolo dell'investigatore | folleto del investigador | Broschüre für die Untersucher einer Studie | 調査者カタログ |
| 3608. investigators' meeting - (n) | réunion des investigateurs | incontro investigatore | reunión de los investigadores | Untersucherkonferenz | 調査者ミーティング |

| English/American | French/Français | Italian/Italiano | Spanish/Español | German/Deutsch | Japanese 日本語 |
|---|---|---|---|---|---|
| 3609. involuntary - (a) | involontaire | involontario | involuntario | unwillkürlich; unfreiwillig | 不随意の、不本意の |
| 3610. involuntary guarding - (n) | défense involontaire | protezione involontaria | defensa involuntaria | unwillkürliche Abwehrspannung | 不随意防御 |
| 3611. involuntary movement - (n) | mouvement involontaire | movimento involontario | movimiento involuntario | unwillkürliche Bewegung | 不随意運動 |
| 3612. involuntary muscle - (n) | muscle involontaire | muscolo involontario | músculo involuntario | glatte Muskulatur | 不随意筋 |
| 3613. involution - (n) | involution | involuzione | involución | Involution; Rückbildung | 退縮 |
| 3614. inward - (a) | interne | interno | interno; interior | innere; innerlich | 内部の |
| 3615. iodine - (n) | iode | iodio | yodo | Jod | 沃化物 |
| 3616. ion - (n) | ion | ione | ion | Ion | イオン |
| 3617. ion channel - (n) | canal ionique | canale ionico | canal iónico | Ionenkanal | イオン経路 |
| 3618. ion exchange chromatography - (n) | chromatographie par échange ionique | cromatografia a scambio ionico | cromatografía de intercambio iónico | Ionenaustausch-chromatographie | イオン交換クロマトグラフィ |
| 3619. ion pump - (n) | pompe ionique | pompa ionica | bomba iónica | Ionenpumpe | イオンポンプ |
| 3620. ionic - (a) | ionique | ionico | iónico | ionisch | イオンの |
| 3621. ionizing radiation - (n) | radiation ionisante | radiazione ionizzante | radiación ionizante | ionisierende Strahlung | 電離線 |
| 3622. iontophoresis - (n) | ionophorèse | ionoforesi | iontoforesis | Iontophorese | イオン導入 [法] |
| 3623. ipsilateral - (a) | ipsilatéral; homolatéral | ipsilaterale; omolaterale | ipsilateral | ipsilateral | 同側にある |
| 3624. irate - (a) | furieux; courroucé | irato | colérico; enojado | zornig; wütend | 怒った |
| 3625. iris - (n) | iris | iride | iris | Iris | 虹彩 |
| 3626. iron - (n) | fer | ferro | hierro | Eisen | 鉄 |
| 3627. irradiate - (v) | irradier | irradiare; illuminare | irradiar | bestrahlen | 照射する |
| 3628. irradiation - (n) | irradiation | irradiazione | irradiación | Bestrahlung | 照射 |
| 3629. irrational - (a) | irrationnel | irrazionale | irracional | irrational | 不合理な |
| 3630. irregular - (a) | irrégulier | irregolare | irregular | irregulär; unregelmäßig | 不規則な |
| 3631. irreversible - (a) | irréversible | irreversibile | irreversible | irreversibel | 不可逆性の |

| English/American | French/Français | Italian/Italiano | Spanish/Español | German/Deutsch | Japanese日本語 |
|---|---|---|---|---|---|
| 3632. irrigate - (v) | irriguer | irrigare | irrigar | spülen; auswaschen | 洗浄する |
| 3633. irrigation - (n) | irrigation | irrigazione | irrigación | Irrigation; Spülung | 洗浄 |
| 3634. irritability - (n) | irritabilité | irritabilità | irritabilidad | Irritabilität; Reizbarkeit | 感応性 |
| 3635. irritation - (n) | irritation | irritazione | irritación | Irritation; Reizung | 過敏 |
| 3636. ischemia (ischaemia) - (n) | ischémie | ischemia | isquemia | Ischämie | 虚血 |
| 3637. ischium - (n) | ischion | ischio | isquión | Sitzbein; Os ischii | 坐骨 |
| 3638. islet cell - (n) | cellule des flots de Langerhans | cellula delle isole pancreatiche | célula de las islas de Langerhans | Inselzelle | [膵] 島細胞 |
| 3639. isoantibody - (n) | isoanticorps | isoanticorpo | isoanticuerpo | Isoantikörper; Alloantikörper | 同種抗体 |
| 3640. isoantigen - (n) | isoantigène | isoantigene | isoantigeno | Isoantigen; Alloantigen | 同種抗原 |
| 3641. isoelectric focusing - (n) | focalisation isoélectrique | focalizzazione isoelettrica | enfoque isoeléctrico | isoelektrische Einstellung | 等電焦点 |
| 3642. isoenzyme - (n) | iso-enzyme | isoenzima | isoenzima | Isoenzym | アイソザイム |
| 3643. isogeneic - (a) | isogénique | isogenico | isogénico | isogen | 同遺伝子系 |
| 3644. isolation - (n) | isolation; isolement | isolamento | aislamiento | Isolierung; Isolation | 隔離、分離 |
| 3645. isomer - (n) | isomère | isomero | isómero | Isomer | 異性体 |
| 3646. isomerism - (n) | isomérie | isomeria | isomerismo | Isomerie | 異性 |
| 3647. isometric - (a) | isométrique | isometrica | isométrico | isometrisch | 等長の |
| 3648. isotonic - (a) | isotonique | isotonico | isotónico | isoton | 等張の |
| 3649. isotope - (n) | isotope | isotopo | isótopo | Isotop | 同位体 |
| 3650. issue - (n) | sécrétion; édition | secrezione; edizione | secreción; edición | Ausfluß; Ausgabe | 打膿、排出、問題点 |
| 3651. isthmus - (n) | isthme | istmo | istmo | Isthmus | 峡部 |
| 3652. itch - (n) | démangeaison | prurito | picazón | Jucken | 疥癬 |
| 3653. itch - (v) | éprouver des démangeaisons | prudere; pizzicare | picar | jucken | むずむずする |
| 3654. itching - (n) | démangeaison | prurito; pizzicore | picazón | Juckreiz; Pruritus | 掻痒 |

186

| English/American | French/Français | Italian/Italiano | Spanish/Español | German/Deutsch | Japanese/日本語 |
|---|---|---|---|---|---|
| 3655. jaundice - (n) | ictère; jaunisse | ittero | ictericia | Gelbsucht; Ikterus | 黄疸 |
| 3656. jaw - (n) | mâchoire | mascella; mandibola | mandibula | Kiefer; Kinnbacke | 顎骨 |
| 3657. jejunal - (a) | jéjunal | digiuno | yeyunal; del yeyuno | jejunal | 空腸の |
| 3658. jejunoileal - (a) | jéjuno-iléal | ileodigiunale | yeyunoileal | jejunoileal | 空回腸の |
| 3659. jejunum - (n) | jéjunum | digiuno | yeyuno | Jejunum; Leerdarm | 空腸 |
| 3660. jerk - (n) | secousse; réflexe tendineux | scossa; riflesso | sacudida | Reflexbewegung; Muskelzuckung | 攣縮 |
| 3661. jerk - (v) | se mouvoir soudainement; donner une secousse | strappare | sacudir | zucken | 痙動する |
| 3662. joint - (n) | articulation | articolazione | articulación | Verbindung; Gelenk | 関節 |
| 3663. joint crepitus - (n) | crépitation articulaire | crepito articolare | crepitación de la articulación | Gelenkkrepitation | 関節摩擦音 |
| 3664. joint development - (n) | développement commun | sviluppo congiunto | desarrollo conjunto | gemeinschaftliche Weiterentwicklung | 共同開発 |
| 3665. joint evaluation - (n) | évaluation commune | valutazione congiunta | evaluación conjunta | gemeinsame Bewertung | 共同評価 |
| 3666. journal - (n) | journal; revue | periodico; diario | periódico; diario | Zeitschrift; Tagebuch | 定期刊行物、日誌 |
| 3667. judgment - (n) | jugement | giudizio | juicio; sentencia | Urteilsvermögen; Urteil | 判断 |
| 3668. jugular - (a) | jugulaire | giugulare | yugular | jugular | 頸および喉の |
| 3669. jugular vein - (n) | veine jugulaire | vena giugulare | vena yugular | Vena jugularis | 頸静脈 |
| 3670. jugular venous distension - (n) | distension de la veine jugulaire | distensione venosa giugulare | distensión de la vena yugular | Jugularvenenerweiterung | 頸静脈膨張 |
| 3671. junction - (n) | jonction | giunzione | junción | Verbindung; Knotenpunkt | 接合部 |
| 3672. juvenile - (a) | juvénile | giovanile | juvenil | jugendlich | 少年少女の |
| 3673. juxtapose - (v) | juxtaposer | giustapporre | yuxtaponer | nebeneinanderstellen | 並列する |

187

| English/American | French/Français | Italian/Italiano | Spanish/Español | German/Deutsch | Japanese/日本語 |
|---|---|---|---|---|---|
| 3674. karyotype - (n) | caryotype | cariotipo | cariotipo | Karyotyp; Karygramm | 核型 |
| 3675. karyotype - (v) | effectuer un caryotype | fare il cariotipo | cariotipear; hacer cariotipos | karyotypisieren | 核型する |
| 3676. karyotyping - (n) | caryotypage | cariotipo | cariotipaje | Karyogramm | 核型 |
| 3677. keloid - (n) | kéloïde; chéloïde | cheloide | queloide | Keloid | ケロイド |
| 3678. keratin - (n) | kératine | cheratina | queratina | Keratin | ケラチン |
| 3679. keratinocyte - (n) | kératinocyte | cheratinocita | queratinocito | Keratinozyt | ケラチノサイト |
| 3680. ketoacidosis - (n) | céto-acitose | chetoacidosi | ceto-acidosis | Ketoazidose | ケト酸症 |
| 3681. ketone - (n) | cétone | chetone | cetona; quetona | Keton | ケトン |
| 3682. ketosis - (n) | cétose | chetosi | cetosis; quetosis | Ketose | ケトーシス |
| 3683. keypunching - (n) | perforation à clavier | perforazione manuale | perforación por teclado | manuelles Lochen; Handlochen | キーパンチで穴を開けること |
| 3684. kidney - (n) | rein | rene | riñón | Niere | 腎臓 |
| 3685. kidney stone - (n) | calcul rénal | calcolo renale | cálculo renal | Nierenstein | 腎臓結石 |
| 3686. kill - (v) | tuer | uccidere | matar | töten | 殺す |
| 3687. killer cell - (n) | cellule K | cellula killer | célula killer | Killerzelle | キラー細胞 |
| 3688. kilogram - (n) | kilogramme | chilogrammo | kilogramo | Kilogramm | キログラム |
| 3689. kinetic profile - (n) | profil cinétique | profilo cinetico | perfil cinético | kinetisches Profil | 運動プロファイル |
| 3690. kinetics - (n) | cinétique | cinetica | cinética | Kinetik | 運動 |
| 3691. knee - (n) | genou | ginocchio | rodilla | Knie | 膝 |
| 3692. knee jerk - (n) | réflexe rotulien | riflesso patellare | contracción del cuadriceps femoral | Kniesehnenreflex | 膝蓋腱 |
| 3693. knuckle - (n) | articulation du doigt; jointure | nocca | nudillo | Knöchel; Fingerknöchel | 指関節 |
| 3694. kyphosis - (n) | cyphose | cifosi | cifosis | Kyphose | 亀背 |

| English/American | French/Français | Italian/Italiano | Spanish/Español | German/Deutsch | Japanese/日本語 |
|---|---|---|---|---|---|
| 3695. lab - (n) | labo; laboratoire | laboratorio | laboratorio | Labor | 研究室 |
| 3696. label - (n) | étiquette | etichetta | etiqueta | Etikett | ラベル |
| 3697. labeled strength - (n) | force désignée; force étiquetée | concentrazione dichiarata sull'etichetta | fuerza marcada; fuerza designada | gekennzeichnete Stärke | 表示どおりの効力 |
| 3698. labelling (labeling) of clinical material - (n) | étiquetage du matériel clinique | etichettatura di materiale clinico | marcación del material clínico | Etikettierung von klinischen Probematerialien | 臨床試験物質の分類 |
| 3699. labia - (n) | lèvres | labbra | labios | Lippen; Labien | 唇 |
| 3700. labile - (a) | labile | labile | lábil | labil | 不安定な |
| 3701. labor - (n) | travail | parto; doglie; lavoro | labor; trabajo de parto | Geburt; Arbeit | 分娩，労働 |
| 3702. laboratory - (n) | laboratoire | laboratorio | laboratorio | Labor | 実験室 |
| 3703. labyrinth - (n) | labyrinthe | labirinto | laberinto | Labyrinth | 迷路 |
| 3704. lacerate - (v) | lacérer | lacerare | lacerar | einreißen; zerreißen | 裂く |
| 3705. lacrimal - (a) | lacrymal | lacrimale | lacrimal; lagrimal | Tränen- | 涙の |
| 3706. lacrimation - (n) | lacrimation | lacrimazione | lacrimación; lagrimeo | Tränenbildung; Tränensekretion | 流涙 |
| 3707. lactase deficiency - (n) | déficience en lactase | deficit di lattasi | deficiencia lactasa | Laktasemangel | 乳酸障害 |
| 3708. lactation - (n) | lactation | lattazione; allattamento | lactación | Milchsekretion | 乳汁分泌 |
| 3709. lactose - (n) | lactose | lattosio | lactosa | Laktose | 乳糖 |
| 3710. lamella - (n) | lamelle | lamella | lamela | Lamelle | 層板 |
| 3711. lameness - (n) | claudication | zoppicatura | cojera | Lahmheit | 跛行 |
| 3712. lamina - (n) | lame | lamina | lámina | Lamina | 層 |
| 3713. lancet - (n) | lancette | lancetta | lanceta | Lanzette | ランセット |
| 3714. language - (n) | langage; langue | linguaggio; lingua | lenguaje; idioma | Sprache | 言語 |
| 3715. laparoscopy - (n) | laparoscopie | laparoscopia | laparoscopia | Laparoskopie | 腹腔鏡検査 [法] |
| 3716. laparotomy - (n) | laparotomie | laparotomia | laparotomía | Laparotomie | 開腹術 |
| 3717. large cell - (n) | grande cellule | grande cellula | célula grande | große Zelle | 大細胞 |

189

| English/American | French/Français | Italian/Italiano | Spanish/Español | German/Deutsch | Japanese/日本語 |
|---|---|---|---|---|---|
| 3718. large intestine - (n) | gros intestin | intestino crasso | intestino grueso | Dickdarm | 大腸 |
| 3719. larva - (n) | larve | larva | larva | Larve | 幼虫 |
| 3720. laryngeal - (a) | laryngien; laryngé | laringeo | laríngeo | laryngeal; laryngealis | 喉頭の |
| 3721. laryngitis - (n) | laryngite | laringite | laringitis | Laryngitis | 喉頭炎 |
| 3722. laryngoscopy - (n) | laryngoscopie | laringoscopia | laringoscopia | Laryngoskopie; Kehlkopfspiegelung | 喉頭鏡検査 [法] |
| 3723. larynx - (n) | larynx | laringe | laringe | Larynx; Kehlkopf | 喉頭 |
| 3724. laser - (n) | laser | laser | láser | Laser | レーザー |
| 3725. laser surgery - (n) | chirurgie au laser | chirurgia con laser | cirugía con láser | Laserchirurgie | レーザー外科 |
| 3726. lassitude - (n) | lassitude | stanchezza | lasitud | Erschöpfung; Müdigkeit | 倦怠 |
| 3727. latent - (a) | latent | latente | latente; no manifiesto | latent | 潜在性の |
| 3728. latent period - (n) | période de latence | periodo di latenza | período de latencia | Latenzzeit | 潜伏期 |
| 3729. late-onset - (a) | de début tardif | inizio tardivo | de comienzo retrasado | Späteinsetzend | 遅い発症の |
| 3730. lateral - (a) | latéral | laterale | lateral | lateral | 外側の |
| 3731. lateral thinking - (n) | pensée latérale | il pensare laterale | pensamiento lateral | unorthodoxe Denkmethode | 片側の思考 |
| 3732. Latin-square - (n) | carré latin | quadrato latino | cuadrado latino | lateinisches Quadrat | ラテン方格 |
| 3733. Latin-square design - (n) | plan carré latin | schema a quadrato latino | diseño del cuadrado latino | Entwurf eines lateinischen Quadrates | ラテン方格デザイン |
| 3734. laugh - (n) | rire | risata | risa | Lachen | 笑い |
| 3735. laugh - (v) | rire | ridere | reír | lachen | 笑う |
| 3736. laughter - (n) | rire | riso; risata | risa | Gelächter | 笑い声 |
| 3737. lavage - (n) | lavage | lavaggio | lavado | Spülung; Lavage | 洗浄 |
| 3738. laxative - (n) | laxatif | lassativo | laxante | Laxans; Abführmittel | 緩下剤 |
| 3739. layer - (n) | couche; strate | strato | capa; estrato | Schicht; Lage | 層 |
| 3740. lazy - (a) | paresseux | pigro; poltrone | perezoso | faul; langsam | 怠惰な |
| 3741. lead - (n) | plomb | piombo | plomo | Blei | 鉛 |
| 3742. leadership - (n) | leadership; direction | comando; guida | dirección; mando | Führung; Leitung | リーダーシップ |

| English/American | French/Français | Italian/Italiano | Spanish/Español | German/Deutsch | Japanese/日本語 |
|---|---|---|---|---|---|
| 3743. leak - (n) | fuite | crepa; fessura | pérdida | Leck; Loch | 漏れ |
| 3744. leak - (v) | fuir; couler | perdere; fuoruscire | perder; derramar | lecken | 漏れる |
| 3745. leakage - (n) | fuite; perte | perdita; fuga | pérdida | Leckage; Lecken | 漏れ |
| 3746. lean - (v) | pencher; appuyer | inclinarsi; inclinare | ladearse; inclinar | lehnen | 傾ける |
| 3747. lean - (a) | maigre; amaigri | magro | flaco; delgado | mager; schlank | やせた |
| 3748. learning - (n) | instruction; apprentissage | apprendimento | el aprender; estudio | Lernen | 学習 |
| 3749. learning disability - (n) | trouble d'apprentissage | difetto di apprendimento | trastorno de aprendizaje | Lernbehinderung | 学習障害 |
| 3750. least squares analysis - (n) | analyse des moindres carrés | analisi dei minimi quadrati | análisis mínimo-cuadrático | Analyse der kleinsten Quadrate | 最小平方根分析 |
| 3751. lecture - (n) | conférence | lezione; conferenza | conferencia | Vortrag; Vorlesung | 講義 |
| 3752. lecture - (v) | faire une conférence | fare lezione | dar una conferencia | einen Vortrag/eine Vorlesung halten | 講義をする |
| 3753. leech - (n) | sangsue | sanguisuga | sanguijuela | Blutegel | 水蛭 |
| 3754. left axis - (n) | axe gauche | asse sinistro | eje izquierdo | linke Achse | 左軸 |
| 3755. left handed - (a) | gaucher | mancino | zurdo | linkshändig | 左利きの |
| 3756. left ventricular end diastolic pressure - (n) | pression télédiastolique ventriculaire gauche | pressione ventricolare sinistra di fine diastole | presión de fin de diástole del ventricular izquierdo | linksventrikulärer enddiastolischer Druck | 左心室拡張期末圧 |
| 3757. left ventricular failure - (n) | insuffisance ventriculaire gauche | insufficienza ventricolare sinistra | insuficiencia del ventrículo izquierdo | Linksherzinsuffizienz; Linksherzversagen | 左心室障害 |
| 3758. leg - (n) | jambe | ramo; gamba | pierna | Bein; Zweig | 脚 |
| 3759. leg of treatment - (n) | bras de traitement | ramo di trattamento | rama de tratamiento | Behandlungszweig | 治療中の足 |
| 3760. legal - (a) | légal | legale | legal | legal; rechtlich | 法律の |
| 3761. legend - (n) | légende | legenda | leyenda | Legende | 伝説 |
| 3762. legislation - (n) | législation | legislazione | legislación | Gesetzgebung | 立法 |
| 3763. legumes - (n) | légumes | leguminose | legumbres | Hülsenfrucht | 豆類 |

191

| English/American | French/Français | Italian/Italiano | Spanish/Español | German/Deutsch | Japanese 日本語 |
|---|---|---|---|---|---|
| 3764. leiomyoma - (n) | léiomyome | leiomioma | leiomioma | Leiomyom | 平滑筋腫 |
| 3765. leisure activities - (n) | loisirs | attività del tempo libero | pasatiempos | Freizeitbeschäftigungen | 娯楽活動 |
| 3766. length of stay - (n) | durée du séjour | durata della degenza | duración de la estadía | Länge des Aufenthalts | 入院期間 |
| 3767. lengthening - (n) | allongement | allungamento | prolongación | Verlängerung | 延長 |
| 3768. lens - (n) | lentille; cristallin | cristallino; lente | lente; cristalino | Linse; Augenlinse | 水晶体、レンズ |
| 3769. lesbian - (a) | lesbien | lesbico | lesbio | lesbisch | 女性間の同性愛の |
| 3770. lesion - (n) | lésion | lesione | lesión | Läsion; Schaden | 病巣 |
| 3771. lethal - (a) | létal; mortel | letale | letal; mortal | letal | 致命的な |
| 3772. lethal dose - (n) | dose létale | dose letale | dosis letal | Letaldosis | 致死量 |
| 3773. lethargy - (n) | léthargie | letargia | letargo | Lethargie | 昏睡 |
| 3774. leucocyte - (n) | leucocyte | leucocita | leucocito | Leukozyt | 白血球 |
| 3775. leucocytosis - (n) | leucocytose | leucocitosi | leucocitosis | Leukozytose | 白血球増多症 |
| 3776. leucopenia - (n) | leucopénie | leucopenia | leucopenia | Leukopenie | 白血球減少症 |
| 3777. leukapheresis - (n) | leucaphérèse | leucaferesi | leucoféresis | Leukopherese | 白血球搬出 |
| 3778. leukemia - (n) | leucémie | leucemia | leucemia | Leukämie | 白血病 |
| 3779. leukocyte - (n) | leucocyte | leucocita | leucocito | Leukozyt | 白血球 |
| 3780. leukopenia - (n) | leucopénie | leucopenia | leucopenia | Leukopenie | 白血球減少症 |
| 3781. levator - (n) | élévateur | elevatore | elevador | Heber | 挙筋 |
| 3782. level - (n) | niveau; hauteur | livello | nivel | Niveau; Grad | レベル |
| 3783. level - (a) | plat | piano; livellato | nivelado | eben | 同等の |
| 3784. level of anesthesia - (n) | niveau d'anesthésie | livello dell'anestesia | nivel de anestesia | Grad der Anästhesie | 麻酔のレベル |
| 3785. level of consciousness - (n) | niveau de conscience | livello di coscienza | nivel de conciencia | Bewußtseinsniveau | 意識のレベル |
| 3786. levo isomer - (n) | isomère levogyre | isomero levogiro | levo isómero | linksdrehendes Isomer | レボアイソマー |
| 3787. liability - (n) | responsabilité | responsabilità | responsabilidad | Verantwortung; Haftung | 義務 |
| 3788. libido - (n) | libido | libido | libido | Libido | 性欲 |

192

| English/American | French/Français | Italian/Italiano | Spanish/Español | German/Deutsch | Japanese/日本語 |
|---|---|---|---|---|---|
| 3789. library - (n) | bibliothèque | biblioteca | biblioteca | Bibliothek | 図書館 |
| 3790. license (licence) - (n) | licence; autorisation | licenza | licencia; permiso | Genehmigung; Erlaubnis | 免許 |
| 3791. licensing activities - (n) | exigences d'autorisation | requisiti di licenza | exigencias de licenciación | Lizenzerteilungs-aktivitäten | 免許を与える機関 |
| 3792. licensing authority - (n) | autorité d'autorisation | autorità che concede licenze | autoridad de licenciación | Lizenzerteilungsamt | 免許を与える権威者 |
| 3793. licensure - (n) | autorisation | certificazione | licenciatura | Lizenzerteilung | 資格試験 |
| 3794. lichen - (n) | lichen | lichene | liquen | Lichen; Flechte | 苔癬 |
| 3795. lid lag - (n) | retard palpébral | ptosi palpebrale | retracción palpebral | Zurückbleiben des Oberlids bei Blicksenkung | 瞼の遅滞 |
| 3796. life - (n) | vie | vita | vida | Leben | 生命 |
| 3797. life change events - (n) | événements modifiant la vie | eventi che combiano la vita | eventos que cambian la vida | lebensverändernde Ereignisse | 人生に変化を与える出来事 |
| 3798. life expectancy - (n) | espérance de vie | attesa di vita | expectativa de vida | Lebenserwartung | 寿命 |
| 3799. life satisfaction - (n) | satisfaction de la vie | soddisfazione nel livello di vita | satisfacción en la vida | Lebenszufriedenheit | 生活満足度 |
| 3800. life style - (n) | style de vie | stile di vita | estilo de vida | Lebensstil | ライフスタイル |
| 3801. life support system - (n) | système de support de la vie | sistema di sopravvivenza | sistema de mantener la vida del enfermo | Lebenserhaltungssystem | 生命補助システム |
| 3802. life survival graph - (n) | graphique de survie | grafico sopravvivenza | gráfico de supervivencia | Überlebenskurve | 生存グラフ |
| 3803. life table - (n) | table de mortalité | tabella di mortalità | tabla de mortalidad | Sterbetafel | 生命表 |
| 3804. lift - (v) | lever | alzare | levantar | heben | 持ち上げる |
| 3805. ligament - (n) | ligament | legamento | ligamento | Ligament; Band | 靭帯 |
| 3806. ligand - (n) | ligand | legante; ligando | ligando | Ligand | 配位子 |

193

| English/American | French/Français | Italian/Italiano | Spanish/Español | German/Deutsch | Japanese日本語 |
|---|---|---|---|---|---|
| 3807. ligate - (v) | lier | legare; allacciare | ligar | binden | 結紮する |
| 3808. ligation - (n) | ligature | legatura; allacciatura | ligación; ligadura | Abbinden; Unterbinden | 結紮 |
| 3809. ligature - (n) | ligature | legatura; allacciatura | ligadura | Ligatur | 結紮糸 |
| 3810. light - (n) | lumière | luce | luz | Licht | 光 |
| 3811. light - (a) | léger; clair | leggero; chiaro | ligero; claro | leicht; hell | 薄い、明るい |
| 3812. light micro-scope - (n) | microscope optique | microscopio ottico | microscopio óptico | Lichtmikroskop | 光学顕微鏡 |
| 3813. light-headed - (a) | pris de vertige | stordito; in preda alle vertigini | mareado | verwirrt; schwindlig | ふらふららする |
| 3814. light-sensitive - (a) | photosensible | fotosensibile | sensible a la luz | lichtempfindlich | 光感受性の |
| 3815. limb - (n) | membre; extrémité | arto; estremità | miembro; extremidad | Extremität | 肢 |
| 3816. limbic system - (n) | système limbique | sistema limbico | sistema límbico | limbisches System | 大脳辺縁系 |
| 3817. limbus - (n) | limbe | limbo | limbo | Rand | 辺縁 |
| 3818. limit of detection - (n) | limite de dépistage | limite di scoperta | límite de detección | Nachweisgrenze | 検出眼界 |
| 3819. limp - (n) | claudication | zoppicatura | cojera | Hinken | 跛行 |
| 3820. limp - (v) | claudiquer; boiter | zoppicare | cojear | hinken | 跛行する |
| 3821. limp - (a) | mou; flasque | floscio | flácido; flojo | schlaff; weich | 跛行性の |
| 3822. line extension - (n) | extension de ligne | estensione filo | extensión linear | Kurvenverlängerung | 延長線 |
| 3823. line graph - (n) | graphique linéaire | grafico lineare | gráfico linear | Liniengraph | 線グラフ |
| 3824. line of equivalence - (n) | ligne de l'equivalence | linea di equivalenza | línea de equivalencia | Äquivalenzlinie | 等量ライン |
| 3825. linear - (a) | linéaire | lineare | lineal | linear | 線状の |
| 3826. linear model - (n) | modèle linéaire | modello lineare | modelo lineal | lineares Modell | リニアモデル |
| 3827. linear relationship - (n) | relation linéaire | relazione lineare | relación lineal | lineare Beziehung | リニア関係 |
| 3828. lingual frenum - (n) | frein de la langue | frenulo linguale | frenillo | Zungenbändchen; Frenulum linguae | 舌小帯 |

194

| English/American | French/Français | Italian/Italiano | Spanish/Español | German/Deutsch | Japanese/日本語 |
|---|---|---|---|---|---|
| 3829. linguistics - (n) | linguistique | linguistica | lingüística | Linguistik; Sprachwissenschaft | 言語学 |
| 3830. lingula - (n) | lingula | lingula | língula | zungenförmiger Lappen | 小舌 |
| 3831. liniment - (n) | liniment | linimento | linimento | Liniment; Einreibemittel | 塗膚剤 |
| 3832. linkage - (n) | liaison; enchaînement | concatenazione | ligadura; encadenamiento | Nexus; Verbindung | 結合 |
| 3833. lip - (n) | lèvre | labbro | labio | Lippe; Labium | 唇 |
| 3834. lipemia - (n) | lipémie | lipemia | lipemia | Lipämie | 脂肪血症 |
| 3835. lipid - (n) | lipide | lipide | lípido | Lipid | 脂質 |
| 3836. lipolysis - (n) | lipolyse | lipolisi | lipólisis | Lipolyse | 脂肪分解 |
| 3837. lipoma - (n) | lipome | lipoma | lipoma | Lipom | 脂肪腫 |
| 3838. lipoprotein - (n) | lipoprotéine | lipoproteina | lipoproteína | Lipoprotien | リポ蛋白 |
| 3839. liposome - (n) | liposome | liposoma | liposoma | Liposom | リポソーム |
| 3840. liquid - (n) | liquide | liquido | líquido | Flüssigkeit | 液体 |
| 3841. liquid - (a) | liquide | liquido | líquido | flüssig | 液体の |
| 3842. list - (n) | liste | lista | lista | Liste | 一覧表 |
| 3843. literature - (n) | littérature; documentation | letteratura; opuscoli | literatura; información | Fachliteratur | 文献 |
| 3844. literature review - (n) | révision de la documentation; revue de la littérature | revisione letteratura | revisión de la literatura | Überprüfung der Fachliteratur | 文献批評 |
| 3845. lithiasis - (n) | lithiase | litiasi | litiasis | Lithiasis; Steinleiden | 結石症 |
| 3846. lithium - (n) | lithium | litio | litio | Lithium | リチウム |
| 3847. litigation - (n) | litige | processo; causa | litigación; litigio | Prozeß; Rechtsstreit | 訴訟 |
| 3848. litmus paper - (n) | papier tournesol | cartina al tornasole | papel de tornasol | Lackmuspapier | リトマス紙 |
| 3849. litter - (n) | portée | lettiga; figliata | camada | Wurf | 同腹児群 |
| 3850. litter - (v) | mettre bas | figliare; partorire | parir | (Junge) werfen | 子を生む |
| 3851. liver - (n) | foie | fegato | hígado | Leber | 肝臓 |
| 3852. liver failure - (n) | insuffisance hépatique | insufficienza epatica | insuficiencia hepática | Leberversagen | 肝不全 |

195

| English/American | French/Français | Italian/Italiano | Spanish/Español | German/Deutsch | Japanese/日本語 |
|---|---|---|---|---|---|
| 3853. liver function - (n) | fonction hépatique | funzionamento epatico | funcionamiento hepático | Leberfunktion | 肝臓機能 |
| 3854. loading dose - (n) | dose du charge | dose di induzione | dosis inicial | Ausgangsdosis s | 負荷投与 |
| 3855. lobar pneumonia - (n) | pneumonie lobaire | polmonite lobare | neumonia lobar | Lobärpneumo-ie | 大葉性肺炎 |
| 3856. lobe - (n) | lobe | lobo | lóbulo | Lappen; Lobus | 葉 |
| 3857. local - (a) | local | locale | local | lokal; örtlich | 局所の |
| 3858. localized - (a) | localisé | localizzato | localizado | lokalisiert; umschrieben | 局在の |
| 3859. locomotion - (n) | locomotion | locomozione | locomoción | Lokomotion; Fortbewegung | ロコモーション |
| 3860. locomotor activity - (n) | activité locomotrice | attività locomotoria | actividad locomotora | lokomotorische Aktivität | 運動活動度 |
| 3861. logarithmic scale - (n) | échelle logarithmique | scala logaritmica | escala logarítmica | logarithmische Skala | 対数スケール |
| 3862. logbook - (n) | registre | giornale di bordo | registro | Protokoll | 日誌 |
| 3863. logging-in - (n) | initialisation d'une session | logging-in; inserire la parola d'ordine in un computer per attivario | inicialización de una sesión | Logon; Anmeldung | ロギングイン |
| 3864. logic - (n) | logique | logica | lógica | Logik | 論理 |
| 3865. logical - (a) | logique | logico | lógica | logisch | 論理的な |
| 3866. logical inconsistencies - (n) | inconsistances de logique | inconsistenze logiche | inconsistencias lógicas | logische Widersprüche | 論理的矛盾 |
| 3867. logistic model - (n) | modèle logistique | modello logistico | modelo logístico | logistisches Modell | 論理模範 |
| 3868. logistics - (n) | logistique | logistica | logística | Logistik | 兵站学 |
| 3869. log-linear model - (n) | modèle linéaire logarithmique | modello logistico-lineare | modelo logarítmico-linear | logarithmisch-lineares Modell | ログリニアモデル |
| 3870. loin - (n) | lombe | fianco; lombi | lomo | Lende; Lumbus | 腰 |
| 3871. lonely - (a) | seul; solitaire | solo; solitario | solo; solitario | einsam | 孤独の |
| 3872. longitudinal - (a) | longitudinal | longitudinale | longitudinal | Längen- | 縦の |

| English/American | French/Français | Italian/Italiano | Spanish/Español | German/Deutsch | Japanese/日本語 |
|---|---|---|---|---|---|
| 3873. long-term, long term - (a) | à long terme | a lungo termine | a largo término | langfristig | 長期の |
| 3874. lordosis - (n) | lordose | lordosi | lordosis | Lordose | 脊柱前弯症 |
| 3875. loss - (n) | perte | perdita | pérdida | Verlust | 損失 |
| 3876. loss of consciousness - (n) | perte de conscience | perdita di coscienza | pérdida del conocimiento | Bewußtseinsverlust | 意識喪失 |
| 3877. loss of weight - (n) | perte de poids | perdita di peso | pérdida de peso | Gewichtsverlust | 体重減少 |
| 3878. lost to follow-up - (n) | perte lors du suivi | uscito dallo studio | pérdida del seguimiento | nicht mehr zur Nachuntersuchung verfügbar | フォローアップできない |
| 3879. lot - (n) | lot | lotto | lote | Charge | ロット |
| 3880. lot number - (n) | nombre du lot | numero di lotto | número del lote | Chargennummer | ロット番号 |
| 3881. lot to lot - (a) | de lot à lot | da lotto a lotto | de lote a lote | von Charge zu Charge | ロットからロットまで |
| 3882. lotion - (n) | lotion | lozione | loción | Lotion | ローション |
| 3883. loudness perception - (n) | perception du bruit | percezione dei rumori | percepción del sonido | Wahrnehmung der Lautstärke | 音の大きさと知覚 |
| 3884. louse - (n) | pou | pidocchio | piojo | Laus | しらみ |
| 3885. low back pain - (n) | lumbago | lombaggine | lumbago | Kreuzschmerz | 腰痛 [症] |
| 3886. low blood pressure - (n) | pression artérielle basse | pressione del sangue bassa | presión arterial baja | niedriger Blutdruck | 低血圧 |
| 3887. low calorie diet - (n) | régime hypocalorique | dieta ipocalorica | dieta baja en calorías | kalorienarme Kost | 低カロリー食 |
| 3888. low carbohydrate diet - (n) | régime faible en hydrates de carbone | dieta a limitato consumo di carboidrati | dieta baja en carbohidratos | kohlenhydratarme Kost | 低含水炭素食 |
| 3889. low cholesterol diet - (n) | régime hypocholestérolémiant | dieta a basso consumo di colesterolo | dieta baja en colesterol | cholesterinarme Kost | 低コレステロール食 |
| 3890. low dose heparin - (n) | héparine à faible dose | eparina a bassa dose | heparina en dosis baja | niedrig dosiertes Heparin | ヘパリン低服用量 |

| English/American | French/Français | Italian/Italiano | Spanish/Español | German/Deutsch | Japanese/日本語 |
|---|---|---|---|---|---|
| 3891. low dose regimen - (n) | régime à dose faible | regime a bassa dose | regimen de dosis baja | Schema mit niedriger Dosierung | 低服用量プロトコール |
| 3892. low fat diet - (n) | régime pauvre en graisse | dieta a limitato consumo di grassi | dieta baja en grasa | fettarme Kost | 低脂肪食 |
| 3893. low grade - (a) | de qualité inférieure; léger | di basso grado | de bajo grado | geringgradig | 低度の |
| 3894. low grade fever - (n) | fièvre légère | febbre di basso grado | febrícula | geringgradiges Feber | 微熱 |
| 3895. low risk group - (n) | groupe à faible risque | gruppo a basso rischio | grupo de bajo riesgo | Gruppe mit niedrgem Risiko | 低リスクグループ |
| 3896. low salt diet - (n) | régime hyposodé | dieta a basso contenuto di sale | dieta hiposódica | salzarme Kost | 低塩食 |
| 3897. low sodium diet - (n) | régime hyposodé | dieta a basso contenuto di sodio | dieta hiposódica | salzarme Kos: | 低塩食 |
| 3898. lower respiratory - (a) | des voies respiratoires inférieures | delle basse vie respiratorie | de las vías aéreas inferiores | die unteren Aterrwege betreffend | 気管支下部の |
| 3899. lozenge - (n) | pastille | pastiglia; pasticca | tableta | Rhombus; Lutschtablette | ひし形錠剤 |
| 3900. lubricant - (n) | lubrifiant | lubrificante | lubricante | Gleitmittel | 潤滑剤 |
| 3901. lucid - (a) | lucide | lucido | lúcido | klar | 正気の |
| 3902. lull - (n) | moment de calme | momento di calma | intervalo | Pause; Stille | 小康 |
| 3903. lull - (v) | calmer; apaiser | calmar; placare | calmar; adormecer | beruhigen | 痛みが鎮まる |
| 3904. lumbar - (a) | lombaire | lombare | lumbar | lumbal | 腰の |
| 3905. lumbar disk - (n) | disque lombaire | disco lombare | disco lumbar | Lumbalbandscheibe | 腰椎 |
| 3906. lumbar puncture - (n) | ponction lombaire | puntura lombare | punción lumbar | Lumbalpunktion | 腰椎穿刺 |
| 3907. lumbosacral plexus - (n) | plexus lombo-sacré | plesso lombosacrale | plexo lumbosacro | Lumbosakralplexus | 腰仙骨神経叢 |
| 3908. lumen - (n) | lumière | lume | lumen | lichte Weite; _umen | 管腔 |
| 3909. luminal - (a) | relatif à la lumière | luminale | luminal | hell; leuchtend | 管腔の |

| English/American | French/Français | Italian/Italiano | Spanish/Español | German/Deutsch | Japanese/日本語 |
|---|---|---|---|---|---|
| 3910. lumi-nescence - (n) | luminescence | luminescenza | luminescencia | Lumineszenz | ルミネセンス |
| 3911. lump - (n) | protubérance; grosseur | massa; nodulo | protuberancia | Klumpen; Schwellung | しこり |
| 3912. lunacy - (n) | aliénation mentale; démence | follia; alienazione mentale | lunatismo; insania | Wahnsinn; Irrsinn | 精神症 |
| 3913. lung - (n) | poumon | polmone | pulmón | Lunge | 肺［臓］ |
| 3914. lung compliance - (n) | compliance pulmonaire | compliance polmonare | adaptabilidad pulmonar | Lungencompliance; Lungendehnbarkeit | 肺のコンプライアンス |
| 3915. lung field - (n) | champ pulmonaire | campo polmonare | campo pulmonar | Lungenfeld | 肺領域 |
| 3916. lung inflation - (n) | inflation du poumon | espansione polmonare | expansión pulmonar | Lungeninsufflation | 肺の膨張 |
| 3917. lung volume - (n) | volume pulmonaire | volume polmonare | volumen pulmonar | Lungenvolumen | 肺の容量 |
| 3918. luteal phase - (n) | phase lutéale | fase luteale | fase luteínica | Lutealphase | 黄体期 |
| 3919. luteinization - (n) | lutéinisation | luteinizzazione | luteinización | Luteinisierung | 黄体形成 |
| 3920. luteinizing hormone - (n) | hormone lutéinisante | ormone luteinizzante | hormona luteinizante | luteinisierendes Hormon | 黄体ホルモン |
| 3921. lying-in - (n) | accouchement; couche | puerperio | puerperio | Entbindung; Wochenbett | 産褥期 |
| 3922. lymph - (n) | lymphe | linfa | linfa | Lymphe; Impfstoff | リンパ液 |
| 3923. lymph gland - (n) | ganglion lymphaticue | linfoghiandola; ghiandola linfatica | ganglio linfático | Lymphknoten | リンパ腺 |
| 3924. lymph node - (n) | ganglion lymphatique | linfonodo | ganglio linfático | Lymphknoten | リンパ節 |
| 3925. lymphaden-opathy - (n) | lymphadénopathie | linfadenopatia | linfadenopatía | Lymphadenopathie | リンパ節症 |
| 3926. lymphatic - (a) | lymphatique | linfatico | linfático | lymphatisch | リンパの |
| 3927. lymphatic system - (n) | système lymphatique | sistema linfatico | sistema linfático | Lymphsystem | リンパ系 |
| 3928. lymphocyte - (n) | lymphocyte | linfocito | linfocito | Lymphozyt | リンパ球 |
| 3929. lymphocyte homing receptor - (n) | récepteur chercheur lymphocytaire | recettore per l'homing dei linfociti | receptor buscador de linfocitos | lymphozytenlenkender Rezeptor | リンパ球ホーミングレセプター |

| English/American | French/Français | Italian/Italiano | Spanish/Español | German/Deutsch | Japanese/日本語 |
|---|---|---|---|---|---|
| 3930. lymphocytic - (a) | lymphocytaire | linfocitario | linfocítico | lymphozytär | リンパ球の |
| 3931. lympho-cytosis - (n) | lymphocytose | linfocitosi | linfocitosis | Lymphozytose | 血中リンパ球増加 [症] |
| 3932. lymphoid - (a) | lymphoïde | linfoide | linfoide | lymphoid; lymphartig | リンパ様の |
| 3933. lymphoma - (n) | lymphome | linfoma | linfoma | Lymphom | リンパ腫 |
| 3934. lymphoprolifera-tive - (a) | lymphoprolifératif | linfoproliferativo | linfoproliferativo | lymphoproliferativ | リンパ球増殖 [性] の |
| 3935. lyophilization - (n) | lyophilisation | liofilizzazione | liofilización | Lyophilisation; Gefriertrocknung | 凍結乾燥 |
| 3936. lyse - (v) | lyser | lisare | desintegrar | auflösen | 溶解する |
| 3937. lysis - (n) | lyse | lisi | lisis | Lyse; Zerfall | 溶解 |
| 3938. lysogeny - (a) | lysogénie | lisogenia | destruido; desintegrado | Lysogenie | 溶原性 |
| 3939. lysosome - (n) | lysosome | lisosoma | lisosoma | Lysosom | リソソーム |
| 3940. lytic - (a) | lytique | litico | lítico | lytisch; lösend | 細胞溶解の |

200

| English/American | French/Français | Italian/Italiano | Spanish/Español | German/Deutsch | Japanese日本語 |
|---|---|---|---|---|---|
| 3941. maceration - (n) | macération | macerazione | maceración | Mazeration | 浸軟 |
| 3942. macro level - (n) | niveau macroscopique | macrolivello | nivel macro | Makro-Ebene | マクロレベル |
| 3943. macro-cephaly - (n) | macrocéphalie | macrocefalia | macrocefalia | Makrozephalie | 大頭 [症] |
| 3944. macrocyte - (n) | macrocyte | macrocita | macrocito | Makrozyt | 大赤血球 |
| 3945. macro-globulin - (n) | macroglobuline | macroglobulina | macroglobulina | Makroglobulin | マクログロブリン |
| 3946. macrophage - (n) | macrophage | macrofago | macrófago | Makrophage | マクロファージ |
| 3947. macrophage colony - (n) | colonie de macrophages | colonia macrofagica | colonia de macrófagos | Makrophagenkolonie | マクロファージコロニー |
| 3948. macular degener-ation - (n) | dégénérescence maculaire | degenerazione maculare | degeneración macular | Makuladegeneration | 黄斑変性 |
| 3949. macule - (n) | macule; macula | macchia; macula | mácula | Makula; Fleck | 斑点 |
| 3950. maculo-papule - (n) | maculo-papule | maculopapule | maculopápula | fleckige Papel | 斑点状丘疹 |
| 3951. mad - (a) | fou; aliéné | matto; pazzo | insano; furioso | geisteskrank | 精神錯乱の |
| 3952. magnesium - (n) | magnésium | magnesio | magnesio | Magnesium | マグネシウム |
| 3953. magnetic resonance imaging [abbr] MRI - (n) | imagerie par résonnance magnétique | risonanza magnetica per imagini | imagen por resonancia magnética | Kernspintomographie | 磁気共鳴影象 |
| 3954. magnitude - (n) | ampleur | grandezza | magnitud | Größe | 大きさ、規模 |
| 3955. mail-order - (a) | commandé par la poste | ordine postale | pedido postal | Versand- | 通信販売 |
| 3956. maintenance - (n) | maintien; entretien | mantenimento; conservazione | mantenimiento | Erhaltung; Instandhaltung | 維持 |
| 3957. maintenance dose - (n) | dose d'entretien | dose di mantenimento | dosis de mantenimiento | Erhaltungsdosis | 維持服用量 |
| 3958. major histocom-patibility complex [abbr] MHC - (n) | complexe majeur d'histocompatibilité | complesso maggiore di istocompatibilità | complejo mayor de histocompatibilidad | Haupthistokompatibilitätskomplex | 主要組織適合遺伝子複合体 |

201

| English/American | French/Français | Italian/Italiano | Spanish/Español | German/Deutsch | Japanese/日本語 |
|---|---|---|---|---|---|
| 3959. makeup session - (n) | session supplémentaire | sessione sostitutiva | sesión suplementaria | nachgeholte Sitzung | 再予約セッション |
| 3960. mal - (n) | mal | male | mal | Mal; Krankheit | 病気 |
| 3961. malab-sorption - (n) | malabsorption | malassorbimento | malabsorción | Malabsorption | 吸収不良 |
| 3962. malacia - (n) | malacie | malacia | malacia | Malazie | 軟化 [症] |
| 3963. maladjusted - (a) | inadapté | maladattato | ajuste defectuoso | verhaltensgestört milieugestört | 適応でさない |
| 3964. malady - (n) | maladie | malattia | enfermedad | Krankheit | 病気 |
| 3965. malaise - (n) | malaise | malessere | malestar | Unwohlsein; Unpaßlichkeit | 不快感 |
| 3966. male - (n) | mâle | maschio | macho | Mann | 男性 |
| 3967. male - (a) | mâle | maschio | macho | männlich | 男性の |
| 3968. male sex organs - (n) | organes génitaux mâles | organi sessuali maschili | órganos sexuales masculinos | männliche Geschlechtsorgane | 男性性器 |
| 3969. malformation - (n) | malformation | malformazione | malformación | Malformation; Fehlbildung | 奇形 |
| 3970. malign - (a) | malin | maligno | maligno | maligne; bösartig | 有害な |
| 3971. malignant - (a) | malin | maligno | maligno | maligne; bösartig | 悪性の |
| 3972. malinger - (v) | simuler la maladie | simulare una malattia | simular enfermedad | Krankheit simulieren | 仮病を使う |
| 3973. malingering - (a) | simulant une maladie | simulazione di una malattia | simulando una enfermedad o defecto | scheinkrank | 仮病の |
| 3974. malnutrition - (n) | malnutrition; sous-alimentation | malnutrizione | malnutrición; desnutrición | Malnutrition; Mangelernährung | 栄養不良 |
| 3975. malocclusion - (n) | malocclusion | malocclusione | maloclusión | Malokklusion; fehlerhafter Gebißschluß | 不正咬合 |
| 3976. malpractice - (n) | négligence professionnelle | negligenza | malpraxis | Kunstfehler; Berufsvergehen | 不正治療 |

202

| English/American | French/Français | Italian/Italiano | Spanish/Español | German/Deutsch | Japanese/日本語 |
|---|---|---|---|---|---|
| 3977. malpractice suit - (n) | poursuite pour négligence professionnelle | azione legale per negligenza | juicio por malpraxis | Berufsvergehensprozeß | 不正治療訴訟 |
| 3978. mammal - (n) | mammifère | mammifero | mamífero | Säugetier | 哺乳類 |
| 3979. mammary - (a) | mammaire | mammario | mamario | mammär | 乳房の |
| 3980. mammogram - (n) | mammogramme | mammogramma | mamograma | Mammogramm | 乳房造影 |
| 3981. mammography - (n) | mammographie | mammografia | mamografía | Mammographie | 乳房造影 [主] |
| 3982. man - (n) | homme; humanité | uomo | hombre | Mann; Mensch | 人 |
| 3983. management - (n) | gestion; administration | gestione; amministrazione | administración; gerencia | Verwaltung; Geschäftsleitung | 管理 |
| 3984. mandible - (n) | mandibule | mandibola | mandíbula | Unterkiefer; Mandibula | 下顎骨 |
| 3985. mandibular joint - (n) | articulation mandibulaire | articolazione mandibolare | articulación mandibular | Mandibulargelenk | 下顎の関節 |
| 3986. maneuver (manoeuvre) - (n) | manoeuvre | manovra | maniobra | Manöver; Handgriff | 操作 |
| 3987. maneuver (manoeuvre) - (v) | manoeuvrer | manovrare | maniobrar | manövrieren | 操作する |
| 3988. mania - (n) | manie | mania | manía | Manie | マニヤ |
| 3989. manic-depressive - (a) | maniaque-dépressif | maniaco-depressiva | maníaco-depresivo | manisch-depressiv | 躁鬱の |
| 3990. manic disorder - (n) | désordre maniaque | disordini maniacali | trastorno maníaco | manische Störung | 躁病 |
| 3991. manifest anxiety scale - (n) | échelle d'anxiété | scala di ansietà | escala de ansiedad | Gradeinteilung manifester Angst | 発現不安尺度 |
| 3992. manifestation - (n) | manifeste manifestation | manifesta manifestazione | manifiesta manifestación | Manifestation; Erscheinungsform | 発現 |
| 3993. manometer - (n) | manomètre | manometro | manómetro | Manometer | 血圧計 |
| 3994. manometry - (n) | manométrie | manometria | manometría | Manometrie | マノメトリー |

203

| English/American | French/Français | Italian/Italiano | Spanish/Español | German/Deutsch | Japanese/日本語 |
|---|---|---|---|---|---|
| 3995. manpower - (n) | main-d'œuvre | forza di lavoro | mano de obra | Arbeitskräfte | 人的資源 |
| 3996. manual - (n) | manuel | manuale | manual | Anleitung; Handbuch | 手引 |
| 3997. manual of operations - (n) | manuel d'utilisation | manuale d'uso | manual de utilización | Anwendungshandbuch | 手術手引書 |
| 3998. manufacturing - (n) | manufacture; fabrication | fabbricazione; produzione | manufacturación; fabricación | Herstellung; Erzeugung | 製造 |
| 3999. mapping - (n) | cartographie | rilevamento; mappatura | mapeo | Mapping; Kartierung | 製図、マッピング |
| 4000. marine toxins - (n) | toxines marines | tossine marine | toxinas marítimas | Meeresorganismustoxine | 海洋性毒素 |
| 4001. marital status - (n) | état matrimonial | stato di famiglia | estado civil | Familienstand | 婚姻状態 |
| 4002. marital therapy - (n) | thérapie maritale | terapia della coppia | terapia matrimonial | Ehetherapie | 結婚療法 |
| 4003. marker - (n) | marqueur; jalon | marcatore; marker | marcador | Marker | 目印 |
| 4004. market - (n) | marché | mercato | mercado | Markt | 市場 |
| 4005. marketed drug - (n) | médicament lancé sur le marché | farmaco in vendita | droga llevada al mercado | auf den Markt gebrachtes Arzneimittel | 市販の薬品 |
| 4006. marketing - (n) | marketing; commercialisation | commercializzazione; marketing | marketing | Marketing | マーケティング |
| 4007. marketing representative - (n) | représentant commercial | rappresentante marketing | representante comercial | Handelsvertreter | マーケティング担当者 |
| 4008. marriage - (n) | mariage | matrimonio | matrimonio | Ehe | 結婚 |
| 4009. marrow - (n) | moelle | midollo | médula ósea | Mark; Knochenmark | 骨髄 |
| 4010. masculine - (a) | masculin | mascolino; maschile | masculino | maskulin; männlich | 男性の |
| 4011. mask - (n) | masque | maschera | máscara | Maske | マスク、顔面包帯 |
| 4012. masking - (n) | couverture | mascheramento | enmascaramiento | Maskierung | マスキング、隠ぺい |
| 4013. masklike facies - (n) | faciès d'allure masquée | faccia "a maschera"; gargolismo | facies de máscara | Maskengesicht | 仮面状顔貌 |
| 4014. masochism - (n) | masochisme | masochismo | masoquismo | Masochismus | マゾヒズム |
| 4015. mass - (n) | masse | massa | masa | Masse | 集団、質量 |

| English/American | French/Français | Italian/Italiano | Spanish/Español | German/Deutsch | Japanese/日本語 |
|---|---|---|---|---|---|
| 4016. mass media - (n) | mass média | mezzi di comunicazione di massa | medios de comunicación | Massenmedien | マスメディア |
| 4017. mass screening - (n) | dépistage de masse | indagine di massa; screening di massa | examen masivo | Massenscreening | 大規模スクリーニング |
| 4018. mass spectrum analysis - (n) | analyse spectrale de masse | analisi spettro di massa | análisis por espectrografía de masas | Massenspektrumanalyse | 質量スペクトル分析 |
| 4019. massage - (n) | massage | massaggio | masaje | Massage | マッサージ, 按摩 |
| 4020. massage - (v) | masser | massaggiare | masajear | massieren | マッサージをる |
| 4021. masseter - (n) | masséter | massetere | masetero | Musculus masseter | 咀嚼筋 |
| 4022. mastectomy - (n) | mastectomie | mastectomia | mastectomía | Mastektomie | 乳房切断 [術] 乳房切除 [術] |
| 4023. mastication - (n) | mastication | masticazione | masticación | Kaubewegung | そしゃく |
| 4024. mastoid - (n) | mastoïde | mastoide | mastoides | Mastoid | 乳様突起 |
| 4025. mastoid - (a) | mastoïdien | mastoideo; della mastoide | mastoideo | Mastoid-; warzenförmig | 乳頭様の. 乳頭様の. |
| 4026. mastoid cells - (n) | cellules mastoïdiennes | cellule mastoidee | celdas mastoideas | Warzenfortsatzzelle | 乳突蜂巣 |
| 4027. mastoid process - (n) | apophyse mastoïde | processo mastoideo | apófisis mastoidea | Warzenfortsatz | 乳 [様] 実 [起] の 乳様突起 |
| 4028. masturbation - (n) | masturbation | masturbazione | masturbación | Onanie; Masturbation | オナニー, 自慰 |
| 4029. matched cases - (n) | cas appariés | casi complementari | casos correlacionados | gepaarte Fälle | マッチしている例, 適合例 |
| 4030. matched pair - (n) | paire appariée | coppia contrapposta | par correlacionado | gepaarte Werte | マッチング対 |
| 4031. matched pair analysis - (n) | analyse de paires appariées | analisi a coppie contrapposte | análisis de pares correlacionados | Analyse der gepaarten Werte | マッチング対分析 |
| 4032. matched-pairs design - (n) | style en paires appariées | progetto a coppie contrapposte | diseño de pares correlacionados | Studienentwurf mit gepaarten Werten | マッチング対デザイン |
| 4033. matching placebo - (n) | placebo apparié | placebo contrapposto | placebo correspondiente | gepaarte Placebo | マッチング偽薬 |

| English/American | French/Français | Italian/Italiano | Spanish/Español | German/Deutsch | Japanese/日本語 |
|---|---|---|---|---|---|
| 4034. maternal - (a) | maternel | materno | maternal; materno | maternal; mütterlich | 母性の |
| 4035. maternal-fetal exchange - (n) | échange fœto-maternel | scambio materno-fetale | intercambio materno-fetal | Austausch zwischen Mutter und Fetus | 母体胎児交換 |
| 4036. maternally acquired immunity - (n) | immunité acquise maternellement | immunità acquisita dalla madre | inmunidad adquirida de la madre | durch die Mutter erworbene Immunität | 母体優得免疫 |
| 4037. maternity - (n) | maternité | maternità | maternidad | Maternität; Mutterschaft | 母性 |
| 4038. mathematical model - (n) | modele mathématique | modello matematico | modelo matemático | mathematisches Modell | 数学のモデル |
| 4039. mathematics - (n) | mathématiques | matematica | matemáticas | Mathematik | 数学 |
| 4040. matrix - (n) | matrice | matrice | matriz | Matrix; Grundsubstanz | 床、基質、マトリックス |
| 4041. matter - (n) | matière; substance | materia; sostanza | materia; sustancia | Masse; Substanz | 物質、物体 |
| 4042. maturation -- (n) | maturation | maturazione | maduración | Maturation; Reifung | 成熟 |
| 4043. mature - (v) | mûrir | maturare | madurar | reifen | 成熟する |
| 4044. mature - (a) | mûr | maturo | maduro | reif | 成熟した |
| 4045. maxilla - (n) | maxillaire | mascella | maxilar | Kiefer; Maxilla | 上顎骨 |
| 4046. maxillary - (a) | maxillaire | mascellare | maxilar | maxillar | 上顎［骨］の |
| 4047. maximum - (n) | maximum | massimo | máximo | Maximum | 最大、最高 |
| 4048. maximum tolerated dose - (n) | dose maximale tolérée | massima dose tollerata | dosis máxima tolerada | maximal tolerierte Dosis | 許容極量 |
| 4049. meal - (n) | repas | pasto | comida | Mahlzeit | 食事 |
| 4050. mean - (a) | moyen | medio | media; promedio | mittel; durchschnittlich | 平均の |
| 4051. means - (n) | moyennes; moyens | mezzo; modo | medios | Mittel; Möglichkeit | 手段 |
| 4052. measure - (n) | mesure | misura | medida | Maß; Maßnahme | 寸法、定量 |
| 4053. measure - (v) | mesurer | misurare | medir | messen | 測定する |
| 4054. measurement - (n) | mensuration | misurazione | mensura | Messung | 測定 |
| 4055. meat - (n) | viande | carne | carne | Fleisch | 肉 |

206

| English/American | French/Français | Italian/Italiano | Spanish/Español | German/Deutsch | Japanese/日本語 |
|---|---|---|---|---|---|
| 4056. meatus - (n) | méat; conduit | meato; passaggio | meato | Gang; Meatus | 道 |
| 4057. mechanical - (a) | mécanique | meccanico | mecánico | mechanisch | 構成の |
| 4058. mechanical device - (n) | appareil mécanique | dispositivo meccanico | dispositivo mecánico | mechanisches Gerät | 機械製造装置 |
| 4059. mechanism - (n) | mécanisme | meccanismo | mecanismo | Mechanismus | メカニズム |
| 4060. mechanism of action - (n) | mécanisme d'action | meccanismo d'azione | mecanismo de acción | Wirkungsweise; Wirkmechanismus | 行動のメカニズム |
| 4061. mechano-receptor - (n) | mécanorécepteur | meccanorecettore | mecanorreceptor | Mechanorezeptor | 機械的受容器、力学的受容器 |
| 4062. meconium - (n) | méconium | meconio | meconio | Mekonium | 胎便 |
| 4063. media - (n) | média; tunique moyenne | mezzi tunica media | medios de comunicación; túnica media | Medien; Tunica media | 中膜、媒所 |
| 4064. media culture - (n) | culture médiatique | coltura di mezzi | media de cultivo | Kulturmedium | 培養、培地 |
| 4065. median - (n) | médiane | mediana | punto medio | Zentralwert; Median | 中央値、中数 |
| 4066. median - (a) | médian | mediano | mediana | mittlere; zentral | 正中位の |
| 4067. median eminence - (n) | éminence médiane | eminenza mediana | eminencia media | zentrale Erhebung | 正中隆起 |
| 4068. mediastinum - (n) | médiastin | mediastino | mediastino | Mediastinum | 縦隔 |
| 4069. mediate - (n) | médiateur | mediatore | mediador | Mediator | 仲介人 |
| 4070. mediate - (v) | servir de médiateur | fare da mediatore | mediar | vermitteln | 仲介する、介在する |
| 4071. medical - (a) | médical | medicale; medico | médico | medizinisch; ärztlich | 医学の、医療の |
| 4072. medical chart - (n) | dossier médical | incartamento clinico | carta médica | medizinische Tabelle | 医療チャート |
| 4073. medical department - (n) | département médical | facoltà medica; ufficio medico | departamento de medicina | medizinische Abteilung | 医学部 |
| 4074. medical device - (n) | appareil médical | dispositivo medico | dispositivo médico | medizintechnisches Gerät | 医療器具 |
| 4075. medical director - (n) | directeur médical | direttore medico | director médico | medizinischer Direktor | 医療ディレクター |

207

| English/American | French/Français | Italian/Italiano | Spanish/Español | German/Deutsch | Japanese/日本語 |
|---|---|---|---|---|---|
| 4076. medical history - (n) | histoire médicale | anamnesi medica | historia médica | Krankengeschichte; Anamnese | 病歴 |
| 4077. medical need - (n) | besoin médical | bisogni sanitari | necesidad médica | medizinische Notwendigkeit | 医療の必要性 |
| 4078. medical practice - (n) | pratique médicale | pratica medica | práctica de medicina | medizinische Praxis; praktische Medizin | （医師の）開業 |
| 4079. medical record - (n) | dossier médical | cartella medica | registro médico | Krankenbericht | 医療記録 |
| 4080. medical report - (n) | rapport médical | rapporto medico | informe médico | Arztbericht | 医療報告書 |
| 4081. medical research organization - (n) | organisation de recherche médicale | organizzazione per la ricerca medica | organización de investigación médica | medizinische Forschungseinrichtung | 医療研究機関 |
| 4082. medical school - (n) | faculté de médecine | facoltà di medicina | facultad de medicina | medizinische Fakultät | 医科大学 |
| 4083. medical specialty - (n) | spécialité médical | specialità clinica | especialidad médica | medizinisches Spezialgebiet | 医療専門 |
| 4084. medically underserved area - (n) | zone médicalement mal desservie | area a scarso sviluppo sanitario | área con atención médica insuficiente | Gebiet mit unzureichender ärztlicher Versorgung | 医療の充実していない地域 |
| 4085. medically uninsured - (a) | sans assurance médicale | privo di assicurazione medica | sin seguro médico | ohne Krankenversicherung | 医療保険のない |
| 4086. medicament - (n) | médicament | medicamento | medicamento | Medikament | 医薬 |
| 4087. medicated - (a) | médicalisé; médicamenteux | medicato | medicado | Arzneistoffe enthaltend | 薬物を添加した |
| 4088. medication - (n) | médication; médicament | medicazione | medicación | Medikation; medikamentöse Behandlung | 投薬［法］、薬剤 |
| 4089. medicinal - (a) | médicinal | medicinale | medicinal | medikamentös; medizinisch | 医薬の |

208

| English/American | French/Français | Italian/Italiano | Spanish/Español | German/Deutsch | Japanese/日本語 |
|---|---|---|---|---|---|
| 4090. medicinal chemistry - (n) | chimie médicinale | chimica medicinale | química medicinal | medizinische Chemie | 薬用化学 |
| 4091. medicinal plant - (n) | plante médicinale | pianta medicinale | planta medicinal | Arzneikraut; Arzneipflanze | 薬草 |
| 4092. medicine - (n) | médecine; drogue | medicina; farmaco | medicina; droga | Medizin | 薬剤, 医学, 医療 |
| 4093. medicine development - (n) | développement en médecine | sviluppo della medicina | desarrollo de la medicina | Medikamententwicklung | 薬品の開発 |
| 4094. medium - (n) | milieu; moyen | mezzo | medio | Mittel; Medium | 培地 |
| 4095. medulla oblongata - (n) | bulbe rachidien | midollo allungato; bolbo | bulbo raquídeo | verlängertes Mark; Nachhirn | 延髄 |
| 4096. meeting - (n) | réunion | riunione | reunión | Versammlung; Besprechung | 会合 |
| 4097. megaloblastic anemia - (n) | anémie mégaloblastique | anemia megaloblastica | anemia megaloblástica | megaloblastische Anämie | 巨赤芽球性貧血 |
| 4098. megalomania - (n) | mégalomanie | megalomania | megalomanía | Megalomanie; Größenwahn | 誇大妄想 |
| 4099. meiosis - (n) | méiose | meiosi | meiosis | Meiose | 減数分裂 |
| 4100. melancholia - (n) | mélancolie | malinconia | melancolía | Melancholie; endogene Depression | メランコリー、うつ病 |
| 4101. melanin - (n) | mélanine | melanina | melanina | Melanin | メラニン |
| 4102. melanocyte - (n) | mélanocyte | melanocito | melanocito | Melanozyt | メラノサイト |
| 4103. melanoma - (n) | mélanome | melanoma | melanoma | Melanom | 黒色腫 |
| 4104. melena - (n) | méléna; melæna | melena | melena | Melaena | メレナ |
| 4105. member - (n) | membre | membro | miembro | Mitglied; Gliedmaße | 会員, 四肢 |
| 4106. member state - (n) | pays membre | paese membro | país miembro | Mitgliedstaat | 会員状態 |
| 4107. membrane - (n) | membrane | membrana | membrana | Membran | 膜 |
| 4108. membrane permeability - (n) | perméabilité membranaire | permeabilità della membrana | permeabilidad de la membrana | Membranpermeabilität | 膜浸透性 |

209

| English/American | French/Français | Italian/Italiano | Spanish/Español | German/Deutsch | Japanese/日本語 |
|---|---|---|---|---|---|
| 4109. membrane potential - (n) | potentiel de membrane | potenziale di membrana | potencial de la membrana | Membranpotential | 膜電位 |
| 4110. membranous - (a) | membraneux; membrané | membranoso | membranoso | membranös; membranartig | 膜性の |
| 4111. memory - (n) | mémoire | memoria | memoria | Gedächtnis | 記憶力 |
| 4112. memory loss - (n) | perte de mémoire | perdita della memoria | pérdida de la memoria | Erinnerungslücke | 記憶力の喪失 |
| 4113. menarche - (n) | ménarche | menarca | menarca | Menarche | 初経、初潮 |
| 4114. Mendelian trait - (n) | trait mendélien | tratto mendeliano | herencia mendeliana | Mendelsches Merkmal | メンデルの形質 |
| 4115. meningeal - (a) | méningé | meningeo | meníngeo | meningeal | [脳軟]髄膜の |
| 4116. meninges [cerebral] - (n) | méninges (cérébrales) | meningi (encefaliche) | meninges (del encéfalo) | Meningen; Gehirnhäute | 脳膜 |
| 4117. meninges [spinal] - (n) | méninges (spinales) | meningi (spinali) | meninges (de la médula espinal) | Rückenmarkshäute | 髄膜 |
| 4118. meningismus, meningism - (n) | méningisme | meningismo | meningismo | Meningismus | 髄膜症 |
| 4119. meningitis - (n) | méningite | meningite | meningitis | Meningitis | 髄膜炎 |
| 4120. meniscus - (n) | ménisque | menisco | menisco | Meniskus | 半月、半月[板] |
| 4121. menopause - (n) | ménopause | menopausa | menopausia | Menopause | 閉経期、月経閉止[期] |
| 4122. menorrhagia - (n) | ménorragie | menorragia | menorragia | Menorrhagie | 月経過多 |
| 4123. menses - (n) | menstrues; menstruation | mestruazione | menstruación | Menses; Menstruation | 月経 |
| 4124. menstrual cycle - (n) | cycle menstruel | ciclo mestruale | ciclo menstrual | Menstruationszyklus | 月経周期 |
| 4125. menstruate - (v) | avoir sa menstruation | mestruare | menstruar | menstruieren | 月経がある |
| 4126. menstruation - (n) | menstruation | mestruazione | menstruación | Menstruation | 月経 |
| 4127. mental - (a) | mental | mentale | mental | psychisch; geistig | 精神[的]の |
| 4128. mental age - (n) | âge mental | età mentale | edad mental | geistes Alter | 精神年令 |
| 4129. mental confusion - (n) | confusion mentale | confusione mentale | confusión mental | geistige Verwirrung | 精神錯乱 |

| English/American | French/Français | Italian/Italiano | Spanish/Español | German/Deutsch | Japanese/日本語 |
|---|---|---|---|---|---|
| 4130. mental deficiency - (n) | déficience mentale | ritardo mentale | deficiencia mental | geistige Retardierung | 精神薄弱 |
| 4131. mental disorder - (n) | désordre mental | disturbo mentale | trastorno mental | Geistesstörung | 精神障害 |
| 4132. mental health - (n) | santé mentale | salute mentale; sanità mentale | salud mental | geistige Gesundheit | 精神衛生 |
| 4133. mental health center - (n) | centre de santé mentale | centro sanità mentale | centro de la salud mental | Zentrum für psychische Krankheiten | 精神衛生センター |
| 4134. mental health service - (n) | service de santé mentale | servizio sanità mentale | servicio de la salud mental | psychisches Gesundheitswesen | 精神衛生サービス |
| 4135. mental illness - (n) | maladie mentale | malattia mentale | enfermedad mental | Geisteskrankheit | 精神病 |
| 4136. mental retardation - (n) | retard mental; arriération mentale | ritardo mentale | retraso mental | geistige Behinderung | 精神薄弱 |
| 4137. mental status - (n) | état mental | stato mentale | estado mental | Geistesstand | 精神状態 |
| 4138. mentor - (n) | mentor | mentore | mentor | Mentor; treuer Ratgeber | 指導者 |
| 4139. mercury - (n) | mercure | mercurio | mercurio | Quecksilber | 水銀 |
| 4140. mercury poisoning - (n) | intoxication au mercure; hydrargyrisme | intossicazione da mercurio; mercurialismo | envenenamiento por mercurio | Quecksilbervergiftung | 水銀中毒 |
| 4141. mesencepha-lon - (n) | mésencéphale | mesencefalo | mesencéfalo | Mesencephalon | 中脳 |
| 4142. mesentery - (n) | mésentère | mesentere | mesenterio | Gekröse; Mesenterium | 腸間膜 |
| 4143. mesmerize - (v) | hypnotiser | mesmerizzare | hipnotizar | hypnotisieren; bannen | 催眠誘導する |
| 4144. mesomorph - (n) | mésomorphe | mesomorfo | mesomorfo | menschlicher Körpertyp mittlerer Größe | 中胚葉型 |
| 4145. mesothelium - (n) | mésothélium | mesotelio | mesotelio | Mesothel | 中皮 |
| 4146. messenger RNA - (n) | ARN messager; acide ribonucléique messager | ARN messaggero | ARN mensajero; ácido ribonucleico mensajero | Boten-RNS; Messenger-Ribonukleinsäure | メッセンジャーＲＮＡ |
| 4147. meta-analysis - (n) | méta-analyse | meta analisi | metanálisis | Meta-analyse | メタ分析 |

211

| English/American | French/Français | Italian/Italiano | Spanish/Español | German/Deutsch | Japanese/日本語 |
|---|---|---|---|---|---|
| 4148. metabolic - (a) | métabolique | metabolico | metabólico | metabolisch; Stoffwechsel- | [物質] 代謝の |
| 4149. metabolic disorder - (n) | désordre métabolique | disordine metabolico; dismetabolismo | trastorno metabólico | Stoffwechselstörung | 代謝障害 |
| 4150. metabolic pathway - (n) | voie métabolique | via metabolica | vía metabólica | Stoffwechselweg | 代謝経路 |
| 4151. metabolism - (n) | métabolisme | metabolismo | metabolismo | Metabolismus; Stoffwechsel | 代謝作用 |
| 4152. metabolite - (n) | métabolite | metabolita | metabolito | Metabolit | 代謝産物 |
| 4153. metabolize - (v) | transformer métaboliquement | metabolizzare | metabolizar | metabolisieren | 代謝する |
| 4154. metacarpal - (a) | métacarpien | metacarpico; metacarpale | metacarpiano | metakarpal | 中手 [骨] の |
| 4155. metal - (n) | métal | metallo | metal | Metall | 金属 |
| 4156. metal - (a) | métallique; de métal | metallico | metálico; de metal | metallisch | 金属の |
| 4157. metallic taste - (n) | goût métal; goût métallique | sapore metallico | gusto metálico | metallischer Geschmack | 金属的な味 |
| 4158. metamorphosis - (n) | métamorphose | metamorfosi | metamorfosis | Metamorphose | 変質 |
| 4159. metaphase - (n) | métaphase | metafase | metafase | Metaphase | 核分裂の中期 |
| 4160. metaphor - (n) | métaphore | metafora | metáfora | Metapher | 隠喩 |
| 4161. metastasis - (n) | métastase | metastasi | metástasis | Metastase | 転移 |
| 4162. metastatic - (a) | métastatique | metastatico | metastático | metastasisch | 転移の |
| 4163. meter - (n) | mètre; compteur | metro; contatore | metro; contador | Meter; Meßgerät | メートル |
| 4164. methemoglobin - (n) | méthémoglobine | metemoglobina | metahemoglobina | Methämoglobin | メトヘモグロビン |
| 4165. method - (n) | méthode | metodo; processo | método | Methode; Verfahren | 方法 |
| 4166. methylation - (n) | méthylation | metilazione | metilación | Methylierung | メチル化 |

212

| English/American | French/Français | Italian/Italiano | Spanish/Español | German/Deutsch | Japanese/日本語 |
|---|---|---|---|---|---|
| 4167. microbe - (n) | microbe | microbo | microbio | Mikrobe; Mikroorganismus | 微生物 |
| 4168. microbial colony count - (n) | décompte des colonies microbiennes | conto colonie microbiche | contec de las colonias microbianas | Anzahl der Bakterienkolonien | 微生物のコロニーカウント |
| 4169. microbial sensitivity test - (n) | épreuve de sensibilité microbienne | test di sensibilità microbica | prueba de sensibilidad microbiana | Test der Bakterienempfindlichkeit | 微生物感受性検査 |
| 4170. microbiologist - (n) | microbiologiste | microbiologo | microbiólogo | Mikrobiologe | 微生物学者 |
| 4171. microbiology - (n) | microbiologie | microbiologia | microbiología | Mikrobiologie | 微生物学 |
| 4172. microbody - (n) | corps microscopique | microcorpo | microcuerpo | Microbody; Zytosom | マイクロボディ |
| 4173. microcephalic - (a) | microcéphale | microcefalo; microcefalico | microcéfalico | kleinköpfig | 小頭[蓋]の |
| 4174. microcirculation - (n) | microcirculation | microcircolazione | microcirculación | Mikrozirkulation | 微小循環 |
| 4175. microcomputer - (n) | micro-ordinateur | microcalcolatore | microcomputadora | Mikrocomputer | マイクロコンピューター |
| 4176. microelectrode - (n) | micro-électrode | microelettrodo | microelectrodo | Mikroelektrode | 微小電極 |
| 4177. microfiche - (n) | microfiche | microfiche; microscheda trasparente | microficha; microcopia | Mikrofiche; Mikrokarte | マイクロフィッシュ |
| 4178. microinjection - (n) | micro-injection | microinoculazione | microinyección | Mikroinjektion | 微小注入 |
| 4179. micron - (n) | micron | micron | micrón | Mikron; Mikrometer | ミクロン |
| 4180. microorganism - (n) | micro-organisme | microrganismo | microorganismo | Mikroorganismus | 微生物 |
| 4181. microscope - (n) | microscope | microscopio | microscopio | Mikroskop | 顕微鏡 |
| 4182. microscopic examination - (n) | examen à microscope | esame al microscopio | examen al microscopio | mikroskopische Untersuchung | 顕微鏡検査 |

| English/American | French/Français | Italian/Italiano | Spanish/Español | German/Deutsch | Japanese/日本語 |
|---|---|---|---|---|---|
| 4183. microscopic hematuria - (n) | hématurie microscopique | ematuria microscopica | hematuria microscópica | Mikrohämaturie | 顕微 [鏡的] 血尿 |
| 4184. microscopy - (n) | microscopie | microscopia | microscopia | Mikroskopie | 顕微鏡検査 [法] |
| 4185. microsome - (n) | microsome | microsoma | microsoma | Mikrosom | 微粒体 |
| 4186. microsphere - (n) | microsphère | microsfera | microsfera | Mikrosphäre | 中心体 |
| 4187. microsurgery - (n) | microchirurgie | microchirurgia | microcirugía | Mikrochirurgie | 顕微手術、顕微外科 |
| 4188. microtome - (n) | microtome | microtomo | micrótomo | Mikrotom | ミクロトーム |
| 4189. microtubule - (n) | microtubule | microtubulo | microtúbulo | Mikrotubulus | 微小管 |
| 4190. micro-vascular - (a) | microvasculaire | microvascolare | microvascular | mikrovascular; Mikrogefäß- | 微小血管の |
| 4191. microvilli - (n) | microvilli | microvilli | microvellosidades | Mikrovilli | 微 [小] 絨毛 |
| 4192. microwave - (n) | micro-onde | microonda | microonda | Mikrowelle | マイクロ波、極超短波 |
| 4193. micturate - (v) | uriner | orinare; urinare | orinar | urinieren | 放尿する |
| 4194. midbrain - (n) | mésencéphale | mesencefalo | mesencéfalo | Mittelhirn; Mesencephalon | 中脳 |
| 4195. midday dose - (n) | dose du midi | dose di mezzogiorno | dosis del medio día | mittägliche Dosis | 日中の投薬 |
| 4196. middle - (a) | (au) milieu; moyen | medio; mediano | medio; central | Mittel- | 中間の |
| 4197. middle ear - (n) | oreille moyenne | orecchio medio | oído medio | Mittelohr | 中耳 |
| 4198. middle-aged - (a) | d'un certain âge; d'âge moyen | di mezza età | de edad media; de mediana edad | in den mittleren Jahren; mittleren Alters | 中年の |
| 4199. midline - (n) | ligne moyenne | linea mediana | línea media | Mittellinie; Med anebene | 中線 |
| 4200. mid-range - (n) | portée moyenne | gamma media | alcance medio | Im mittleren Bere:ch der Spanne | 中間の範囲 |
| 4201. midwife - (n) | sage-femme | ostetrica | comadrona | Hebamme | 助産婦 |
| 4202. migraine - (n) | migraine | emicrania; cefalea | migraña; jaqueca | Migräne | 片頭痛 |
| 4203. migrant - (a) | migrateur | migratore; migrante | migratorio | wandernd; Migrations- | 移住性の |
| 4204. migration - (n) | migration | migrazione | migración | Migration; Wa⁻derung | 移動 |
| 4205. migratory - (a) | migratoire | migratore; migrante | migratorio | wandernd | 移動性の |

214

| English/American | French/Français | Italian/Italiano | Spanish/Español | German/Deutsch | Japanese/日本語 |
|---|---|---|---|---|---|
| 4206. migratory pain - (n) | douleur migratoire | dolore migrante | dolor migratorio | Wanderschmerz | 移動性の痛み |
| 4207. mild - (a) | doux; léger | leggero; moderato; lieve | suave; leve | mild; geringgradig | 柔らかな、軽い |
| 4208. milestone - (n) | borne | pietra miliare | hito | Meilenstein | 画期的事件 |
| 4209. miliary lesion - (n) | lésion miliaire | lesione miliare | lesión miliar | Miliarverletzung; hirsekornartige Läsion | 粟粒病巣 |
| 4210. milieu - (n) | milieu | ambiente | ambiente | Milieu; Umgebung | 環境 |
| 4211. military - (n) | militaire; armée | militare | militar | Militär | 軍隊 |
| 4212. milk - (n) | lait | latte | leche | Milch | 乳 |
| 4213. milligram (milligramme) - (n) | milligramme | milligrammo | miligramo | Milligramm | ミリグラム |
| 4214. millimeter (millimetre) - (n) | millimètre | millimetro | milímetro | Millimeter | ミリメートル |
| 4215. mind - (n) | esprit; pensée | mente | mente | Geist; Gedächtnis | 精神、心 |
| 4216. mineral - (n) | minéral | minerale | mineral | Mineral | 無機質、鉱質 |
| 4217. mineral - (a) | minéral | minerale | mineral | mineralisch | 無機質の |
| 4218. mineralocorticoid - (n) | minéralocorticoïde | mineralocorticoide | mineralocorticoide | Mineralokortikoid | 鉱質コルチコイド |
| 4219. miniaturization - (n) | miniaturisation | miniaturizzazione | miniaturización | Miniaturisierung | 小型化 |
| 4220. minimum - (n) | minimum | minimo | mínimo | Minimum | 最小量 |
| 4221. minor error - (n) | erreur mineuse | errore minore | error mínimo | geringgradiger Fehler | 小さい過ち |
| 4222. minority group - (n) | groupe minoritaire | minoranza | minoría; grupo minoritario | Minderheit | 少数民族、小数者集団 |
| 4223. miosis - (n) | myosis | miosi | miosis | Miose; Miosis | 縮瞳、軽減期 |
| 4224. miotic - (a) | myotique | miotico | miótico | miotisch | 縮瞳の |
| 4225. misanthropy - (n) | misanthropie | misantropia | misantropia | Misanthropie; Menschenfeindlichkeit | 人間嫌い |

215

| English/American | French/Français | Italian/Italiano | Spanish/Español | German/Deutsch | Japanese/日本語 |
|---|---|---|---|---|---|
| 4226. miscarriage - (n) | fausse couche; avortement | aborto; gravidanza interrotta | aborto (espontáneo) | Spontanabort; Fehlgeburt | 流産 |
| 4227. miscegenation - (n) | croisement entre races | incrocio di razze | miscegenación | Rassenmischung | 異種族間結婚 |
| 4228. miscible - (a) | miscible | miscibile; mescolabile | miscible | mischbar | 混和性の |
| 4229. misconduct - (n) | inconduite | cattiva condotta | mala conducta | schlechtes Benehmen; Berufsvergehen | 不正行為 |
| 4230. misinterpretation - (n) | mauvaise interprétation | interpretazione errata | mala interpretación | Fehldeutung; Fehlinterpretation | 誤解、誤訳 |
| 4231. misogamy - (n) | misogamie | misogamia | misogamia | Misogamie; Ehefeindlichkeit | 結婚嫌い |
| 4232. misogyny - (n) | misogynie | misoginia | misoginia | Misogynie; Frauenhaß | 女嫌い |
| 4233. missed visit - (n) | visite manquée | visita mancata | pérdida del turno médico | Untersuchungstermin verpaßter | 来院しなかったこと |
| 4234. misshapen - (a) | difforme; déformé | deforme; malfatto | deforme | unförmig; mißgestaltet | 奇形の |
| 4235. missing - (a) | manquant | mancante | ausente; perdido | fehlend | 行方不明の |
| 4236. mission - (n) | mission | missione | misión | Auftrag | 任務 |
| 4237. misuse - (n) | mauvais usage | uso improprio | mal uso; abuso | Mißbrauch | 誤用 |
| 4238. misuse - (v) | faire mauvais usage | usare impropriamente | maltratar | mißbrauchen | 誤用する |
| 4239. mite - (n) | mite | acaro | ácaro | Milbe | ダニ |
| 4240. mitochondria - (n) | mitochondrie | mitocondri | mitocondria | Mitochondrien | ミトコンドリア |
| 4241. mitochondrial - (a) | mitochondrial | mitocondriale | mitocondrial | mitochondrial | ミトコンドリアの |
| 4242. mitogen - (n) | mitogène | mitogeno | mitógeno | mitogene Substanz | ミトゲン |
| 4243. mitogen receptor - (n) | récepteur mitogène | recettore mitogeno | receptor mitógeno | mitogener Rezeptor | ミトゲンレセプター |
| 4244. mitosis - (n) | mitose | mitosi | mitosis | Mitose | 有糸分裂 |
| 4245. mitotic - (a) | mitotique | mitotico | mitótico | mitotisch | 有糸分裂の |
| 4246. mitotic spindle apparatus - (n) | appareil fusiforme mitotique | apparato di fuso mitotico | aparato del uso mitótico | Mitosespindel; Zellteilungsspindel | ［有糸分裂］紡錘体 |

| English/American | French/Français | Italian/Italiano | Spanish/Español | German/Deutsch | Japanese/日本語 |
|---|---|---|---|---|---|
| 4247. mitral - (a) | mitral | mitrale | mitral | mitral; mitralis | 僧帽弁の、僧帽の |
| 4248. mitral insufficiency - (n) | insuffisance mitrale | insufficienza mitralica | insuficiencia mitral | Mitralklappeninsuffizienz | 僧帽弁閉鎖不全症 |
| 4249. mitral stenosis - (n) | sténose mitrale | stenosi mitralica | estenosis mitral | Mitralstenose | 僧帽弁狭窄症 |
| 4250. mitral valve - (n) | valve mitrale | valvola mitrale | válvula mitral | Mitralklappe | 僧帽弁 |
| 4251. Mittel- schmerz - (n) | crise intermenstruelle | dolore intermestruale | dolor intermenstrual | Mittelschmerz | 中間痛 |
| 4252. mixed - (a) | mélangé; mêlé | misto | mixto; mezclado | gemischt; Misch-gemischter | 混合の |
| 4253. mixed lymphocyte culture test - (n) | épreuve de culture lymphocytaire mixte | test delle colture linfocitarie miste | prueba de cultivo mixto linfocitario | Lymphozyten-Kultur-Test | リンパ球混合培養試験 |
| 4254. mixing - (n) | mélange; préparation | mescolatura | mezcla; preparación | Mischen | 混合 |
| 4255. mobile health unit - (n) | unité mobile de santé | centro mobile per la salute | unidad móvil de atención de la salud | mobile Kranken-versorgungseinheit | 移動保健部 |
| 4256. mobility - (n) | mobilité | mobilità | movilidad | Mobilität; Beweglichkeit | 可動性 |
| 4257. modality - (n) | modalité | modalità | modalidad | Modalität | 様式、感覚 |
| 4258. mode - (n) | mode | moda | modo | Art; Modus | 最頻値、モード |
| 4259. model - (n) | modèle | modello | modelo | Muster; Modell | 標準型、鋳型、モデル |
| 4260. model case - (n) | cas modèle | caso modello | caso modelo | Musterfall | 模範例 |
| 4261. moderate - (v) | modérer | moderare | moderar | mäßigen | 和らげる |
| 4262. moderate - (a) | modéré | moderato | moderado | mäßig; moderat | 適度の |
| 4263. modified - (a) | modifié | modificato | modificado | modifiziert; abgeändert | 修飾された |
| 4264. moist rales - (n) | râles humides | rantoli umidi | estertores húmedos | feuchte Rasselgeräusche | 湿性雑音 |
| 4265. moisture - (n) | humidité | umidità | humedad | Feuchtigkeit | 湿気 |
| 4266. molar - (n) | molaire | molare | molar | Molar; Backenzahn | 摩砕、臼歯、モル濃度 |
| 4267. mold - (n) | moule; moisissure | forma; stampo; muffa | molde; moho | Gußform; Schimmel | カビ、鋳状菌、型 |
| 4268. mole - (n) | môle; mole | nevo; mole; grammomolecola | mola; mol | Muttermal; Nävus; Mole | 黒あざ、モル |

217

| English/American | French/Français | Italian/Italiano | Spanish/Español | German/Deutsch | Japanese/日本語 |
|---|---|---|---|---|---|
| 4269. molecular - (a) | moléculaire | molecolare | molecular | molekular | 分子の |
| 4270. molecular biology - (n) | biologie moléculaire | biologia molecolare | biología molecular | Molekularbiologie | 分子生物学 |
| 4271. molecular weight - (n) | poids moléculaire | peso molecolare | peso molecular | Molekulargewicht | 分子量 |
| 4272. molecule - (n) | molécule | molecola | molécula | Molekül | 分子 |
| 4273. moniliasis - (n) | moniliase | moniliasi | moniliasis | Moniliasis | カンジダ症、モニリア症 |
| 4274. monitor - (n) | moniteur | monitor; schermo | monitor; supervisor | Monitor; Überwacher | 監視、監督者 |
| 4275. monitor - (v) | surveiller | monitorare; controllare | monitorear; supervisar | überwachen | 監視する |
| 4276. monitoring - (n) | monitorage; surveillance continue | monitoraggio; controllo | monitoreo; supervisión | Überwachung | 監視 |
| 4277. monitoring visit - (n) | visite de surveillance | visite di controllo | visita de monitoreo; visita de supervisión | Überwachungsuntersuchung | 監視下の来院（往診） |
| 4278. monitor's visit log - (n) | registre de visites de moniteur | giornale di visite di controllo | registro de visitas de monitoreo | Protokoll der Arztbesuche des Überwachers | 監視者の来院日誌 |
| 4279. monoclonal - (a) | monoclonal | monoclonale | monoclonal | monoklonal | 単［一］クローン［系］の |
| 4280. monoclonal antibody - (n) | anticorps monoclonal | anticorpo monoclonale | anticuerpo monoclonal | monoklonaler Antikörper | モノクローナル抗体 |
| 4281. monocyte - (n) | monocyte | monocita | monocito | Monozyt | 単球、単核細胞 |
| 4282. monomania - (n) | monomanie | monomania | monomanía | Monomanie | モノマニー、偏執狂 |
| 4283. monotherapy - (n) | monothérapie | monoterapia | monoterapia | Monotherapie | 単一薬品による治療 |
| 4284. monounsaturated - (a) | monoinsaturé | monoinsaturo | monoinsaturado | einfach ungesättigt | 単不飽和の |
| 4285. monozygotic - (a) | monozygote | monozigotico | monocigótico | monozygot | 一卵［性］の、単一接合子の |
| 4286. month - (n) | mois | mese | mes | Monat | 月、一か月 |
| 4287. moon face - (n) | faciès lunaire | facies lunare | facies lunar | Vollmondgesicht | 満月状（満月様）顔［貌］ |
| 4288. moral - (a) | moral | morale | moral | moralisch | 精神的な |

| English/American | French/Français | Italian/Italiano | Spanish/Español | German/Deutsch | Japanese/日本語 |
|---|---|---|---|---|---|
| 4289. morale - (n) | moral | morale; spirito | moral | Moral | 鳳紀 |
| 4290. morbid - (a) | morbide; pathologique | morboso; patologico | mórbido | morbid | 病的な |
| 4291. morbid obesity - (n) | obésité morbide; obésité pathologique | obesità patologica | obesidad mórbida | krankhafte Fettsucht | 病的肥満 |
| 4292. morbidity - (n) | morbidité | morbilità | morbididad | Morbidität | 病的状態、罹病率 |
| 4293. morbilliform rash - (n) | éruption morbilliforme | esantema morbilliforme | erupción morbilliforme | masernähnlicher Ausschlag | 麻疹 |
| 4294. morgue - (n) | morgue | obitorio | morgue | Leichenhalle | モルグ、霊安室 |
| 4295. moribund - (a) | moribond | moribondo | moribundo | moribund | 瀕死の |
| 4296. morning - (n) | matin | mattina | mañana | Morgen | 午前 |
| 4297. morning - (a) | matinal | del mattino; mattutino | de mañana; de madrugada | Morgen-; morgendlich | 午前の |
| 4298. moron - (n) | débile | imbecille; cretino | morón | Geistesschwache(r); Debile(r) | 軽愚 |
| 4299. morose - (a) | morose; maussade | cupo; tetro | malhumorado; hosco | verdrießlich; mißmutig | 気難しい |
| 4300. morphogenesis - (n) | morphogénèse | morfogenesi | morfogénesis | Morphogenese | 形態発生 |
| 4301. morphology - (n) | morphologie | morfologia | morfología | Morphologie | 形態学 |
| 4302. mortal - (a) | mortel | mortale | mortal | sterblich; letal | 致死的の |
| 4303. mortality - (n) | mortalité | mortalità | mortalidad | Mortalität; Sterblichkeit | 死 |
| 4304. mortality rate - (n) | taux de mortalité | tasso di mortalità | tasa de mortalidad | Mortalitätsrate; Sterblichkeitsrate | 死亡率 |
| 4305. mortify - (v) | se gangrener | necrotizzare | gangrenarse | absterben lassen; brandig machen | 壊死にかからせる |
| 4306. mosaic - (n) | mosaïque | mosaico | mosaico | Mosaik | モザイク |
| 4307. mosaicism - (n) | mosaïsme | mosaicismo | mosaiquismo | Mosaik | モザイク現象 |
| 4308. mosquito - (n) | moustique | zanzara | mosquito | Moskito; Stechmücke | 蚊 |
| 4309. motility - (n) | motilité | motilità | movilidad | Motilität; Beweglichkeit | ［自動］運動性 |
| 4310. motion - (n) | mouvement | moto | movimiento | Bewegung | 運動、便通 |

219

| English/American | French/Français | Italian/Italiano | Spanish/Español | German/Deutsch | Japanese/日本語 |
|---|---|---|---|---|---|
| 4311. motion perception - (n) | perception du mouvement | percezione di moto | percepción del movimiento | Bewegungs-wahrnehmung | 運動知覚 |
| 4312. motion sickness - (n) | mal des transports | chinetosi; cinetosi | mareo | Kinetose | 動揺病、乗物酔い |
| 4313. motivation - (n) | motivation | motivazione | motivación | Motivierung; Stimulierung | 動機付け |
| 4314. motor - (a) | moteur | motorio | motor | motorisch | 運動の |
| 4315. motor neuron - (n) | neurone moteur | motoneurone | neurona motora | motorisches Neuron; Motoneuron | 運動神経 |
| 4316. motor paralysis - (n) | paralysie motrice | paralisi motoria | parálisis motora | motorische Lähmung | 運動麻痺 |
| 4317. motor system - (n) | système moteur | sistema motorio | sistema motor | motorisches System | 運動系 |
| 4318. mottled - (a) | tacheté | variegato | manchado | gesprenkelt | 斑紋のある |
| 4319. mourn - (v) | pleurer | lamentare | lamentar | trauern; betrauern | 喪に服する |
| 4320. mouse - (n) | souris | topo; sorcio | ratón | Maus | ハツカネズミ |
| 4321. mouth - (n) | bouche | bocca | boca | Mund | 口 |
| 4322. mouth-to-mouth resuscitation - (n) | respiration bouche à bouche | respirazione bocca a bocca | respiración boca a boca | Mund-zu-Mund-Beatmung | マウスツーマウス人工呼吸法 |
| 4323. movement - (n) | mouvement | moto | movimiento | Bewegung | 動作、排便 |
| 4324. movement disorder - (n) | désordre du mouvement | disordine motorio | trastorno del movimiento | Bewegungsstörung | 運動障害 |
| 4325. moving average - (n) | moyenne mobile | media di movimento | promedio variable | gleitender Durchschnitt | 移動平均［法］ |
| 4326. mu receptor - (n) | récepteur mu | recettore mu | receptor mu | mu-Rezeptor | ミュウレセプター |
| 4327. muco-cutaneous - (a) | muco-cutané | mucocutaneo | mucocutáneo | mukokutan | 粘膜皮膚の |
| 4328. mucoprotein - (n) | mucoprotéine | mucoproteina | mucoproteína | Mukoprotein | ムコ蛋白、粘［性］蛋白 |
| 4329. mucosa - (n) | muqueuse | mucosa | mucosa | Mukosa; Schleimhaut | 粘膜 |
| 4330. mucous - (a) | muqueux | mucoso | mucoso | mukös | 粘液［性］の |

220

| English/American | French/Français | Italian/Italiano | Spanish/Español | German/Deutsch | Japanese/日本語 |
|---|---|---|---|---|---|
| 4331. mucous membrane - (n) | membrane muqueuse | membrana mucosa | membrana mucosa | Schleimhaut | 粘膜 |
| 4332. mucus - (n) | mucus | muco | moco | Mukus; Schleim | 粘液 |
| 4333. mucus discharge - (n) | écoulement de mucus | secrezione mucosa | drenaje de moco | Schleimabsonderung | 粘液性排出物 |
| 4334. muffled heart sounds - (n) | bruits cardiaques assourdis | suoni cardiaci ottusi | ruidos cardiacos distantes | gedämpfte Herztöne | 聞き取れない心音 |
| 4335. multi infarct dementia - (n) | démence par infarcissements multiples | demenza da multi-infarto | demencia por múltiples infartos | Multiinfarktdemenz | 多発脳梗塞性痴呆 |
| 4336. multicenter - (a) | multicentrique | multicentro | multicentrico | an mehreren Zentren | マルチセンター |
| 4337. multicenter trial - (n) | essai multicentrique | prova multicentrica | prueba en multi-centros | multizentrische Studie | マルチセンター試験 |
| 4338. multidose drug trial - (n) | essai médicamenteux multidose | studio farmaco multidose | prueba medicamentosa de múltiples dosis | Versuch mit mehreren Dosierungen | 複数投与の薬品試験 |
| 4339. multidose vial - (n) | ampoule multidose | flacone multidose | ampolla de múltiples dosis | Multidosisphiole | 複数投与分の薬の入ったガラス瓶 |
| 4340. multienzyme complex - (n) | complexe multienzymatique | complesso multienzimatico | complejo multienzimático | Multienzymkomplex | 多酵素複合体 |
| 4341. multigravida - (n) | multipare | plurigravida | multigrávida; plurigrávida | Multigravida | 経妊婦 |
| 4342. multinational - (n) | multinationale | multinazionale | multinacional | multinationaler Konzern | 多国籍企業 |
| 4343. multinational - (a) | multinational | multinazionale | multinacional | multinational | 多国籍の |
| 4344. multinational company - (n) | compagnie multinationale | compagnia multinazionale; società multinazionale | compañía multinacional | multinationale Firma | 多国籍企業 |
| 4345. multipara - (n) | multipare | multipara | multipara | Multipara | 経産婦 |
| 4346. multiple - (a) | multiple | multiplo | múltiple | mehrfach | 多発 [性] の |

221

| English/American | French/Français | Italian/Italiano | Spanish/Español | German/Deutsch | Japanese/日本語 |
|---|---|---|---|---|---|
| 4347. multivariate analysis - (n) | analyse multivariée | analisi multivariata | análisis multivariante | Multivariatanalyse | 多変量解析 |
| 4348. multivariate methods - (n) | méthodes multivariées | metodi multivariati; metodi plurivariati | métodos multivariantes | multivariate Methoden | 多変量方法 |
| 4349. municipal - (a) | municipal | municipale; comunale | municipal | städtisch | 市政の |
| 4350. mural - (a) | mural | murale | mural | mural | 壁の、壁在［性］の |
| 4351. murine - (a) | murin | murino | murino | murin | ネズミの |
| 4352. murmur - (n) | murmure; souffle | soffio | soplo | Geräusch | 雑音 |
| 4353. muscle - (n) | muscle | muscolo | músculo | Muskel | 筋 |
| 4354. muscular - (a) | musculaire | muscolare | muscular | muskular; Muskel- | 筋［性］の |
| 4355. muscular rigidity - (n) | rigidité musculaire | rigidità muscolare | rigidez muscular | Muskelsteife; Muskelhypertonie | 筋硬直 |
| 4356. musculature - (n) | musculature | muscolatura; sistema muscolare | musculatura | Muskulatur | 筋系 |
| 4357. musculoskeletal - (n) | musculosquelettique | muscoloscheletrico | musculoesquelético | muskuloskeletal; Muskel-Skelett- | 筋骨格の |
| 4358. mutagen - (n) | mutagène | agente mutageno; mutageno | mutágeno | Mutagen | 突然変異原、変異誘発物質（因子） |
| 4359. mutagenesis - (n) | mutagénèse | mutagenesi | mutagénesis | Mutagenese | ［突然］変異誘発 |
| 4360. mutagenicity test - (n) | épreuve de mutagénicité | test mutagenetico | prueba de mutagenicidad | Mutagenitätstest | ［突然］変異発性試験 |
| 4361. mutant - (n) | mutant | mutante | mutante | Mutante | ［突然］変異体 |
| 4362. mutant - (a) | mutant | di mutazione | mutante | mutiert | ［突然］変異体の |
| 4363. mutate - (v) | subir une mutation | mutare | mutar | mutieren | ［突然］変異をおこす |
| 4364. mutation - (n) | mutation | mutazione | mutación | Mutation | ［突然］変異 |
| 4365. mute - (a) | muet | muto | mudo | stumm | 唖の |
| 4366. mutilate - (v) | mutiler | mutilare | mutilar | mutilieren; verstümmeln | 断節する |

| English/American | French/Français | Italian/Italiano | Spanish/Español | German/Deutsch | Japanese/日本語 |
|---|---|---|---|---|---|
| | reconnaissance mutuelle | riconoscimento reciproco | reconocimiento mutuo | beiderseitiges Erkennen | 相互認識 |
| 4367. mutual recognition - (n) | | | | | |
| 4368. myalgia - (n) | myalgie | mialgia | mialgia | Myalgie | 筋 [肉] 痛 |
| 4369. myasthenia - (n) | myasthénie | miastenia | miastenia | Myasthenie | 筋無力症 |
| 4370. mycology - (n) | mycologie | micologia | micologia | Mykologie | [真] 菌学 |
| 4371. mycosis - (n) | mycose | micosi | micosis | Mykose | 真菌症 |
| 4372. mydriasis - (n) | mydriase | midriasi | midriasis | Mydriasis | 散瞳、瞳孔散大 |
| 4373. myelin - (n) | myéline | mielina | mielina | Myelin | ミエリン |
| 4374. myelin sheath - (n) | couche de myéline | guaina mielinica | vaina de la mielina | Myelinscheide | ミエリン鞘 |
| 4375. myelinated nerve fiber - (n) | fibre nerveuse myélinisée | fibra nervosa mielinica | fibra nerviosa mielinizada | markhaltige Nervenfaser | 有髄神経繊維 |
| 4376. myelocyte - (n) | myélocyte | mielocita | mielocito | Myelozyt | 骨髄球、ミエロサイト |
| 4377. myelodysplastic syndrome - (n) | syndrome myélodysplastique | sindrome mielodisplastica | sindrome mielodisplástico | myelodysplastisches Syndrom | 脊髄形成異常症 |
| 4378. myeloid leukemia - (n) | leucémie myéloïde | leucemia mieloide | leucemia mieloidea | myeloide Leukämie | 骨髄球性白血病 |
| 4379. myeloma - (n) | myélome | mieloma | mieloma | Myelom; Plasmozytom | 骨髄腫 |
| 4380. myocardial - (a) | myocardique | miocardico | miocárdico | myokardial | 心筋 [層] の |
| 4381. myocardial infarction - (n) | infarctus du myocarde | infarto miocardico | infarto de miocardio | Myokardinfarkt; Herzinfarkt | 心筋梗塞 [症] |
| 4382. myocardial ischemia - (n) | ischémie myocardique | ischemia miocardica | isquemia miocárdica | Myokardischämie | 心筋虚血 |
| 4383. myocarditis - (n) | myocardite | miocardite | miocarditis | Myokarditis | 心筋炎 |
| 4384. myocardium - (n) | myocarde | miocardio | miocardio | Myokard | 心筋層 |
| 4385. myoclonic - (a) | myoclonique | mioclonico | mioclónico | myoklonisch | 間代性筋痙攣の、ミオクロ [ー] ヌスの |
| 4386. myofascial pain syndrome - (n) | syndrome de douleur myofasciale | sindrome dolore miofasciale | sindrome de dolor miofascial | myofasziales Schmerzsyndrom | 筋筋膜疼痛症候群 |

223

| English/American | French/Français | Italian/Italiano | Spanish/Español | German/Deutsch | Japanese/日本語 |
|---|---|---|---|---|---|
| 4387. myoglobin - (n) | myoglobine | mioglobina | mioglobina | Myoglobin | ミオグロビン |
| 4388. myopathy - (n) | myopathie | miopatia | miopatia | Myopathie; Muskelerkrankung | ミオパシー、筋障害 |
| 4389. myopia - (n) | myopie | miopia | miopia | Myopie; Kurzsichtigkeit | 近視 |
| 4390. myxedema - (n) | myxœdème | mixedema | mixedema | Myxödem | 粘膜水腫 |

224

| English/American | French/Français | Italian/Italiano | Spanish/Español | German/Deutsch | Japanese/日本語 |
|---|---|---|---|---|---|
| 4391. n of one trial - (n) | n d'une étude | n di un studio | n de un ensayo | n eines Versuches | 単一サンプルの試験 |
| 4392. nadir - (n) | nadir | nadir | nadir | Nadir; Tiefstpunkt | 天底 |
| 4393. nail - (n) | ongle | unghia | uña | Nagel | 爪 |
| 4394. name - (n) | nom | nome | nombre | Name; Bezeichnung | 名称 |
| 4395. name recognition - (n) | reconnaissance de nom | riconoscimento del nome | reconocimiento de nombre | Namenerkennung | 名前の認識 |
| 4396. narcissism - (n) | narcissisme | narcisismo | narcisismo | Narziß mus | 自己愛、ナルシシズム |
| 4397. narcolepsy - (n) | narcolepsie | narcolessia | narcolepsia | Narkolepsie | ナルコレプシー、睡眠発作 |
| 4398. narcosis - (n) | narcose | narcosi | narcosis | Narkose | 麻酔、昏迷、ナルコーシス |
| 4399. narcotic - (n) | narcotique | narcotico | narcótico | Opiat | 麻酔薬、麻薬 |
| 4400. narcotic - (a) | narcotique | narcotico | narcótico | narkotisch | 麻酔性の |
| 4401. narrowing - (n) | rétrécissement | restringimento | estrechamiento | Verengung | 狭くすること |
| 4402. nasal - (a) | nasal | nasale; del naso | nasal | nasal | 鼻の、鼻側の |
| 4403. nasal passage - (n) | voie nasale | passaggio nasale | fosa nasal | Nasenweg | 鼻道 |
| 4404. nasal septum - (n) | septum nasal | setto nasale | tabique nasal | Nasenseptum | 鼻中隔 |
| 4405. nasal stuffiness - (n) | congestion nasale | congestione nasale | congestión nasal | Nasenverstopfung | 鼻づまり |
| 4406. nascent - (a) | naissant | nascente | naciente | wachsend; entstehend | 生まれようとする、発生期の |
| 4407. nasogastric tube - (n) | tube nasogastrique | tubo nasogastrico | tubo nasogástrico | Nasen-Magen-Sonde | 経鼻胃管 |
| 4408. nasopharyngeal - (a) | nasopharyngien | rinofaringeo | nasofaríngeo | nasopharyngeal | 鼻咽頭の |
| 4409. national health program - (n) | programme de sarté national | programma per la salute nazionale | programa de salud nacional | nationales Gesundheits-fürsorgprogramm | 国家健康プログラム |

| English/American | French/Français | Italian/Italiano | Spanish/Español | German/Deutsch | Japanese/日本語 |
|---|---|---|---|---|---|
| 4410. nationality - (n) | nationalité | nazionalità | nacionalidad | Staatsangehörigkeit; Nationalität | 国籍 |
| 4411. natriuresis - (n) | natriurèse | natriuria | natriuresis | Natriurese | ナトリウム排泄増加 |
| 4412. natriuretic factor - (n) | facteur natriurétique | fattore natriuretico | factor natriurético | natriuretischer Faktor | ナトリウム排泄増加性因子 |
| 4413. natural - (a) | naturel | naturale | natural | natürlich | 自然の |
| 4414. natural disaster - (n) | catastrophe naturelle | disastro naturale | desastre de la naturaleza | Naturkatastrophe | 自然災害 |
| 4415. natural history of disease - (n) | anamnèse naturelle de maladies | anamnesi naturale di malattie | anamnesis natural de enfermedades | normaler Krankheitsverlauf | 病気の一定期間における |
| 4416. natural immunity - (n) | immunité naturelle | immunità naturale | inmunidad natural | angeborene Immunität | 自然な進展 自然免疫 |
| 4417. natural killer cell - (n) | cellule naturelle killer | cellula natural killer | célula natural killer | natürliche Killerzelle | N K細胞 |
| 4418. natural product - (n) | produit naturel | prodotto naturale | producto natural | Naturprodukt | 自然製品 |
| 4419. natural resources - (n) | ressources naturelles | risorse naturale | recursos naturales | Bodenschätze | 自然原料 |
| 4420. natural selection - (n) | sélection naturelle | selezione naturale | selección natural | natürliche Selektion | 自然選択 |
| 4421. nausea - (n) | nausée | nausea | náusea | Brechreiz; Nausea | 悪心、吐気 |
| 4422. navel - (n) | nombril | ombelico | ombligo | Nabel | 臍 |
| 4423. nearsighted - (a) | myope | miope | miope | kurzsichtig | 近視の |
| 4424. nebulizer - (n) | nébuliseur | nebulizzatore; atomizzatore | nebulizador; atomizador | Vernebler | 噴霧器、ネブライザ |
| 4425. neck - (n) | cou | collo | cuello | Hals | 頸 [部] |
| 4426. necrolysis - (n) | nécrolyse | necrolisi | necrólisis | Nekrolyse | 表皮壊死症 |
| 4427. necropsy - (n) | nécropsie | necropsia; necroscopia | necropsia | Nekropsie | 検死 |

226

| English/American | French/Français | Italian/Italiano | Spanish/Español | German/Deutsch | Japanese/日本語 |
|---|---|---|---|---|---|
| 4428. necrosis - (n) | nécrose | necrosi | necrosis | Nekrose | 壊死 |
| 4429. needle - (n) | aiguille | ago | aguja | Nadel | 針 |
| 4430. needle biopsy - (n) | biopsie à l'aiguille | biopsia per ago | biopsia por punción | Nadelbiopsie | 穿刺針生検 |
| 4431. needle histogram - (n) | histogramme à l'aiguille | istogramma a picchi | histograma de punción | Nadelhistogramm | 穿刺針ヒストグラム |
| 4432. needlestick injury - (n) | blessure par aiguille | lesione dalla puntura di un ago | picadura de aguja | Nadelstichverletzung | 穿刺による傷 |
| 4433. negative - (a) | négatif | negativo | negativo | negativ | 陰性の、否定の |
| 4434. negotiations - (n) | négociations | negoziati | negociaciones | Verhandlungen | 交渉 |
| 4435. neonatal - (a) | néonatal | neonatale | neonatal | neonatal; neugeboren | 新生児 [期] の |
| 4436. neonatology - (n) | néonatalogie | neonatologia | neonatología | Neonatologie | 新生児学 |
| 4437. neoplasm - (n) | néoplasme; néoplasie | neoplasma; neoplasia | neoplasma; neoplasia | Neoplasma; Tumor | 腎症、ネフロパシー |
| 4438. neoplastic cell transformation - (n) | transformation cellulaire néoplasique | trasformazione cellulare neoplastica | transformación de la célula neoplásica | neoplastische Zelltransformation | 細胞の癌化 |
| 4439. neovascularization - (n) | néovascularisation | neovascolarizzazione | neovascularización | Gefäßneubildung | 新生血管形成 |
| 4440. nephritis - (n) | néphrite | nefrite | nefritis | Nephritis | 腎炎 |
| 4441. nephrology - (n) | néphrologie | nefrologia | nefrología | Nephrologie | 腎臓病学 |
| 4442. nephron - (n) | néphron | nefrone | nefrona | Nephron | ネフロン |
| 4443. nephropathy - (n) | néphropathie | nefropatia | nefropatía | Nephropathie | 腎症、ネフロパシー |
| 4444. nephrotoxicity - (n) | néphrotoxicité | nefrotossicità | nefrotoxicidad | Nephrotoxizität | 腎毒性 |
| 4445. nerve - (n) | nerf | nervo | nervio | Nerv | 神経 |
| 4446. nerve block - (n) | anesthésie du nerf | blocco del nervo | bloqueo del nervio | Nervenblockade | 神経ブロック |
| 4447. nerve cell - (n) | cellule nerveuse | cellula nervosa | célula nerviosa | Nervenzelle | 神経細胞 |
| 4448. nerve conduction study - (n) | étude de conduction nerveuse | studio delle conduzione nervosa | estudio de la conducción nerviosa | Untersuchung zur Nervenleitung | 神経伝導研究 |
| 4449. nerve ending - (n) | terminaison nerveuse | terminazione nervosa | terminación nerviosa | Nervenendigung | 神経終末 |

227

| English/American | French/Français | Italian/Italiano | Spanish/Español | German/Deutsch | Japanese/日本語 |
|---|---|---|---|---|---|
| 4450. nerve fiber - (n) | fibre nerveuse | fibra nervosa | fibra nerviosa | Nervenfaser | 神経繊維 |
| 4451. nerve impulse - (n) | influx nerveux | impulso nervoso | impulso nervioso | Nervenimpuls | 神経衝動 |
| 4452. nerve root - (n) | racine nerveuse | radice nervosa | raíz nerviosa | Nervenwurzel | 神経根 |
| 4453. nervous - (a) | nerveux | nervoso | nervioso | nervös | 神経の |
| 4454. nervous breakdown - (n) | dépression nerveuse | esaurimento nervoso | colapso nervioso | Nervenzusammenbruch | 神経衰弱 |
| 4455. nervous system - (n) | système nerveux | sistema nervoso | sistema nervioso | Nervensystem | 神経系統 |
| 4456. nervousness - (n) | nervosité | nervosismo | nerviosismo | Nervosität | 神経質 |
| 4457. network - (n) | réseau | rete | red | Netz; Netzwerk | ネットワーク |
| 4458. neural - (a) | neural | neurale | neural | neural | 神経の |
| 4459. neural computer network - (n) | réseau d'ordinateurs | rete neurale di computer | red de computadoras | Computernetzwerk | 神経コンピューターネットワーク |
| 4460. neural tube defect - (n) | défaut du tube neural | difetto del tubo neurale | defecto del tubo neural | Neuralrohrdefekt | 神経管欠損 |
| 4461. neuralgia - (n) | névralgie | nevralgia | neuralgia | Neuralgie | 神経痛 |
| 4462. neurogenic bladder - (n) | vessie neurogène | vescica neurogena | vejiga neurogénica | neurogene Blase | 神経因性膀胱 [障害] |
| 4463. neuroleptic - (n) | neuroleptique | neurolettico | neuroléptico | Neuroleptikum | 神経弛緩薬 |
| 4464. neurologic - (a) | neurologique | neurologico | neurológico | neurologisch | 神経学の |
| 4465. neurological - (a) | neurologique | neurologico | neurológico | neurologisch | 神経学の |
| 4466. neurology - (n) | neurologie | neurologia | neurología | Neurologie | 神経学 |
| 4467. neuroma - (n) | névrome | neuroma | neuroma | Neurom | 神経腫 |
| 4468. neuromuscular - (a) | neuromusculaire | neuromuscolare | neuromuscular | neuromuskulär | 神経筋の |
| 4469. neuromuscular junction - (n) | jonction neuromusculaire | giunzione neuromuscolare | unión neuromuscular | neuromuskuläre Verbindung | 神経筋接合部 |
| 4470. neuron - (n) | neurone | neurone | neurona | Neuron | ニューロン、神経単位 |

| English/American | French/Français | Italian/Italiano | Spanish/Español | German/Deutsch | Japanese/日本語 |
|---|---|---|---|---|---|
| 4471. neuronal - (a) | neuronal | neuronale | neuronal | neuronal | ニューロンの |
| 4472. neuropathy - (n) | neuropathie | neuropatia | neuropatia | Neuropathie | 神経病 |
| 4473. neuroscience - (n) | neuroscience | neuroscienza | neurociencia | Neurowissenschaft | 神経科学 |
| 4474. neuro-secretory - (a) | neurosécrétoire | neurosecretore | neurosecretorio | neurosekretorisch | 神経分泌の |
| 4475. neurosis - (n) | névrose | nevrosi | neurosis | Neurose | 神経症、ノイローゼ |
| 4476. neurosurgery - (n) | neurochirurgie | neurochirurgia | neurocirugía | Neurochirurgie | 神経外科 |
| 4477. neurotic - (n) | névrotique | nevrotico | neurótico | Neurotiker | 神経症患者 |
| 4478. neurotic - (a) | névrotique | nevrotico | neurótico | neurotisch | 神経病の |
| 4479. neurotoxin - (n) | neurotoxine | neurotossina | neurotoxina | Neurotoxin | 神経毒 |
| 4480. neuro-transmitter - (n) | neurotransmetteur | neurotrasmittitore | neurotransmisor | Neurotransmitter | 神経伝達物質 |
| 4481. neutral - (a) | neutre | neutro | neutro | neutral; wirkungslos | 中性の |
| 4482. neutralization - (n) | neutralisation | neutralizzazione | neutralización | Neutralisierung | 中和 |
| 4483. neutralizing antibody - (n) | anticorps neutralisant | anticorpo neutralizzante | anticuerpo neutralizante | neutralisierender Antikörper | 中和抗体 |
| 4484. neutron - (n) | neutron | neutrone | neutrón | Neutron | 中性子、ニュートロン [症] |
| 4485. neutropenia - (n) | neutropénie | neutropenia | neutropenia | Neutropenie | 好中球減少 [症] |
| 4486. neutrophil - (n) | neutrophile | leucocita neutrofilo | neutrófilo | neutrophiler Leukozyt | 好中球 |
| 4487. nevus - (n) | naevus | nevo; neo | nevus; nevo | Nävus; Muttermal | 母斑 |
| 4488. new chemical entity - (n) | nouvelle entité chimique | nuova entità chimica | nueva entidad química | neue chemische Entität | 新化学実体 |
| 4489. newborn - (a) | nouveau-né | neonato | recién nacido | neugeboren | 新生児の |
| 4490. niche drug - (n) | médicament à usage spécifique | farmaco di uso specifico | medicamento de uso específico | Medikament mit spezifischer Anwendung | ニッシェ |
| 4491. night - (n) | nuit | notte | noche | Nacht | 夜 |
| 4492. night blindness - (n) | héméralopie | nictalopia | ceguera nocturna | Nachtblindheit; Nyktalopie | 夜盲症 |

229

| English/American | French/Français | Italian/Italiano | Spanish/Español | German/Deutsch | Japanese/日本語 |
|---|---|---|---|---|---|
| 4493. night sweat - (n) | sueur nocturne | sudorazione notturna | sudor nocturno | Nachtschweiß | 寝汗 |
| 4494. nightmare - (n) | cauchemar | incubo | pesadilla | Alptraum | 悪夢 |
| 4495. night-time - (n) | nuit | notte; ore notturne | noche | Nacht | 夜間 |
| 4496. nipple - (n) | mamelon | capezzolo | pezón | Mamille; Brustwarze | 乳頭、乳首 |
| 4497. nitrogen - (n) | azote | azoto | nitrógeno | Stickstoff | 窒素 |
| 4498. nociception - (n) | nociception | nocicezione | nocicepción | Nozizeption | 侵害受容 |
| 4499. nociceptor - (n) | nocicepteur | nocicettore | nociceptor | Noziceptor | 侵害受容器 |
| 4500. nocturia - (n) | nycturie | nocturia; nicturia | nocturia | Nykturie | 夜間多尿［症］ |
| 4501. nocturnal - (a) | nocturne; de nuit | notturno; della notte | nocturno | nächtlich | 夜行性の |
| 4502. nodal rhythm - (n) | rythme nodal | ritmo nodale | ritmo nodal | Knotenrhythmus | 結節リズム |
| 4503. node - (n) | nœud | nodo | nudo | Knoten; Nodus | 結節、節 |
| 4504. nodular goiter - (n) | goitre nodulaire | gozzo nodulare; struma nodosa | bocio nodular | Struma nodularis | 結節性甲状腺腫 |
| 4505. nodule - (n) | nodule | nodulo | nódulo | Knötchen; Nod_lus | 小［結］節 |
| 4506. noise - (n) | bruit | rumore | ruido | Geräusch; Rauschen | 雑音 |
| 4507. noisy data - (n) | données parasitaires | dati parassiti | datos parasíticos | gestörte Daten | 不完全データ |
| 4508. nomenclature - (n) | nomenclature | nomenclatura | nomenclatura | Nomenklatur | 組織的命名法 |
| 4509. nominal - (a) | nominal | nominale | nominal | nominell | 名目上の |
| 4510. nominal data - (n) | données nominales | dati nominali | datos nominales | Nominaldaten | 名目データ |
| 4511. nomogram - (n) | nomogramme | nomogramma | nomograma | Nomogramm | ノモグラム |
| 4512. noncompetitive antagonist - (n) | antagoniste non-compétitif | antagonista non competitivo | antagonista no competitivo | nichtkompetitive  Antagonist | 非競合的拮抗質 |
| 4513. noncompli-ance - (n) | opposition; refus | inadempienza | no cumplimiento; falta de cumplimiento | Nichteinhaltung | 不服従 |
| 4514. nondepolarizing agent - (n) | agent non-dépolarisant | agente non depolarizzante | sustancia que no despolariza | nicht depolarisie-rendes Mittel | 非減極薬 |
| 4515. nondrug - (n) | non-médicament | non-droga | no droga | nicht systematisch getestetes Medikament | 薬品でないもの |

| English/American | French/Français | Italian/Italiano | Spanish/Español | German/Deutsch | Japanese/日本語 |
|---|---|---|---|---|---|
| 4516. nonesterified - (a) | non-estérifié | non esterificato | no esterificado | unverestert | エステル化していない |
| 4517. nonevaluable - (a) | non-évaluable | non valutabile | no evaluable | unauswertbar; nicht abschätzbar | 評価できない |
| 4518. non-insulin dependent - (n) | non-insulinodépendant | non dipendente da insulina | no dependiente de la insulina | insulinunabhängig | インスリン非依存性の |
| 4519. noninvasive procedure - (n) | procédure non-invas.ve | procedura non invadente | procedimiento no invasor | nichtinvasives Verfahren | 非侵襲的手法 |
| 4520. nonlinear relationship - (n) | relation non-linéaire | relazione non lineare | relación no lineal | nichtlineare Beziehung | 非線形関係 |
| 4521. nonparametric test - (n) | épreuve non-paramétrique | test non parametrico | prueba no paramétrica | parameterfreies Testverfahren | 非パラメトリック検査 |
| 4522. nonpenetrat-ing - (a) | non-pénétrant | non penetrante | que no penetra | nicht penetrierend | 非浸透性の |
| 4523. nonprescrip-tion - (a) | sans ordonnance | farmaco non prescritto | sin receta | rezeptfrei | 処方箋なしで買える |
| 4524. nonrandom - (a) | non-aléatoire | non a caso | no al azar | nicht zufällig | 無作為抽出でない |
| 4525. non-responder - (n) | non-répondeur | non rispondente | que no responde | Nicht-Responder | 無反応物 |
| 4526. nonspecific factor - (n) | facteur non-spécifique | fattore non specifico | factores no específicos | unspezifischer Faktor | 一般的な要因 |
| 4527. non-steroidal - (a) | non-stéroïdien | non steroideo | no esteroidal | nicht-steroidal | ステロイドでない |
| 4528. nonsupportive results - (n) | résultats sans fondement | risultati non favorevoli | resultados que no respaldan | nicht stützende Ergebnisse | 支援的でない結果 |
| 4529. nonunion - (n) | non-union | frattura non rimarginata | desunión | Nichtvereinigung | 偽関節 |
| 4530. nonverbal communica-tion - (n) | communication non-verbale | comunicazione extraverbale | comunicación no verbal | non-verbale Kommunikation | 非言語的コミュニケーション |
| 4531. nonviable - (a) | non-viable | non vitale | no viable | nicht lebensfähig | 成育不能の |

231

| English/American | French/Français | Italian/Italiano | Spanish/Español | German/Deutsch | Japanese/日本語 |
|---|---|---|---|---|---|
| 4532. noontime - (n) | midi | mezzogiorno | mediodía | Mittagszeit | 正午 |
| 4533. noradrenaline - (n) | noradrénaline | noradrenalina | noradrenalina | Noradrenalin | ノルアドレナリン |
| 4534. nor-adrenergic - (a) | noradrénergique | noradrenergico | noradrenérgico | noradrenerg | ノルアドレナリン作用性の |
| 4535. norepineph-rine - (n) | norépinéphrine | norepinefrina | norepinefrina | Norepinephrin | ノルエピネフリン |
| 4536. normal - (a) | normal | normale | normal | normal | 正常な |
| 4537. normal distribution - (n) | distribution normale | distribuzione normale | distribución normal | Normalverteilung | 正規分布 |
| 4538. normal limits - (n) | limites normales | limiti normali | limites normales | Normalbereich | 正常限界 |
| 4539. normal range - (n) | variations normales | gamma normale | gama normal | Referenzbereich; Normalbreite | 正常範囲 |
| 4540. normalized value - (n) | valeur normalisée | valore normalizzato | valor normalizado | normalisierter Wert | 標準化された値 |
| 4541. normo-chromic - (a) | normochrome | normocromico | normocrómico | normochrom | 正色素性の |
| 4542. normocytic - (a) | normocytaire | normocitico | normocítico | normozytär | 正球性の |
| 4543. normotensive - (a) | normotensif | normoteso | normotenso | normoton | 正常血圧[性]の |
| 4544. northern blot - (n) | analyse Northern blot | analisi di Northern blot | análisis Northern blot | Northern-Blot | ノザンブロット |
| 4545. nose - (n) | nez | naso | nariz | Nase | 鼻 |
| 4546. nosebleed - (n) | saignement de nez; épistaxis | emorragia nasale; epistassi | hemorragia nasal | Nasenbluten; Epistaxis | 鼻血 |
| 4547. nosocomial - (a) | nosocomial | nosocomiale; ospedaliero | nosocomial; hospitalario | nosokomial | 病院の |
| 4548. nosocomial infection - (n) | infection nosocomiale | infezione nosocomiale | infección nosocomial; infección hospitalaria | nosokomiale Infektion; Hospitalismus | 院内感染 |
| 4549. nosology - (n) | nosologie | nosologia | nosología | Nosologie | 疾病分類学 |
| 4550. notification - (n) | notification; annonce | notificazione | notificación; aviso | Meldung | 通知 |

| English/American | French/Français | Italian/Italiano | Spanish/Español | German/Deutsch | Japanese/日本語 |
|---|---|---|---|---|---|
| 4551. no-treatment group - (n) | groupe sans traitement | gruppo senza trattamento | grupo que no recibe tratamiento | nicht behandelte Gruppe | 無治療グループ |
| 4552. novel approach - (n) | nouvelle approche | nuovo approccio | procedimiento nuevo | neuartiger Ansatz | 新奇なアプローチ |
| 4553. noxious - (a) | nocif; nuisible | nocivo; dannoso | nocivo; pernicioso | schädlich | 有害な |
| 4554. nuchal rigidity - (n) | rigidité de la nuque | rigidità nucale | rigidez de la nuca | Nackensteife | 項部強直 |
| 4555. nuclear - (a) | nucléaire | nucleare | nuclear | nuklear; atomar | 核の |
| 4556. nuclear magnetic resonance [abbr] NMR- (n) | résonance magnétique nucléaire | risonanza magnetica nucleare | resonancia magnética nuclear | kernmagnetische Resonanz | 核磁気共鳴 |
| 4557. nuclear reactor - (n) | réacteur nucléaire | reattore nucleare | reactor nuclear | Kernreaktor, Atomreaktor | 原子炉 |
| 4558. nucleic acid - (n) | acide nucléique | acido nucleico | ácido nucléico | Nukleinsäure | 核酸 |
| 4559. nucleolus - (n) | nucléole | nucleolo | nucléolo | Nukleolus | 核小体 |
| 4560. nucleosome - (n) | nucléosome | nucleosoma | nucleosoma | Nukleosom | ヌクレオソーム |
| 4561. nucleus - (n) | nucléus | nucleo | núcleo | Kern; Nucleus | 核 |
| 4562. nude - (a) | nu | nudo | desnudo | nackt | 裸の |
| 4563. null hypothesis - (n) | hypothèse nulle | ipotesi nulla | hipótesis nula | Nullhypothese | 帰無仮説 |
| 4564. numb - (v) | engourdir; endormir | intirizzire; intorpidire | adormecer; anestesiar | betäuben | 麻痺させる |
| 4565. numb - (a) | engourdi; endormi | intirizzito; intorpidito | adormecido | betäubt; gefühllos | 麻痺した |
| 4566. number - (n) | numéro | numero | número | Zahl; Anzahl | 数 |
| 4567. numbness - (n) | engourdissement | intirizzimento; intorpidimento | adomercimiento | Taubheitsgefühl; Betäubung | 麻痺 |
| 4568. numerical analysis - (n) | analyse numérique | analisi numerica | análisis numérico | numerische Analyse | 数値解析 |
| 4569. numerical data - (n) | données numériques | dati numerici | datos numéricos | numerische Daten | 数的データ |

233

| English/American | French/Français | Italian/Italiano | Spanish/Español | German/Deutsch | Japanese/日本語 |
|---|---|---|---|---|---|
| 4570. numerical score - (n) | résultat numérique | risultato numerico | puntuación numérica | numerisches Ergebnis | 点数 |
| 4571. nurse - (n) | infirmier | infermiera; nurse | enfermera | Krankenschwester; Krankenpfleger | 看護婦 |
| 4572. nurse practitioner - (n) | infirmier praticien | infermiera specializzata | auxiliar de enfermería | selbstständiger Krankenpfleger | 実践看護婦 |
| 4573. nursery - (n) | chambre des enfants; garderie | sala neonati | guardería | Neugeborenerstation | 託児所、育児室 |
| 4574. nursing - (n) | profession d'infirmier | professione infermiera | enfermería | Krankenpflege; Säugen | 看護 |
| 4575. nursing home - (n) | maison de soins infirmiers; centre d'accueil | casa di cura; casa di riposo | asilo de ancianos; clínica | Altersheim | 療養院、個人病院 |
| 4576. nutrient - (n) | substance nutritive | sostanza nutriente | nutriente | Nährstoff | 栄養物 |
| 4577. nutriment - (n) | nourriture | nutrimento | nutrimento | Nahrung; Nahrungsmittel | 栄養物 |
| 4578. nutrition - (n) | nutrition | nutrizione | nutrición | Ernährung | 栄養 |
| 4579. nutritional - (a) | nutritionnel | nutrizionale; nutritivo | nutricional | nahrhaft | 栄養の |
| 4580. nutritional disorder - (n) | désordre nutritionnel | disordini della nutrizione | trastorno de la nutrición | Ernährungsstörung | 栄養障害 |
| 4581. nutritional status - (n) | état nutritionnel | stato nutritivo | estado nutricional | Ernährungszustand | 栄養状態 |
| 4582. nutritionist - (n) | nutritionniste | dietista; dietologo | nutricionista | Ernährungs- wissenschaftler | 栄養士 |
| 4583. nutritive value - (n) | valeur nutritive | valore nutritivo | valor nutritivo | Nährwert | 栄養価 |
| 4584. nylon - (n) | nylon | nylon | nilón | Nylon | ナイロン |
| 4585. nystagmus - (n) | nystagmus | nistagmo | nistagmo | Nystagmus | 眼振 |

234

| English/American | French/Français | Italian/Italiano | Spanish/Español | German/Deutsch | Japanese/日本語 |
|---|---|---|---|---|---|
| 4586. obese - (a) | obèse | obeso | obeso | fettleibig | 肥満の |
| 4587. obesity - (n) | obésité | obesità | obesidad | Fettsucht; Obesität | 肥満 [症] |
| 4588. objective - (n) | objectif | oggettivo | objetivo | Ziel; Objektiv | 目的 |
| 4589. objective measurement - (n) | mesure objective | misuramento oggettivo | medida objetiva | objektive Messung | 客観的測定 |
| 4590. obligations of investigators - (n) | obligations des investigateurs | obblighi degli investigatori | obligaciones de los investigadores | Verpflichtungen der Untersucher | 調査者の義務 |
| 4591. obligations of sponsors - (n) | obligations des répondants | obblighi degli sponsors | obligaciones de los patrocinadores | Verpflichtungen der Sponsoren | 主催者の義務 |
| 4592. oblique - (a) | oblique | obliquo | oblicuo; inclinado | schräg | 斜の |
| 4593. observation - (n) | observation | osservazione | observación | Beobachtung | 観察、診察 |
| 4594. observation period - (n) | période d'observation; période de surveillance | periodo di osservazione | periodo de observación | Beobachtungszeitraum | 観察期間 |
| 4595. observational study - (n) | étude d'observation | studio di osservazione | estudio observacional | empirische Studie | 観察研究 |
| 4596. observational unit - (n) | unité d'observation | gruppo di osservazione | unidad de observación | Beobachtungseinheit | 観察室、観察ユニット |
| 4597. observed sample size - (n) | taille d'un échantillon observé | misura campione osservato | tamaño de la muestra observada | beobachtete Stichprobengröße | 観察された試験数 |
| 4598. observer - (n) | observateur | osservatore | observador | Untersucher; Beobachter | 観察者間のばらつき |
| 4599. obsession - (n) | obsession | ossessione | obsesión | Obsession; Zwangsvorstellung | 強迫観念 |
| 4600. obsessive - (a) | obsessionnel | ossessivo | obsesivo | zwanghaft | 強迫的な |
| 4601. obsessive compulsive disorder - (n) | désordre obsédant; névrose obsessionnelle | nevrosi ossessivo-compulsiva | trastorno obsesivo-compulsivo | Zwangserkrankung | 強迫精神病 |
| 4602. obstetrical - (a) | obstétrical | ostetrico | obstétrico | geburtshilflich | 産科学の |
| 4603. obstetrics - (n) | obstétrique | ostetricia | obstetricia | Geburtshilfe | 産科学 |
| 4604. obstruction - (n) | obstruction | ostruzione | obstrucción | Hindernis; Verstopfung | 閉塞 [症] |

235

| English/American | French/Français | Italian/Italiano | Spanish/Español | German/Deutsch | Japanese日本語 |
|---|---|---|---|---|---|
| 4605. obstructive - (a) | obstructif | ostruttivo; da ostruzione | obstructivo | obstruktiv | 閉塞［症］の |
| 4606. obturation - (n) | obturation | otturazione; otturatore | obturación | Obturation; Verschließung | 閉鎖、閉鎖 |
| 4607. occipital - (a) | occipital | occipitale | occipital | okzipital | 後頭部の |
| 4608. occiput - (n) | occiput | occipite | occipucio | Okziput; Hinterhaupt | 後頭部 |
| 4609. occlusion - (n) | occlusion | occlusione | oclusión | Okklusion; Verschluß | 閉鎖 |
| 4610. occlusive - (a) | occlussif | occlusivo | oclusivo | abschließend; okklusiv | 閉塞の |
| 4611. occult - (a) | occulte | occulto | oculto | okkult; verborger | 潜んだ、不顕性の |
| 4612. occult blood - (n) | sang occulte | sangue occulto | sangre oculta | okkultes Blut | 潜血 |
| 4613. occupation - (n) | occupation; profession | professione; occupazione | ocupación; profesión | Beruf | 職業 |
| 4614. occupational - (a) | professionnel; du métier | professionale | ocupacional; profesional | beruflich | 職業の |
| 4615. occupational health - (n) | santé professionnelle | salute professionale | salud ocupacional | Arbeitsmedizin | 職業的健康 |
| 4616. occupational health risk - (n) | risque à la santé professionnelle | rischio della salute professionale | riesgo a la salud ocupacional | berufliches Gesundheitsrisiko | 職業的健康のリスク |
| 4617. occupational therapy - (n) | thérapie occupationnelle | terapia occupazionale | terapia ocupacional | Arbeitstherapie; Beschäftigungstherapie | 作業療法 |
| 4618. ocular - (n) | oculaire | oculare | ocular | Okular | 目 |
| 4619. ocular - (a) | oculaire | oculare | ocular | okular | 眼の |
| 4620. ocular convergence - (n) | convergence oculaire | convergenza oculare | convergencia ocular | okuläre Konvergenz | 眼収束 |
| 4621. oculomotor - (a) | oculomoteur | oculomotore | oculomotor | okulomotorisch | 動眼神経の |
| 4622. odd - (a) | impair; étrange | dispari; insolito | impar; extraño | ungerade; merkwürdig | 奇数の、奇妙な |
| 4623. odds ratio - (n) | risque relatif | rapporto di previsione | relación de probabilidades | Chancenverhältnis | 蓋然性の比率 |
| 4624. odontometry - (n) | odontométrie | odontometria | odontometría | Kieferheilkunde | オドントメトリー、歯の測定［法］ |
| 4625. odor - (n) | odeur | odore | olor | Geruch | 臭気 |

| English/American | French/Français | Italian/Italiano | Spanish/Español | German/Deutsch | Japanese／日本語 |
|---|---|---|---|---|---|
| 4626. offense - (n) | offense; infraction | infrazione; trasgressione; violazione | ofensa; infracción | Vergehen; Verstoß | 罪, 立腹, 攻撃 |
| 4627. office visit - (n) | visite au cabinet | visita in studio | visita al consultorio | Arztbesuch | 来院 |
| 4628. official - (a) | officiel | ufficiale | oficial | amtlich | 公式の |
| 4629. offsite - (a) | extérieur; au loin | fuori sito | fuera del sitio | vom Standort entfernt | 構外の |
| 4630. offspring - (n) | descendant | discendente | descendiente | Nachkommenschaft; Abkömmling | 子孫 |
| 4631. oil - (n) | huile | olio | aceite | Öl | 油 |
| 4632. ointment - (n) | onguent; pommade | unguento; pomata | ungüento; pomada | Salbe | 軟膏 |
| 4633. old - (a) | vieux | vecchio | viejo | alt | 老いた |
| 4634. old age - (n) | vieillesse | età avanzata | vejez | hohes Alter | 老年 |
| 4635. olfactory - (a) | olfactif | olfattivo; olfattorio | olfatorio | olfaktorisch | 嗅覚の |
| 4636. olfactory bulb - (n) | bulbe olfactif | bulbo olfattivo | bulbo olfatorio | Riechkolben; Bulbus olfactorius | 嗅球 |
| 4637. oligemia (oligaemia) - (n) | oligémie | oligoemia | oligohemia | Oligämie | 血液過少（減少）［症］, 乏血［症］ |
| 4638. oliguria - (n) | oligurie | oliguria | oliguria | Oligurie | 尿量過少（減少）［症］, 乏尿［症］ |
| 4639. omentum - (n) | épiploon | omento; epiploon | epiplón | Omentum; Netz | 膜, 網 |
| 4640. once a day - (adv) | une fois par jour | una volta al giorno | una vez al día | einmal pro Tag | 一日一回 |
| 4641. oncogene - (n) | oncogène | oncogene | oncogén | Onkogen | 腫瘍遺伝子 |
| 4642. oncogenesis - (n) | oncogénèse | oncogenesi | oncogénesis | Onkogenese | 腫瘍形成 |
| 4643. oncologic - (a) | oncologique | oncologico | oncológico | onkologisch | 腫瘍学の |
| 4644. oncology - (n) | oncologie | oncologia | oncología | Onkologie | 腫瘍学 |
| 4645. one-compartment model - (n) | modèle à un compartiment | modello a un compartimento | modelo de un sólo compartimiento | Modell mit einem Kompartiment | 一区切りの模型 |
| 4646. one-sided hypothesis test - (n) | épreuve d'hypothèse unilatérale | prova di ipotesi unilaterale | prueba de hipótesis unilateral | einseitiger Hypothesentest | 一方的な仮定の検査 |

237

| English/American | French/Français | Italian/Italiano | Spanish/Español | German/Deutsch | Japanese/日本語 |
|---|---|---|---|---|---|
| 4647. one-tailed test - (n) | épreuve d'un bras | prova a unico ramo | prueba a una rama | einseitiger Test | 一方的な検査 |
| 4648. online system - (n) | système en direct | sistema in linea | sistema en línea | Online-System | オンラインシステム |
| 4649. onset - (n) | début | insorgenza | comienzo | Beginn; Ausbruch vor Ort | 開始、発病 |
| 4650. onsite - (a) | sur place | sul posto | en sitio | | その場で |
| 4651. oocyte - (n) | ovocyte | oocita; ovocita | oocito | Oozyte | 卵母細胞 |
| 4652. oogenesis - (n) | ovogénèse | oogenesi; ovogenesi | oogénesis | Oogenese | 卵子発生 |
| 4653. oophorectomy - (n) | ovariectomie | ooforectomia; ovariectomia | ooforectomía | Oophorektomie | 卵巣摘除 [術] |
| 4654. oozing - (a) | suintant | trasudante | sudante | sickernd; nässend | 徐々に流出する |
| 4655. opaque - (a) | opaque | opaco | opaco | opak; undurchsichtig | 不透明の |
| 4656. open - (v) | ouvrir | aprire; liberare | abrir | öffnen | 開く |
| 4657. open - (a) | ouvert | aperto; libero | abierto | offen | 公開の |
| 4658. open angle glaucoma - (n) | glaucome à angle ouvert | glaucoma ad angolo aperto | glaucoma de ángulo abierto | Weitwinkelglaukom | 開放 [隅] 角緑内障 |
| 4659. open clinical trial - (n) | essai clinique ouvert | studio clinico aperto | ensayo clínico abierto | offene klinische Studie | 公開臨床試験 |
| 4660. open fracture - (n) | fracture ouverte | frattura aperta | fractura expuesta | offener Bruch | 開放骨折 |
| 4661. open label trial - (n) | essai d'étiquette ouverte | studio a etichetta aperta | ensayo de etiqueta abierta | Studie mit enthülltem Etikett | 公けの薬品試験 |
| 4662. open study - (n) | étude ouverte | studio aperto | estudio abierto | offene randomis-erte Studie | 公開研究 |
| 4663. opening - (n) | ouverture | apertura | abertura | Öffnung | 開始 |
| 4664. opening snap - (n) | claquement d'ouverture | schiocco di apterura | chasquido de apertura | Mitralöffnungston | 開弁期弾発音 |
| 4665. operable - (a) | opérable | operabile | operable | operierbar | 手術可能の |
| 4666. operant conditioning - (n) | conditionnement opérant | condizionamento operante | condicionamiento operante | operante Konditionierung | オペラント条件付け |
| 4667. operating procedure - (n) | procédure opératoire | procedura di una operazione | procedimiento de operación | Betriebsverfahren | 手術の手順 |

238

| English/American | French/Français | Italian/Italiano | Spanish/Español | German/Deutsch | Japanese/日本語 |
|---|---|---|---|---|---|
| 4668. operating room (operating theatre) - (n) | salle d'opération | sala operatoria | quirófano; sala de operaciones | Operationssaal | 手術室 |
| 4669. operation - (n) | opération | operazione | operación | Operation; Betrieb | 外科手術 |
| 4670. operational definition - (n) | définition opérationnelle | definizione operatorio | definición operacional | Betriebsdefinition | 実用上の定義 |
| 4671. operative - (a) | opératif, d'opération | operatorio; operante | operatorio; operativo | operativ; wirksam | 手術の |
| 4672. operon - (n) | opéron | operon; operone | operón | Operon | オペロン |
| 4673. ophthalmic - (a) | ophthalmique | oftalmico; ottico | oftálmico | ophthalmisch | 眼の |
| 4674. ophthalmology - (n) | opthalmologie | oftalmologia | oftalmología | Ophthalmologie; Augenheilkunde | 眼科学 |
| 4675. ophthalmoscopy - (n) | ophthalmoscopie | oftalmoscopia | oftalmoscopia | Ophthalmoskopie | 検眼鏡検査 [法] |
| 4676. opiate - (n) | opiacé | oppiaceo; oppioide | opiáceo | Opiat | アヘン [製] 剤; アヘン誘導体 |
| 4677. opiate - (a) | opiacé | oppiato; soporifero | opiáceo | Opiat | 麻酔させる、催眠の |
| 4678. opinion - (n) | opinion | opinione; consiglio | opinión | Meinung; Gutachten | 意見 |
| 4679. opinion leader - (n) | faiseur d'opinion | formatore d'opinione | creador de opinión | Meinungsbildner | 意見リーダー |
| 4680. opisthotonos - (n) | opisthotonos | opistotono | opistótonos | Opisthotonus | 後弓反張 |
| 4681. opportunistic infection - (n) | infection opportuniste | infezione opportunistica | infección oportunista | opportunistische Infektion | 日和見感染 |
| 4682. optic - (a) | optique | ottico | óptica | optisch | 視覚の |
| 4683. optical - (a) | optique | ottico | óptico | optisch | 光の |
| 4684. optical density - (n) | densité optique | densità ottica | densidad óptica | optische Dichte | 光学濃度 |
| 4685. optical disk - (n) | disque optique | disco ottico | disco óptico | Optikuspapille; optischer Festspeicher | 光ディスク |

| English/American | French/Français | Italian/Italiano | Spanish/Español | German/Deutsch | Japanese/日本語 |
|---|---|---|---|---|---|
| 4686. optical rotation - (n) | rotation optique | rotazione ottica | rotación óptica | optische Drehung | 旋光度 |
| 4687. optician - (n) | opticien | ottico | óptico | Optiker | 光学器械技術者 |
| 4688. optics - (n) | optique | ottica | óptica | Optik | 光学 |
| 4689. optimal dose - (n) | dose optimale | dose ottimale | dosis óptima | Optimaldosis | 最適服用量 |
| 4690. optometry - (n) | optométrie | optometria | optometría | Optometrie | 検眼 |
| 4691. oral - (a) | oral; buccal | orale; buccale | oral; bucal | oral; mündlich | 口の |
| 4692. oral administration - (n) | administration orale | somministrazione orale | administración oral | orale Verabreichung | 経口的投与 |
| 4693. oral contraceptive - (n) | contraceptif oral | anticontracettivo orale | contraceptivo oral | orales Kontrazeptivum | 経口避妊薬 |
| 4694. oral diagnosis - (n) | diagnostic oral | diagnosi orale | diagnóstico oral | mündliche Diagrose | 口頭診断 |
| 4695. oral drug delivery - (n) | système de livraison medicamenteux oral | somministrazione orale | administración de una droga por via oral | orale Pharmakotherapie | 経口薬品投与 |
| 4696. oral informed consent - (n) | consentement éclairé verbal | consenso orale informato | consentimiento informado oral | mündliche Einverständniserklärung | 口語告知の同意 |
| 4697. orbit - (n) | orbite | orbità | órbita | Augenhöhle | 眼窩 |
| 4698. orbital - (a) | orbitaire | orbitale | orbital | orbital; orbitalis | 眼窩の |
| 4699. orchitis - (n) | orchite | orchite | orquitis | Orchitis | 睾丸炎 |
| 4700. order - (n) | ordre | ordine | orden | Ordnung; Reihenfolge | 目、命令 |
| 4701. orderly - (n) | aide-infirmier | inserviente | asistente | Krankenpflegehelfer; Sanitäter | 看護夫 |
| 4702. ordinal - (a) | ordinal | ordinale | ordinal | ordinal | 目の、順序の |
| 4703. ordinate - (n) | ordonnée | ordinata | ordenada | Ordinate | 縦座標 |
| 4704. organ - (n) | organe | organo | órgano | Organ | 器官 |
| 4705. organelle - (n) | organelle | organello; organulo | organela | Organelle | オルガネラ |
| 4706. organic - (a) | organique | organico | orgánico | organisch | 有機の |

| English/American | French/Français | Italian/Italiano | Spanish/Español | German/Deutsch | Japanese/日本語 |
|---|---|---|---|---|---|
| 4707. organic chemistry - (n) | chimie organique | chimica organica | química orgánica | organische Chemie | 有機化学 |
| 4708. organism - (n) | organisme | organismo | organismo | Organismus | 生物、生体、有機体 |
| 4709. organization - (n) | organisation | organizzazione | organización | Organisation | 組織 |
| 4710. organizational structure - (n) | structure organisationnelle | struttura organizzativa | estructura organizativa | Organisationsaufbau | 組織構造 |
| 4711. orgasm - (n) | orgasme | orgasmo | orgasmo | Orgasmus | 性恍惚期 |
| 4712. oriental - (a) | oriental | orientale | oriental | orientalisch | 東洋の |
| 4713. orientation - (n) | orientation | orientamento | orientación | Orientierung; Ausrichtung | 見当識、配位 |
| 4714. orifice - (n) | orifice | orifizio | orificio | Körperöffnung; Orifizium | 口、開口 [部] |
| 4715. oropharyngeal - (a) | oropharyngé | orofaringeo | orofaríngeo | oropharyngeal | 口腔咽頭の |
| 4716. oropharynx - (n) | oropharynx | orofaringe; mesofaringe | orofaringe | Oropharynx | 口腔咽頭部 |
| 4717. orphan drug - (n) | médicament non parrainé | farmaco orfano | fármaco huérfano | Orphan-Drug; in geringer Menge hergestelltes Arzneimittel | スポンサーなしの新薬品 |
| 4718. orthodontic appliance - (n) | appareil d'orthodontie | strumento ortodontico | aparato de ortodoncia | zahn- und kieferregulierendes Gerät | 歯科矯正器具 |
| 4719. orthodontics - (n) | orthodontie | ortodontia; ortognatodonzia | ortodoncia | Orthodontie; Kieferorthopädie | 歯科矯正学 |
| 4720. orthomolecular therapy - (n) | thérapie orthomoléculaire | terapia ortomolecolare | terapia ortomolecular | orthomolekulare Therapie | 正常生体分子療法 |
| 4721. orthopedic - (a) | orthopédique | ortopedico | ortopédico | orthopädisch | 整形外科の |
| 4722. orthopnea - (n) | orthopnée | ortopnea | ortopnea | Orthopnoe | 坐位呼吸 |
| 4723. orthostasis - (n) | orthostase | ortostasi | ortostasis | Orthostase | 起立 |
| 4724. orthostatic hypotension - (n) | hypotension orthostatique | ipotensione ortostatica | hipotensión ortostática | orthostatische Hypotonie | 起立性低血圧 [症] |

| English/American | French/Français | Italian/Italiano | Spanish/Español | German/Deutsch | Japanese/日本語 |
|---|---|---|---|---|---|
| 4725. orthotic device - (n) | appareil orthoptique | meccanismo ortotico | aparato ortótico | orthotisches Gerät | 歯科矯正器具 |
| 4726. oscillograph - (n) | oscillographe | oscillografo | oscilógrafo | Oszillograph | オシログラフ |
| 4727. oscilloscope - (n) | oscilloscope | oscilloscopio | osciloscopio | Oszilloskop | オシロスコープ |
| 4728. osmolality - (n) | osmolalité | osmolalità | osmolalidad | Osmolalität | 重量オスモル濃度 |
| 4729. osmolar concentration - (n) | concentration osmolaire | concentrazione osmolare | concentración osmolar | osmolare Konzentration | 浸透圧濃度 |
| 4730. osmolarity - (n) | osmolarité | osmolarità | osmolaridad | Osmolarität | 容量オスモル濃度 |
| 4731. osmotic pressure - (n) | pression osmotique | pressione osmotica | presión osmótica | osmotischer Druck | 浸透圧 |
| 4732. osseous - (a) | osseux | osseo | óseo | knöchern; osseous | 骨［性］の |
| 4733. ossification - (n) | ossification | ossificazione | osificación | Ossifikation; Knochenbildung | 骨形成、骨化 |
| 4734. osteitis - (n) | ostéite | osteite | osteitis | Ostitis | 骨炎 |
| 4735. osteoarthritis - (n) | ostéo-arthrite | osteoartrite | osteoartritis | Osteoarthritis | 変形性関節症 |
| 4736. osteoarthropathy - (n) | ostéo-arthropathie | osteoartropatia | osteoartropatia | Osteoarthropathie | 骨関節症 |
| 4737. osteoblast - (n) | ostéoblaste | osteoblasto | osteoblasto | Osteoblast | 骨芽細胞 |
| 4738. osteoclast - (n) | ostéoclaste | osteoclasto | osteoclasto | Osteoklast | 破骨細胞、破骨器 |
| 4739. osteoma - (n) | ostéome | osteoma | osteoma | Osteom | 骨腫 |
| 4740. osteomyelitis - (n) | ostéomyélite | osteomielite | osteomielitis | Osteomyelitis | 骨髄炎 |
| 4741. osteopathic medicine - (n) | médecine ostéopathique | medicina osteopatica | medicina osteopática | osteopathische Medizin | 整骨医学 |
| 4742. osteopathy - (n) | ostéopathie | osteopatia | osteopatia | Osteopathie | オステオパシー |
| 4743. osteoporosis - (n) | ostéoporose | osteoporosi | osteoporosis | Osteoporose | オステオポローシス |
| 4744. osteosarcoma - (n) | ostéosarcome | osteosarcoma | osteosarcoma | Osteosarkom | 骨肉腫 |
| 4745. osteotomy - (n) | ostéotomie | osteotomia | osteotomia | Osteotomie | 骨切り術 |

242

| English/American | French/Français | Italian/Italiano | Spanish/Español | German/Deutsch | Japanese/日本語 |
|---|---|---|---|---|---|
| 4746. ostomy - (n) | ostomie | ostomia | ostomía | Stomaanlage | 口、小孔、造孔 [術] |
| 4747. otic - (a) | otique | otico | ótico | -ohrig | 耳の |
| 4748. otitis - (n) | otite | otite | otitis | Otitis | 耳炎 |
| 4749. otitis externa - (n) | otite externe | otite esterna | otitis externa | Otitis externa; Entzündung des äußeren Ohranteiles | 外耳炎 |
| 4750. otitis media - (n) | otite moyenne | otite media | otitis media | Mittelohrentzündung | 中耳炎 |
| 4751. otolaryn- gology - (n) | otolaryngologie | otorinolaringoiatria | otorrinolaringología | Otolaryngologie | 耳鼻咽喉科学 |
| 4752. otoscope - (n) | otoscope | otoscopio | otoscopio | Otoskop; Ohrentrichter | 耳鏡、耳聴管 |
| 4753. outbreak - (n) | éruption | esplosione (di un' epidemia) | erupción; epidemia | Ausbruch | 突発 |
| 4754. outcome - (n) | résultat; conséquence | risultato | resultado | Ergebnis | 結果 |
| 4755. outcomes research - (n) | recherche des résultats | ricerca dei risultati | investigación de los resultados | Erforschung des besten Ergebnisses | 結果の研究 |
| 4756. outlier - (n) | valeur aberrante | valore erratico | valor erróneo | Ausreißer | 群はずれの データポイント |
| 4757. outline - (n) | plan | schema | trazado | Umriß; Entwurf | 概要 |
| 4758. outline - (v) | exposer à grands traits; résumer | delineare; schizzare | explicar en términos generales; resumir | umreißen | 概要する |
| 4759. outpatient - (n) | malade en consultation externe | paziente d'ambulatorio; paziente esterno | paciente ambulatorio | ambulanter Patient | 外来患者 |
| 4760. outpatient clinic - (n) | service de consultation externe; clinique externe | clinica per pazienti d'ambulatorio | consultorios externos | Poliklinik | 外来患者診療所 |
| 4761. output - (n) | production | produzione | producción | Ausgabe; Ertrag | 出力 |
| 4762. ovarian - (a) | ovarien | ovarico | ovárico | ovarial | 卵巣の |
| 4763. ovary - (n) | ovaire | ovaia; ovario | ovario | Eierstock; Ovar | 卵巣 |
| 4764. over the counter drug - (n) | médicament sans ordonnance | farmaco senza prescrizione | medicamento sin receta | freiverkäufliches Medikament | 処方箋なしで買える薬品 |

243

| English/American | French/Français | Italian/Italiano | Spanish/Español | German/Deutsch | Japanese/日本語 |
|---|---|---|---|---|---|
| 4765. over the counter name - (n) | nom générique | nome generico | nombre genérico | allgemein verwendeter Name | 処方箋なしで買える薬品名 |
| 4766. overall health - (n) | santé générale; santé globale | stato generale delle salute | salud general | allgemeine Gesundheit | 総合的健康 |
| 4767. overdose - (n) | dose excessive; surdose | dose eccessiva; iperdosaggio | sobredosis | Überdosis | 薬の過量 |
| 4768. overdose - (v) | prendre une dose excessive; surdoser | sovradosare | tomar una sobredosis | überdosieren | 過剰に薬を服用する |
| 4769. overhead cost - (n) | frais généraux | costi fissi | gastos generales | allgemeine Unkosten | 間接費 |
| 4770. overlay - (n) | surcharge; addition | sovrapposizione | sobrepeso | Überzug | 重畳 |
| 4771. overreporting - (n) | excès de reportage | reportage eccessiva | exceso de reportaje | Übertriebene Angabe von Krankheitsfällen | 過剰報告 |
| 4772. overt symptom - (n) | symptôme évident | sintomo evidente | síntoma evidente | offensichtliches Symptom | 明白な徴候 |
| 4773. overweight - (n) | obèse; surpoids | obesità; peso eccessivo | obesidad; sobre peso | Übergewicht | 肥満 |
| 4774. oviduct - (n) | oviducte | ovidotto | oviducto | Eileiter; Tuba uterina | 卵管 |
| 4775. ovulate - (v) | ovuler | ovulare | ovular | ovulieren | 排卵する |
| 4776. ovulation - (n) | ovulation | ovulazione | ovulación | Ovulation | 排卵 |
| 4777. ovum - (n) | ovule | uovo; cellula uovo | óvulo | Ei; Ovum | 卵 |
| 4778. oxidant - (n) | oxydant | ossidante | oxidante | Oxidant; Oxidationsmittel | 酸化剤 |
| 4779. oxidation - (n) | oxydation | ossidazione | oxidación | Oxidation | 酸化 |
| 4780. oxidation reduction - (n) | oxydoréduction; réduction oxydative | ossidoriduzione | reducción oxidación | Oxydoreduktion | 酸化還元 |
| 4781. oximetry - (n) | oxymétrie | ossimetria | oximetría | Oximetrie; Sauerstoffmessung | 酸素測定 [法] |
| 4782. oxygen - (n) | oxygène | ossigeno | oxígeno | Sauerstoff | 酸素 |
| 4783. oxygen inhalation therapy - (n) | oxygénothérapie | terapia di inalazione ossigeno | terapia de inhalación de oxígeno | Sauerstoffinhalations-therapie | 酸素吸入療法 |

244

| English/American | French/Français | Italian/Italiano | Spanish/Español | German/Deutsch | Japanese/日本語 |
|---|---|---|---|---|---|
| 4784. oxygenate - (v) | oxygéner | ossigenare | oxigenar | oxygenieren; mit Sauerstoff anreichern | 酸化する |
| 4785. oxygenation - (n) | oxygénation | ossigenazione | oxigenación | Oxygenation; Sauerstoffzufuhr | 酸素付加 |
| 4786. oxyhemo- globin - (n) | oxyhémoglobine | ossiemoglobina | oxihemoglobina | Oxyhämoglobin | 酸化ヘモグロビン |
| 4787. ozone - (n) | ozone | ozono | ozono | Ozon | オゾン |

| English/American | French/Français | Italian/Italiano | Spanish/Español | German/Deutsch | Japanese/日本語 |
|---|---|---|---|---|---|
| 4788. pacemaker - (n) | stimulateur cardiaque | stimolatore cardiaco; pacemaker | marcapasos | Schrittmacher | 歩調を定めるもの |
| 4789. packaging - (n) | emballage | imballaggio | envasado | Verpackung | 包装 |
| 4790. page proof - (n) | épreuve en page | bozze impaginati | prueba de plana | Korrekturfahne | ページ校正 |
| 4791. pain - (n) | douleur | dolore | dolor | Schmerz; Geburtswehen | 痛み |
| 4792. pain fibers - (n) | fibres de la douleur | fibre dolorifiche | fibras del dolor | Schmerzfasern | 痛覚神経線維 |
| 4793. pain free walking distance - (n) | distance de marche sans douleur | distanza coperta senza dolore | distancia que puede caminar sin dolor | schmerzfreie Gehdistanz | 無痛歩行距離 |
| 4794. pain measurement - (n) | mesure de la douleur | misura del dolore | medición del dolor | Schmerzmessung | 痛みの測定 |
| 4795. pain threshold - (n) | seuil de tolérance à la douleur | soglia del dolore | umbral del dolor | Schmerzgrenze | 痛みのいき値 |
| 4796. painful - (a) | douloureux | doloroso; dolente | doloroso | schmerzhaft | 痛い |
| 4797. painless - (a) | indolore; sans douleur | indolore | sin dolor; indoloro | schmerzlos | 無痛の |
| 4798. paired t-test - (n) | épreuve statistique T pairé | t-test accoppiato | prueba t en pares | t-Test für gepaarte Stichproben | ペアードt テスト |
| 4799. pairing - (n) | appariement | accoppiamento | apareamiento | Paarung; Begattung | 対合 |
| 4800. palatable - (a) | agréable au goût | gradevole al palato | sabroso; apetitoso | genießbar; schmackhaft | 美味の |
| 4801. palate - (n) | palais | palato | paladar | Gaumen; Palatum | 口蓋 |
| 4802. palliate - (v) | pallier | palliare | paliar | lindern | 緩和する、軽減する |
| 4803. palliative - (n) | palliatif | palliativo | paliativo | Palliativum | 緩和剤 |
| 4804. palliative - (a) | palliatif | palliativo | paliativo | palliativ | 待機の |
| 4805. pallor - (n) | pâleur | pallore | palidez | Blässe; Pallor | 蒼白 |
| 4806. palm - (n) | paume | palma | palma | Hohlhand | 手掌 |
| 4807. palmar erythema - (n) | érythème palmaire | eritema palmare | eritema palmar | Palmarerythem | 手掌紅斑 |
| 4808. palmar reflex - (n) | réflexe palmaire | riflesso palmare | reflejo palmar | Palmarreflex | 手掌反射 |
| 4809. palpable - (a) | palpable | palpabile | palpable | palpabel | 触知可能の、明白な |

| English/American | French/Français | Italian/Italiano | Spanish/Español | German/Deutsch | Japanese/日本語 |
|---|---|---|---|---|---|
| 4810. palpation - (n) | palpation | palpazione | palpación | Palpation | 触診 [法]、触感 |
| 4811. palpebral - (a) | palpébral | palpebrale | palpebral | palpebral | 眼瞼の |
| 4812. palpitate - (v) | palpiter | palpitare | palpitar | palpitieren | 動悸がする、脈打つ |
| 4813. palpitation - (n) | palpitation | palpitazione | palpitación | Palpitation | 動悸、心悸亢進 |
| 4814. palsy - (n) | paralysie | paralisi | parálisis | Lähmung; Paralyse | 麻痺 |
| 4815. panacea - (n) | panacée | panacea | panacea | Allheilmittel | 万能薬 |
| 4816. pancreas - (n) | pancréas | pancreas | páncreas | Pankreas; Bauchspeicheldrüse | 膵臓 |
| 4817. pancreatitis - (n) | pancréatite | pancreatite | pancreatitis | Pankreatitis | 膵 [臓] 炎 |
| 4818. pancytopenia - (n) | pancytopénie | pancitopenia | pancitopenia | Panzytopenie | 汎血球減少 [症] |
| 4819. pandemic - (n) | pandémie | pandemia | pandémico | Pandemie | 汎発性流行病 |
| 4820. pandemic - (a) | pandémique | pandemico | pandémico | pandemisch | 汎発性流行病の |
| 4821. panel - (n) | commission; assemblée | commissione; lista | panel. lista | Arztregister; Gremium | 委員会 |
| 4822. panel discussion - (n) | réunion-débat; débat en commission | discussione di gruppo | discusión de panel | Podiumsdiskussion | 討論会 |
| 4823. panel study - (n) | étude de commission | studio di un gruppo di esperti | estudio de panel | Forumsstudie | パネルスタディ |
| 4824. panic - (n) | panique | panico | pánico | Panik | パニック、恐慌 |
| 4825. panic - (v) | paniquer; s'affoler | gettare nel panico | aterra; infundir pánico | in Panik geraten | 狼狽する |
| 4826. panic - (a) | panique; affolé | panico | lleno de pánico; asustado | panisch; ängstlich | 狼狽した |
| 4827. panoramic radiography - (n) | radiographie panoramique | radiografia panoramica | radiografía panorámica | Panoramaaufnahme | パノラマラジオグラフィ、パノラマX線撮影 [法] |
| 4828. pant - (v) | haleter | sbuffare; ansimare | jadear | keuchen | 息切れする |
| 4829. Pap smear - (n) | épreuve Pap; frottis vaginal | Pap test; striscio vaginale | prueba Pap; frotis de Pap | Papanicolaou-Abstrich | 子宮癌検診 |
| 4830. paper - (n) | papier; document | foglio; documento | papel; documento | Papier; Abhandlung | 紙、論文 |
| 4831. paper trail - (n) | documentation écrite | documentazione scritta | documentación escrita | schriftliche Belege | 文書 |

247

| English/American | French/Français | Italian/Italiano | Spanish/Español | German/Deutsch | Japanese/日本語 |
|---|---|---|---|---|---|
| 4832. papillary - (a) | papillaire | papillare | papilar | papillär | 乳頭[状]の |
| 4833. papilledema - (n) | papilledème; œdème de la papille | papilledema | papiledema | Papillenödem; Stauungspapille | 乳頭水腫（浮腫） |
| 4834. papilloma - (n) | papillome | papilloma | papiloma | Papillom | 乳頭腫 |
| 4835. papule - (n) | papule | papula | pápula | Papula; Papel | 丘疹 |
| 4836. para-- (prefix) | pare; para | para- | para- | para- | パラ、傍、近傍の |
| 4837. paradoxical pulse - (n) | pouls paradoxal | polso paradosso | pulso paradójico | Pulsus paradoxus | 奇脈 |
| 4838. paraffin - (n) | paraffine | paraffina | parafina | Paraffin | パラフィン |
| 4839. paraffin embedding - (n) | paraffinage; enrobage de paraffine | inclusione in paraffina | inclusión en parafina | Einbettung in Paraffin | パラフィン包埋 |
| 4840. parallel - (a) | parallèle | parallelo | paralelo | parallel | 平行の |
| 4841. paralysis - (n) | paralysie | paralisi | parálisis | Paralyse; Lähmung | 麻痺 |
| 4842. paralyze - (v) | paralyser | paralizzare | paralizar | paralysieren; lähmen | 麻痺させる |
| 4843. paramedical staff - (n) | personnel paramédical | staff paramedico | personal paramédico | paramedizinisches Personal | 準医療スタッフ |
| 4844. parameter - (n) | paramètre | parametro | parámetro | Parameter | パラメーター |
| 4845. parametric test - (n) | examen paramétrique | test parametrico | prueba paramétrica | parametrischer Test | パラメトリック検査 |
| 4846. paranasal sinus - (n) | sinus paranasal | seno paranasale | seno paranasal | Nasennebenhöhle | 副鼻腔 |
| 4847. paranoia - (n) | paranoïa | paranoia | paranoia | Paranoia | パラノイア、妄想症 |
| 4848. paranoid - (a) | paranoïde | paranoide | paranoide | paranoid | パラノイア様の、妄想[性]の |
| 4849. paraparesis - (n) | paraparésie | paraparesi | paraparesia | Paraparese | 不全対麻痺 |
| 4850. paraplegia - (n) | paraplégie | paraplegia | paraplejía | Paraplegie | 対麻痺 |
| 4851. parapsychology - (n) | parapsychologie | parapsicologia | parapsicología | Parapsychologie | 超心理学 |
| 4852. parasite - (n) | parasite | parassita | parásito | Parasit | 寄生生物 |

248

| English/American | French/Français | Italian/Italiano | Spanish/Español | German/Deutsch | Japanese/日本語 |
|---|---|---|---|---|---|
| 4853. parasitic - (a) | parasitaire | parassitario | parasitario | parasitär | 寄生生物の、寄生性の |
| 4854. parasitology - (n) | parasitologie | parassitologia | parasitología | Parasitologie | 寄生生物学、寄生虫学 |
| 4855. parasympa-thetic - (a) | parasympathique | parasimpatico | parasimpático | parasympathisch | 副交感神経の |
| 4856. parasympathetic nervous system - (n) | système nerveux parasympathique | sistema nervoso parasimpatico | sistema nervioso parasimpático | parasympathisches Nervensystem | 副交感神経系 |
| 4857. parasympatholyt-ic - (a) | parasympatholytique | parasimpaticolitico | parasimpaticolítico | parasympathikolytisch | 副交感神経遮断薬の |
| 4858. parasympatho-mimetics - (n) | parasympathomimétique | parasimpaticomimetico | parasimpaticomimético | Parasympathiko-mimetikum | 副交感神経興奮剤 |
| 4859. parathyroid - (n) | parathyroide | paratiroide | paratiroideo | Nebenschilddrüse | 上皮小体 |
| 4860. parathyroid - (a) | parathyroidien | paratiroide; paratiroideo | paratiroideo | parathyreoidal | 甲状腺傍の |
| 4861. parathyroid gland - (n) | glande parathyroide | ghiandola paratiroidea | glándula paratiroidea | Nebenschilddrüse | 皮小体 |
| 4862. parent - (n) | parent (père/mère) | genitore | padre (madre/padre) | Elternteil | 親 |
| 4863. parent drug - (n) | drogue mère | farmaco primario | droga madre | Vorläufermedikament | 新開発製品の元の薬品 |
| 4864. parent institution - (n) | institution mère | istituzione madre | institución matriz | Hauptinstitution | 親会社 |
| 4865. parenteral - (a) | parentéral | parenterale | parenteral | parenteral | 非経口の、腸管外の |
| 4866. parenteral dosage form - (n) | formulation parenterale | dosaggio in forma parenterale | forma de dosis parenteral | parenterale Verabreichungsform | 静脈内点滴の薬の形態 |
| 4867. parenteral nutrition - (n) | alimentation parenterale | nutrizione parenterale | nutrición parenteral | parenterale Ernährung | 非経口栄養 |
| 4868. parenting - (n) | élever un enfant | l'essere genitore | cuidado de los hijos | elterliche Pflege | 子育て |
| 4869. paresis - (n) | parésie | paresi | paresia | Parese | 不全麻痺、進行麻痺 |
| 4870. paresthesia - (n) | paresthésie | paresthesia | parestesia | Parästhesie | 感覚異常 [症] |
| 4871. parietal - (a) | pariétal | parietale | parietal | parietal | 壁の、壁在の、壁側の |

| English/American | French/Français | Italian/Italiano | Spanish/Español | German/Deutsch | Japanese/日本語 |
|---|---|---|---|---|---|
| 4872. parity - (n) | parité; égalité | parità | paridad; igualdad | Gebärfähigkeit; Ähnlichkeit | 同等 |
| 4873. parotid - (n) | parotide | parotide | parótida | Parotis; Ohrspeicheldrüse | 耳下腺 |
| 4874. parotid gland - (n) | glande parotide | ghiandola parotide | glándula parótida | Ohrspeicheldrüse | 耳下腺 |
| 4875. paroxysm - (n) | paroxysme | parossismo | paroxismo | Paroxysmus; Anfall | 痙攣、発作 |
| 4876. paroxysmal - (a) | paroxystique | parossistico | paroxístico | paroxysmal | 発作［性］の |
| 4877. paroxysmal nocturnal dyspnea - (n) | dyspnée nocturne paroxystique | dispnea notturna parossistica | disnea nocturna paroxística | paroxysmale nächtliche Dyspnoe | 発作性夜間呼吸困難 |
| 4878. parthenogenesis - (n) | parthénogénèse | partenogenesi | partenogénesis | Parthenogenese; Jungfernfruchtbarkeit | 単為生殖、処女生殖 |
| 4879. partial - (a) | partiel | parziale | parcial | teilweise; partiell | 部分的な |
| 4880. partial agonist - (n) | agoniste partiel | agonista parziale | agonista parcial | partieller Agonist | 不完全作動物質、不完全作用薬 |
| 4881. partial responder - (n) | répondeur partiel | rispondente parziale | que responde parcialmente | partieller Responder | 不完全反応者 |
| 4882. partial thromboplastin time - (n) | temps de thromboplastine partiel | tempo di tromboplastina parziale | tiempo de tromboplastina parcial | partielle Thromboplastinzeit | 部分トロンボプラスチン時間 |
| 4883. participant - (n) | participant | partecipante | participante | Teilnehmer | 参加者 |
| 4884. participation - (n) | participation | partecipazione | participación | Beteiligung | 参加 |
| 4885. particle accelerator - (n) | accélérateur de particules | acceleratore di particelle | acelerador de particulas | Teilchenbeschleuniger | 粒子加速器 |
| 4886. particle size - (n) | grosseur de la particule | dimensione della particella | tamaño de la particula | Partikelgröße | 粒子の大きさ |
| 4887. partition coefficient - (n) | coefficient de partage | coefficiente di ripartizione | coeficiente de partición | Verteilungskoeffizient | 分配係数 |
| 4888. parts of a study - (n) | parties d'une étude | parti di uno studio | partes de un estudio | Teile einer Studie | 研究の部分 |

| English/American | French/Français | Italian/Italiano | Spanish/Español | German/Deutsch | Japanese/日本語 |
|---|---|---|---|---|---|
| 4889. parts per... - (n) | parties par .... | parti per ... | partes por... | Teile pro ... | ...分の... |
| 4890. parturient paresis - (n) | parésie parturiente | paresi della partoriente | paresia; parturiente | Schwangerschaftsparese | 分娩性蹲躄 |
| 4891. parturition - (n) | parturition | parto | parturición; parto | Geburt; Partus | 分娩、出産 |
| 4892. pass - (n) | passage; passe | passo | pasillo; conducto | Übergang | 通過 |
| 4893. pass - (v) | passer; évacuer | evacuare; espellere | pasar; evacuar | ausscheiden; weitergeben | 通過する、省く |
| 4894. passage - (n) | passage; conduit | passaggio | pasaje; conducto | Passage; Gang | 通過、排泄、通路 |
| 4895. passive - (a) | passif | passivo | pasivo | passiv | 受け身の |
| 4896. passive immunity - (n) | immunité passive | immunità passiva | inmunidad pasiva | passive Immunität | 受動免疫 |
| 4897. passive transfer - (n) | transfert passif | trasferimento passivo | transferencia pasiva | passive Übertragung | 移動性転嫁 |
| 4898. past medical history - (n) | histoire médicale | anamnesi remota | historia médica | medizinische Vorgeschichte | 過去の病歴 |
| 4899. past trends - (n) | tendances passées | tendenze passate | tendencias pasadas | frühere Tendenzen | 過去の傾向 |
| 4900. pasteuri-zation - (n) | pasteurisation | pastorizzazione | pasteurización | Pasteurisation | 低温殺菌 [法] |
| 4901. patch test - (n) | épreuve épidermique | test intradermico; test epicutaneo | prueba de parche | Patchtest | パッチテスト |
| 4902. patella - (n) | patella; rotule | patella; rotula | patela | Kniescheibe; Patella | 膝蓋骨 |
| 4903. patellar reflex - (n) | réflexe patellaire; réflexe rotulien | riflesso patellare | reflejo patelar | Patellarsehnenreflex; Quadrizepssehnenreflex | 膝蓋反射 |
| 4904. patency - (n) | perméabilité | pervietà | patente | Durchgängigkeit | 開存性 |
| 4905. patent - (n) | brevet d'invention | brevetto d'invenzione | patente | Patent | 特許 |
| 4906. patent ductus arteriosus - (n) | canal artériel perméable | dotto arterioso pervio | ductus arterioso patente | offener ductus arteriosus | 動脈管開存 |
| 4907. patent protection - (n) | protection de brevet | protezione brevetto | protección de patente | Patentschutz | 特許の保護 |

251

| English/American | French/Français | Italian/Italiano | Spanish/Español | German/Deutsch | Japanese/日本語 |
|---|---|---|---|---|---|
| 4908. paternal - (a) | paternel | paterno; da padre | paternal; paterno | väterlich | 父 [性] の |
| 4909. paternity - (n) | paternité | paternità | paternidad | Vaterschaft | 父性 |
| 4910. pathogen - (n) | pathogène | organismo patogeno; agente patogeno | patógeno | pathogener Mikroorganismus; Krankheitserreger | 病原体 |
| 4911. pathogenesis - (n) | pathogenèse | patogenesi | patogénesis | Pathogenese | 病院 [論]、病原 [論] |
| 4912. pathogenetic - (a) | pathogénique | patogeno; patogenetico | patogenético | pathogenetisch | 発病 [性] の |
| 4913. pathogno-monic - (a) | pathognomonique | patognomonico | patognomónico | pathognomonisch | [疾病] 特有証候の |
| 4914. pathological - (a) | pathologique | di patologia; patologico | patológico | pathologisch | 病理学の、病的の |
| 4915. pathological changes - (n) | changements pathologiques | cambi patologici | cambios patológicos | krankhafte Veränderungen | 病理学的変化 |
| 4916. pathological fracture - (n) | fracture pathologique | frattura patologica | fractura patológica | pathologische Fraktur | 病的骨折 |
| 4917. pathology - (n) | pathologie | patologia | patología | Pathologie | 病理学 |
| 4918. pathophysiolo-gy - (n) | pathophysiologie | patofisiologia | fisiopatología | Pathophysiologie | 病態生理学 |
| 4919. pathway - (n) | sentier; voie | via traiettoria | curso; vía | Weg; Bahn | 経路 |
| 4920. patient - (n) | patient; malade | paziente | paciente | Patient | 患者 |
| 4921. patient - (a) | patient; endurant | paziente; che ha pazienza | paciente | geduldig | 忍耐強い |
| 4922. patient compli-ance - (n) | conformité du patient | fedeltà del paziente alla terapia | cumplimiento del paciente | Patientencompliance | 患者の承諾 |
| 4923. patient diary - (n) | journal du patient | diario del paziente | diario del paciente | Patiententagebuch | 患者の日誌 |
| 4924. patient discharge - (n) | congé du patient; sortie | dimissione del paziente | dar de alta al paciente | Entlassung | 患者の退院 |
| 4925. patient eligibility - (n) | éligibilité du patient | eleggibilità del paziente | elegibilidad del paciente | Patienteneignung | 患者の適格性 |

| English/American | French/Français | Italian/Italiano | Spanish/Español | German/Deutsch | Japanese/日本語 |
|---|---|---|---|---|---|
| 4926. patient enrollment - (n) | enrôlement du patient; recrutement du patient | registrazione del paziente | inscripción del paciente | Patientenanmeldung | 患者登録 |
| 4927. patient examination - (n) | examen du patient | esame del paziente | examen del paciente | Patientenuntersuchung | 患者検査 |
| 4928. patient identification number - (n) | numéro d'identification du patient | numero di identificazione de la paziente | número de identificación del paciente | Patientenidentifikations-nummer | 患者認識番号 |
| 4929. patient number - (n) | numéro du patient | numero del paziente | número de paciente | Patientennummer | 患者番号 |
| 4930. patient outcome - (n) | résultat de patient | risultato di paziente | evolución de paciente | Ergebnis einer Patientenbehandlung | 患者の結果 |
| 4931. patient package insert - (n) | feuillet d'information pour le patient | foglietto illustrativo per il paziente | información para el paciente | Verpackungsbeilage für Patienten | 患者の受け取る パッケージの添付書 |
| 4932. patient quota - (n) | quota des patients | quota pazienti | cuota de pacientes | Patientenanzahl pro Zeiteinheit | 患者割当 |
| 4933. patient recruitment - (n) | recrutement des patients | reclutamento di pazienti | selección de pacientes | Patientenanwerbung (für eine Studie) | 患者を集めること |
| 4934. patient register - (n) | registre des patients | registro dei pazienti | registro de pacientes | Patientenregister | 患者登録 |
| 4935. patient relations - (n) | rapport avec le patient | relazione con il paziente | relaciones con el paciente | Beziehung zum Patienten | 患者関係 |
| 4936. patient screening log - (n) | registre de dépistage des patients | giornale delle valutazioni dei pazienti | registro de exploración de pacientes | Patientenscreening-logbuch | 患者スクリーニング記録簿 |
| 4937. patient visit - (n) | visite de patient | esame del paziente | visita de paciente | Patientenbesuch | 患者の来院 |
| 4938. patient's perspective - (n) | perspective du pat ent | prospettiva del paziente | perspectiva del paciente | Perspektive des Patienten | 患者の見通し |
| 4939. pattern - (n) | modèle; dessin | modello; schema | modelo; diseño | Muster; Modell | [原] 型、模様 |
| 4940. pattern of response - (n) | modèle de réponse | modalità della risposta | modelo de respuesta | Erwiederungsmuster | 反応の型式 |
| 4941. payment - (n) | paiement; versement | pagamento | pago | Zahlung | 支払 |

253

| English/American | French/Français | Italian/Italiano | Spanish/Español | German/Deutsch | Japanese/日本語 |
|---|---|---|---|---|---|
| 4942. peak - (n) | pic; maximum | picco; massimo | punto; máximo | Spitze; Höhepunkt | 先端、最高点 |
| 4943. peak - (v) | atteindre un maximum; atteindre le sommet | raggiungere un massimo | alcanzar su punto más alto; llevar al máximo | Höhepunkt erreichen | やせ衰える |
| 4944. peak plasma level - (n) | niveau plasmatique maximal | livello plasmatico massimo | nivel de plasma más alto | Höhepunkt des Blutspiegels | プラズマレベルの最高点 |
| 4945. peak response - (n) | réponse maximale | risposta massimale | máxima respuesta | maximale Reaktion | 最高点の反応 |
| 4946. pectoral - (a) | pectoral | pettorale | pectoral | zur Brust gehörend; pectoralis | 胸の、胸筋の |
| 4947. pedal edema - (n) | oedème du pied | edema pedale | edema de los tobillos | Fußödem | 足の浮腫 |
| 4948. pediatric (paediatric) - (a) | pédiatrique | pediatrico | pediátrico | pädiatrisch | 小児科の |
| 4949. pediatrician - (n) | pédiatre | pediatra | pediatra | Kinderarzt | 小児科医 |
| 4950. pedigree - (n) | arbre généalogique; ascendance | pedigree; albero genealogico | genealogía; linaje | Stammbaum | 家系図、起源 |
| 4951. peer - (n) | pair; pareil | pari; uguale | par; igual | Gleiche(r); Gleichrangige(r) | 同輩 |
| 4952. peer review - (n) | révision par des pairs | analisi da parte dei colleghi | revisión hecha por colegas | Überprüfung durch Gleichrangige | スタッフ間での批評 |
| 4953. pelvic - (a) | pelvien | pelvico | pélvico | das Becken betreffend | 骨盤の |
| 4954. pelvis - (n) | pelvis; bassin | pelvi | pelvis | Becken; Nierenbecken | 骨盤 |
| 4955. pending - (a) | pendant; en attente | in corso | pendiente | anhängend; bevorstehend | 未定の |
| 4956. penetrating eye injury - (n) | blessure oculaire pénétrante | lesione penetrante dell'occhio | lesión ocular penetrante | penetrierende Augenverletzung | 貫通眼障害 |
| 4957. penetration - (n) | pénétration | penetrazione | penetración | Penetration | 貫通 |
| 4958. penis - (n) | pénis | pene | pene | Penis | 陰茎 |
| 4959. pension - (n) | pension | pensione | pensión | Pension; Rente | 保護金、年金 |

254

| English/American | French/Français | Italian/Italiano | Spanish/Español | German/Deutsch | Japanese/日本語 |
|---|---|---|---|---|---|
| 4960. people year - (n) | année-personne | anno-uomo | año-gente | Menschenjahr | 一人の人が一年間同じに行動をしたときに起こる確率、頻度、死亡率、等 |
| 4961. peptic - (a) | peptique; gastrique | peptico | péptico | peptisch | 消化性潰瘍の |
| 4962. peptic ulcer - (n) | ulcère gastrique | ulcera peptica | úlcera péptica | peptisches Ulkus | 消化性潰瘍 |
| 4963. peptide - (n) | peptide | peptide | péptido | Peptid | ペプチド |
| 4964. peptide fragment - (n) | fragment peptidique | frammento peptidico | fragmento de péptido | Peptidfragment | ペプチドフラグメント |
| 4965. peptide mapping - (n) | cartographie peptidique | rilevamento di un peptide | mapeo de péptidos | Peptidmapping; Peptidkartierung | ペプチドマッピング |
| 4966. percent - (n) | pour cent; pourcentage | percento; percentuale | por ciento; porcentaje | Prozent | パーセント |
| 4967. percent change - (n) | pourcentage du changement | percentuale di cambio | cambio porcentual | Prozent der Änderung | パーセント変化 |
| 4968. percent of maximal response - (n) | pourcentage de la réponse maximale | percentuale di risposta massima | porcentaje de respuesta máxima | Prozent der maximalen Reaktion | 最高反応のパーセント |
| 4969. percent of total - (n) | pourcentage du total | percento del totale | porcentaje del total | Prozent der Gesamtsumme | 全体の一率 |
| 4970. percentage - (n) | pourcentage | percentuale | porcentaje | Anteil | 百分率 |
| 4971. percentile - (n) | percentile | percentile | percentil | Perzentile | パーセンタイル |
| 4972. perception - (n) | perception | percezione | percepción | Wahrnehmung | 知覚、認知 |
| 4973. perceptual - (a) | perceptif | percettivo | perceptual | perzeptiv | 知覚の |
| 4974. percuss - (v) | percuter | percuotere | percutir | perkutieren; klopfen | 打診する |
| 4975. percussion - (n) | percussion | percussione | percusión | Perkussion | 打診 [法]、軽打打診摩 |
| 4976. percussion tenderness - (n) | douleur à la percussion | sensibilità alla percussione | sensibilidad a la percusión | durch Perkussion verursachte Empfindlichkeit | 打診圧痛 |
| 4977. perennial - (n) | perpétuel | perenne | perenne | mehrjährig | 多年性植物 |

| English/American | French/Français | Italian/Italiano | Spanish/Español | German/Deutsch | Japanese日本語 |
|---|---|---|---|---|---|
| 4978. perennial allergic rhinitis - (n) | rhinite allergique perpétuelle | rinite allergica perenne | rinitis alérgica perenne | Rhinopathin vasomotorica | 万年アレルギー性鼻炎 |
| 4979. perforation - (n) | perforation | perforazione | perforación | Perforation | 穿孔 |
| 4980. performance - (n) | rendement; exécution | rendimento; prestazione | rendimiento; cumplimiento | Leistung; Durchführung | 達成度 |
| 4981. performance appraisal - (n) | évaluation du rendement; évaluation de l'exécution | valutazione delle prestazioni | evaluación del rendimiento | Leistungsbewertung | 達成度の評価 |
| 4982. performance test - (n) | épreuve d'exécution | test di prestazione | prueba de rendimiento | Leistungstest | 作為試験 |
| 4983. perfusion - (n) | perfusion | perfusione | perfusión | Perfusion; Durchblutung | 浸流 |
| 4984. periapical - (a) | peri-apical | periapicale | periapical | periapikal | 歯根尖[端]周囲の |
| 4985. pericardial - (a) | péricardique | pericardico | paricárdico | perikardial | 心臓の、心臓周囲の |
| 4986. pericardial effusion - (n) | épanchement péricardique | effusione pericardica | derrame pericárdico | Perikarderguß | 心臓滲出物 |
| 4987. pericardium - (n) | péricarde | pericardio | pericardio | Perikard; Pericardium | 心膜 |
| 4988. perimeter - (n) | périmètre | perimetro | perímetro | Perimeter | 周界、[周辺]視野計 |
| 4989. perinatal - (a) | périnatal | perinatale | perinatal | perinatal | 周産(周生)期の |
| 4990. perineal - (a) | périnéal | perineale | perineal | perineal | 会陰の |
| 4991. perineum - (n) | périnée | perineo | perineo | Perineum | 会陰 |
| 4992. period - (n) | période; phase | periodo; fase | periodo; fase | Zeitraum; Phase | 期間、周期 |
| 4993. period of a study - (n) | période d'une étude | durata di uno studio | periodo del estudio | Zeitraum einer Studie | 研究期間 |
| 4994. periodic - (a) | périodique | periodico | periódico | periodisch | 周期的な |
| 4995. periodical - (n) | périodique | periodico | periódica | Zeitschrift | 定期刊行物 |
| 4996. periodicity - (n) | périodicité | periodicità | periodicidad | Periodizität; Regelmäßigkeit | 周期性 |
| 4997. periodontal, peridental - (a) | périodontal; péridentaire | periodontale; parodontale | periodontal; peridental | paradontal; periodontal | 歯周の、歯根膜の |

| English/American | French/Français | Italian/Italiano | Spanish/Español | German/Deutsch | Japanese/日本語 |
|---|---|---|---|---|---|
| 4998. periodontics - (n) | périodontie | periodonzia; paradontologia | periodoncia | Periodontologie | 歯周病学 |
| 4999. periorbital - (a) | périorbitaire | periorbitale | periorbitario | periorbital | 眼窩骨膜の、眼窩周囲の |
| 5000. periosteum - (n) | périoste | periostio | periostio | Periost; Periostenum | 骨膜 |
| 5001. peripheral - (a) | périphérique | periferico | periférico | peripher | 末梢［性］の、周辺の |
| 5002. peripheral nerve - (n) | nerf périphérique | nervo periferico | nervio periférico | peripherer Nerv | 末梢神経 |
| 5003. peripheral visual field - (n) | champ visuel périphérique | campo visivo periferico | campo visual periférico | peripheres Gesichtsfeld | 末梢視野 |
| 5004. peristalsis - (n) | péristaltisme | peristalsi | peristaltismo | Peristaltik | 蠕動 |
| 5005. peristaltic sounds - (n) | bruits péristaltiques | rumori peristaltici | sonidos peristálticos | Darmgeräusche | 蠕動音 |
| 5006. peristaltic wave - (n) | onde péristaltique | onda peristaltica | onda peristáltica | peristaltische Welle | 蠕動波 |
| 5007. peritoneal - (a) | péritonéal | peritoneale | peritoneal | peritoneal | 腹膜の |
| 5008. peritoneum - (n) | péritoine | peritoneo | peritoneo | Peritoneum; Bauchfell | 腹膜 |
| 5009. peritonitis - (n) | périonite | peritonite | peritonitis | Peritonitis | 腹膜炎 |
| 5010. permanent tooth - (n) | dent permanente | dente permanente | diente permanente | bleibender Zahn | 永久歯 |
| 5011. permeability - (n) | perméabilité | permeabilità | permeabilidad | Permeabilität | 透過性 |
| 5012. permeable - (a) | perméable | permeabile | permeable | permeabel | 透過し得る |
| 5013. pernicious - (a) | pernicieux | pernicioso | pernicioso | perniziös | 悪性の、壊滅の |
| 5014. peroral - (a) | par voie buccale; par la bouche | perorale; per os | peroral; per os | peroral | 経口［的］の |
| 5015. peroxide - (n) | peroxyde | perossido | peróxido | Peroxid | 過酸化物 |
| 5016. person - (n) | personne; individu | persona; individuo | persona; individuo | Person | 人 |
| 5017. personal - (a) | personnel; individuel | personale; individuale | personal; individual | persönlich | 個人の |
| 5018. personality - (n) | personnalité | personalità | personalidad | Persönlichkeit; Charakter | 人格 |

| English/American | French/Français | Italian/Italiano | Spanish/Español | German/Deutsch | Japanese/日本語 |
|---|---|---|---|---|---|
| 5019. personnel - (n) | personnel | personale | personal | Personal | 人員 |
| 5020. personnel turnover - (n) | roulement de personnel | ricambio del personale | cambio de personal | Rate der Neu- und Wiedereinstellung von Arbeitskräfter | 人事移動 |
| 5021. perspiration - (n) | transpiration | perspirazione | perspiración | Perspiration; Schwitzen | 発汗、蒸散、汗 |
| 5022. Pert chart - (n) | dossier de Pert | tabella Pert | diagrama Pert | Pert-Diagramm | 管理図式 |
| 5023. perversion - (n) | perversion | perversione | perversión | Perversion | 倒錯 [症] |
| 5024. perverted - (a) | pervers | pervertito | pervertido | pervers; widernatürlich | 異常な |
| 5025. pessary - (n) | pessaire | pessario | pesario | Pessar | ペッサリー、膣坐薬 |
| 5026. pesticide - (n) | pesticide | pesticida | pesticida | Pestizid; Schädlingsbekämpfungsmittel | 農薬、殺虫剤 |
| 5027. pestilence - (n) | peste | peste; pestilenza | pestilencia | Pest; Pestilenz | ペスト、悪疫、流行病 |
| 5028. Pet scan - (n) | scan par tomographie d'émission positronique | Pet scan; tomografia ad emissione di positroni | tomografía por emisión de positrones | Pet-Scan; Positronenemissionstomographie | 陽電子射出断層撮影 [法] |
| 5029. petechia, (pl.) petechiae - (n) | pétéchie | petecchia | petequia | Petechie | 点状出血 |
| 5030. petit mal - (n) | petit mal | piccolo male | pequeño mal | Petit mal; kleiner epileptischer Anfall | 小発作 |
| 5031. petrolatum - (n) | pétrolatum | petrolato | petrolado | Petrolatum; Paraffinöl | ワセリン |
| 5032. phagocyte - (n) | phagocyte | fagocita | fagocito | Phagozyt | [貪] 食細胞 |
| 5033. phagocytosis - (n) | phagocytose | fagocitosi | fagocitosis | Phagozytose | 食 [菌] 作用、[貪] 食作用 [能] |
| 5034. phagosome - (n) | phagosome | fagosoma | fagosoma | Phagosom | 食胞 |
| 5035. phalanx - (n) | phalange | falange | falange | Phalanx | 指 (趾) 節骨 |
| 5036. phallic - (a) | phallique | fallico | fálico | phallisch | 陰茎の、ファルスの |
| 5037. phantom limb - (n) | membre fantôme | arto fantasma | miembro fantasma | Phantomglied | 幻 [影] 肢 |
| 5038. pharmaceutic - (a) | pharmaceutique | farmaceutico | farmacéutico | pharmazeutisch | 薬学の、製薬の |
| 5039. pharmaceutical - (a) | pharmaceutique | farmaceutico | farmacéutico | pharmazeutisch | 薬学の、製薬の |

| English/American | French/Français | Italian/Italiano | Spanish/Español | German/Deutsch | Japanese/日本語 |
|---|---|---|---|---|---|
| 5040. pharmaceutical company - (n) | compagnie pharmaceutique | ditta farmaceutica | compañía farmacéutica | Pharmaunternehmen | 製薬会社 |
| 5041. pharmaceutical industry - (n) | industrie pharmaceutique | industria farmaceutica | industria farmacéutica | Arzneimittelindustrie | 製薬産業 |
| 5042. pharmaceuticals - (n) | pharmaceutiques | prodotti farmaceutici | fármacos | Arzneimittel | 製薬 |
| 5043. pharmaceutics - (n) | pharmacie | farmacia; arte farmaceutica | farmacia | Pharmazie | 製剤学、薬剤学 |
| 5044. pharmacist - (n) | pharmacien | farmacista | farmacéutico | Apotheker | 薬剤師 |
| 5045. pharmacodynamics - (n) | pharmacodynamie | farmacodinamica | farmacodinamia | Pharmakodynamik | 薬理力学 |
| 5046. pharmacoeconomics - (n) | pharmacoéconome | farmaeconomica | farmacoeconomía | Pharmakowirtschaft | 薬理経済学 |
| 5047. pharmacoepidemiology - (n) | pharmacoépidémiologie | farmaco-epidemiologia | farmacoepidemiología | Pharmakoepidemiologie | 薬物流行病学 |
| 5048. pharmacogenetics - (n) | pharmacogénétique | farmacogenetica | farmacogenética | Pharmakogenetik | 薬理遺伝学 |
| 5049. pharmacognosy - (n) | pharmacognosie | farmacognosia | farmacognosia | Pharmakognosie | 生薬学 |
| 5050. pharmacokinetic study - (n) | étude pharmacocinétique | studio farmacocinetico | estudio farmacocinético | pharmakokinetische Studie | 薬物動態 [学] の研究 |
| 5051. pharmacokinetics - (n) | pharmacocinétique | farmacocinetica | farmacocinética | Pharmakokinetik | 薬物動態 [学] |
| 5052. pharmacological activity - (n) | activité pharmacologique | attività farmacologica | actividad farmacológica | pharmakologische Aktivität | 薬理活性 |
| 5053. pharmacologist - (n) | pharmacologiste | farmacologo | farmacólogo | Pharmakologe | 薬理学者 |
| 5054. pharmacology - (n) | pharmacologie | farmacologia | farmacología | Pharmakologie | 薬理学、薬物学 |

| English/American | French/Français | Italian/Italiano | Spanish/Español | German/Deutsch | Japanese/日本語 |
|---|---|---|---|---|---|
| 5055. pharmaco-peia - (n) | pharmacopée | farmacopea | farmacopea | Pharmakopöe; Arzneibuch | 薬局方 |
| 5056. pharmaco-therapy - (n) | pharmacothérapie | farmacoterapia | farmacoterapia | Pharmakotherapie | 薬物療法 |
| 5057. pharmaco-vigilance - (n) | pharmacovigilance | farmacovigilanza | farmacovigilancia | Überwachung der Pharmakonwirkung | 薬物使用の管理 |
| 5058. pharmacy - (n) | pharmacie | farmacia | farmacia | Apotheke; Pharmazie | 調剤、薬局 |
| 5059. pharmacy refill - (n) | renouvellement pharmaceutique | ricambio farmaci | recambio de una receta farmacéutica | Wiedereinlösen eines Rezepts | 薬局補充 |
| 5060. pharma-politics - (n) | avis pharmaceutique | farmapolitica | farmacopolitica | Pharmapolitik | 薬理政治学 |
| 5061. pharyngeal - (a) | pharyngien | faringeo | faríngeo | pharyngeal | 咽頭の |
| 5062. pharynx - (n) | pharynx | faringe | faringe | Rachen; Pharynx | 咽頭 |
| 5063. phase - (n) | phase | fase | fase | Phase; Periode | 位相 |
| 5064. phase 1 - (n) | première phase; phase 1 | prima fase; fase 1 | primera fase; fase 1 | Phase 1; erste Phase | 第一次 |
| 5065. phase 1 study - (n) | étude de première phase | studio in prima fase | estudio de primera fase | Phase-1-Studie; Studie der ersten Phase | 第一次研究 |
| 5066. phase 1 unit - (n) | unité de première phase | gruppo in prima fase | unidad de primera fase | Phase-1-Einheit; Einheit der ersten Phase | 第一次ユニット |
| 5067. phenomenon - (n) | phénomène | fenomeno | fenómeno | Phänomen | 現象、徴候 |
| 5068. phenotype - (n) | phénotype | fenotipo | fenotipo | Phänotyp | 表現型 |
| 5069. pheromone - (n) | phéromone | feromone | feromona | Pheromon | フェロモン |
| 5070. phlebitis - (n) | phlébite | flebite | flebitis | Phlebitis | 静脈炎 |
| 5071. phlebotomy - (n) | phlébotomie | flebotomia | flebotomía | Venenpunktion; Phlebotomie | 静脈切開 |
| 5072. phlegm - (n) | flegme | flemma | flema | Phlegma | 粘液分泌過多、粘液質 |
| 5073. phobia - (n) | phobie | fobia | fobia | Phobie | 恐怖［症］ |
| 5074. phobic disorder - (n) | désordre phobique | disordini fobici | trastorno fóbico | Phobieerkrankung | 恐怖症 |

260

| English/American | French/Français | Italian/Italiano | Spanish/Español | German/Deutsch | Japanese日本語 |
|---|---|---|---|---|---|
| 5075. phonation - (n) | phonation | fonazione | fonación | Phonation | 発声 |
| 5076. phonetics - (n) | phonétique | fonetica | fonética | Phonetik | 音声学 |
| 5077. phonocardio-graphy - (n) | phonocardiographie | fonocardiografia | fonocardiografía | Phonokardiographie | 心音図検査 [法] |
| 5078. phosphorus - (n) | phosphore | fosforo | fósforo | Phosphor | リン |
| 5079. photic stimulation - (n) | stimulation photique | stimolazione fotica | estimulo fótico | Photostimulation | 光刺激 |
| 5080. photochemis-try - (n) | photochimie | fotochimica | fotoquímica | Photochemie | 光化学 |
| 5081. photocopy - (n) | photocopie | fotocopia | fotocopia | Fotokopie | 写真複写 |
| 5082. photocopy - (v) | photocopier | fotocopiare | fotocopiar | Fotokopieren | 写真複写する |
| 5083. photograph - (n) | photographie | fotografia | fotografía | Fotografie; Aufnahme | 写真 |
| 5084. photograph - (v) | photographier | fotografare | fotografiar | fotographieren | 写真にとる |
| 5085. photophobia - (n) | photophobie | fotofobia | fotofobia | Photophobie | 羞明、光恐怖 [症] まぶしがり [症] |
| 5086. photosensi-tive - (a) | photosensible | fotosensibile | fotosensible | lichtempfindlich | 感光性の |
| 5087. photosensitivi-ty - (n) | photosensibilité | fotosensibilità | fotosensibilidad | Lichtempfindlichkeit | 光感受性 |
| 5088. photosensitizing agent - (n) | agent photosensibilisateur | agente fotosensitivo | agente fotosensibilizador | Photosensibilisator | 感光剤 |
| 5089. phototherapy - (n) | photothérapie | fototerapia | fototerapia | Phototherapie; Lichttherapie | 光線療法 |
| 5090. phrenic - (a) | phrénique | frenico | frénico | diaphragmatisch; Geist-Phrenologie | 横隔膜の |
| 5091. phrenology - (n) | phrénologie | frenologia | frenología | Phrenologie | 骨相学 |
| 5092. physical - (a) | physique | fisico | físico | physisch; körperlich | 身体的な |
| 5093. physical activity - (n) | activité physique | attività fisica | actividad física | körperliche Aktivität | 身体活動 |

261

| English/American | French/Français | Italian/Italiano | Spanish/Español | German/Deutsch | Japanese/日本語 |
|---|---|---|---|---|---|
| 5094. physical dependence - (n) | dépendance physique | dipendenza fisica | dependencia física | körperliche Abhängigkeit | 身体依存 |
| 5095. physical exam - (n) | examen physique | esame obiettivo | examen físico | körperliche Untersuchung | 身体検査 |
| 5096. physical exercise - (n) | exercice physique | esercizio fisico | ejercicio físico | körperliche Bewegung | 身体運動 |
| 5097. physical fitness - (n) | forme physique | salute fisica | buen estado físico | körperliche Gesundheit; Fitneß | 身体健康 |
| 5098. physical restraint - (n) | contrainte physique | limitazione fisica | restricción física | körperliche Einschränkung | 身体拘束 |
| 5099. physical sign - (n) | signe physique | segno fisico | signo físico | körperliches Symptom | 身体的徴候 |
| 5100. physical stability - (n) | stabilité physique | stabilità fisica | estabilidad física | physische Stabilität | 身体安定 |
| 5101. physical symptoms - (n) | symptômes physiques | sintomi fisici | síntomas físicos | körperliche Symptome | 身体的徴候 |
| 5102. physical therapy - (n) | physiothérapie; thérapie physique | fisioterapia | terapia física | physikalische Therapie | 身体療法 |
| 5103. physician - (n) | médecin | medico | médico | Arzt | 医者 |
| 5104. physician-patient relationship - (n) | relation médecin-patient | rapporto medico-paziente | relación médico-paciente | Arzt-Patient-Verhältnis | 医師と患者の関係 |
| 5105. physics - (n) | physique | fisica | física | Physik | 物理学 |
| 5106. physiognomy - (n) | physionomie | fisiognomia; fisionomia | fisiognomía | Physiognomie | 人相学、人相 |
| 5107. physiologic monitoring - (n) | surveillance physiologique | monitoraggio dei parametri fisiologici | monitoreo fisiológico | physiologische Überwachung | 生理的監視 |
| 5108. physiological - (a) | physiologique | fisiologico | fisiológico | physiologisch | 生理学の |
| 5109. physiological marker - (n) | marqueur physiologique | segno fisiologico; marker fisiologico | marcador fisiológico | physiologische Marker | 生理的マーカー |
| 5110. physiological training - (n) | entraînement physiologique | allenamento fisiologico | entrenamiento fisiológico | physiologisches Training | 生理的訓練 |

262

| English/American | French/Français | Italian/Italiano | Spanish/Español | German/Deutsch | Japanese 日本語 |
|---|---|---|---|---|---|
| 5111. physiology - (n) | physiologie | fisiologia | fisiología | Physiologie | 生理学 |
| 5112. physiothera-py - (n) | physiothérapie | fisioterapia | fisioterapia | Physiotherapie | 物理療法 |
| 5113. pia mater - (n) | pie-mère | pia madre; pia meninge | piamadre | weiche Hirnhaut; Pia mater | 軟膜 |
| 5114. pica - (n) | pica; picacisme | pica; picacismo | pica | Pica; Pikazismus | 異食 [症] |
| 5115. picogram - (n) | picogramme | picogrammo | picogramo | Pikogramm | ピコグラム |
| 5116. pictorial displays - (n) | affiches illustrées | esposizione di immagini | muestras pictóricas; muestras gráficas | Bildanzeigen | 写真又は絵の表示 |
| 5117. pie chart - (n) | graphique circulaire; diagramme circulaire | diagramma a settori | gráfico de sectores | Kreisdiagramm; Tortendiagramm | 円グラフ |
| 5118. pie graph - (n) | graphique circulaire | grafico a settori | gráfico de sectores | Kreisdiagramm; Tortendiagramm | 円グラフ |
| 5119. pigment - (n) | pigment | pigmento | pigmento | Pigment | 色素 |
| 5120. pigmentation - (n) | pigmentation | pigmentazione | pigmentación | Pigmentierung; Pigmentation | 色素沈着 |
| 5121. pigmented nevus - (n) | nævus pigmentaire | nevo pigmentato | nevus pigmentado | Pigmentnävus | 色素性母斑 |
| 5122. piles - (n) | hémorroïdes | emorroidi | hemorroides | Hämorrhoiden | 痔 |
| 5123. pill - (n) | pilule | pillola | píldora | Pille | 丸薬 |
| 5124. pill board - (n) | pilulier | tavoletta di conta delle pillole | tabla de píldoras | Pillentablett | 丸薬をとりわける板 |
| 5125. pill count - (n) | comptage de pilules | conta delle pillole | conteo de píldoras | Pillenzahl | 丸薬数 |
| 5126. pill rolling tremor - (n) | mouvement d'émiettement des parkinsoniens | tremore di movimento di contare monete | temblor ce enfermedad de Parkinson | Pillendrehertremor | 丸薬丸め運動 |
| 5127. pilomotor - (a) | pilomoteur | pilomotore | pilomotor | pilomotorisch | 毛髪運動の |
| 5128. pilot project - (n) | projet-pilote | progetto pilota | proyecto piloto | Versuchsprojekt; Pilotprojekt | パイロットプロジェクト |

263

| English/American | French/Français | Italian/Italiano | Spanish/Español | German/Deutsch | Japanese/日本語 |
|---|---|---|---|---|---|
| 5129. pilot scale production - (n) | production d'échelle pilote | produzione in scala ridotta | producción en escala piloto | Herstellung auf Versuchsbasis | 小規模生産 |
| 5130. pilot trial - (n) | essai pilote | prova pilota | prueba pilota | Pilotstudie; Vorversuch | 初期試験 |
| 5131. pimple - (n) | bouton | pustola; papula | pústula pequeña; grano | Pustel; Pickel | 丘疹、面ぽう |
| 5132. pineal - (a) | pinéal | pineale | pineal | Pineal- | 松果状の |
| 5133. pineal body - (n) | corps pinéal; épiphyse | corpo pineale; epifisi | cuerpo pineal; glándula pineal | Zirbeldrüse; Epiphyse | 松果体 |
| 5134. pink eye - (n) | conjonctivite aiguë contagieuse; oeil rouge | congiuntivite batterica acuta | conjuntivitis aguda infecciosa | akute Konjunktivitis; rotes Auge | 伝染性角膜炎、急性カタル性結膜炎 |
| 5135. pinprick sensation - (n) | sensation à la piqûre | sensazione da puntura di spillo | sensación de pinchazo | Nadelstichempfindung | 針で差す痛み |
| 5136. pipe smoking - (n) | fumer la pipe | fumare la pipa | fumar una pipa | Pfeifenrauchen | パイプ喫煙 |
| 5137. pipeline - (n) | conduite; canalisation | condotta | tubería; cañería | (Rohr)leitung | 輸送管 |
| 5138. pipette - (n) | pipette | pipetta | pipeta | Pipette | ピペット |
| 5139. pit - (n) | puits; cicatrice | fossa; fossetta; fovea | fóvea; indentación | Grube; Fossa | 小窩、擦痕 |
| 5140. pitch perception - (n) | perception de la tonalité | percezione del timbro | percepción de tono | Tonwahrnehmung | ピッチ知覚 |
| 5141. pitfall - (n) | piège; trappe | trappola | trampa; escollo | Falle; Fallstrick | 落とし穴 |
| 5142. pitting - (n) | formation de concavités; formation de godet | formazione di depressioni | formación de pequeñas impresiones | Eindellung; Dellenbildung | くぼみ、点食 |
| 5143. pitting edema - (n) | oedème à godet | edema depressibile | edema depresible | nicht wegdrückbares Ödem | 正蝕水腫（浮腫） |
| 5144. pituitary - (n) | glande pituitaire; hypophyse | pituitario; ipofisario | pituitaria; hipófisis | Hypophyse | 脳下垂体 |
| 5145. pituitary adrenal system - (n) | système hypophyso-surrénal | sistema ipofisi-surrenale | sistema adreno-hipofisario | Hypophysen-Nebennieren-System | 脳下垂体副腎系 |
| 5146. pituitary gland - (n) | glande pituitaire; hypophyse | ghiandola pituitaria; ipofisi | glándula pituitaria; hipófisis | Hirnanhangdrüse; Hypophyse | 下垂体 |

264

| English/American | French/Français | Italian/Italiano | Spanish/Español | German/Deutsch | Japanese/日本語 |
|---|---|---|---|---|---|
| 5147. pituitary hormone - (n) | hormone pituitaire; hormone hypophysaire | ormone pituitario | hormona pituitaria | Hypophysenhormon | 下垂体ホルモン |
| 5148. pivotal trial - (n) | essai central | studio chiave | estudio fundamental | zentrale Probe; zentrale Studie | 主要試験 |
| 5149. placebo - (n) | placebo | placebo | placebo | Placebo | 偽薬 |
| 5150. placebo controlled trial - (n) | essai contrôlé avec placebo | prova controllata con placebo | estudio controlada por placebo | placebokontrollierter Versuch | 偽薬対照試験 |
| 5151. placebo effect - (n) | effet placebo | effetto placebo | efecto placebo | Placeboeffekt | 偽薬効果 |
| 5152. placenta - (n) | placenta | placenta | placenta | Plazenta | 胎盤 |
| 5153. plague - (n) | peste | peste | plaga; peste | Pest; Seuche | 悪疫、ペスト |
| 5154. planimetric analysis - (n) | analyse planimétrique | analisi planimetrica | análisis planimétrico | planimetrische Analyse | 面積分析 |
| 5155. planner - (n) | planificateur | programmatore | planificador | Planer | 企画者 |
| 5156. plant - (n) | plante | pianta | planta | Pflanze | 植物 |
| 5157. plantar - (a) | plantaire | plantare | plantar | plantar | 足底の |
| 5158. plaque - (a) | plaque | placca | placa | Plakette; Zahnbelag | 斑、局面、プラク |
| 5159. plasma - (n) | plasma | plasma | plasma | Plasma | 血漿、プラズマ |
| 5160. plasma cell - (n) | cellule plasmatique | plasmacellula | célula plasmática | Plasmazelle | 形質細胞、プラスマ細胞 |
| 5161. plasma level - (n) | niveau plasmatique | livello plasmatico | nivel plasmático | Plasmaspiegel | プラスマレベル |
| 5162. plasmapheresis - (n) | plasmaphérèse | plasmaferesi | plasmaféresis | Plasmapherese | 血漿瀉血、血漿搬出 |
| 5163. plasmid - (n) | plasmide | plasmide | plásmido | Plasmid | プラスミド |
| 5164. plasmin - (n) | plasmine | plasmina | plasmina | Plasmin | プラスミン |
| 5165. plastic - (n) | plastique | plastica | plástico | Plastik; Kunststoff | プラスチック、可塑物 |
| 5166. plastic - (a) | plastique; en plast que | plastico; di plastica | plástico; de plástico | plastisch | プラスチックの、可塑性の |
| 5167. plastic surgery - (n) | chirurgie plastique | chirurgia plastica | cirugía plástica | plastische Chirurgie | 形成外科 [学] |

265

| English/American | French/Français | Italian/Italiano | Spanish/Español | German/Deutsch | Japanese/日本語 |
|---|---|---|---|---|---|
| 5168. plasticity - (n) | plasticité | plasticità | plasticidad | Plastizität | 形成性、[可] 塑性 |
| 5169. plate - (n) | plaque; dentier | placca;piastra | placa; lámina plana | Platte | 板、金属板、平板 |
| 5170. platelet - (n) | plaquette | piastrina | plaqueta | Plättchen; Thrombozyt | 血小板、小板 |
| 5171. platelet adhesion - (n) | adhésion plaquettaire | adesione piastrinica | adhesión plaquetaria | Thrombozytenadhäsivität | 血小板粘着 |
| 5172. platelet aggregation - (n) | agrégation plaquettaire | aggregazione piastrinica | agregación plaquetaria | Thrombozytenaggregation | 血小板凝集 |
| 5173. platelet count - (n) | compte plaquettaire | conta piastrinica | conteo plaquetario | Thrombozytenzahl | 血小板数 |
| 5174. platinum - (n) | platine | platino | platino | Platin | 白金 |
| 5175. plausibility check - (n) | vérification de plausibilité | controllo di plausibilità | comprobaciones de admisibilidad | Plausibilitätskontrolle | 概当性検査 |
| 5176. play - (v) | jouer | giocare | jugar | spielen | 自由に動き回る |
| 5177. plethora - (n) | pléthore | pletora | plétora | Plethora | 多血 [症] |
| 5178. plethysmography - (n) | pléthysmographie | pletismografia | pletismografía | Plethysmographie | プレチスモグラフィ |
| 5179. pleura - (a) | plèvre | pleura | pleura | Pleura- | 胸膜 |
| 5180. pleural cavity - (n) | cavité pleurale | cavità pleurica | cavidad pleural | Pleuraspalte; Pleurahöhle | 胸腔胸腔 |
| 5181. pleural effusion - (n) | effusion pleurale | essudato pleurico | derrame pleural | Pleuraerguß | 胸膜滲出液 |
| 5182. pleurisy - (n) | pleurésie | pleurite | pleuresía | Pleuritis; Rippenfellentzündung | 胸膜炎 |
| 5183. plexus - (n) | plexus | plesso | plexo | Geflecht; Plexus | 叢 |
| 5184. pneumococcus - (n) | pneumocoque | pneumococco | neumococo | Pneumokokkus | 肺炎球菌 |
| 5185. pneumonia - (n) | pneumonie | polmonite | neumonía | Lungenentzündung; Pneumonie | 肺炎 |
| 5186. pneumonitis - (n) | pneumonite | polmonite | neumonitis | Pneumonitis; Lungenentzündung | 肺 [臓] 炎、肺実質炎 |

266

| English/American | French/Français | Italian/Italiano | Spanish/Español | German/Deutsch | Japanese/日本語 |
|---|---|---|---|---|---|
| 5187. pneumo-thorax - (n) | pneumothorax | pneumotorace | neumotórax | Pneumothorax | 気胸 [送] 、気胸 [術] |
| 5188. pocket - (n) | poche | sacco; sacca | cavidad; espacio sacular | Tasche; Hohlraum | 嚢、ポケット |
| 5189. podiatry - (n) | podologie | podiatria | podiatría | Fußpflege | 足瘀字 |
| 5190. poikilocytosis - (n) | poikilocytose | poichilocitosi | poiquilocitosis | Poikilozytose | 変形赤血球症 |
| 5191. point graphs - (n) | graphiques punctiformes | grafici puntiformi | gráficos puntiformes | Punktdiagramme | 点グラフ |
| 5192. point mutation - (n) | mutation punctiforme | mutazione puntiforme | mutación puntiforme | Punktmutation | 点 [突然] 変異 |
| 5193. point tenderness - (n) | sensibilité à un point; précis | dolorabilità puntiforme | sensibilidad al punto preciso | Druckschmerzhaftigkeit | 点圧痛 |
| 5194. poison - (n) | poison | veleno | veneno | Gift | 毒 |
| 5195. poison - (v) | empoisonner | avvelenare | envenenar | vergiften | 毒する |
| 5196. poison control center - (n) | centre anti-poison | centro controllo veleni | centro de toxicología | Vergiftungsberatungsstelle | 毒物規制センター |
| 5197. poisoning - (n) | empoisonnement | avvelenamento | envenenamiento | Vergiftung | 中毒 |
| 5198. policy - (n) | politique; ligne de conduite | politica; linea di condotta | política; normas de conducta | Politik; Praktiken | 方針 |
| 5199. policy issue - (n) | question de politique générale; question de conduite générale | problema linea di condotta | punto político; tema político | Verfahrensfrage | 政策問題 |
| 5200. polishing - (n) | action de polir | lucidatura | pulimento | Politur | 研磨、磨くこと |
| 5201. politics - (n) | politique | politica | política | Politik | 政治 |
| 5202. pollen - (n) | pollen | polline | polen | Pollen | 花粉 |
| 5203. pollutant - (n) | polluant | sostanza inquinante | contaminante | Schmutzstoff; Schadstoff | 汚染物質、汚染物質 |
| 5204. pollution - (n) | pollution | inquinamento | polución | Verschmutzung; Verunreinigung | 汚染 |
| 5205. polyarthritis - (n) | polyarthrite | poliartrite | poliartritis | Polyarthritis | 多発 [性] 関節炎 |
| 5206. polycystic - (a) | polycystique | policistico | policístico | polyzystisch | 多嚢胞の |

267

| English/American | French/Français | Italian/Italiano | Spanish/Español | German/Deutsch | Japanese/日本語 |
|---|---|---|---|---|---|
| 5207. polycythemia - (n) | polycythémie | policitemia | policitemia | Polyzythämie | 赤血球増加［症］ |
| 5208. polydipsia - (n) | polydipsie | polidipsia | polidipsia | Polydipsie | 多渇症 |
| 5209. polygraph - (n) | polygraphe | poligrafo | poligrafo | Mehrfachschreiber; Lügendetektor | ポリグラフ、多用途［記録］計 |
| 5210. polymer - (n) | polymère | polimero | polímero | Polymer | 重合体、ポリマー |
| 5211. polymyositis - (n) | polymyosite | polimiosite | polimiositis | Polymyositis | 多発［性］筋炎 |
| 5212. polyneuritis - (n) | polynévrite | polineurite | polineuritis | Polyneuritis | 多発［性］神経炎 |
| 5213. polyp - (n) | polype | polipo | pólipo | Polyp | ポリープ |
| 5214. polyphagia - (n) | polyphagie | polifagia | polifagia | Polyphagie | 多食［症］、大食性 |
| 5215. polypharma-cy - (n) | polypharmacie | prescrizione multipla; terapia combinata | polifarmacia | Mehrfachkombinations-therapie | 多薬療法 |
| 5216. polyploidy - (n) | polyploïdie | poliploidia | poliploide | Polyploidie | 倍数性 |
| 5217. polyunsaturat-ed - (a) | poly-insaturé | polinsaturo | polinsaturado | mehrfach ungesättigt | 多不飽和の |
| 5218. polyuria - (n) | polyurie | poliuria | poliuria | Polyurie | 多尿［症］ |
| 5219. pons - (n) | pont | ponte | puente | Pons; Brücke | 橋 |
| 5220. poor - (a) | pauvre; maigre | povero; insufficiente | pobre; malo | arm; schlecht | 欠けている、貧弱な |
| 5221. popliteal - (a) | poplité | poplitea | poplíteo | popliteal | 膝窩の |
| 5222. population - (n) | population | popolazione | población | Population; Bevölkerung | 母集団 |
| 5223. pore - (n) | pore | poro | poro | Öffnung; Pore | 孔 |
| 5224. porous - (a) | poreux | poroso | poroso | porös | 多孔性の |
| 5225. porphyrin - (n) | porphyrine | porfirina | porfirina | Porphyrie | ポルフィリン |
| 5226. portal - (n) | porte | porta | puerta; portal | Pforte | 門戸 |
| 5227. portal system - (n) | système porte | sistema portale | sistema portal | Pfortadersystem | 門脈系 |
| 5228. portal vein - (n) | veine porte | vena porta | vena porta | Pfortader | 門脈 |
| 5229. portfolio - (n) | portefeuille; portefolio | cartella | carpeta; cartera | (Akten)mappe; Kollektion | 書類入れ |
| 5230. position - (n) | position | posizione | posición | Lage; Einstellung | 胎向、体位 |
| 5231. position - (v) | positionner | piazzare; mettere in posizione | posicionar | positionieren; plazieren | 位置させる |

268

| English/American | French/Français | Italian/Italiano | Spanish/Español | German/Deutsch | Japanese/日本語 |
|---|---|---|---|---|---|
| 5232. positive - (a) | positif | positivo | positivo | positiv | 陽性の |
| 5233. positive pressure respiration - (n) | respiration à pression positive | respirazione a pressione positiva | respiración de presión positiva | Überdruckbeatmung | 陽圧呼吸 |
| 5234. posology - (n) | posologie | posologia | posología | Dosierung; Posologie | 薬量学 |
| 5235. possibly drug related - (a) | peut-être relié à la drogue | possibilmente correlato al farmaco | posiblemente relacionado con droga | vielleicht medikamentös bedingt | おそらく薬物関連の |
| 5236. post- anesthesia - (n) | post-anesthésie | post anestesia | posanestesia | Postnarkose | 麻酔後 |
| 5237. postcoital - (a) | post-coit | postcoitale | poscoito | postkoital | 性交後の |
| 5238. postdose - (n) | post-dose | postdose | posdosis | Nachdosis | 服用後 |
| 5239. poster - (n) | affiche | manifesto; affisso | póster; cartel | Poster; Plakat | ポスター |
| 5240. posterior - (a) | postérieur | posteriore | posterior | hinterer; posterior | 後部の |
| 5241. postganglion- ic - (a) | post-gangionnaire | postgangliare | posganglionar | postganglionär | 神経節後の |
| 5242. posthumous - (a) | posthume | postumo | póstumo | posthum | 死後の |
| 5243. postictal - (a) | post-convulsion; après une convulsion | post ictale | posictal | postiktal; nach dem Anfall | 発作後の |
| 5244. postmarket- ing - (n) | postmarketing; post- mise en marché | postmarketing | posmarketing | Nach dem Marketing | マーケティングの後 |
| 5245. postmarketing surveillance - (n) | surveillance post-mise en marché | sorveglianza successiva al marketing | vigilancia de posmarketing | Überwachung nach dem Marketing | マーケティングの後の監視 |
| 5246. postmenopau- sal - (a) | post-ménopausique | postmenopausa | posmenopáusico | postmenopausal | 閉経後の |
| 5247. postmortem - (a) | post mortem | post-mortem; dopo il decesso | postmortem | post mortem; postmortal | 死後の |
| 5248. postnasal - (a) | post-nasal | retronasale | posnasal | postnasal | 鼻後方の |
| 5249. postnatal - (a) | post-natal | postnatale | posnatal | postnatal | 生後の |
| 5250. postoperative - (a) | postopératoire | postoperatorio | posoperatorio | postoperativ | 術後 [性] の、[手] 術後の |

269

| English/American | French/Français | Italian/Italiano | Spanish/Español | German/Deutsch | Japanese/日本語 |
|---|---|---|---|---|---|
| 5251. postpartum - (a) | post partum | successivo al parto | post partum; posparto | postpartal; nachgeburtlich | 産後の、分娩後の |
| 5252. postprandial - (a) | postprandial | postprandiale | posprandial | postprandial | 食後の |
| 5253. postpubertal, postpuberal - (a) | postpubère | postpuberale | pospuberal | postpuberal | 思春期後の |
| 5254. poststudy phase - (n) | phase après l'étude | fase successiva allo studio | fase pos estudio | Phase nach der Studie | 研究後期間 |
| 5255. postsynaptic - (a) | postsynaptique | postsinaptico | postsináptico | postsynaptisch | シナプス後［部］の |
| 5256. posttreatment - (n) | post-traitement | trattamento successivo | postratamiento | Nachbehandlung | 治療後 |
| 5257. posttreatment - (a) | post-traitement | da trattamento successivo | postratamiento | Nachbehandlungs- | 治療後の |
| 5258. posttrial - (n) | post-essai | post-prova | posensayo | Nachversuchsphase | 試験後 |
| 5259. posttrial - (a) | post-essai | da post-prova | posensayo | Nachversuchs- | 試験後の |
| 5260. postulate - (n) | postulat | postulato | postulado | Postulat | 仮定、仮説 |
| 5261. postulate - (v) | postuler | postulare | postular | fordern | 仮定する |
| 5262. postural - (a) | postural | posturale | postural | Lage-; Stellungs- | 体位の、体位性の |
| 5263. postural hypotension - (n) | hypotension posturale | ipotensione posturale | hipotensión postural | orthostatische Hypotonie | 体位性低圧［症］ |
| 5264. postural tone - (n) | tonus postural | tono posturale | tono postural | Haltungstonus | 体位緊張 |
| 5265. posture - (n) | posture | postura | postura | Körperhaltung; Körperstellung | 体位 |
| 5266. potable - (a) | potable | potabile | potable | trinkbar | 飲用の |
| 5267. potassium - (n) | potassium | potassio | potasio | Kalium | カリウム |
| 5268. potassium channel - (n) | canal potassique | canale del potassio | canal de potasio | Kaliumkanal | カリウムチャンネル |
| 5269. potency - (n) | puissance | potenza | potencia | Potenz; Wirkpotential | 潜在能力、勢力、効力 |
| 5270. potential - (n) | potentiel | potenziale | potencial | Potential | 電位［差］、ポテンシャル |
| 5271. potential - (a) | potentiel | potenziale | potencial | potentiell | 潜在［性］の、潜能的 |
| 5272. potentiation - (n) | potentiation | potenziamento | potenciación | Potenzierung | 相乗作用 |

| English/American | French/Français | Italian/Italiano | Spanish/Español | German/Deutsch | Japanese/日本語 |
|---|---|---|---|---|---|
| 5273. potentiometry - (n) | potentiométrie | potenziometria | potenciometría | Potentiometrie | 電位差計 |
| 5274. potion - (n) | potion | pozione | poción | Arzneitrank | 頓服水剤 |
| 5275. pouch - (n) | poche | borsa | saco; bolsa | Sack; Tasche | 嚢、窩 |
| 5276. pound - (n) | livre | libbra | libra | Pfund | ポンド |
| 5277. poverty - (n) | pauvreté | povertà | pobreza | Armut | 貧困 |
| 5278. powder - (n) | poudre | polvere | polvo | Puder; Pulver | 粉末、散剤、粉剤 |
| 5279. power - (n) | puissance; force | potenza; efficacia | potencia | Macht | 拡大能、仕事率 |
| 5280. pox - (n) | vérole | esantema; eruzione papulosa | viruela | Pocken; Blattern | 痘、膿疹 |
| 5281. practical considerations - (n) | considérations pratiques | considerazioni pratiche | consideraciones prácticas | praktische Gesichtspunkte | 実用的考慮 |
| 5282. practice - (n) | pratique | professione | práctica | Praxis | 診療、開業 |
| 5283. practice guidelines - (n) | principes directeurs de la pratique | linee di condotta professionali | pautas de la práctica | Richtlinien für die Praxis | 診療ガイドライン |
| 5284. practice management - (n) | gestion de la pratique | gestione della professione | administración de la práctica | Verwaltung der Praxis | 診療管理 |
| 5285. practitioner - (n) | médecin | medico | médico | praktischer Arzt; Praktiker | 開業医 |
| 5286. preanesthetic - (a) | préanesthésique | preanestetico | preanestésico | pränarkotisch | 麻酔前の |
| 5287. precancerous - (a) | précancéreux | precanceroso | precanceroso | präkanzerös | 前癌の |
| 5288. precaution - (n) | précaution | precauzione | precaución | Vorsichtsmaßnahme | 予防策 |
| 5289. preceding - (a) | précédent | precedente | precedente; anterior | vorangegangen; vorhergehend | 先行する |
| 5290. preceptorship - (n) | préceptorat | ufficio di precettore | posición de preceptor | Lehramt; Lehrstelle | 指導者 |
| 5291. precipitant - (n) | précipitant | precipitante | precipitante | Fällungsmittel | 沈殿剤 |
| 5292. precipitation - (n) | précipitation | precipitazione | precipitación | Präzipitation; Ausfällung | 沈殿［析出］、沈降［反応］ |
| 5293. precision - (n) | précision | precisione | precisión | Präzision; Genauigkeit | 精度 |
| 5294. preclinical - (a) | préclinique | preclinico | preclínico | vorklinisch | 前臨床の、症状発現前の |
| 5295. precocious - (a) | précoce | precoce | precoz | frühreif; vorzeitig | 早熟の、早発の |

271

| English/American | French/Français | Italian/Italiano | Spanish/Español | German/Deutsch | Japanese/日本語 |
|---|---|---|---|---|---|
| 5296. precocious puberty - (n) | puberté précoce | pubertà precoce | pubertad precoz | Pubertas praecox | 早発思春期、性的早熟 |
| 5297. precordial thrust - (n) | coup précordial | itto precordiale | impulso precordial | präkordialer Faustschlag | 前胸部刺傷 |
| 5298. precursor - (n) | précurseur | precursore | precursor | Vorläufer; Vorstacium | 前駆物質、前駆体 |
| 5299. prediabetic - (a) | prédiabétique | prediabetico | prediabético | prädiabetisch | 糖尿病前症の |
| 5300. prediction - (n) | prédiction | predizione | pronóstico | Voraussage | 予言 |
| 5301. predictive - (a) | prédictif | predittivo | utilizable como pronóstico | prophezeiend; vorhersagend | 予言の |
| 5302. predisposition - (n) | prédisposition | predisposizione | predisposición | Anfälligkeit; Empfänglichkeit | 素因、素質 |
| 5303. preeclampsia - (n) | pré-éclampsie | pre-eclampsia | preeclampsia | Präeklampsie | 子癇前症 |
| 5304. preferred term - (n) | terme préféré | termine preferito | término preferido | bevorzugter Ausdruck | 希望期間 |
| 5305. preganglionic - (a) | préganglionnaire | pregangliare | preganglionar | präganglionär | [神経] 節前の |
| 5306. pregnancy - (n) | grossesse | gravidanza | embarazo | Schwangerschaft | 妊娠 |
| 5307. pregnancy test - (n) | épreuve de grossesse | test di gravidanza | prueba del embarazo | Schwangerschaftstest | 妊娠反応 |
| 5308. pregnancy waiver - (n) | renonciation en cas de grossesse | rinuncia in caso di gravidanza | renuncia en caso de embarazo | Verzichterklärung bei Schwangerschaft | 妊娠棄権証書 |
| 5309. pregnant - (a) | enceinte | gravida | embarazada; grávida | schwanger | 妊娠している |
| 5310. preimplantation - (a) | préimplantation | preimpianto | preimplantación | vorzeitig implantiert | 移植前の |
| 5311. preinfusion - (n) | préinfusion | preinfusione | preinfusión | Vorinfusion | 注入前 |
| 5312. preinjection - (n) | préinjection | preiniezione | preinyección | Vorinjektion | 注射前 |
| 5313. prejudice - (n) | préjudice | pregiudizio; preconcetto | prejuicio; parcialidad | Vorurteil; Voreingenommenheit | 偏見 |
| 5314. preliminary data - (n) | données préliminaires | dati preliminari | datos preliminares | vorläufige Daten | 予備データ |

272

| English/American | French/Français | Italian/Italiano | Spanish/Español | German/Deutsch | Japanese/日本語 |
|---|---|---|---|---|---|
| 5315. premarketing - (n) | prémarketing; avant la mise en marché | premarketing | premarketing | Vormarketing | マーケティング前 |
| 5316. premature - (a) | prématuré | prematuro | prematuro | vorzeitig; nicht ausgereift | 早熟の |
| 5317. premature beat - (n) | battement prématuré; extrasystole | battito prematuro; extrasistole | latido prematuro | Extrasystolen | 期外収縮、早期収縮 |
| 5318. premature labor - (n) | travail prématuré | parto prematuro | parto prematuro | Frühgeburt | 早産 |
| 5319. premature withdrawal - (n) | retrait prématuré | sospensione prematura | supresión prematura | vorzeitiger Abbruch der Studie | 早期撤回 |
| 5320. prematurity - (n) | prématurité | prematurità | premadurez | Unreife | 早熟、早期接触 |
| 5321. premedi-cation - (n) | prémédication | premedicazione | premedicación | Prämedikation | 前投薬、プレメディケイション |
| 5322. prenatal - (a) | prénatal | prenatale | prenatal | pränatal | 出生前の |
| 5323. preoperative - (a) | préopératoire | preoperatorio | preoperatorio | präoperativ | 手術前の |
| 5324. prepackaged medication - (n) | médication pré-emballée | farmaco preconfezionato | medicamento preempaquetado | fertig verpackte Medikation | 包装済み医薬品 |
| 5325. preparation - (n) | préparation | preparato | preparación | Vorbereitung; Präparat | 準備 |
| 5326. prepuberal - (a) | prépubère | prepuberale | prepuberal | präpuberal | 思春期前の |
| 5327. prerandomization visit - (n) | visite avant la randomisation | visita fatta prima della randomizzazione | visita previa a la randomización | Untersuchung vor der Randomisierung | 無作為化前の検査 |
| 5328. presbyopia - (n) | presbyopie | presbiopia; presbitismo | presbiopia | Presbyopie; Alterssichtigkeit | 老眼、老視 |
| 5329. preschool child - (n) | enfant d'âge préscolaire | bambino in età prescolare | un preescolar | Kind im Vorschulalter | 未就学児童 |
| 5330. prescriber - (n) | préscripteur | chi prescrive | recetador | Verschreiber; Rezeptaussteller | 処方者 |
| 5331. prescribing pattern - (n) | modèle de prescription | metodo di prescrizione | modelo de receta | Verschreibungsmuster | 処方パターン |
| 5332. prescription - (n) | prescription; ordonnance | prescrizione; ricetta | prescripción; receta | Verordnung; Rezept | 処方箋、処方 |

273

| English/American | French/Français | Italian/Italiano | Spanish/Español | German/Deutsch | Japanese/日本語 |
|---|---|---|---|---|---|
| 5333. prescription medicine - (n) | médication sur ordonnance | farmaco su prescrizione | medicina bajo receta | verschreibungspflichtiges Medikament | 処方薬薬 |
| 5334. preselection - (n) | présélection | preselezione | preselección | Vorauswahl | 予備選択 |
| 5335. presenile dementia - (n) | démence présénile | demenza presenile | demencia presenil | präsenile Demenz | 初老期痴呆 |
| 5336. present - (a) | présent | attuale | actual | gegenwärtig | 現在の |
| 5337. presentation - (n) | présentation | presentazione | presentación | Einstellung; Vorstellung | 発表 |
| 5338. presenting - (a) | présentant | presentante | presentando | darstellend | 代表する |
| 5339. preservation - (n) | préservation; conservation | preservazione; conservazione | preservación; conservación | Konservierung; Haltbarmachen | 保存 |
| 5340. preservative - (n) | préservatif; conservateur | preservativo; agente conservativo | preservativo; agente de conservación | Konservierungsmittel | 保存薬、防腐薬 |
| 5341. preservative - (a) | préservatif; préservateur | preservativo; conservativo | preservativo | konservierend | 保存の |
| 5342. press conference - (n) | conférence de presse | conferenza stampa | conferencia de prensa | Pressekonferenz | 記者会見 |
| 5343. press release - (n) | communiqué de presse | comunicato stampa | comunicado de prensa | Pressemitteilung | プレスリリース |
| 5344. pressor - (n) | presseur | pressorio | presor | Pressor | 昇圧剤 |
| 5345. pressoreceptor - (n) | pressorécepteur | pressorecettore | presorreceptor | Pressorezeptor; Barozeptor | 圧受容器 |
| 5346. pressure - (n) | pression | pressione | presión | Druck | 圧、圧力、圧迫 |
| 5347. pressure group - (n) | groupe de pression | gruppo di pressione | grupo de presión | Interessengruppe | 圧力団体 |
| 5348. pressure sore - (n) | escarre de décubitus | ulcera da decubito | llaga por presión | Druckgeschwür; Dekubitus | とこずれ |
| 5349. pressure transducer - (n) | transducteur de pression | trasduttore a pressione | transductor de presión | Druckgeber; Druckumformer | 圧力変換器 |
| 5350. presynaptic - (a) | présynaptique | presinaptico | presináptico | präsynaptisch | シナプス前［部］の |
| 5351. pretreatment - (n) | prétraitement | pretrattamento | pretratamiento | Vorbehandlung | 前処理 |

274

| English/American | French/Français | Italian/Italiano | Spanish/Español | German/Deutsch | Japanese/日本語 |
|---|---|---|---|---|---|
| 5352. pretrial - (n) | avant l'essai | studio iniziale; pretrial | previo a la prueba | Vorversuchs- | 試験前 |
| 5353. prevalence - (n) | prévalence | prevalenza | prevalencia | Prävalenz | 有病率、有病割合 |
| 5354. prevention - (n) | prévention | prevenzione | prevención | Vorbeuge; Prophylaxe | 予防 |
| 5355. preventive - (a) | préventif | preventivo | preventivo | präventiv | 予防的な |
| 5356. preventive medicine - (n) | médicament préventif | medicina preventiva | medicina preventiva | vorbeugende Medizin | 予防薬 |
| 5357. pre-existing - (a) | préexistant | pre-esistente | preexistente | vorherexistierend | 先在の |
| 5358. price competition - (n) | compétition de prix | concorrenza nel prezzo | competencia en precios | Preiskonkurrenz | 価格競争 |
| 5359. pricing studies - (n) | études de prix | analisi dei costi | estudios de precios | Preisstudien | 価格決定研究 |
| 5360. primal - (a) | primal | primario; primitivo | primal | zuerst; primär | 主要な |
| 5361. primary - (a) | primaire | primario | primario; principal | primär; ursprünglich | 初期の |
| 5362. primary care - (n) | soins primaires | assistenza primaria | atención primaria | Grundversorgung | 一次医療 |
| 5363. primary dentition - (n) | dentition primaire | dentizione decidua | dentición primaria | erste Dentition; Milchzahngebiß | 第一生歯 |
| 5364. primary event - (n) | événement primaire | evento primario | evento principal | Hauptereignis; Primärereignis | 最初の出来事 |
| 5365. primary lesion - (n) | lésion primaire | lesione primaria | lesión principal | Primäraffekt | 原発巣 |
| 5366. primary objective - (n) | objectif primaire | obiettivo primario | objetivo principal | Primärziel; Hauptziel | 主要目的 |
| 5367. primary prevention - (n) | prévention primaire | prevenzione primaria | prevención primaria | Primärprävention | 初期予防 |
| 5368. primary prevention trial - (n) | essai de prévention | studio di prevenzione | prueba de prevención | primäre Präventionsstudie | 初期予防試験 |
| 5369. primate - (n) | primate | primate | primate | Primat | 霊長類 |
| 5370. primipara - (n) | primipare | primipara | primipara | Primipara; Erstgebärende | 初産婦 |

275

| English/American | French/Français | Italian/Italiano | Spanish/Español | German/Deutsch | Japanese/日本語 |
|---|---|---|---|---|---|
| 5371. principal investigator - (n) | investigateur principal | investigatore principale | investigador principal | Hauptuntersucher | 主任研究者 |
| 5372. principle - (n) | principe | principio | principio | Prinzip | 原理、原則、成分 |
| 5373. prior - (a) | précédent | precedente | previa | früher | 以前の |
| 5374. prioritization - (n) | établir la priorité | prioritizzazione | prioritización | Ordnung nach Priorität | 優先化 |
| 5375. priority - (n) | priorité | priorità | prioridad | Priorität | 優先 |
| 5376. prisoner - (n) | prisonnier | prigioniero | prisionero | Häftling; Sträfling | 囚人 |
| 5377. private - (a) | privé | privato | privado | privat | 個人の |
| 5378. private practice - (n) | pratique privée | studio privato | practica privada | Privatpraxis | 個人開業 |
| 5379. private sector - (n) | secteur privé | settore privato | sector privado | privater Sektor | 私立の部分 |
| 5380. proarrhythmic - (n) | proarythmique | proaritmico | proarrítmico | Arrhythmikum | 不整脈を起こしやすい状態 |
| 5381. probability - (n) | probabilité | probabilità | probabilidad | Wahrscheinlichkeit | 確率 |
| 5382. probably drug related - (n) | probablement relié à la drogue | probabilmente correlato al farmaco | probablemente relacionado con droga | wahrscheinlich medikamentös bedingt | おそらく薬物に関連の |
| 5383. probe - (n) | sonde | sonda | sonda | Sonde; Sondierung | 消息子、ゾンデ |
| 5384. probe - (v) | sonder | sondare | sondear | sondieren | 探る |
| 5385. problem - (n) | problème | problema | problema | Problem | 問題 |
| 5386. problem solving - (n) | résolution de problème | soluzione del problema | resolución de problema | Problemlösung | 問題解決 |
| 5387. problem-oriented record - (n) | dossier des problèmes | cartella clinica dei problemi | registro de los problemas | problembezogenes Protokoll | 問題指向型記録 |
| 5388. procedure - (n) | procédure | procedura | procedimiento | Verfahren; Vorgehen | 手順 |
| 5389. process - (n) | processus; procédé | processo | proceso | Prozeß; Verfahren | 過程 |
| 5390. processing - (n) | traitement; transformation | elaborazione; trattamento | procesamiento; elaboración | Entwicklung; Verarbeitung | 処理 |
| 5391. proconvulsant - (n) | proconvulsivant | proconvulsivante | proconvulsionante | krampfauslösendes Medikament | 痙攣を起こしやすい状態 |

| English/American | French/Français | Italian/Italiano | Spanish/Español | German/Deutsch | Japanese/日本語 |
|---|---|---|---|---|---|
| 5392. procreation - (n) | procréation | procreazione | procreación | Zeugung; Fortpflanzung | 生殖 |
| 5393. proctoscope - (n) | rectoscope | proctoscopio; rettoscopio | proctoscopio | Proktoskop | 直腸鏡 |
| 5394. proctosig-moidoscopy - (n) | rectosigmoidoscopie | retto-sigmoidoscopia | proctosigmoidoscopia | Proktosigmoidoskopie | 直腸 S 状結腸鏡検査［法］ |
| 5395. prodrome - (n) | prodrome | prodromo | pródromo | Prodrom | 前駆症［状］, 前徴 |
| 5396. prodrug - (n) | promédicament | profarmaco | profármaco | Arzneimittelvorstufe | プロドラッグ |
| 5397. producing - (n) | production; fabrication | produttore | productor | Herstellung; Produktion | 生成, 積 |
| 5398. product - (n) | produit; résultat | prodotto; risultato | producto; resultado | Produkt; Resultat | 産物, 生成物 |
| 5399. product develop-ment - (n) | développement de produit | sviluppo del prodotto | desarrollo del producto | Produktentwicklung | 製品開発 |
| 5400. product differenti-ation - (n) | différenciation de produit | differenziazione del prodotto | diferenciación del producto | Produktspezialisierung | 製品区別 |
| 5401. product license - (n) | autorisation de produit | brevetto di un prodotto | licencia de fabricación | Produktzulassung | 製品許可書 |
| 5402. product license application - (n) | application pour autorisation d'un produit | domanda per autorizzazione di un prodotto | solicitud de licencia del producto | Produktzulassungsantrag | 製品許可書出願 |
| 5403. product safety - (n) | sécurité de produit | sicurezza del prodotto | seguridad del producto | Sicherheit des Produkts | 製品の安全性 |
| 5404. product surveil-lance - (n) | surveillance de produit | sorveglianza di un prodotto | monitoreo del producto | Produktüberwachung | 製品の監視 |
| 5405. production - (n) | production; fabrication | produzione | producción; fabricación | Produktion; Herstellung | 生産 |
| 5406. production facility - (n) | installation de production | impianti per la produzione | facilidad de fabricación | Produktionsanlage | 製造施設 |
| 5407. production lot - (n) | lot de production; lot de fabrication | lotto di produzione | lote de fabricación | Produktionscharge | 製品のロット |
| 5408. professional - (a) | professionnel | professionale | profesional | beruflich; fachmännisch | 専門の |
| 5409. professional practice - (n) | pratique professionnelle | studio professionale | práctica profesional | Facharztpraxis | 専門診療 |

277

| English/American | French/Français | Italian/Italiano | Spanish/Español | German/Deutsch | Japanese日本語 |
|---|---|---|---|---|---|
| 5410. professor - (n) | professeur | professore | profesor | Professor; Dozent | 教授 |
| 5411. progestation-al - (a) | progestatif | progestativo | progestacional | progesteronartig | 妊娠のための、プロゲステロンの |
| 5412. progestogen - (n) | progestogène | progestinico | progestógeno | Gestagen | プロゲストーゲン |
| 5413. prognosis - (n) | pronostic | prognosi | pronóstico; prognosis | Prognose | 予後 |
| 5414. prognostic - (a) | pronostique | prognostica | pronóstico | prognostisch | 予後の |
| 5415. program (programme) - (n) | programme | programma | programa | Programm | プログラム |
| 5416. program - (v) | programmer | programmare | programar | programmieren | プログラムする |
| 5417. programming language - (n) | langage de programmation | linguaggio di programmazione | lenguaje de programación | Programmiersprache | プログラミング言語 |
| 5418. progress note - (n) | note de progrès | annotazione della evoluzione | nota de evolución | Notiz über den Fortschritt | 進行記録 |
| 5419. progressive - (a) | progressif | progressivo | progresivo | progressiv | 進行 [性] の、直進 [性] の |
| 5420. prohibited - (a) | prohibé | proibito | prohibido | verboten | 禁止された |
| 5421. prohibition - (n) | prohibition | proibizione | prohibición | Verbot; Prohibition | 禁止 |
| 5422. project - (n) | projet | progetto; piano | proyecto | Projekt | プロジェクト |
| 5423. project - (v) | projeter; faire des plans | fare un piano | proyectar | projizieren; planen | 立案する |
| 5424. projection - (n) | projection | proiezione | proyección | Projektion; Verlagerung | 突出、投射 |
| 5425. projector - (n) | projecteur | proiettore | proyector | Projektor | プロジェクター |
| 5426. prolapse - (n) | prolapsus | prolasso | prolapso | Prolaps; Vorfall | 脱 [出症] |
| 5427. proliferation - (n) | prolifération | proliferazione | proliferación | Proliferation | 増殖、繁殖 |
| 5428. prolong - (v) | prolonger | prolungare | prolongar | verlängern; ausdehnen | 延期する |
| 5429. prolongation - (n) | prolongation | prolungamento | prolongación | Verlängerung | 延長 |
| 5430. prominence - (n) | proéminence | prominenza | prominencia | Vorsprung | 隆起 |
| 5431. promoter - (n) | promoteur | promotore | promotor | Förderer | 助成者、プロモーター |
| 5432. promotion - (n) | promotion | promozione | promoción | Promotion; Förderung | 増進 |

| English/American | French/Français | Italian/Italiano | Spanish/Español | German/Deutsch | Japanese 日本語 |
|---|---|---|---|---|---|
| 5433. pronation - (n) | pronation | pronazione | pronación | Pronation | 回内［運動］ |
| 5434. prone - (a) | prédisposé; prostré | disposto; prostrato | ser propenso a; estar postrado | zu etwas neigend | 腹臥の、うつむきになる |
| 5435. propagate - (v) | propager | propagare | propagar | fortpflanzen; fortleiten | 生殖する |
| 5436. property - (n) | propriété | proprietà | propiedad | Eigenschaft | 性質 |
| 5437. prophase - (n) | prophase | profase | profase | Prophase | 前期 |
| 5438. prophylactic - (n) | prophylactique | profilattico | profiláctico | prophylaktisches Mittel | 予防薬 |
| 5439. prophylactic - (a) | prophylactique | profilattico | profiláctico | prophylaktisch | 予防の |
| 5440. prophylaxis - (n) | prophylaxie | profilassi | profilaxis | Prophylaxe; Vorbeugung | 予防［法］ |
| 5441. proportion surviving - (n) | proportion survivance | proporzione sopravvivente | porción sobreviviente | Überlebensrate | 生残名割合 |
| 5442. proprietary - (a) | de propriété; breveté | brevettato; di proprietà | propietario | geschützt | 所有の |
| 5443. proprietary medicine - (n) | médecine brevetée | medicinale brevettato | remedio de patente | geschütztes Handelspräparat | 特許薬品 |
| 5444. proprietary name - (n) | marque brevetée | marchio brevettato | nombre de patente | geschützter Name | 商品名 |
| 5445. proprioception - (n) | proprioception | propriocezione | propiocepción | Propriozeption | 固有受容性 |
| 5446. proptosis - (n) | proptose | proptosi | proptosis | Vorfall; Exophthalmus | 突出、脱出 |
| 5447. propulsion - (n) | propulsion | propulsione | propulsión | Propulsion; Antepulsion | 前方突進 |
| 5448. propulsive gait - (n) | démarche propulsive | andatura propulsiva | marcha propulsora | propulsiver Gang | 前方突進歩行 |
| 5449. prospective - (a) | prospectif | prospettico; probabile | prospectivo; probable | voraussichtlich | 予期している |
| 5450. prospective study - (n) | étude prospective | studio prospettico | estudio prospectivo | prospektive Studie | 予期研究 |
| 5451. prostate - (n) | prostate | prostata | próstata | Prostata | 前立腺 |
| 5452. prosthesis - (n) | prothèse | protesi | prótesis | Prothese | プロテーゼ、人工器官 |
| 5453. prostrate - (a) | prostré; étendu | prostrato | postrado | ausgestreckt | 衰えた |

279

| English/American | French/Français | Italian/Italiano | Spanish/Español | German/Deutsch | Japanese/日本語 |
|---|---|---|---|---|---|
| 5454. prostration - (n) | prostration | prostrazione | postración | Prostration | 疲労状い、へばり |
| 5455. protease - (n) | protéase | proteasi | proteasa | Protease; Proteinase | プロテアーゼ、蛋白［質］分解酵素 |
| 5456. protection - (n) | protection | protezione | protección | Schutz; Schutzvorrichtung | 保護 |
| 5457. protective device - (n) | appareil protecteur | dispositivo di protezione | dispositivo protector | Schutzvorrichtung | 保護装置 |
| 5458. protein - (n) | protéine; protide | proteina | proteína | Protein; Eiweiß | 蛋白質 |
| 5459. protein binding - (n) | liaison protéique | legame alle proteine | fijación a proteínas | Proteinbindung | 蛋白質結合 |
| 5460. protein denaturation - (n) | dénaturation protéique; dénaturation protidique | denaturazione delle proteine | desnaturalización de proteínas | Proteindenaturierung | 蛋白質変性 |
| 5461. protein structure - (n) | structure protéique | struttura di una proteina | estructura de la proteína | Proteinstruktur | 蛋白質の構造 |
| 5462. proteinase - (n) | protéinase | proteinasi | proteinasa | Proteinase | プロテアーゼ、蛋白分解酵素 |
| 5463. proteinuria - (n) | protéinurie | proteinuria | proteinuria | Proteinurie | 蛋白尿 |
| 5464. proteolysis - (n) | protéolyse | proteolisi | proteólisis | Proteolyse | 蛋白分解 |
| 5465. prothrombin - (n) | prothrombine | protrombina | protrombina | Prothrombin | プロトロンビン |
| 5466. prothrombin time - (n) | temps de prothrombine | tempo di protrombina | tiempo de protrombina | Prothrombinzet | プロトロンビン時間 |
| 5467. proto-oncogene - (n) | protooncogène | proto-oncogene | protooncogén | Protoonkogen | プロトオンコジーン |
| 5468. protocol - (n) | protocole | protocollo | protocolo | Protokoll | プロトコル |
| 5469. protocol amendment - (n) | modification de protocole | emendamento del protocollo | enmienda al protocolo | Protokolländerung; -ergänzung | プロトコル修正 |
| 5470. protocol deviation - (n) | déviation de protocole | deviazione dal protocollo | desviación del protocolo | Protokollabweichung | プロトコルからはずれていること |

280

| English/American | French/Français | Italian/Italiano | Spanish/Español | German/Deutsch | Japanese/日本語 |
|---|---|---|---|---|---|
| 5471. protocol number - (n) | numéro de protocole | numero di protocollo | número del protocolo | Protokollnummer | プロトコル番号 |
| 5472. protocol review committee - (n) | comité de revue de protocole | commissione per la revisione dei protocolli clinici | comité de revisión del protocolo | Protokollüberprüfungs-ausschuß | プロトコル点検委員会 |
| 5473. protocol violation - (n) | violation du protocole | violazione del protocollo | violación del protocolo | Protokollverletzung; -übertretung | プロトコル違反 |
| 5474. proton - (n) | proton | protone | protón | Proton | 陽子 |
| 5475. proton pump - (n) | pompe à proton | pompa protonica | bomba de protón | Protonenpumpe | 陽子ポンプ |
| 5476. protoplasm - (n) | protoplasme | protoplasma | protoplasma | Protoplasma | 原形質 |
| 5477. protozoa - (n) | protozoaires | protozoa; protozoi | protozoa | Protozoen | 原生動物 |
| 5478. protozoan - (n) | protozoaire | protozoario | protozoario | Protozoon | 原生動物の |
| 5479. protruding tongue - (n) | langue saillante | lingua protrudente | lengua saliente; lengua protuberante | herausgestreckte Zunge | 突出している舌 |
| 5480. protrusion - (n) | protubérance | protrusione | protrusión | Protrusion; Vorwölbung | 突出、前突 |
| 5481. proud - (a) | orgueilleux; fier | soddisfatto; orgoglioso | orgulloso | stolz | 誇らしい |
| 5482. province - (n) | province | provincia | provincia | Provinz | 領域 |
| 5483. provitamin - (n) | provitamine | provitamina | provitamina | Provitamin | プロビタミン |
| 5484. provocation test - (n) | épreuve de provocation | test provocatorio | prueba de provocación | Provokationstest | 誘発検査 |
| 5485. proximal - (a) | proximal | prossimale | proximal | proximal; ungefähr | 近位の |
| 5486. pruritus - (n) | prurit | prurito | prurito | Pruritus; Hautjucken | かゆみ [症] |
| 5487. pseudomembranous enterocolitis - (n) | pseudomembraneuse | pseudomembranosa | seudomembranosa | pseudomembranöse Enterokolitis | 偽膜性腸炎 |
| 5488. pseudo- - (prefix) | pseudo- | pseudo- | seudo | Pseudo- | 偽性の |
| 5489. psyche - (n) | psychisme; psyché | psiche | psique | Psyche | 精神 |
| 5490. psychedelic - (a) | psychédélique | psichedelico | psicodélico | psychedelisch | サイケデリックな |

281

| English/American | French/Français | Italian/Italiano | Spanish/Español | German/Deutsch | Japanese/日本語 |
|---|---|---|---|---|---|
| 5491. psychiatric - (a) | psychiatrique | psichiatrico | psiquiátrico | psychiatrisch | 精神医学の |
| 5492. psychiatric status rating scale - (n) | échelle d'état psychiatrique | grado delle stato psichiatrico | escala del estado psiquiátrico | Beurteilungssystem für den psychiatrischen Zustand | 精神状態判断尺度 |
| 5493. psychiatry - (n) | psychiatrie | psichiatria | psiquiatría | Psychiatrie | 精神医学 |
| 5494. psychic - (a) | psychique | psichico | psíquico | psychisch | 精神的な、心的な |
| 5495. psychoanalysis - (n) | psychanalyse | psicanalisi | psicoanálisis | Psychoanalyse | 精神分析 [学] |
| 5496. psychoanalytic - (a) | psychanalytique | psicanalitico | psicoanalítico | psychoanalytisch | 精神分析 [学] の |
| 5497. psychological - (a) | psychologique | psicologico | psicológico | psychologisch | 心理学の、心 [理] 的の |
| 5498. psychological interview - (n) | entrevue psychologique | colloquio psicologico | entrevista psicológica | psychologische Befragung | 心理学的面接 |
| 5499. psychology - (n) | psychologie | psicologia | psicología | Psychologie | 心理学 |
| 5500. psychometric evaluation - (n) | évaluation psychométrique | valutazione psicometrica | evaluación psicométrica | psychometrische Bewertung | 心理測定評価 |
| 5501. psychometrics - (n) | psychométrie | psicometria | psicometría | Psychometrie | 心理測定 [学] |
| 5502. psychomotor - (a) | psychomoteur | psicomotorio | psicomotor | psychomotorisch | 精神運動の |
| 5503. psychopathology - (n) | psychopathologie | psicopatologia | psicopatología | Psychopathologie | 精神病理学 |
| 5504. psychopharmacology - (n) | psychopharmacologie | psicofarmacologia | psicofarmacología | Psychopharmakologie | 精神薬理学 |
| 5505. psychosexual - (a) | psychosexuel | psicosessuale | psicosexual | psychosexuell | 精神、性的の |
| 5506. psychosis - (n) | pyschose | psicosi | psicosis | Psychose | 精神病 |
| 5507. psychosocial - (a) | psychosocial | psicosociale | psicosocial | psychosozial | 心理、社会的の |
| 5508. psychosomatic - (a) | psychosomatique | psicosomatico | psicosomático | psychosomatisch | 心身の、精神身体の |

| English/American | French/Français | Italian/Italiano | Spanish/Español | German/Deutsch | Japanese日本語 |
|---|---|---|---|---|---|
| 5509. psycho-surgery - (n) | psychochirurgie | psicochirurgia | psicocirugía | Psychochirurgie | 精神外科 |
| 5510. psycho-therapy - (n) | psychothérapie | psicoterapia | psicoterapia | Psychotherapie | 心理療法、精神療法 |
| 5511. psychotic - (a) | psychotique | psicotico | psicótico | psychotisch | 精神病 [性] の |
| 5512. psychotic affective disorder - (n) | désordre affect f | disordine psicotico-affettivo | trastorno afectivo psicótico | psychotische Affektstörung | 精神病性情動障害 |
| 5513. psychotic disorder - (n) | désordre psychotique | disordine psicotico | trastorno psicótico | psychotische Störung | 精神病 |
| 5514. psychotropic - (a) | psychotrope | psicotropico | psicotrópico | psychotrop | 精神作用 [性] の |
| 5515. ptosis - (n) | ptose | ptosi | ptosis | Ptosis; Senkung | 下垂 [症] |
| 5516. puberty - (n) | puberté | pubertà | pubertad | Pubertät | 青春期 |
| 5517. pubic bone - (n) | os pubien | osso del pube | hueso pubis | Schambein | 恥骨 |
| 5518. pubis - (n) | pubis | pube | pubis | Schamhaar; Schambein | 恥骨、陰毛 |
| 5519. public - (a) | publique | pubblico | público | öffentlich | 公共の |
| 5520. public health - (n) | santé publique | sanità pubblica | salud pública | Gesundheitswesen; Volksgesundheit | 公衆衛生 |
| 5521. public policy - (n) | politique publique | linea di condotto pubblico | política pública | öffentliche Belange; öffentliches Interesse | 公共政策 |
| 5522. public relations - (n) | relations publiques | relazioni pubbliche | relaciones públicas | öffentliche Meinungspflege; Öffentlichkeitsarbeit | ピーアール、宣伝活動 |
| 5523. public sector - (n) | secteur publique | settore pubblico | sector público | öffentlicher Bereich | 公立の部分 |
| 5524. publication - (n) | publication | pubblicazione | publicación | Veröffentlichung | 公表 |
| 5525. publishing - (n) | publication | editoria | publicación | Veröffentlichen | 出版 |
| 5526. pudendal - (a) | relatif aux organes génitaux | pudendo | pudendo | Scham- | 外陰部の |
| 5527. puerile - (a) | puéril | puerile | pueril | kindisch | 幼児の |

283

| English/American | French/Français | Italian/Italiano | Spanish/Español | German/Deutsch | Japanese/日本語 |
|---|---|---|---|---|---|
| 5528. puerperal - (a) | puerpéral | puerperale | puerperal | puerperal | 産褥の |
| 5529. puerperal fever - (n) | fièvre puerpérale | febbre puerperale | fiebre puerperal | Kindbettfieber | 産褥熱 |
| 5530. pulmonary - (a) | pulmonaire | polmonare | pulmonar | pulmonal; Lungen- | 肺の |
| 5531. pulmonary capillary wedge pressure - (n) | pression capillaire pulmonaire | pressione d'incuneamento polmonare | presión capilar pulmonar | Lungenkapilla-verschlußdruck | 肺毛細管楔入圧 |
| 5532. pulmonary function test - (n) | épreuve de fonction pulmonaire | test di funzionalità polmonare | prueba de función pulmonar | Lungenfunktionstest | 肺機能検査 |
| 5533. pulmonary surfactant - (n) | surfactant pulmonaire | surfactante polmonare | surfactante pulmonar | Surfactant-Faktor | 肺の界面活性物質 |
| 5534. pulmonary valve - (n) | valve pulmonaire | valvola polmonare | válvula pulmonar | Pulmonalklappe | 肺動脈弁 |
| 5535. pulmonary vascular resistance - (n) | résistance vasculaire pulmonaire | resistenza polmonare vascolare | resistencia vascular pulmonar | Lungengefäßwiderstand | 肺血管抵抗 |
| 5536. pulmonary wedge pressure - (n) | pression capillaire pulmonaire bloquée | pressione arteriosa polmonare | presión pulmonar | Pulmonalarterien-verschlußdruck | 肺楔入圧 |
| 5537. pulp - (n) | pulpe | polpa | pulpa | Pulpa | 骨髄［質］ |
| 5538. pulsatile flow - (n) | flot pulsatile | flusso pulsante | flujo pulsátil | pulsierender Fuß | 拍動性の流れ |
| 5539. pulsation - (n) | pulsation | pulsazione | pulsación | Pulsation | 脈動、拍動 |
| 5540. pulse - (n) | pouls | polso | pulso | Puls | 脈拍、脈 |
| 5541. pulse - (v) | pulser | pulsare | pulsar | pulsieren | 脈打つ |
| 5542. pulse pressure - (n) | pression du pouls | pressione pulsatoria | presión del pulso | Pulsdruck | 脈圧 |
| 5543. pulse wave - (n) | onde du pouls | onda di pulsazione | onda del pulso | Pulswelle | 脈波 |
| 5544. pump - (n) | pompe | pompa | bomba | Pumpe | ポンプ |
| 5545. pump - (v) | pomper | pompare | bombear | pumpen | ポンプの作用をする |

| English/American | French/Français | Italian/Italiano | Spanish/Español | German/Deutsch | Japanese/日本語 |
|---|---|---|---|---|---|
| 5546. punctate rash - (n) | éruption punctiforme | eczema puntiforme | erupción punteada | punktförmiger Ausschlag | 小斑点の皮疹 |
| 5547. puncture - (n) | ponction | puntura | punción | Punktion; Punktur | 穿刺 |
| 5548. punishment - (n) | punition | punizione | castigo | Strafe | 罰 |
| 5549. pupil - (n) | pupille | pupilla | pupila | Pupille | 瞳孔 |
| 5550. pupillary reflex - (n) | réflexe pupillaire | riflesso pupillare | reflejo pupilar | Pupillenreflex; Lichtreflex | 瞳孔反射 |
| 5551. purgative - (n) | purgatif | purgante; purga | purgante | Purgativum; Abführmittel | 下剤 |
| 5552. purgative - (a) | purgatif | purgativo | purgativo | purgativ; abführend | 下剤の |
| 5553. purinergic receptor - (n) | récepteur purinergique | recettore purinergico | receptor purinérgico | purinergischer Rezeptor | プリン作動性レセプター |
| 5554. purity - (n) | pureté | purezza | pureza | Reinheit | 純度、武純 |
| 5555. purpura - (n) | purpura | porpora | púrpura | Purpura | 紫斑、紫斑病 |
| 5556. purulent - (a) | purulent | purulento | purulento | purulent | 化膿 [性] の |
| 5557. pus - (n) | pus | pus | pus | Eiter; Pus | 膿 |
| 5558. pustule - (n) | pustule | pustola | pústula | Pustel; Pustula | 膿疱、プステル |
| 5559. putrefaction - (n) | putréfaction | putrefazione | putrefacción | Fäulnisvorgang; Verwesung | 腐敗 |
| 5560. putrid - (a) | putride | putrido | pútrido | verfaulend | 腐敗性の、腐敗の |
| 5561. p-value - (n) | valeur de p (probabilité) | valore p; p-value | valor p | p-Wert | p－値 |
| 5562. pyelonephritis - (n) | pyélonéphrite | pielonefrite | pielonefritis | Pyelonephritis | 腎盂腎炎 |
| 5563. pyemia - (n) | pyémie; pyohémie | piemia | piemia | Pyämie | 膿血 [症] |
| 5564. pyloric antrum - (n) | antre pylorique | antro pilorico | antro pilórico | Antrum pyloricum | 幽門洞 |
| 5565. pylorus - (n) | pylore | piloro | píloro | Magenpförtner; Pylorus | 幽門 |
| 5566. pyogenic - (a) | pyogène | piogenico; piogeno | piogénico | eiterbildend; pyogen | 化膿 [性] の |
| 5567. pyramid chart - (n) | graphique en pyramide | diagramma piramidale | diagrama piramidal | Pyramidendiagramm | ピラミッド形のグラフ |
| 5568. pyramid histogram - (n) | histogramme en pyramide | istogramma a piramide | histograma piramidal | Pyramidenhistogramm | ピラミッド形の ヒストグラム |

285

| English/American | French/Français | Italian/Italiano | Spanish/Español | German/Deutsch | Japanese/日本語 |
|---|---|---|---|---|---|
| 5569. pyramidal tract - (n) | voie pyramidale | tratto piramidale | tracto piramidal | Pyramidenbahn | 錐体路 |
| 5570. pyrexia - (n) | pyrexie | piressia | pirexia | Pyrexie; Fieber | 発熱 |
| 5571. pyrogen - (n) | pyrogène | pirogeno | pirógeno | Pyrogen | 発熱物質 |
| 5572. pyuria - (n) | pyurie | piuria | piuria | Pyurie | 膿尿 |

| English/American | French/Français | Italian/Italiano | Spanish/Español | German/Deutsch | Japanese 日本語 |
|---|---|---|---|---|---|
| 5573. quack - (n) | charlatan; toubib | sedicente medico; imbroglione | curandero | Quacksalber; Kurpfuscher | やぶ医者 |
| 5574. quadrant - (n) | quadrant | quadrante | cuadrante | Quadrant | 四分円 [部分] |
| 5575. quadriplegia - (n) | quadriplégie | quadriplegia | cuadriplejia | Tetraplegie | 四肢麻痺 |
| 5576. qualitative - (a) | qualitatif | qualitativo | cualitativo | qualitativ | 定性の |
| 5577. quality - (n) | qualité | qualità | calidad | Qualität | 性質 |
| 5578. quality adjusted life year - (n) | année de vie ajustée à la qualité | anni di sopravvivenza/ qualità di vita | año de vida ajustado a la calidad | Lebensjahre mit guter Lebensqualität | 生活度に適合した年月 |
| 5579. quality assurance - (n) | assurance de qualité | verifica di qualità | garantía de calidad | Qualitätssicherung | 品質保証 |
| 5580. quality control - (n) | contrôle de qualité | controllo di qualità | control de calidad | Qualitätskontrolle | 品質管理 |
| 5581. quality of life - (n) | qualité de vie | qualità della vita | calidad de vida | Lebensqualität | 生活度 |
| 5582. qualm - (n) | malaise; nausée | senso di nausea | bascas; náusea | Schwächeanfall; Angstgefühl | 眩暈 |
| 5583. quantitative - (a) | quantitatif | quantitativo | cuantitativo | quantitativ | 定量の |
| 5584. quarantine - (n) | quarantaine | quarantena | cuarentena | Quarantäne | 検疫 |
| 5585. quarantine - (v) | mettre en quarantaine | mettere in quarantena | poner en cuarentena | unter Quarantäne stellen; isolieren | 検疫する |
| 5586. quench - (v) | assouvir; étancher | inibire; bloccare | apagar | abschrecken; abkühlen | 消滅させる |
| 5587. questionnaire - (n) | questionnaire | questionario | cuestionario | Fragebogen | 質問書、調査票 |
| 5588. quick and dirty study - (n) | étude vite faite | studio veloce e sommario | estudio rápido e improlijo | auf die Schnelle durchgeführte Studie | 雑な初期的研究 |
| 5589. quiescent - (a) | passif; immobile | latente | quieto; inactivo | inaktiv; asymptomatisch | 静隠の |
| 5590. quiet - (a) | tranquille; silencieux | quieto; silenzioso | silencioso; callado | ruhig; still | 静かな |
| 5591. quirk - (n) | bizarrerie; excentricité | stravaganza | peculiaridad | Laune; Zucken | 急変 |
| 5592. quiver - (n) | tremblement; frisson | fremito; tremito | temblor; estremecimiento | Zittern; Zuckung | 震え |
| 5593. quorum - (n) | quorum | quorum | quórum | Quorum | 定足数 |
| 5594. quota - (n) | quota; quote-part | parte quota; aliquota | cuota | Quote | 割当 |

| English/American | French/Français | Italian/Italiano | Spanish/Español | German/Deutsch | Japanese/日本語 |
|---|---|---|---|---|---|
| 5595. rabid - (a) | enragé | rabbico; idrofobo | rabioso | tollwütig; wütend | 狂犬病の |
| 5596. race - (n) | race | razza | raza | Rasse | 人種 |
| 5597. radial keratotomy - (n) | kératotomie radiale | cheratotomia radiale | queratotomía radial | radiale Keratotomie | 放射状角膜切開 |
| 5598. radiant - (a) | radieux; rayonnant | radiante | radiante | strahlend | 放射能物質、光点 |
| 5599. radiating pain - (n) | douleur irradiante | dolore irradiante | dolor irradiado | ausstrahlender Schmerz | 放散痛 |
| 5600. radiation - (n) | radiation | radiazione | radiación | Strahlung | 放射、照射 |
| 5601. radiation induced - (a) | induit par la radiation | indotto da radiazione | inducido por radiación | strahleninduziert | 放射線誘発の |
| 5602. radiation sensitizing agent - (n) | agent radiosensibilisateur | agente sensibilizzante alle radiazioni | agente sensibilizador de radiación | strahlensensibilisierendes Mittel | 放射線感受作剤 |
| 5603. radiation therapy - (n) | radiothérapie | radioterapia | radioterapia | Strahlentherapie | 放射線療法 |
| 5604. radical - (n) | radical | radicale | radical | Radikal | 基、ラジカル |
| 5605. radical - (a) | radical | radicale | radical | radikal | 根本的の |
| 5606. radical mastectomy - (n) | mastectomie radicale | mastectomia radicale | mastectomía radical | radikale Mastektomie | 定型的[根治的]乳房切断[術] |
| 5607. radio wave - (n) | onde radioélectrique; onde radio | onda radio; radioonda | onda radioeléctrica | Funkwelle; Radiowelle | 無線波 |
| 5608. radioactive - (a) | radioactif | radioattivo | radioactivo | radioaktiv | 放射性の |
| 5609. radioactive tracer - (n) | traceur radioactif | tracciante radioattivo | trazador radioactivo | Radioindikator | 放射能トレーサ |
| 5610. radioactive uptake - (n) | captation radioactive | captazione radioattiva | captación radioactiva | Aufnahme radioaktiver Substanzen | 放射能吸収 |
| 5611. radiobiology - (n) | radiobiologie | radiobiologia | radiobiología | Radiobiologie; Strahlenbiologie | 放射線生物学 |
| 5612. radiocontrast medium - (n) | agent de radiocontraste | mezzo di contrasto radioattivo | medio de radiocontraste | Radiokontrastmedium | 放射造影剤 |

288

| English/American | French/Français | Italian/Italiano | Spanish/Español | German/Deutsch | Japanese/日本語 |
|---|---|---|---|---|---|
| 5613. radiograph - (n) | radiographie | radiografia | radiografía | Röntgenaufnahme | X線写真 |
| 5614. radiographic - (a) | radiographicue | radiografico | radiográfico | radiografisch | X線写真の |
| 5615. radiography - (n) | radiographie | radiografia | radiografía | Radiographie | X線撮影の |
| 5616. radioimmunoas- say - (n) | essai immunologique | radioimmunoassay; test radioimmunologico | radioinmunoanálisis | Radioimmunoassay | ラジオイムノアッセイ [法] |
| 5617. radioimmuno- detection - (n) | détection radioimmuno ogique | evidenziazione con metodo radioimmunologico | radioinmunodetección | Radioimmunodetektion | 放射性免疫検出 |
| 5618. radioisotope - (n) | radioisotope | radioisotopo | radioisótopo | Radioisotop | 放射性同位元素 |
| 5619. radiolabeled - (a) | marqué radioactivement | radiomarcato | marcado radioactivamente | mit radioaktiver Markierung | 放射性標識の |
| 5620. radioligand - (n) | ligand radioacif | radioligando | radioligando | radioaktiver Ligand | 放射リガンド |
| 5621. radiologist - (n) | radiologue; radiologiste | radiologo | radiólogo | Radiologe | 放射線科医 |
| 5622. radiology - (n) | radiologie | radiologia | radiología | Radiologie | 放射線 [医] 学 |
| 5623. radiometry - (n) | radiométrie | radiometria | radiometría | Radiometrie | 線量測定 [法] |
| 5624. radionuclide - (n) | radionucléide | radionuclide | radionúclido | Radionuklid | 放射性核種 |
| 5625. radiopaque - (a) | radio-opaque | radiopaco | radiopaco | strahlenundurchlässig | 放射能不透過性の |
| 5626. radiosensitive - (a) | radiosensible | radiosensibile | radiosensible | strahlenempfindlich | 放射能感受性の |
| 5627. radiosensi- tizer - (n) | radiosensibilisateur | radiosensibilizzatore | radiosensibilizador | Radiosensibilisator | 放射能感受性物質 |
| 5628. radiosurgery - (n) | radiochirurgie | radiochirurgia | radiocirugía | Hochfrequenzchirurgie | 放射線三術 |
| 5629. radiotherapy - (n) | radiothérapie | radioterapia | radioterapia | Radiotherapie; Strahlentherapie | 放射線治療 |
| 5630. radius - (n) | radius; rayon | radio; raggio | radio | Radius | 半径、橈骨 |
| 5631. radon - (n) | radon | radon | radón | Radon | ラドン |
| 5632. rage - (n) | rage; fureur | rabbia; furore | rabia; ira | Wut | 激怒、怒り、狂暴 |
| 5633. raised lesion - (n) | lésion surélevée | lesione rilevata | lesión levantada | erhobene Läsion | 隆起病巣 |
| 5634. rales - (n) | râles | rantoli | estertores | Rasselgeräusche; Atemgeräusche | ラッセル |

| English/American | French/Français | Italian/Italiano | Spanish/Español | German/Deutsch | Japanese 日本語 |
|---|---|---|---|---|---|
| 5635. Raman spectrum analysis - (n) | analyse spectrale Raman | spettrofotometria di Raman | análisis de espectro de Raman | Raman-Spektralanalyse | ラマンスペクトル分析 |
| 5636. random - (a) | aléatoire; au hasard | a caso; casuale | al azar | zufällig; ungeordnet | 無作為抽出の |
| 5637. random allocation - (n) | allocation au hasard | assegnazione casuale | asignación al azar | zufällige Zuteilung | 無作為抽出割当 |
| 5638. random numbers - (n) | nombres aléatoires | numeri casuali | números al azar | Zufallszahlen | 乱数 |
| 5639. random sample - (n) | échantillon aléatoire | esempio casuale | muestra seleccionada al azar | Zufallsstichprobe | 無作為抽出検体 |
| 5640. random screening - (n) | dépistage aléatoire | preselezione casuale | examen al azar | Zufallsauslese | 無作為スクリーニング |
| 5641. randomization (randomi-sation) - (n) | randomisation; arrangement au hasard | randomizzazione; scelta a caso | randomización; aleatorización | Randomisierung | 無作為化 |
| 5642. randomization code - (n) | code de randomisation | codice di randomizzazione | código de aleatorización | Randomisierungskode | 無作為コード |
| 5643. randomization schedule - (n) | programme de randomisation | scheda di randomizzazione | programa de aleatorización | Randomisierungszeitplan | 無作為化スケジュール |
| 5644. randomization visit - (n) | visite de randomisation | visita di randomizzazione | visita de aleatorización | randomisierte Untersuchung | 無作為抽出観察 |
| 5645. randomize - (v) | randomiser | randomizzare | randomizar; aleatorizar | randomisieren | 無作為化する |
| 5646. randomized controlled trial - (n) | essai contrôlé et randomisé | sperimentazione randomizzata controllata | estudio controlado y randomizado | randomisierte kontrollierte Studie | 無作為コントロール試験 |
| 5647. range - (n) | gamme; amplitude | gamma; ampiezza | extensión; distribución | Bereich | 範囲、分布域 |
| 5648. range of motion - (n) | étendue de mouvement | gamma di movimento | límite de movimiento | Bewegungsausmaß | 動作範囲 |
| 5649. rank - (n) | rang; ordre | rango | rango; orden | Rang; Reihe | 等級 |

| English/American | French/Français | Italian/Italiano | Spanish/Español | German/Deutsch | Japanese日本語 |
|---|---|---|---|---|---|
| 5650. rank correlation - (n) | corrélation par rangs | cograduazione | correlación por rangos | Rangkorrelation | 順位相関 |
| 5651. rank order - (n) | ordre de rangs | ordine di grado | orden de rangos | Rangordnung | 等級順序 |
| 5652. rape - (n) | viol | violenza sessuale; stupro | violación | Vergewaltigung | 強姦、強姦行為 |
| 5653. rapid eye movements [abbr] REM - (n) | mouvements oculaires rapides | movimenti oculari rapidi | movimientos oculares rápidos | schnelle Augenbewegungen | 急速眼球運動 |
| 5654. rapid speech - (n) | élocution rapide | parlata veloce | habla rápida | schnelle Sprache | 早口 |
| 5655. rare disease - (n) | maladie rare | malattia rara | enfermedad poco común | seltene Krankheit | まれな病気 |
| 5656. rash - (n) | éruption; exanthème | rash; eruzione cutanea | erupción cutánea | Ausschlag; Exanthem | 発疹、皮疹 |
| 5657. rat - (n) | rat | ratto | rata | Ratte | ラット |
| 5658. rate - (n) | taux | tasso | tasa | Häufigkeit; Anteil | 割合、率 |
| 5659. rate of enrollment - (n) | taux d'inscription | tasso di scrizione | tasa de inscripción | Patientenbeitrittsrate | 登録率 |
| 5660. rate of hospitalization - (n) | taux d'hospitalisation | tasso di ospedalizzazione | tasa de hospitalización | Krankenhauseinweisungsrate | 入院率 |
| 5661. rate of infusion - (n) | vitesse d'infusion | velocità di infusione | velocidad de infusión | Infusionsgeschwindigkeit | 浸出率 |
| 5662. rating scale - (n) | échelle d'évaluation | scala di valutazione | escala de calificación | Beurteilungssystem | 評価の尺度 |
| 5663. ratio - (n) | ratio; proportion | rapporto | relación; proporción | Verhältnis | 割合、比 |
| 5664. ration - (n) | ration | razione | ración | Ration | 定量 |
| 5665. rational - (a) | rationnel | razionale | racional | rational | 合理的な、有理的な |
| 5666. rationale - (n) | raisonnement | ragione fondamentale | razón fundamental | Grund | 原理 |
| 5667. rationalization - (n) | rationalisation | razionalizzazione | racionalización | Rationalisierung | 合理化 |
| 5668. rationing - (n) | rationnement | razionamento | racionamiento | Rationierung | 制限すること |
| 5669. rave - (v) | délirer | delirare | delirar | phantasieren | 狂乱する |
| 5670. raw data - (n) | données non traitées | dati originali | datos no procesados | unaufbereitete Daten; Rohdaten | 基本データ |
| 5671. raw score - (n) | pointage brut | punteggio originale | puntaje en bruto | Rohwert | 基本スコア |

| English/American | French/Français | Italian/Italiano | Spanish/Español | German/Deutsch | Japanese/日本語 |
|---|---|---|---|---|---|
| 5672. reabsorption - (n) | réabsorption | riassorbimento | reabsorción | Rückresorption | 再吸収 |
| 5673. reaction - (n) | réaction | reazione | reacción | Reaktion | 反応 |
| 5674. reactivation - (n) | réactivation | riattivazione | reactivación | Reaktivierung | 再活性化 |
| 5675. reactive - (a) | réactif | reattivo | reactivo | reaktiv | 反応の |
| 5676. reading - (n) | lecture | lettura | lectura | Ablesung; Lesen | 示度数、読書 |
| 5677. readmission - (n) | réadmission | riammissione | readmisión | Wiederzulassung | 再入院 |
| 5678. reagent - (n) | réactif | reagente; reattivo | reactivo | Reagenz | 試薬 |
| 5679. reality testing - (n) | épreuve de réalité | prova della realtà | comprobación de la realidad | Realitätsprüfung | 現実検討 |
| 5680. reallocation - (n) | redistribution | nuova assegnazione | reasignación; redistribución | Neuverteilung | 再割当 |
| 5681. rearrange-ment - (n) | réarrangement | riordinamento; riassetto | reorganización | Neuordnung | 再配列 |
| 5682. rebound - (n) | rebondissement; rebond | rimbalzo; rebound | rebote; contragolpe | Rückstoß | 反動 |
| 5683. rebound - (v) | rebondir; reprendre | rimbalzare | rebotar | zurückprallen | はね返る |
| 5684. rebound tenderness - (n) | douleur de rebond | dolorabilità di rimbalzo | dolor de rebote | Loslaßschmerz | 反跳圧痛、反動痛 |
| 5685. recall - (n) | rappel; souvenir | ricordo; memoria | llamada, recuerdo | Erinnerung | 想起、追想 |
| 5686. receptor - (n) | récepteur | recettore | receptor | Rezeptor; Empfänger | レセプター、受容体 |
| 5687. recess - (n) | recessus; fossette | recesso | recessus; receso | Ausbuchtung; Recessus | 陥凹 |
| 5688. recessive - (a) | récessif | recessivo | recesivo | rezessiv | 退縮の、劣性の |
| 5689. rechallenge - (n) | stimulation répétée; provocation répétée | ricarica; riprovocazione | estimulo repetido; provocación repetida | wiederholte Provokation | 再挑戦 |
| 5690. recipe - (n) | recette | ricetta | récipe; receta | Rezept | 処方箋 |
| 5691. reclining - (a) | à bascule; étendu | inclinato; clinato | acostado; tumbado | zurückliegend, rekliniert | よりかかる |
| 5692. recognition - (n) | reconnaissance | riconoscimento | reconocimiento | Erkennung | 認識 |
| 5693. recombinant DNA - (n) | ADN recombinant | ADN ricombinante | ADN recombinante | rekombinierte DNS | 組換えDNA |
| 5694. reconstitution - (n) | reconstitution | ricostituzione | reconstitución | Wiederaufbau | 再形成 |

| English/American | French/Français | Italian/Italiano | Spanish/Español | German/Deutsch | Japanese/日本語 |
|---|---|---|---|---|---|
| 5695. reconstruction - (n) | reconstruction | ricostruzione | reconstrucción | Wiederherstellung | 再建 |
| 5696. record - (n) | registre; enregistrement | nota; documento | registro | Aufzeichnung; Unterlage | 記録 |
| 5697. record - (v) | enregistrer | registrare | registrar | registrieren; aufzeichnen | 記録する |
| 5698. record linkage - (n) | liaison des dossiers | collegamento di dati | enlace de los registros | Verbindung von Unterlagen | 記録結合 |
| 5699. record review - (n) | révision de dossiers | revisione di dati | revisión de registros | Unterlagenüberprüfung | 記録再検討 |
| 5700. recovery - (n) | rétablissement; guérison | guarigione; ristabilimento | recuperación; restablecimiento | Erholung; Erholungsphase | 回復 |
| 5701. recovery room - (n) | chambre de récupération | sala di recupero | sala de posoperatorio | Aufwachstation | 回復室 |
| 5702. recreation - (n) | récréation | ricreazione | recreación | Erholung | 改造、娯楽 |
| 5703. recrudescence - (n) | recrudescence | recrudescenza | recrudecimiento | Wiederauftreten; Rekrudeszenz | 再燃 |
| 5704. recruitment - (n) | recrutement | reclutamento | inscripción; reclutamiento | Rekruitment; Rekrutierung | 漸増員 |
| 5705. recruitment log - (n) | registre de recrutement | lista di reclutamento | registro de reclutamiento | Rekrutierungslogbuch | 募集日誌 |
| 5706. recruitment period - (n) | période de recrutement | periodo di reclutamento | periodo de reclutamiento | Rekrutierungszeit | 募集期間 |
| 5707. rectal - (a) | rectal | rettale | rectal | rektal | 直腸の |
| 5708. rectal exam - (n) | examen rectal | esame rettale | examen rectal | rektale Untersuchung | 直腸検査 |
| 5709. rectum - (n) | rectum | retto | recto | Rektum | 直腸 |
| 5710. recumbent - (a) | couché; étendu | reclinato | recumbente | liegend | 横臥の |
| 5711. recuperate - (v) | se rétablir; se remettre | guarire | recuperar | erholen | 回復する |
| 5712. recurrence - (n) | récurrence; récidive | ricorrenza | recurrencia | Wiederauftreten; Rezidiv | 再発、反復 |
| 5713. recurrent - (a) | récurrent | ricorrente | recurrente | rekurrierend; wiederkehrend | 再発［性］の、反回の |
| 5714. red blood cell - (n) | globule rouge | globulo rosso | glóbulo rojo | Erythrozyt | 赤血球 |

293

| English/American | French/Français | Italian/Italiano | Spanish/Español | German/Deutsch | Japanese/日本語 |
|---|---|---|---|---|---|
| 5715. red cell count - (n) | numération des globules rouges; hémogramme | conto dei globuli rossi | recuento de glóbulos rojos | Erythrozytenzahl; -zählung | 赤血球数 |
| 5716. reduce - (v) | réduire | ridurre | reducir | reduzieren; abnehmen | 還元する、整復する |
| 5717. reducing diet - (n) | régime de réduction | dieta dimagrante | dieta de reducción | Reduktionskost | 体重減量食 |
| 5718. reduction - (n) | réduction | riduzione | reducción | Abnahme; Reduktion | 還元、整復 |
| 5719. reevaluation - (n) | réévaluation | rivalutazione | reevaluación | Wiederholung der Auswertung | 再評価 |
| 5720. reference - (n) | référence | riferimento; referenza | referencia; remisión | Hinweis; Literaturangabe | 参照、身元保証人 |
| 5721. reference range - (n) | gamme de référence | gamma di riferimento | gama de referencias | Referenzbereich | 参照の範囲 |
| 5722. reference standard - (n) | norme de référence | standard di riferimento | estándar de referencia | Referenzmaßstab | 参照の標準 |
| 5723. reference value - (n) | valeur de référence | valore di riferimento | valor de referencia | Referenzwert | 参照値 |
| 5724. referral - (n) | recommandation | riferimento | remisión | Empfehlung | 照会 |
| 5725. referred pain - (n) | douleur référée | dolore riferito; dolore trasferito | dolor referido | fortgeleiteter Schmerz | 関連痛 |
| 5726. reflex - (n) | réflexe | riflesso | reflejo | Reflex | 反射 [現象]、反射 |
| 5727. reflex arc - (n) | arc réflexe | arco riflesso | arco reflejo | Reflexbogen | 反射弓 |
| 5728. reflux - (n) | reflux | riflusso | reflujo | Reflux | 逆流、還流 |
| 5729. refraction - (n) | réfraction | rifrazione | refracción | Refraktion | 屈折 |
| 5730. refractive error - (n) | erreur de réfraction | errore di rifrazione | error de refracción | Brechungsfehler | 屈折誤差 |
| 5731. refractory - (a) | réfractaire | refrattario | refractario | obstinat; widerspenstig | 難治 [性] の |
| 5732. refrigerated storage - (n) | entreposage réfrigéré; emmagasinage réfrigéré | magazzino frigorifero | almacenamiento refrigerado | gekühlte Lagerung | 冷蔵保存 |
| 5733. refusal - (n) | refus | rifiuto | negativa; denegación | Ablehnung; Weigerung | 拒絶 |
| 5734. refuser - (n) | refusant | chi rifiuta | rehusador; rechazador | Verweigerer | 拒絶者 |
| 5735. regeneration - (n) | régénération | rigenerazione | regeneración | Regeneration | 再生 |

294

| English/American | French/Français | Italian/Italiano | Spanish/Español | German/Deutsch | Japanese/日本語 |
|---|---|---|---|---|---|
| 5736. regimen - (n) | régime | regime | régimen | Regimen; Therapieplan | 生活規則，摂生 |
| 5737. region - (n) | région | regione | región | Bereich; Region | 部位，領域 |
| 5738. regional - (a) | régional | regionale | regional | regional | 部位の，領域の |
| 5739. regional blood flow - (n) | flot sanguin régional | flusso sanguineo regionale | flujo sanguíneo regional | regionale Durchblutung | 局所血流量 |
| 5740. regional ileitis - (n) | iléite régionale; maladie de Crohn | ileo-colite granulomatosa; morbo di Crohn | ileitis regional; enfermedad de Crohn | regionale Enteritis; Crohn-Krankheit | 限局性回腸炎 |
| 5741. regional lymphadenopathy - (n) | lymphadénopathie régionale | linfadenopatia locale | linfadenopatia regional | regionale Lymphadenopathie | 局所リンパ節症 |
| 5742. registered nurse - (n) | infirmière diplômée | infermiera diplomata | enfermera diplomada | staatlich geprüfter Krankenpfleger | 登録正看護婦 |
| 5743. registration - (n) | enregistrement; inscription | registrazione; iscrizione | registro; inscripción | Registrierung; Eintragung | 登録 |
| 5744. registry - (n) | registre | registrazione | registro | Register | 登録［簿］ |
| 5745. regress - (v) | régresser | regredire | regresar | zurückentwickeln | 後退する |
| 5746. regression - (n) | régression | regressione | regresión | Regression; Rückbildung | 後退，回帰，退行 |
| 5747. regression analysis - (n) | analyse de régression | analisi di regressione | análisis de regresión | Regressionsanalyse | 回帰分析 |
| 5748. regression line - (n) | ligne de régression | linea di regressione | línea de regresión | Regressionsgerade | 回帰直線 |
| 5749. regression to the mean - (n) | régression à la moyenne | regressione alla media | regresión hacia la media | Regression zum Durchschnitt | 平均への回帰 |
| 5750. regular - (a) | régulier | regolare | regular | normal; regelrecht | 定期的な |
| 5751. regulation - (n) | régulation; réglage | regolazione; norma | regulación | Regelung; Vorschrift | 規定 |
| 5752. regulator - (n) | régulateur | chi regola | regulador | Regler | 調節器 |

| English/American | French/Français | Italian/Italiano | Spanish/Español | German/Deutsch | Japanese/日本語 |
|---|---|---|---|---|---|
| 5753. regulatory - (a) | régulateur | regolatore | reguladora | Aufsichts-; Ausführungs- | 調節する |
| 5754. regulatory dossier - (n) | dossier régulateur | dossier regolatorio | carpeta reguladora | Durchführungsdossier | 原則記録 |
| 5755. regulatory submission - (n) | soumission régulatrice | presentazione regolatoria | sumisión reguladora | Durchführungsvorlage | 原則に従った投稿 |
| 5756. regurgitation - (n) | régurgitation | rigurgito | regurgitación | Regurgitation Rückfließen | 逆流 |
| 5757. rehabilitation - (n) | réhabilitation | riabilitazione | rehabilitación | Rehabilitation; Wiederherstellung | リハビリテーション |
| 5758. rehydration - (n) | rehydration | reidratazione | rehidratación | Rehydration | 再水和 |
| 5759. reimbursement - (n) | remboursement | rimborso | reembolso | Rückerstattung; Entschädigung | 返済 |
| 5760. reinfarction - (n) | réinfarcissement | reinfarto | que vuelve a infartarse | Reinfarkt | 再硬鑑 |
| 5761. reinfection - (n) | réinfection | reinfezione | reinfección | Reinfektion | 再感染 |
| 5762. reinforcement - (n) | renforcement | rinforzo | reforzamiento | Verstärkung | 強化 |
| 5763. rejection - (n) | rejet | rigetto | rechazo | Ablehnung; Zurückweisung | 拒絶 [反応] |
| 5764. relapse - (n) | rechute; récidive | ricaduta; recidiva | recaída; relapso | Rezidiv; Rückfall | 再発、回帰 |
| 5765. relapse - (v) | rechuter; récidiver | riammalarsi | relapsar; recaer | rezidivieren | 再発する |
| 5766. relapse incidence - (n) | incidence des récidives | incidenza di ricadute | incidencia de recaídas | Rückfallsinzidenz | 再発率 |
| 5767. relapsing fever - (n) | fièvre récurrente | febbre ricorrente | fiebre recurrente | rekurrierendes Fieber | 回帰熱 |
| 5768. relations - (n) | parents | parente | parentescos | Verwandtschaft | 親族 [血縁] 関係 |
| 5769. relative - (n) | parent | parente | pariente | Verwandte- | 親類 |
| 5770. relative - (a) | relatif | relativo | relativo | relativ | 相対的な |

296

| English/American | French/Français | Italian/Italiano | Spanish/Español | German/Deutsch | Japanese/日本語 |
|---|---|---|---|---|---|
| 5771. relative bioavailability - (n) | biodisponibilité relative | biodisponibilità relativa | biodisponibilidad relativa | relative Bioverfügbarkeit | 相対的生物学的利用能 |
| 5772. relative humidity - (n) | humidité relative | umidità relativa | humedad relativa | relative Feuchtigkeit | 相対湿度 |
| 5773. relative potency - (n) | puissance relative | potenza relativa | potencia relativa | relative Potenz; relative Wirksamkeit | 相対効能 |
| 5774. relative risk - (n) | risque relatif | rischio relativo | riesgo relativo | relatives Risiko | レラティブリスク |
| 5775. relax - (v) | relâcher; relaxer | rilassare | relajar | relaxieren; entspannen | 弛緩する |
| 5776. relaxant - (n) | relaxant | spasmolitico | relajante | Relaxans | 弛緩薬 |
| 5777. relaxation - (n) | relaxation; relâchement | rilassamento | relajación | Relaxation; Entspannung | 弛緩 |
| 5778. relaxation technique - (n) | technique de relaxation | tecnica di rilassamento | técnica de relajación | Relaxationstechnik | 弛緩技術 |
| 5779. relaxing factor - (n) | facteur de relaxation | fattore rilassante | factor de relajación | entspannender Faktor | 弛緩因子 |
| 5780. reliability - (n) | fiabilité | attendibilità; affidabilità | confiabilidad; fiabilidad | Zuverlässigkeit | 信頼度、信頼性 |
| 5781. relief - (n) | soulagement | sollievo | alivio | Entlastung; Erleichterung | 軽減 |
| 5782. religion - (n) | religion | religione | religión | Religion | 宗教 |
| 5783. REM sleep - (n) | sommeil REM | sonno REM | sueño de REM | REM-Schlaf | REM睡眠 |
| 5784. remainder - (n) | reste | resto | residuo | Rückstand | 残余 |
| 5785. remedial - (a) | réparateur; curatif | che porta rimedio | curativo | heilsam | 治療の、治効の |
| 5786. remedy - (n) | remède | rimedio | remedio | Heilmittel; Arzneimittel | 治療薬 |
| 5787. remineralization - (n) | reminéralisation | remineralizzazione | remineralización | Remineralisierung | 無機質補充 |
| 5788. remission - (n) | rémission | remissione | remisión | Remission | 緩解、軽快、緩解期 |
| 5789. remittent - (a) | rémittent | remittente | remitente | remittierend | 弛緩性の |
| 5790. remote data entry - (n) | entrée de données à distance | ingresso di dati a distanza | entrada remota de datos | Datenferneingabe | 遠隔データ入力 |
| 5791. removal - (n) | élimination; enlèvement | rimozione; estirpazione | eliminación; extirpación | Entfernung; Beseitigung | 除去 |

| English/American | French/Français | Italian/Italiano | Spanish/Español | German/Deutsch | Japanese/日本語 |
|---|---|---|---|---|---|
| 5792. renal - (a) | rénal | renale | renal | renal; Nieren- | 腎［臓］の、腎性の |
| 5793. renal failure - (n) | insuffisance rénale | insufficienza renale | insuficiencia renal | Nierenversagen | 腎不全 |
| 5794. renal pelvis - (n) | bassinet | pelvi renale | pelvis renal | Nierenbecken | 腎盂 |
| 5795. renal tubules - (n) | tubules rénaux | tubuli renali | túbulos renales | Nierentubuli | 尿細管 |
| 5796. renewal - (n) | renouvellement; reprise | rinnovo | renovación; reanudación | Erneuerung | 再生 |
| 5797. renovascular hypertension - (n) | hypertension rénovasculaire | ipertensione renovascolare | hipertensión renovascular | renovaskulärer Hochdruck | 腎血管性高血圧［症］ |
| 5798. reoperation - (n) | réoperation | rioperazione | reoperación | wiederholte Operation | 再手術 |
| 5799. repair - (n) | réparation | riparazione | reparación | Reparation; Instandsetzung | 修復 |
| 5800. repeat - (n) | répétition | ripetizione | repetición | Wiederholung | 反復 |
| 5801. repeat - (v) | répéter | ripetere | repetir | wiederholen | 反復する |
| 5802. repeated observation - (n) | observation répétée | osservazione ripetuta | observación repetida | wiederholte Beobachtung | 反復観察 |
| 5803. reperfusion - (n) | reperfusion | riperfusione | reperfusión | Reperfusion | 再灌流 |
| 5804. reperfusion injury - (n) | dommage de reperfusion | lesione da riperfusione | lesión por reperfusión | Wiederdurchblutung Reperfusionsschädigung | 再灌流による障害 |
| 5805. replacement - (n) | remplacement | sostituzione | repuesto; sustitución | Ersatz | 置換 |
| 5806. replacement therapy - (n) | thérapie de remplacement | terapia sostitutiva | terapia de sustitución | Substitutionsbehandlung | 代償療法、置換療法 |
| 5807. replication - (n) | réplication | replicazione | replicación | Replikation; Wiederholung | 再現、反復 |
| 5808. repolarization - (n) | repolarisation | ripolarizzazione | repolarización | Repolarisierung; Erregungsrückbildung | 再分極 |
| 5809. report - (n) | rapport | rapporto | informe | Bericht | 報告 |
| 5810. report - (v) | rapporter | riferire | informar | berichten | 報告する |
| 5811. reporting - (n) | reportage | relazione | reportaje | Dokumentation; Bericht | 報告すること |

| English/American | French/Français | Italian/Italiano | Spanish/Español | German/Deutsch | Japanese/日本語 |
|---|---|---|---|---|---|
| 5812. representative - (a) | représentatif | rappresentativo | representante | repräsentativ | 代表的な |
| 5813. repress - (v) | réprimer | reprimere | reprimir | unterdrücken; verdrängen | 抑圧する |
| 5814. repression - (n) | répression | repressione | represión | Unterdrückung; Repression | 抑圧 |
| 5815. reproducibility - (n) | reproductibilité | riproducibilità | reproducibilidad | Reproduzierbarkeit | 生殖可能なこと |
| 5816. reproducible - (a) | reproductible | riproducibile | reproducible | reproduzierbar | 再生できる |
| 5817. reproduction - (n) | reproduction | riproduzione | reproducción | Reproduktion; Fortpflanzung | 再現、生殖 |
| 5818. reproduction study - (n) | étude de reproduction | studio di riproduzione | estudio de reproducción | Reproduktionsstudie | 生殖研究 |
| 5819. reproductive organ - (n) | organe de reproduction | organo riproduttore | órgano de reproducción | Genitalorgan | 生殖器 |
| 5820. repulsive - (a) | répulsif | repulsivo; ripulsivo | repulsivo | widerlich; abstoßend | 反発する |
| 5821. requirement - (n) | exigence | requisito | requisito | Erfordernis | 必要条件 |
| 5822. rescue - (n) | sauvetage; secours | salvataggio | rescate; salvamento | Rettung | 救出 |
| 5823. research - (n) | recherche | ricerca; investigazione | investigación | Forschung | 研究 |
| 5824. research - (v) | rechercher | indagare; svolgere ricerche | investigar | forschen | 研究する |
| 5825. research and development - (n) | recherche et développement | ricerca e sviluppo | investigación y desarrollo | Forschung und Entwicklung | 研究及び開発 |
| 5826. research tool - (n) | instrument de recherche | mezzo di ricerca | instrumento de investigación | Forschungswerkzeug | 研究手段 |
| 5827. resect - (v) | réséquer | resecare; risecare | resecar | resezieren | 切除する |
| 5828. resectable - (a) | résécable | resecabile | resecable | resezierbar | 切除できる |
| 5829. resection - (n) | résection | resezione | resección; escisión | Resektion | 切除 [術] |
| 5830. reservoir - (n) | réservoir | riserva | reservorio | Reservoir | レザバー、貯蔵所 |

299

| English/American | French/Français | Italian/Italiano | Spanish/Español | German/Deutsch | Japanese/日本語 |
|---|---|---|---|---|---|
| 5831. residence - (n) | résidence; séjour | residenza; abitazione | residencia | Wohnheim; Wohnung | 居住 |
| 5832. residency - (n) | internat | stadio di un medico interno | internado | Assistenzzeit | 専門医学実習期間 |
| 5833. residential - (a) | résidentiel | residenziale | residencial | Wohn- | 居住の |
| 5834. residual - (a) | résiduel | residuo | residual | residual; Res- Rückstand; Res. | 残留 [性] の 残留物 |
| 5835. residue - (n) | résidu | residuo | residuo | Unverwüstlichkeit; Elastizität | 弾性エネルギー、弾力性 |
| 5836. resilience - (n) | ressort; élasticité | resilienza; elasticità | resiliencia | | |
| 5837. resin - (n) | résine | resina | resina | Harz | 樹脂、レジン |
| 5838. resistance - (n) | résistance | resistenza | resistencia | Resistenz; Widerstand | 抵抗 [性] |
| 5839. resolution - (n) | résolution | risoluzione | resolución | Auflösung; Auflösungsvermögen | 消散、分解能 |
| 5840. resolve - (v) | résoudre | risolvere; risolversi | resolver | auflösen | 消散する、散らす |
| 5841. resonance - (n) | résonance | risonanza | resonancia | Resonanz; Schall | 共鳴 |
| 5842. resorption - (n) | résorption | riassorbimento | reabsorción | Resorption | 吸収 |
| 5843. resource - (n) | ressource | risorsa | recurso | Quelle; Mittel | 資源 |
| 5844. resource allocation - (n) | allocation des ressources | distribuzione delle risorse | asignación de recursos | (Hilfs)mittelzuteilung | 資源割当 |
| 5845. respiration - (n) | respiration | respirazione | respiración | Respiration; Atmrung | 呼吸 |
| 5846. respirator - (n) | respirateur; appareil respiratoire | respiratore | respirador | Respirator; Beatmungsgerät | レスピレーター、人工呼吸器 |
| 5847. respiratory - (a) | respiratoire | respiratorio | respiratorio | respiratorisch | 呼吸 [性] の |
| 5848. respiratory acidosis - (n) | acidose respiratoire | acidosi respiratoria | acidosis respiratoria | respiratorische Azidose | 呼吸性アシドーシス |
| 5849. respiratory airflow - (n) | flot respiratoire | flusso d'aria respiratoria | flujo respiratorio | Expirationsstärke | 呼吸による空気流 |
| 5850. respiratory alkalosis - (n) | alcalose respiratoire | alcalosi respiratoria | alcalosis respiratoria | respiratorische Alkalose | 呼吸性アルカローシス |

| English/American | French/Français | Italian/Italiano | Spanish/Español | German/Deutsch | Japanese/日本語 |
|---|---|---|---|---|---|
| 5851. respiratory depression - (n) | dépression respiratoire | depressione respiratoria | depresión respiratoria | Atemdepression | 呼吸低下 |
| 5852. respiratory depth - (n) | amplitude respiratoire | profondità del respiro | profundidad respiratoria | Atemtiefe | 呼吸深度 |
| 5853. respiratory syncytial virus - (n) | virus respiratoire syncytial, VRS | virus respiratorio sinciziale | virus sincitial respiratorio | RS-Virus | R S ウイルス |
| 5854. respiratory system - (n) | système respiratoire | apparato respiratorio | sistema respiratorio | Atemtrakt | 呼吸器系 |
| 5855. respiratory tract - (n) | voies respiratoires; voies aériennes | vie respiratorie | tracto respiratorio | Respirationstrakt; Atemwege | 気道 |
| 5856. responder - (n) | répondeur | chi risponde | respondedor; contestador | Responder | 応答者 |
| 5857. response - (n) | réponse; réaction | risposta; reazione | respuesta; reacción | Antwort; Reaktion | 応答、反応 |
| 5858. rest - (n) | repos | riposo | reposo | Ruhe; Erholung | 安静 |
| 5859. rest - (v) | reposer | riposarsi | reposar; descansar | ruhen | 休養する |
| 5860. resting stage - (n) | phase de repos | stadio di riposo | etapa de descanso | Erholungsphase | 静止状態 |
| 5861. restless legs - (n) | syndrome des jambes sans repos; syndrome d'Ekbom | sindrome delle gambe irrequiete; sindrome di Ekbom | piernas inquietas; síndrome de Ekbom | Wittmaack-Ekbom-Syndrom | 不穏下肢 |
| 5862. restlessness - (n) | agitation; inquiétude | irrequietezza | inquietud; agitación | Unruhe; Ruhelosigkeit | 不安 |
| 5863. restorative - (n) | reconstituant; fort fiant | ricostituente | reconstituyente; regenerador | starkendes Mittel | 強壮薬 |
| 5864. restorative - (a) | reconstituant; fortifiant | ricostituente | reconstituyente | restorativ; stärkend | 回復推進の |
| 5865. restraint - (n) | contrainte | costrizione | restricción | Zwangsmaßnahme; Einschränkung | 抑制、拘束 |
| 5866. restricted diet - (n) | diète restrictive | dieta limitata | dieta restringida | beschränkte Diät | 制限食 |
| 5867. restriction - (n) | restriction; limitation | restrizione; limitazione | restricción; limitación | Restriktion; Beschränkung | 制限 |

301

| English/American | French/Français | Italian/Italiano | Spanish/Español | German/Deutsch | Japanese/日本語 |
|---|---|---|---|---|---|
| 5868. restrictive labeling - (n) | étiquetage restrictif | etichetta indicante limite d'uso | etiqueta restrictiva | Kennzeichnung der Anwendungs-einschränkungen | 限定分類薬品の使用上注意 |
| 5869. result - (n) | résultat | risultato | resultado | Ergebnis; Resultat | 結果 |
| 5870. resuscitate - (v) | ressusciter; réanimer | rianimare | resucitar | wiederbeleben | 蘇生する |
| 5871. resuscitation - (n) | ressuscitation; réanimation | rianimazione | resucitación | Reanimation; Wiederbelebung | 蘇生 [法]、救急蘇生 [法] |
| 5872. resuscitation orders - (n) | ordres de ressuscitation; ordres de réanimation | ordine di rianimare | órdenes de resucitación | Anordnung über Wiederbelebungs-maßnahmen | 蘇生命令 |
| 5873. retardation - (n) | retardement | ritardo | retraso | Retardierung, Verzögerung | 遅延、遅滞 |
| 5874. retarded - (a) | retardé; arriéré | ritardato | retardado; retrasado | zurückgeblieben | 遅延の |
| 5875. retch - (v) | avoir des nausées | vomitare | vomitar | würgen; brechen | 吐き気を催す、むかつく |
| 5876. retching - (n) | nausée | conato di vomito | esfuerzo; por vomitar | Würgen; Erbrechen | むかつき、レッチング |
| 5877. retention - (n) | rétention | ritenzione | retención | Retention; Zurückhalten | 遺残、貯留 |
| 5878. reticular - (a) | réticulaire | reticolare | reticular | retikular | 網様の、細網 [状] の |
| 5879. reticulocyte - (n) | réticulocyte | reticolocito | reticulocito | Retikulozyt | 網 [状] 赤血球 |
| 5880. reticulocytosis - (n) | réticulocytose | reticolocitosi | reticulocitosis | Retikulozytcse | 網 [状] 赤血球増加 [症] |
| 5881. reticuloendothelial - (a) | réticulo-endothélial | reticoloendoteliale | reticuloendotelial | Retikuloendothel- | [細] 網内 [皮] 細胞の |
| 5882. retina - (n) | rétine | retina | retina | Netzhaut; Retina | 網膜 |
| 5883. retinal - (a) | rétinien | retinico | retinal | retinal; Netzhaut- | 網膜の |
| 5884. retinoid - (a) | rétinoïde | retinoide | retinoide | retinoid | レチノイド |
| 5885. retinopathy - (n) | rétinopathie | retinopatia | retinopatía | Retinopathie | 網膜症、網膜障害 |
| 5886. retirement - (n) | retraite | ritiro | retiro | Ruhestand | 退去 |
| 5887. retraction - (n) | rétraction | retrazione | retracción | Retraktion; Schrumpfung | 退縮、後退 |

| English/American | French/Français | Italian/Italiano | Spanish/Español | German/Deutsch | Japanese/日本語 |
|---|---|---|---|---|---|
| 5888. retrieval - (n) | récupération; recouvrement | reperimento; ricupero | recuperación | Wiederauffinden | 想起 |
| 5889. retro- - (prefix) | rétro- | retro- | retro- | Retro-; zurück | 後方の、後部の |
| 5890. retroflexion - (n) | rétrofléxion | retroflessione | retroflexión | Retroflexion | 後屈する |
| 5891. retrograde - (v) | rétrograder | regredire | degenerar | regredieren | 退化する、後方に動く |
| 5892. retrograde - (a) | rétrograde | retrogrado | retrógrado | retrograd | 退行［性］の、逆行する |
| 5893. retrogress - (v) | rétrogresser | regredire | retroceder | sich zurückentwickeln | 退化する、逆行する、退行する |
| 5894. retroperitoneal - (a) | rétropéritonéal | retroperitoneale | retroperitoneal | retroperitoneal | 腹膜後の |
| 5895. retrospective - (a) | rétrospectif | retrospettivo | retrospectivo | retrospektiv | 回想の、追想的 |
| 5896. retrospective study - (n) | étude rétrospect ve | studio retrospettivo | estudio retrospectivo | retrospektive Studie | 回顧研究 |
| 5897. retrosternal - (a) | rétrosternal | retrosternale | retroesternal | retrosternal | 胸骨後［方］の |
| 5898. retroversion - (n) | rétroversion | retroversione | retroversión | Retroversion | 後傾「症」、後反 |
| 5899. retrovirus - (n) | rétrovirus | retrovirus | retrovirus | Retrovirus | レトロウイルス |
| 5900. returned drug log - (n) | registre des drogues retournées | elenco farmaci restituiti | registro de drogas devueltas | Logbuch der zurückgegebenen Medikamente | 返却薬物日誌 |
| 5901. revascularization - (n) | révascularisation | rivascolarizzazione | revascularización | Revaskularisation | 血管再生、脈管再生 |
| 5902. reversal dose - (n) | dose de revirement | dose di rovesciamento | dosis de reversión | einen Effekt rückgängigmachende Dosis | 逆の服用 |
| 5903. reverse transcriptase - (n) | transcriptase de réversion | trascrittasi inversa | transcriptasa inversa | reverse Transkriptase | 逆トランスクリプターゼ |
| 5904. reversible effect - (n) | effet réversible | effetto reversibile | efecto reversible | reversibler Effekt | 可逆効果 |
| 5905. reversion - (n) | réversion | reversione | reversión | Reversion; Atavismus | 先祖返り、隔世遺伝 |
| 5906. review - (n) | révision; examen | recensione; revisione | revisión; examen | Überblick; Überprüfung | 再検討 |

303

| English/American | French/Français | Italian/Italiano | Spanish/Español | German/Deutsch | Japanese日本語 |
|---|---|---|---|---|---|
| 5907. review - (v) | réviser; examiner | recensire | repasar; examinar | überprüfen; besprechen | 再検討する |
| 5908. review of literature - (n) | examen de la littérature | ricerca bibliografica | revista de literatura | Fachliteraturüberblick | 文献の再検討 |
| 5909. review of systems - (n) | examen des systèmes | revisione dei sistemi | revisión de los sistemas | Systemenüberblick | システムの再検討 |
| 5910. revive - (v) | réanimer | rianimare; risuscitare | resucitar | wiederbeleben; erneuern | 生き返る |
| 5911. revolve - (v) | tourner | rotare; girare | girar; dar vueltas | drehen; rotieren | 回転する |
| 5912. revulsion - (n) | révulsion | revulsione | revulsión | Ableitung; Revulsion | 誘導、誘出法 |
| 5913. reward - (n) | récompense | compenso | recompensa | Belohnung | 診査料、[検査] 報酬 |
| 5914. reward - (v) | récompenser | ricompensare | recompensar | belohnen | 報いる |
| 5915. rhabdomyo-sarcoma - (n) | rhabdomyosarcome | rabdomiosarcoma | rabdomiosarcoma | Rhabdomyosarkom | 横紋筋肉腫 |
| 5916. rheology - (n) | rhéologie | reologia | reologia | Rheologie | レオロジー |
| 5917. rheumatic - (a) | rhumatismal | reumatico | reumático | rheumatisch | リウマチ [性] の |
| 5918. rheumatic fever - (n) | fièvre rhumatismale | febbre reumatica | fiebre reumática | rheumatisches Fieber | リウマチ熱 |
| 5919. rheumatic heart disease - (n) | cardiopathie rhumatismale | miocardite reumatica | cardiopatía reumática | rheumatische Herzkrankheit | リウマチ性心臓疾患 |
| 5920. rheumatism - (n) | rhumatisme | reumatismo | reumatismo | Rheuma; Rheumatismus | リウマチ |
| 5921. rheumatoid arthritis - (n) | arthrite rhumatismale | artrite reumatoide | artritis reumatoide | rheumatoide Arthritis | リウマチ様関節炎 |
| 5922. rheumatology - (n) | rhumatologie | reumatologia | reumatologia | Rheumatologie | リウマチ [病] 学 |
| 5923. rhinitis - (n) | rhinite | rinite | rinitis | Rhinitis; Nasenschleim-hautentzündung | 鼻炎 |
| 5924. rhinoplasty - (n) | rhinoplastie | rinoplastica | rinoplastia | Rhinoplastik; Nasenplastik | 鼻形成 [術]、造鼻術 |
| 5925. rhinorrhea - (n) | rhinorrhée | rinorrea | rinorrea | Rhinorrhö | 鼻漏 |
| 5926. rhinovirus - (n) | rhinovirus | rhinovirus; rinovirus | rinovirus | Rhinovirus | ライノウイルス |

| English/American | French/Français | Italian/Italiano | Spanish/Español | German/Deutsch | Japanese/日本語 |
|---|---|---|---|---|---|
| 5927. rhonchus - (n) | ronchis | ronco | ronquido | Rhonchus; Rasselgeräusch | ヲ音、水包音 |
| 5928. rhythm - (n) | rythme | ritmo | ritmo | Rhythmus | リズム |
| 5929. rib - (n) | côte | costola; costa | costilla | Rippe | 肋骨 |
| 5930. ribonucleic acid [abbr] RNA - (n) | acide ribonucléique, ARN | acido ribonucleico, ARN | ácido ribonucleico, ARN | Ribonukleinsäure, RNS | リボ核酸 |
| 5931. ribosomal DNA - (n) | ADN ribosomique | ADN ribosomiale | ADN ribosomal | ribosomale DNS | リボソームDNA |
| 5932. ribosome - (n) | ribosome | ribosoma | ribosoma | Ribosom | リボソーム |
| 5933. Rickettsia - (n) | Rickettsie | Rickettsia | Rickettsia | Rickettsie | リケッチア属 |
| 5934. ridge - (n) | crête | cresta; sperone | arruga | Kamm; Crista | 隆線、稜 |
| 5935. Rift Valley fever - (n) | fièvre de la vallée de Rift | febbre della valle di Rift | fiebre del valle de Rift | Rift-Tal-Fieber | リフトバレー熱 |
| 5936. right axis - (n) | axe droit | asse destro | eje derecho | rechte Achse | 右軸 |
| 5937. right handed - (a) | droitier | destrimano | diestro | rechtshändig | 右手利きの |
| 5938. rigidity - (n) | rigidité; raideur | rigidità; rigor | rigidez | Rigidität; Steife | 硬直、固縮、硬さ |
| 5939. rigor - (n) | rigueur; rigidité | rigor; rigidità | rigor; rigidez | Rigor; Rigidität | 硬直 |
| 5940. rigor mortis - (n) | rigidité cadavérique | rigor mortis; rigidità cadaverica | rigidez cadavérica | Rigor mortis | 死体硬直 |
| 5941. ring - (n) | anneau; noyau cyclique | anello | anillo | Ring; Annulus | 輪、環 |
| 5942. risk - (n) | risque | rischio | riesgo | Risiko | 危険 |
| 5943. risk - (v) | risquer | rischiare | arriesgar | riskieren | 危険にさらす |
| 5944. risk benefit ratio - (n) | rapport bénéfice/risque | rapporto rischio-beneficio | relación riesgo-beneficio | Risiko-Vorteil-Verhältnis | リスクと恩恵の割合 |
| 5945. risk factor - (n) | facteur de risque | fattore di rischio | factor de riesgo | Risikofaktor | リスクファクター |
| 5946. risk factor analysis - (n) | analyse des facteurs de risque | analisi del fattore di rischio | análisis de los factores de riesgo | Risikofaktoranalyse | リスクファクター分析 |
| 5947. risk group - (n) | groupe à risque | gruppo a rischio | grupo a riesgo | Risikogruppe | リスクグループ |
| 5948. risk reduction - (n) | réduction du risque | riduzione del rischio | reducción de riesgo | Risikoreduktion | リスク削減 |

| English/American | French/Français | Italian/Italiano | Spanish/Español | German/Deutsch | Japanese/日本語 |
|---|---|---|---|---|---|
| 5949. RNA splicing - (n) | assemblage d'ARN | splicing dell'ARN | empalme de ARN | RNS-Spleißen | RNAスプライシング |
| 5950. robotics - (n) | robotique | robotica | robótica | Robotertechnik | ロボット工学 |
| 5951. robustness - (n) | robustesse | robustezza | robustez | Widerstandsfähigkeit; Robustheit | 強健 |
| 5952. rodent - (n) | rongeur | roditore | roedor | Nagetier | 齧歯動物 |
| 5953. rodent - (a) | rongeur | roditore | roedor | nagend; fressend | 齧歯類の |
| 5954. roentgen - (n) | Roentgen; Röntgen | röntgen | roentgen | Röntgen | レントゲン |
| 5955. rolling average - (n) | moyenne mobile | media volvente | promedio oscilante | sich verändernder Durchschnitt | 累積平均 |
| 5956. root - (n) | racine | radice | raíz | Wurzel; Radix | 根 |
| 5957. root canal - (n) | canal radiculaire | canale radicolare | conducto radicular | Wurzelkanal | 根管 |
| 5958. rosette formation - (n) | formation en rosette | formazione di rosetta | formación en roseta | Rosettenbildung | ロゼット形成 |
| 5959. rotating tourniquet - (n) | tourniquet; garrot | pinza emostatica rotante | torniquete rotatorio | rotierende Aderpresse | 回転止血帯 |
| 5960. rotation - (n) | rotation | rotazione | rotación | Rotation; Umdrehung | 回転、循環 |
| 5961. rotator cuff - (n) | coiffe des rotateurs | cuffia dei muscoli rotatori della spalla | manguito rotatorio del hombro | Rotatorenmanschette | 回旋筋腱盖 |
| 5962. rote behavior - (n) | comportement routinier | comportamento automatico | conducta aprendida de memoria | mechanisches Verhalten | 機械的行動 |
| 5963. roughage - (n) | matière cellulosique | sostanza ricca di fibre | sustancia celulósica | Ballaststoff; Schlacke | 粗質物 |
| 5964. rouleau - (n) | rouleau; pile de globules rouges | impilamento dei globuli rossi | apilamiento de los glóbulos rojos; rollo | Rolle; Rundfalte | 連銭状 |
| 5965. rounding off - (n) | arrondissement | arrotondamento | redondeo | Abrunden | 四捨五入 |
| 5966. round table - (n) | table ronde | tavola rotonda | mesa redonda | runder Tisch | 円卓 |
| 5967. route - (n) | route; voie | via | via | Weg; Route | 経路 |
| 5968. route of administration - (n) | voie d'administration | via di somministrazione | via de administración | Verwaltungsweg | 投与経路 |

306

| English/American | French/Français | Italian/Italiano | Spanish/Español | German/Deutsch | Japanese/日本語 |
|---|---|---|---|---|---|
| 5969. route of elimina- tion - (n) | voie d'élimination | via di eliminazione | vía de eliminación | Ausscheidungsweg | 排他経路 |
| 5970. routine - (n) | routine | routine | rutina | Routine | 定期の課程 |
| 5971. routine - (a) | routinier | corrente; normale | rutina | routinemäßig; alltäglich | 定期的な |
| 5972. routine monitoring visit - (n) | visite de contrôle routine | visita di controllo normale | visita de monitoreo de rutina | routinemäßiger Überwachungsbesuch | 定期的（監視）診療 |
| 5973. row - (n) | rang; rangée | fila; riga | fila; hilera | Reihe | 列 |
| 5974. rudimentary - (a) | rudimentaire | rudimentale | rudimentario | rudimentär | 痕跡の、不全の |
| 5975. rule out - (v) | exclure; éliminer | escludere | excluir; descartar | ausschließen | 除外する |
| 5976. rump - (n) | derrière; postérieur | natiche; sedere | nalgas; trasero | Steiß | 臀部 |
| 5977. run-in period - (n) | période initiale | fase iniziale | período inicial | Einlaufzeit | 初期期間 |
| 5978. rupture - (n) | rupture; déchirement | rottura; ernia | ruptura | Ruptur; Riß | ヘルニア，裂傷 |
| 5979. rural - (a) | rural | rurale | rural | ländlich | 地方の |

307

| English/American | French/Français | Italian/Italiano | Spanish/Español | German/Deutsch | Japanese日本語 |
|---|---|---|---|---|---|
| 5980. sac - (n) | sac; poche | sacca; borsa | saco | Sack, Saccus | 嚢, 包 |
| 5981. saccade - (n) | saccade | movimento saccadico | movimiento sacádico | Sakkade | 目の断続的運動 |
| 5982. sacral spine - (n) | épine sacrée | spina sacrale | espina sacra | Sakralwirbel | 仙骨棘 |
| 5983. sacroiliac - (a) | sacro-iliaque | sacroiliaco | sacroilíaco | sakroiliakal | 仙腸骨の |
| 5984. sacrolumbar - (a) | sacro-lombaire | sacrolombare | sacrolumbar | sacrolumbal; lumbosacral | 仙腰[椎]の |
| 5985. sacrum - (n) | sacrum | sacro | sacro | Sakrum; Os sacrum | 仙骨 |
| 5986. sadism - (n) | sadisme | sadismo | sadismo | Sadismus | サディズム |
| 5987. sadomasochism - (n) | sadomasochisme | sadomasochismo | sadomasoquismo | Sadomasochismus | サドマゾヒズム |
| 5988. safe - (a) | en sécurité | sicuro | seguro | sicher | 安全な |
| 5989. safety - (n) | sécurité | salvezza; sicurezza | seguridad | Sicherheit | 安全性 |
| 5990. safety committee - (n) | comité de sécurité | comitato di sicurezza | comité de seguridad | Sicherheitsausschuß | 安全委員会 |
| 5991. safety evaluation - (n) | évaluation de sécurité | valutazione di sicurezza | evaluación de seguridad | Sicherheitsbewertung | 安全性評価 |
| 5992. safety index - (n) | index de sécurité | indice di sicurezza | índice de seguridad | Sicherheitsindex | 安全指数 |
| 5993. safety monitoring committee - (n) | comité de surveillance de la sécurité | comitato controllo della sicurezza | comité de monitoreo de seguridad | Sicherheitsüberwachungsausschuß | 安全監視委員会 |
| 5994. safety profile - (n) | profil de sécurité | profilo di sicurezza | perfil de seguridad | Sicherheitsprofil | 安全プロフィール |
| 5995. safety variable - (n) | variable de sécurité | variabile di sicurezza | variable de seguridad | Sicherheitsvariable | 安全変数 |
| 5996. sagittal - (a) | sagittal | sagittale | sagital | sagittal | 矢状[方向]の |
| 5997. sales representative - (n) | représentant de commerce | rappresentante | representante de ventas | Vertreter | 販売員 |
| 5998. saline - (n) | salin | soluzione salina | salino | Salzlösung | 食塩水 |
| 5999. saline control - (n) | contrôle salin | controllo di sale | control salino | salinische Kontrolle | 食塩水のコントロール |
| 6000. saliva - (n) | salive | saliva | saliva | Speichel; Saliva | 唾液 |
| 6001. salivary - (a) | salivaire | salivare | salival | Speichel-; Sialo- | 唾液の |

308

| English/American | French/Français | Italian/Italiano | Spanish/Español | German/Deutsch | Japanese/日本語 |
|---|---|---|---|---|---|
| 6002. salivary gland - (n) | glande salivaire | ghiandola salivare | glándula salival | Speicheldrüse | 唾液腺 |
| 6003. salt - (n) | sel | sale | sal | Salz | 塩、食塩 |
| 6004. salt-free diet - (n) | diète sans sel | dieta iposodica | dieta libre de sal | salzfreie Diät | 無塩食 |
| 6005. salutary - (a) | salutaire | salutare | saludable | heilsam | 健康的な |
| 6006. salvage therapy - (n) | thérapie de sauvetage | terapia di recupero | tratamiento de rescate | Rettungstherapie; Bergung | 救助療法 |
| 6007. salve - (n) | baume | unguento; pomata | ungüento | Salbe | 軟膏 [剤] |
| 6008. sample - (n) | échantillon | campione | muestra | Probe; Stichprobe | 試料、標本 |
| 6009. sample size - (n) | taille d'un échantillon | dimensione di campione | tamaño de la muestra | Stichprobengröße | 試料数 |
| 6010. sample size calculation - (n) | calcul de la taille d'un échantillon | calcolo delle dimensioni di campione | cálculo del tamaño de la muestra | Berechnung der Stichprobengröße | 試料数の計算 |
| 6011. sample size requirement - (n) | exigence de la taille d'un échantillon | requisito per il dimensione di campione | requisito del tamaño de la muestra | erforderliche Stichprobengröße | 必要な試料数 |
| 6012. sampling - (n) | échantillonnage; prise d'échantillons | campionamento; campionatura | muestreo | Probenentnahme; Stichprobenerhebung | 試料採集 |
| 6013. sanatorium - (n) | sanatorium | sanatorio | sanatorio | Sanatorium | サナトリウム、療養所 |
| 6014. sane - (a) | sain; raisonnable | sano di mente | sensato; cuerdo | geistig gesund; zurechnungsfähig | 正気の、健全な |
| 6015. sanguine - (a) | sanguin; rubicond | sanguigno | sanguíneo; pletórico | plethorisch; blutreich | 血色のよい |
| 6016. sanitary - (a) | sanitaire; hygiénique | sanitario; igienico | sanitario | sanitär; hygienisch | 衛生の、保健の |
| 6017. sanitary napkin - (n) | serviette hygiénique; serviette sanitaire | assorbente igienico | paño higiénico | Damenbinde | 生理用ナプキン |
| 6018. sanitation - (n) | assainissement | misure sanitarie; igiene | saneamiento; sanidad | Sanitation; Sanierung | 衛生 |
| 6019. sanitize - (v) | aseptiser | rendere igienico | sanear | entkeimen; sterilisieren | 衛生的にする |
| 6020. sanity - (n) | santé d'esprit | sanità mentale | cordura | geistige Gesundheit | 正気、健全 |
| 6021. sarcoma - (n) | sarcome | sarcoma | sarcoma | Sarkom | 肉腫 |
| 6022. sarcoplasmic reticulum - (n) | sarcoplasmique | reticolo sarcoplasmatico | retículo sarcoplásmico | sarkoplasmatisches Retikulum | 筋小胞体 |

| English/American | French/Français | Italian/Italiano | Spanish/Español | German/Deutsch | Japanese/日本語 |
|---|---|---|---|---|---|
| 6023. satellite center - (n) | centre satellite | centro satellite | centro satélite | Satellitenzentrum | サテライトセンター |
| 6024. satellite DNA - (n) | ADN satellite | ADN satellite | ADN satélite | Satelliten-DNS | サテライトDNA |
| 6025. satellite site - (n) | emplacement satellite | sito satellite | sitio satélite | Satellitenort | サテライト場所 |
| 6026. satiation - (n) | satiété | saziamento | saciedad | Sättigung | 飽和 |
| 6027. satiety - (n) | satiété | sazietà | saciedad | Sattheit | 飽満 |
| 6028. satiety response - (n) | réponse de satiété | risposta di sazietà | respuesta a la saciedad | Sättigungsreaktion | 飽満反応 |
| 6029. satisfaction - (n) | satisfaction | soddisfazione | satisfacción | Befriedigung | 満足 |
| 6030. saturated - (a) | saturé | saturo | saturado | gesättigt | 飽和の |
| 6031. scab - (n) | croûte; escarre | escara | costra | Kruste; Schorf | 痂皮、かさぶた |
| 6032. scald - (n) | échaudure | scottatura | escaldadura | Verbrühung; Verbrennung | 熱傷、頭皮結痂疹 |
| 6033. scald - (v) | échauder | scottare | escaldar | verbrühen | 熱傷させる |
| 6034. scale - (n) | échelle; écaille | gamma; squama | escala; escama | Skala; Schuppe | 目盛り、鱗 |
| 6035. scale-up - (n) | augmentation proportionnelle | aumento proporzionale | aumento proporcional | (maßstäbliches) Vergrößern | 一定比率の増加 |
| 6036. scalp - (n) | cuir chevelu | cuoio capelluto | cuero cabelludo | Kopfhaut | 頭皮 |
| 6037. scalpel - (n) | scalpel | bisturi | escalpelo | Skalpell | 小刀、メス |
| 6038. scaly - (a) | écailleux | squamoso | escamoso | schuppig | 鱗屑のある、落屑性の |
| 6039. scan - (n) | scanographie | scintigrafia | gammagrama | Abtastung | スキャン |
| 6040. scan - (v) | faire une scanographie | scandire; esplorare | hacer una gammagrama | abtasten | スキャンする |
| 6041. scanning - (n) | scanographie | scintigrafia | gammagrama | Scanning; Abtastung | スキャニング、スキャン |
| 6042. scanning electron microscope - (n) | microscope électronique de balayage | microscopio elettronico a scansione | microscopio electrónico de barrido | Rasterelektronenmikroskop | 走査[型]電子顕微鏡 |
| 6043. scanning speech - (n) | scansion; parole scandée | parola scandita (sillaba per sillaba) | escansión | skandierende Sprache | 断続性言語、分節言語 |
| 6044. scapula - (n) | omoplate | scapola | escápula | Skapula; Schulterblatt | 肩甲骨 |

310

| English/American | French/Français | Italian/Italiano | Spanish/Español | German/Deutsch | Japanese/日本語 |
|---|---|---|---|---|---|
| 6045. scar - (n) | cicatrice | cicatrice | cicatriz; escara | Narbe | 瘢痕 |
| 6046. scar - (v) | cicatriser | cicatrizzarsi; cicatrizzare | cicatrizar | vernarben | 瘢痕を残す |
| 6047. scatology - (n) | scatologie | scatologia | escatología | Skatologie | 糞便学 |
| 6048. scatterplot - (n) | dispersion graphique | grafico a valori sparsi | dispersión gráfica | Korrelationsdiagramm; Streuungsdiagramm | スキャッターブロット |
| 6049. scavenger cell - (n) | phagocyte | macrofago; scavenger | fagocito | Phagozyt | 食細胞 |
| 6050. schedule - (n) | programme; plan | programma | programa | Zeitplan | スケジュール |
| 6051. scheduling - (n) | établissement d'un programme | programmare | programación | Terminplanung | 予定をたてること |
| 6052. schema - (n) | schéma | schema | esquema | Schema | 計画、概要 |
| 6053. schematic - (a) | schématique | schematico | esquemático | schematisch | 模型の、図解の |
| 6054. schematic diagram - (n) | schéma | diagramma schematico | diagrama esquemático | schematisches Diagramm | 図解 |
| 6055. schizoid - (a) | schizoïde | schizoide | esquizoide | schizoid | 分裂症質の |
| 6056. schizophre- nia - (n) | schizophrénie | schizofrenia | esquizofrenia | Schizophrenie | 精神分裂病 |
| 6057. schizophren- ic - (a) | schizophrène | schizofrenico | esquizofrénico | schizophren | 分裂病性の、分裂病的な |
| 6058. schizotypal personality - (n) | personnalité schizo'de | personalità schizotipica | personalidad esquizoide | schizotype Persönlichkeit | 分裂型人格 |
| 6059. school - (n) | école; université | scuola; universitario | escuela; universidad | Schule; Universität | 学校、学部 |
| 6060. sciatic - (a) | sciatique | sciatico | ciática | ischial | 坐骨の、坐骨神経の |
| 6061. science - (n) | science | scienza | ciencia | Wissenschaft | 科学 |
| 6062. scientific - (a) | scientifique | scientifico | científico | wissenschaftlich | 科学の |
| 6063. scientific misconduct - (n) | inconduite scientifique | cattiva condotta scientifica | mala conducta científica | wissenschaftlicher Fehltritt | 科学的不正 |
| 6064. scientist - (n) | scientifique | scienziato | científico | Wissenschaftler | 科学者 |
| 6065. sclera - (n) | sclérotique | sclera | esclerótica | Sklera | 強膜 |

311

| English/American | French/Français | Italian/Italiano | Spanish/Español | German/Deutsch | Japanese/日本語 |
|---|---|---|---|---|---|
| 6066. scoliosis - (n) | scoliose | scoliosi | escoliosis | Skoliose | [脊柱] 側弯 [症] |
| 6067. scotoma, (pl.) scotomata - (n) | scotome | scotoma | escotoma | Skotom | [視野] 暗点 |
| 6068. scratch - (n) | excoriation; égratignure | graffio | rasguño | Kratzen; Kratzwunde | 擦傷 |
| 6069. scratch - (v) | excorier; égratigner | graffiare | rasguñar; rayar | kratzen | ひっかく |
| 6070. screen - (n) | écran | schermo | pantalla | Schirm | 遮へい板、スクリーン |
| 6071. screen - (v) | sélectionner | preselezionare | seleccionar | einer Auswahlprüfung unterziehen | 検査する、評価する |
| 6072. screening - (n) | examen et interrogatoire | screening; indagine di massa | examen masivo | Screening; Reihenuntersuchung | スクリーニング、判別検査 |
| 6073. screening examination - (n) | visite de dépistage | esame iniziale del paziente | examen de seleccionar | Suchtest | スクリーニング検査 |
| 6074. screening period - (n) | période de dépistage | periodo de screening | periodo de seleccionar | Screeningzeit | スクリーニング期間 |
| 6075. scrotum - (n) | scrotum | scroto | escroto | Skrotum | 陰嚢 |
| 6076. search categories - (n) | catégories de recherche | categorie di ricerca | categorías de investigación | Suchkategorien | 調査カテゴリー |
| 6077. season - (n) | saison | stagione | estación | Jahreszeit | 季節 |
| 6078. seasonal - (a) | saisonnier | stagionale | estacional | jahreszeitlich bedingt | 季節的 |
| 6079. sebaceous gland - (n) | glande sébacée | ghiandola sebacea | glándula sebácea | Talgdrüse; Haarbalgdrüse | 皮脂腺 |
| 6080. second line therapy - (n) | thérapie de deuxième ligne | terapia di seconda linea | terapia de segunda línea | Therapie der 2. Wahl | 第二線の療法 |
| 6081. second messenger system - (n) | système de second messager | sistema del secondo messaggero | sistema de mensajero segundo | System des zweiten Messengers | セカンドメッセンジャーシステム |
| 6082. second order kinetics - (n) | cinétique de deuxième ordre | cinetica di secondo ordine | cinética de segundo orden | Kinetik der zweiten Ordnung | 第二次関数の逆動 |
| 6083. secondary - (a) | secondaire | secondario | secundario | sekundär; Zweit- | 二次の |

312

| English/American | French/Français | Italian/Italiano | Spanish/Español | German/Deutsch | Japanese/日本語 |
|---|---|---|---|---|---|
| 6084. secondary care - (n) | soins secondaires | cura secondaria | atención secundaria | fachärztliche Betreuung | 二次医療 |
| 6085. secondary event - (n) | événement secondaire | evento secondario | evento secundario | Sekundärereignis | 第二次の出来事 |
| 6086. secondary lesion - (n) | lésion secondaire | lesione secondaria | lesión secundaria | Sekundärläsion | 二次傷害 |
| 6087. secondary objective - (n) | objectif secondaire | oggetto secondario | objetivo secundario | Sekundärziel | 二次目的 |
| 6088. secondary outcome - (n) | résultat secondaire | risultato secondario | resultado secundario | Sekundärresultat | 二次結果 |
| 6089. secrete - (v) | sécréter | secernere | secretar | sekretieren; sezernieren | 分泌する |
| 6090. secretion - (n) | sécrétion | secrezione | secreción | Sekretion; Ausscheidung | 分泌、分泌物 |
| 6091. secretory rate - (n) | taux de sécrétion | rata di secrezione | índice secretorio | Sekretionsrate | 分泌率 |
| 6092. section - (n) | section; partie | sezione; parte | sección | Schnitt; Sektion | 切開 [術] 切断 |
| 6093. section - (v) | couper en sections; diviser | sezionare | seccionar; dividir en secciones | schneiden; durchtrennen | 解体する |
| 6094. sedation - (n) | sédation | sedazione | sedación | Sedierung | 鎮静 |
| 6095. sedative - (a) | sédatif | sedativo | sedante | Sedativum | 鎮静薬 |
| 6096. sedentary - (a) | sédentaire | sedentario | sedentario | sitzend; seßhaft | 坐業の、坐位の |
| 6097. sediment - (n) | sédiment | sedimento | sedimento | Sediment; Niederschlag | 沈渣 |
| 6098. seduction - (n) | séduction | seduzione | seducción | Verführung; Versuchung | 誘惑 |
| 6099. seeding trial - (n) | essai d'ensemencement | test di germinazione: test di inseminazione | ensayo de siembra | Einsaatversuch | 基本となる試験 |
| 6100. segment - (n) | segment | segmento | segmento | Segment; Abschnitt | 区 [域] |
| 6101. segmental - (a) | segmentaire | segmentale | segmentario | segmental | 分節 [性] の |
| 6102. segmentation - (n) | segmentation | segmentazione | segmentación | Segmentierung; Unterteilung | 分節、分割 |
| 6103. segregation - (n) | ségrégation | segregazione | segregación | Segregation; Aufspaltung | 分離、隔離 |

| English/American | French/Français | Italian/Italiano | Spanish/Español | German/Deutsch | Japanese/日本語 |
|---|---|---|---|---|---|
| 6104. seizure - (n) | crise; attaque | attacco; crisi | convulsión; ataque | Anfall; Krampf | 発作、痙攣 |
| 6105. selection - (n) | sélection | selezione | selección | Selektion; Auswahl | 選択 |
| 6106. selective - (a) | sélectif | selettivo | selectivo | selektiv | 選択的 |
| 6107. selectivity - (n) | sélectivité | selettività | selectividad | Selektivität | 選択性 |
| 6108. self-administration - (n) | auto-administration | autosomministrazione | autoadministración | Selbstapplikation | 自己投薬 |
| 6109. self-assessment - (n) | auto-évaluation | autovalutazione | autoevaluación | Selbsteinschätzung | 自己評価 |
| 6110. self-care - (n) | soins auto-administrés; autosoins | cura di sé | cuidado propio | Selbstversorgung | 自己看護 |
| 6111. self-concept - (n) | perception de soi | concetto di sé | noción de si mismo; concepto propio | Selbstkonzept | 自己概念 |
| 6112. self-destruction - (n) | autodestruction | autodistruzione | autodestrucción | Selbstzerstörung | 自滅、自殺 |
| 6113. self-examination - (n) | auto-examen | autoesame | autoexamen | Selbstuntersuchung | 自己検査 |
| 6114. self-hypnosis - (n) | auto-hypnose | autoipnosi | autohipnosis | Autohypnose | 自己催眠 |
| 6115. self-limited - (a) | auto-limité | autolimitante | autolimitado | selbstbegrenzt; selbstlimitiert | 自己限定 [性] の |
| 6116. self-medication - (n) | automédication | automedicamento | automedicación | Selbstmedikation | 自己投薬 |
| 6117. self-monitoring - (n) | auto-surveillance | autosupervisione | supervisión propia | Selbstkontrolle | 自己監視 |
| 6118. self-stimulation - (n) | auto-stimulation | autostimolazione | autoestimulación; estimulación propia | Eigenstimulation | 自己刺激 |
| 6119. semantics - (n) | sémantique | semantica | semántica | Semantik | 意味論 |
| 6120. semen - (n) | semence | seme | semen | Samen | 精液、種子 |
| 6121. semicircular canals - (n) | canaux semi-circulaires | canali semicircolari | canales semicirculares | Bogengänge | 骨半規管 |

314

| English/American | French/Français | Italian/Italiano | Spanish/Español | German/Deutsch | Japanese/日本語 |
|---|---|---|---|---|---|
| 6122. semi-dependent - (a) | semi-dépendant | semidipendente | semidependiente | halbabhängig | 半依存的 |
| 6123. semi-logarithmic - (a) | semilogarithmique | semilogaritmico | semilogaritmico | halblogarithmisch | 半対数的 |
| 6124. seminal fluid - (n) | liquide séminal | liquido seminale | flujo seminal | Samenflüssigkeit | 精液 |
| 6125. seminal vesicle - (n) | vésicule séminale | vescicola seminale | vesícula seminal | Samenblase | 精嚢 |
| 6126. seminar - (n) | séminaire | seminario | seminario | Seminar | セミナー |
| 6127. semipermeable - (a) | semi-perméable | semipermeabile | semipermeable | semipermeabel | 半透 [性] の |
| 6128. semisynthetic - (a) | semi-synthétique | semisintetico | semisintético | halbsynthetisch | 半合成の |
| 6129. senescence - (n) | sénescence; vieillissement | senescenza | senescencia; envejecimiento | Seneszenz; Altern | 老化. 老齢化 |
| 6130. senile - (a) | sénile | senile | senil | senil | 老人 [性] の. 老年 [性] の |
| 6131. senile dementia - (n) | démence sénile | demenza senile | demencia senil | senile Demenz | 老年 (老人) 痴呆 |
| 6132. sensation - (n) | sensation | sensazione | sensación | Sensation; Sinnesempfindung | 感覚 |
| 6133. sense - (n) | sens | senso | sentido | Sinn | 感覚. 知覚 |
| 6134. sense - (v) | sentir | sentire | sentir | empfinden | 感知する |
| 6135. sense organ - (n) | organe sensoriel | organo di senso | órgano de los sentidos | Sinnesorgan | 感覚器 |
| 6136. sensitive - (a) | sensitif | sensibile | sensitivo | sensitiv; empfindlich | 知覚しうる |
| 6137. sensitivity - (n) | sensibilité | sensibilità | sensitividad; sensibilidad | Empfindlichkeit | 感受性. 感度 |
| 6138. sensorium - (n) | sensorium | sensorio | sensorio | Sensorium; Sinnesapparat | 感覚器. 感覚神経中枢 |
| 6139. sensory receptor - (n) | récepteur sensoriel | recettore sensoriale | receptor sensitivo | sensorischer Rezeptor | 感覚受容器 |

315

| English/American | French/Français | Italian/Italiano | Spanish/Español | German/Deutsch | Japanese/日本語 |
|---|---|---|---|---|---|
| 6140. sensory threshold - (n) | seuil sensoriel | soglia sensoriale | umbral sensitivo | Empfindungswahrnehmungsschwelle | 感覚いき値 |
| 6141. separated - (a) | séparé | separato | separado | getrennt | 分離した |
| 6142. separation - (n) | séparation | separazione | separación | Separation; Trennung | 分離、離開 |
| 6143. sepsis - (n) | septicémie | sepsi | sepsis | Sepsis | 敗血症、セプシス |
| 6144. septal defect - (n) | anomalie septale | difetto del setto | defecto del septum | Septumdefekt | 中隔欠損 |
| 6145. septal deviation - (n) | déviation septale | deviazione del setto | desviación del septum | Septumdeviation | 中隔偏差 |
| 6146. septic - (a) | septique | settico | séptico | septisch | 敗血[症][性]の |
| 6147. septic shock - (n) | choc septique | shock settico | choque séptico | septischer Schock | 敗血性ショック |
| 6148. septicemia - (n) | septicémie | setticemia | septicemia | Septikämie | 敗血症 |
| 6149. septum - (n) | septum; cloison | setto | septum | Septum; Scheidewand | 中隔、隔壁 |
| 6150. sequel - (n) | suite; conséquence | seguito | secuela | Folge; Konsequenz | 結果、続き |
| 6151. sequela - (n) | séquelle; phénomène secondaire | sequela | secuela | Folgezustand | 後遺症、続発症 |
| 6152. sequence - (n) | suite; ordre | sequenza | secuencia | Sequenz | 続発、連鎖 |
| 6153. sequence homology - (n) | homologie de concordance | omologia di sequenza | homología secuencial | Sequenzhomologie | 配列相同性 |
| 6154. sequential - (a) | séquentiel | sequenziale | secuencial | sequentiell | 続発性の |
| 6155. sequential analysis - (n) | analyse séquentielle | analisi sequenziale | análisis secuencial | sequentielle Analyse | 連続分析 |
| 6156. sequential design - (n) | plan séquentiel | disegno sequenziale | diseño secuencial | sequentieller Entwurf | 連続設計 |
| 6157. serial tracings - (n) | tracés sériées | tracciati seriali | rastreos en series | Serienaufzeichnungen | 連続追跡 |
| 6158. serial values - (n) | valeurs sériées | valori seriali | valores en serie | aufeinanderfolgende Werte | 連続値 |
| 6159. serious - (a) | sérieux; grave | serio; grave | serio; grave | ernst; schwer | 重大な |

| English/American | French/Français | Italian/Italiano | Spanish/Español | German/Deutsch | Japanese/日本語 |
|---|---|---|---|---|---|
| 6160. serious adverse event - (n) | événement adverse grave | evento seriamente avverso | evento adverso significativo | ernsthaft schädliches Ereignis | 重大な悪い出来事 |
| 6161. serodiagnosis - (n) | sérodiagnostic | sierodiagnosi | serodiagnóstico | Serodiagnostik | 血清 [学的] 診断 [法] |
| 6162. seroepidemiologic method - (n) | méthode séro-épidémiologique | metodo sieroepidemiologico | método seroepidemielógico | seroepidemiologische Methode | 血清疫学的手法 |
| 6163. serology - (n) | sérologie | sierologia | serología | Serologie | 血清学 |
| 6164. seropositive - (a) | séro-positif | sieropositivo | seropositivo | seropositiv | セロポジティブの |
| 6165. seropositivity - (n) | séro-positivité | sieropositività | seropositividad | Seropositivität | セロポジティブ |
| 6166. seroprevalence - (n) | séro-prévalence | sieroprevalenza | seroprevalente | Seroprävalenz | セロポジティブの頻度 |
| 6167. seropurulent - (a) | séropurulent | sieropurulento | seropurulento | eitrig-serös | 漿液膿性の |
| 6168. serotonergic - (a) | sérotoninergique | serotoninergico | serotoninérgico | serotonerg | セロトニン [様] の |
| 6169. serotyping - (n) | sérotype | determinare il sierotipo | serotipo | Serotypisierung | 血清型 |
| 6170. serous effusion - (n) | épanchement séreux | versamento sieroso | derrame seroso | seröser Erguß | 漿液性浸出物 |
| 6171. serous membrane - (n) | membrane séreuse | membrana sierosa | membrana serosa | Tunica serosa | 漿膜 |
| 6172. serrated - (a) | dentelé | dentellato | serrado | gezackt | 鋸 [歯] 状の |
| 6173. serum - (n) | sérum | siero | suero | Serum | 漿液、血液、血清 |
| 6174. serum albumin - (n) | séralbumine | sieroalbumina | seroalbúmina | Serumalbumin | 血清アルブミン |
| 6175. serum electrolytes - (n) | électrolytes sériques | elettroliti siericchi | electrólitos de suero | Serumelektrolyte | 血清電解質 |
| 6176. serum sickness - (n) | maladie du sérum | malattia da siero | enfermedad del suero | Serumkrankheit | 血清病 |
| 6177. session - (n) | session | sessione | sesión | Sitzung | セッション |
| 6178. severe - (a) | sévère; grave | severo; grave | severo; grave | schwer; heftig | 重大な |
| 6179. severity - (n) | sévérité; gravité | gravità | severidad; gravedad | Ernsthaftigkeit; Schwere | 重大性 |

| English/American | French/Français | Italian/Italiano | Spanish/Español | German/Deutsch | Japanese/日本語 |
|---|---|---|---|---|---|
| 6180. sewage - (n) | vidange; eaux d'égout | fogna; fognatura | cloacas; aguas residuales | Abwasser | 下水 |
| 6181. sex - (n) | sexe | sesso | sexo | Geschlecht; Sexualität | 性 |
| 6182. sex chromosome - (n) | chromosome sexuel | cromosoma del sesso | cromosoma sexual | Geschlechtschromosom | 性染色体 |
| 6183. sex hormone - (n) | hormone sexuelle | ormone sessuale | hormona sexual | Geschlechtshormon | 性ホルモン |
| 6184. sex ratio - (n) | proportion sexuelle | rapporto tra sessi | proporción sexual | Geschlechtsverteilung; Geschlechtsverhältnis | 性別割合 |
| 6185. sex-linked - (a) | lié au sexe | legato al sesso | ligado al sexo | geschlechtsgebunden | 伴性の |
| 6186. sexual - (a) | sexuel | sessuale | sexual | sexuell; Geschlechts- | 性 [的] の、性に関する |
| 6187. sexual dysfunction - (n) | dysfonction sexuelle | disfunzione sessuale | disfunción sexual | sexuelle Funktionsstörung | 性機能障害 |
| 6188. sexual history - (n) | histoire sexuelle | storia sessuale | historial sexual | sexuelle Vorgeschichte | 性歴 |
| 6189. sexual intercourse - (n) | rapport sexuel; coït | rapporto sessuale; coito | coito; intercambio | Geschlechtsverkehr; Koitus | 性交 |
| 6190. sexual organs - (n) | organes sexuels | organi sessuali | órganos sexuales | Geschlechtsorgane | 性器 |
| 6191. sexual partner - (n) | partenaire sexuel | partner sessuale | sexual; pareja | Sexualpartner, Intimpartner | 性交のパートナー |
| 6192. sexual potency - (n) | puissance sexuelle | potenza sessuale | potencia sexual | sexuelle Potenz | 性効能 [力] |
| 6193. sexual relationship - (n) | liaison sexuelle | relazione sessuale | relación sexual | sexuelles Verhältnis | 性関係 |
| 6194. sexually transmitted disease [abbr] STD - (n) | maladie transmise sexuellement | malattia a trasmissione sessuale | enfermedad de transmisión sexual | Geschlechtskrankheit | 性感染症 |
| 6195. shading - (n) | ombrification | gradazione | sombreado | Shading; Abstufung | 描影法 |
| 6196. shadow - (n) | ombre | ombra | sombra | Schatten; Verschattung | 影、[陰] 影、非有色細胞 |
| 6197. shake - (v) | agiter; trembler | tremare; agitare | agitar | schütteln | 震える |

| English/American | French/Français | Italian/Italiano | Spanish/Español | German/Deutsch | Japanese/日本語 |
|---|---|---|---|---|---|
| 6198. shallow respiration - (n) | respiration superficielle | respirazione debole | respiración superficial | flache Atmung | 浅い呼吸 |
| 6199. sham operation - (n) | opération simulée | operazione simulata | operación simulada | Scheinoperation | 模擬手術 |
| 6200. sham procedure - (n) | procédure simulée | procedura simulata | procedimiento simulado | fingierte Behandlung | 模擬手順 |
| 6201. shape - (n) | forme | forma | forma | Form | 形状 |
| 6202. shape - (v) | former | formare | dar forma a | formen | 形づくる |
| 6203. sharp - (a) | affilé; aigu | affilato; appuntito | afilado; agudo | scharf | 鋭い |
| 6204. sheath - (n) | gaine | guaina | vaina | Scheide; Hülle | 鞘、鞘膜 |
| 6205. shedding - (n) | élimination; perte | il perdere | derramamiento | Shedding; Abstoßung | 脱皮、脱落 |
| 6206. sheet - (n) | drap; feuille | foglio | sábana; hoja | Blatt; dünne Schicht | 一枚の紙、敷布 |
| 6207. shelf life - (n) | durée de conservation | durata di immagazzinamento | caducidad | Lagerfähigkeit | 貯蔵寿命 |
| 6208. shell - (n) | couche externe | guscio; strato esterno | capa externa | Schale; Rinde | 外皮 |
| 6209. shin - (n) | crête du tibia | cresta tibiale | tibia; espinilla | Schienbein; Tibiavorderseite | 脛（すね） |
| 6210. shipment - (n) | embarquement | imbarco; spedizione | embarque | Sendung; Ladung | 船積み |
| 6211. shiver - (v) | trembler; frissonner | rabbrividire | temblar; estremecerse | zittern | 戦慄み |
| 6212. shivering - (a) | frissonnant; tremblant | brivido | temblando | zitternd | 震える |
| 6213. shock - (n) | choc | shock | choque | Schock | ショック |
| 6214. short - (a) | court; petit | corto; piccolo | corto; bajo | kurz; klein | 短い |
| 6215. short-of-breath - (a) | à court de souffle; dyspnéique | respiro corto | falta de aliento; dificultad respiratoria | kurzatmig | 息切れする |
| 6216. short term - (a) | de durée courte | di breve durata | a corto plazo | kurzfristig | 短期の |
| 6217. shortsightedness - (n) | myopie | miopia | miopía; corto de vista | Kurzsichtigkeit | 近視 |
| 6218. shoulder - (n) | épaule | spalla | hombro | Schulter | 肩 |
| 6219. shrivel - (v) | se ratatiner; se flétrir | raggrinzarsi | arrugar | schrumpfen; verwelken | 縮む |

| English/American | French/Français | Italian/Italiano | Spanish/Español | German/Deutsch | Japanese/日本語 |
|---|---|---|---|---|---|
| 6220. shudder - (n) | frisson; frémissement | fremito; brivido | estremecimiento; escalofrío | Schütteln; Zittern | 身震い |
| 6221. shunt - (n) | shunt; dérivation | shunt; by-pass | shunt; anastomosis | Shunt; Nebenschluß | シャント |
| 6222. sialography - (n) | sialographie | scialografia | sialografía | Sialographie | 唾液腺造影（撮影）[法] |
| 6223. sibling - (n) | fratrie; frère/sœur | fratello/sorella | hermano/hermana | Geschwister | 兄弟姉妹 |
| 6224. sickle cell - (n) | drépanocyte; hématie falciforme | eritrocita falciforme | drepanocito | Sichelzelle | 鎌状赤血球 |
| 6225. sickle cell anemia - (n) | drépanocytose; anémie à hématies falciformes | anemia falciforme | drepanocitosis | Sichelzellanämie | 鎌状赤血球貧血症 |
| 6226. sickness - (n) | maladie; mal | malattia; infermità | enfermedad | Erkrankung; Krankheit | 病気、疾病 |
| 6227. side - (n) | côté; flanc | fianco; lato | lado | Seite; Körperhälfte | 側 |
| 6228. side effect - (n) | effet secondaire | effetto collaterale | efecto secundario | Nebenwirkung | 副作用 |
| 6229. sigh - (n) | soupir | sospiro | suspiro | Seufzer | ため息 |
| 6230. sight - (n) | vue; vision | vista; visione | vista; visión | Sehvermögen; Sicht | 視覚、視力 |
| 6231. sigmoid - (a) | sigmoïde | sigmoideo | sigmoide | sigmoid | S状の |
| 6232. sigmoid colon - (n) | côlon sigmoïde | colon sigmoideo | colon sigmoide | Sigma; Sigmoid | S状結腸 |
| 6233. sigmoidoscope - (n) | sigmoïdoscope | sigmoidoscopio | sigmoidoscopio | Sigmoidoskop | S状結腸鏡 |
| 6234. sigmoidoscopy - (n) | sigmoïdoscopie | sigmoidoscopia | sigmoidoscopia | Sigmoidoskopie | S状結腸鏡検査 [法] |
| 6235. sign - (n) | signe; symptôme | segno; sintomo | signo; síntoma | Zeichen; Symptom | 徴候、符号 |
| 6236. sign language - (n) | langage gestuel | linguaggio segno | lenguaje por señas | Zeichensprache | 指話 |
| 6237. sign test - (n) | épreuve de signes | test dei segni | prueba de signos | Zeichentest | 指話のテスト |
| 6238. signal - (n) | signal | segnale | señal | Signal; Anzeichen | 信号 |
| 6239. signal peptide - (n) | séquence signal | sequenza segnale | secuencia señal | Signalsequenz | シグナルペプチド |
| 6240. signature - (n) | signature | firma; segnatura | signatura; firma | Unterschrift; Signatur | 用法指示 |

| English/American | French/Français | Italian/Italiano | Spanish/Español | German/Deutsch | Japanese/日本語 |
|---|---|---|---|---|---|
| 6241. significance - (n) | signification; importance | significato; importanza | significado | Signifikanz; Bedeutung | 有意性 |
| 6242. significant - (a) | significatif; important | importante | significante | bedeutend; wichtig | 有意な |
| 6243. significantly different - (a) | avec une différence significative | significamente differente | significativamente diferente | signifikant verschieden | 顕著に異なる |
| 6244. signs and symptoms - (n) | signes et symptômes | segni e sintomi | signos y síntomas | Zeichen und Symptome | 所見と症状 |
| 6245. silent - (a) | silencieux | silente | silencioso | stumm; ruhig | 無症候性の |
| 6246. silicon implant - (n) | implant de silicone | impianto di silicone | injerto de silicio | Silikonimplantat | シリコン移植 |
| 6247. silver staining - (n) | coloration à l'argent | colorazione all'argento | tinción de plata | Silberfärbung | 銀染色 |
| 6248. silver standard - (n) | étalon argent | standard di argento; standard di riferimento | patrón de plata | 'Silberstandard'; zweitbeste Behandlung | 銀本位制 |
| 6249. simple - (a) | simple | semplice | simple | unkompliziert; einfach | 単純な、単一の |
| 6250. simulate - (v) | simuler | simulare | simular | simulieren | 擬態する |
| 6251. simultaneous - (a) | simultané | simultaneo | simultáneo | gleichzeitig; simultan | 同時の |
| 6252. sinew - (n) | tendon | tendine | fibra | Sehne | 腱 |
| 6253. singe - (v) | brûler légèrement | bruciacchiare | chamuscar | sengen | 焦がす |
| 6254. single - (a) | seul; unique | solo; singolo | solo; único | einfach; einmalig | 単一の |
| 6255. single blind - (a) | à l'insu; aveugle | a singolo-cieco | ciego simple | einfach blind | 一重盲検の |
| 6256. single center trial - (n) | essai dans un seul centre | studio monocentrico | estudio en un sólo centro | an nur einem Ort durchgeführte Studie | 単一センター試験 |
| 6257. single chain - (n) | chaîne unique | catena singola | cadena única | Einzelkette; Einzelstrang | 単一チェーン |
| 6258. single patient - (n) | patient unique | paziente singolo | único paciente | Einzelpatient | 一人の患者 |
| 6259. single study site - (n) | centre d'étude unique | posto per studio singolo | sitio de un sólo estudio | ein Durchführungsort der Studie | 単一研究場所 |
| 6260. sinistral - (a) | sinistre | sinistro | sinistral | links; Links- | 左側の |
| 6261. sinoatrial node - (n) | noeud sino-auriculaire; noeud sinusal | nodo senoatriale; nodo del seno | nodo sinoauricular | Sinusknoten | 洞房結節 |
| 6262. sinus - (n) | sinus | seno | seno | Sinus; Nebenhöhle | 洞 |

321

| English/American | French/Français | Italian/Italiano | Spanish/Español | German/Deutsch | Japanese/日本語 |
|---|---|---|---|---|---|
| 6263. sinusitis - (n) | sinusite | sinusite | sinusitis | Sinusitis | 副鼻腔炎、静脈洞炎 |
| 6264. site - (n) | site; lieu | posizione; località | sitio; local | Bereich;Stelle | 部位 |
| 6265. site audit - (n) | vérification de l'essai au site | verifica al luogo | revisión del ensayo al sitio | Überprüfung einer Probe vor Ort | 場所監査 |
| 6266. site directed mutagenesis - (n) | mutagénèse de site | mutagenesi selettiva | mutagénesis de sitio | ortsgerichtete Mutagenese | 部位特異的変異 |
| 6267. site selection - (n) | sélection du site | selezione di posti | selección del sitio | Ortauswahl | 場所選択 |
| 6268. site visit - (n) | visite de site | visita di posto | visita al emplazamiento | Ortsbesichtigung | 場所審査 |
| 6269. site visit report - (n) | rapport de la visite de site | resoconto di posti | informe de la visita al sitio | Ortsbesichtigungsbericht | 場所審査報告書 |
| 6270. sitting - (n) | séance; posture assise | seduta | sentada; sesión | Sitzung | 抱卵期 |
| 6271. sitting - (a) | assis | seduta | sentado | sitzend | 抱卵期の |
| 6272. situs - (n) | situs | situs | situs | Lage; Position | 位置 |
| 6273. sitz bath - (n) | bain de siège | vasca a sedile | baño de asiento | Sitzbad | 座浴 |
| 6274. size - (n) | taille; dimension | dimensione; grandezza | tamaño | Größe | 寸法 |
| 6275. skeleton - (n) | squelette | scheletro | esqueleto | Skelett | 骨格 |
| 6276. skew - (a) | oblique; biaisé | asimmetrico; obliquo | distorsionado; desviado | schräg | 非対称 |
| 6277. skill - (n) | habilité; aptitude | abilità | habilidad; destreza | Fähigkeit; Geschicklichkeit | 技術 |
| 6278. skin - (n) | peau | pelle; cute | piel | Haut | 皮膚 |
| 6279. skin deposit - (n) | dépôt cutané | deposito cutaneo | depósito en la piel | Hautvorrat (zur Transplantation) | 皮膚沈着 |
| 6280. skin eruption - (n) | éruption cutanée | eruzione cutanea | erupción de la piel | Hautausschlag | 皮疹 |
| 6281. skin graft - (n) | greffe cutanée | innesto di cute | injerto de piel | Hauttransplantat | 植皮［片］、皮膚移植［片］ |
| 6282. skin test - (n) | épreuve cutanée | cutireazione; test cutaneo | prueba cutánea | Hauttest | 皮膚試験 |
| 6283. skin turgor - (n) | turgescense cutanée | turgore delle pelle | turgor de la piel | Hautturgor | 皮膚緊満 |

322

| English/American | French/Français | Italian/Italiano | Spanish/Español | German/Deutsch | Japanese/日本語 |
|---|---|---|---|---|---|
| 6284. skinfold thickness - (n) | épaisseur d'un pli cutané | spessore dello strato sottocutaneo | grosor del pliego de la piel | Hautfaltendicke | 皮膚をつまんだ時の厚さ |
| 6285. skull - (n) | crâne | cranio | cráneo | Schädel | 頭蓋 |
| 6286. slant - (n) | inclinaison; biais | pendenza; inclinazione | inclinación | Neigung; Schräge | 傾斜 |
| 6287. slash - (n) | entaille; taillade | taglio; sfregio | cuchillada | Schnitt | 深い切り傷 |
| 6288. slash - (v) | entailler; taillader | tagliare | acuchillar | zerfetzen | 切りさく |
| 6289. sleep - (n) | sommeil | sonno; dormire | sueño | Schlaf | 睡眠、眠り |
| 6290. sleep - (v) | dormir | dormire | dormir | schlafen | 眠る |
| 6291. sleep dysfunction - (n) | dysfonctionnement du sommeil | disordine del ritmo sonno-veglia | trastorno en el sueño | Schlafstörung | 睡眠不全 |
| 6292. sleep stages - (n) | phases de sommeil | stadi del sonno | etapas del sueño | Schlafstadien | 睡眠段階 |
| 6293. sleep walking - (n) | somnambulisme | sonnambulismo | sonambulismo | Schlafwandeln; Somnambulismus | 夢遊病 |
| 6294. sleeplessness - (n) | insomnie | insonnia | insomnio | Schlaflosigkeit; Insomnie | 不眠［症］ |
| 6295. slide - (n) | glissade; diapositive | scivolata; vetrino | portaobjeto; diapositiva | Gleiten; Objektträger | すべること、スライドガラス |
| 6296. slide - (v) | glisser | scivolare | resbalar | gleiten; rutschen | 滑る |
| 6297. sling - (n) | écharpe | bandaggio a triangolo | cabestrillo | Schlinge; Binde | 三角布 |
| 6298. slipped disk - (n) | hernie du disque | ernia del disco | hernia del disco | Bandscheibenprolaps | 椎間板ヘルニア |
| 6299. slit - (n) | fente; incision | fenditura; incisione | abertura; incisión | Schlitze; Spalte | スリット、細隙 |
| 6300. slit - (v) | fendre; faire une incision | fendere; incidere | cortar; hender | aufschlitzen | 細長く切る |
| 6301. slit lamp examination - (n) | examen avec une lampe à fente | esame con luce incidente | examen por lámpara de hendidura | Spaltlampenuntersuchung | 細隙灯検査 |
| 6302. slough - (n) | croûte; dépouille | escara; crosta | costra | Schorf | 脱落組織、かさぶた |
| 6303. slow - (a) | lent | lento | lento | langsam | 遅い |
| 6304. slow onset - (n) | début lent | inizio lento | de comienzo lento | schleichender Beginn | 遅延開始 |
| 6305. slow speech - (n) | élocution lente | parlata lenta | de habla lenta | Bradylalie | 遅い話した |
| 6306. sluggish - (a) | paresseux; lent | pigro; lento | perezoso; lento | träge | 不活発な |

| English/American | French/Français | Italian/Italiano | Spanish/Español | German/Deutsch | Japanese/日本語 |
|---|---|---|---|---|---|
| 6307. small intestine - (n) | intestin grêle | intestino tenue | intestino delgado | Dünndarm | 小腸 |
| 6308. smear - (n) | frottis | striscio | frotis | Abstrich | 塗抹［標本］、スミア |
| 6309. smear - (v) | préparer un frottis | fare uno striscio di | preparar un frotis de | schmieren; ausstreichen | 塗る |
| 6310. smell - (n) | odeur; odorat | odore; olfatto | olor; olfato | Geruch; Geruchssinn | 嗅覚、におい |
| 6311. smell - (v) | sentir | sentire odore di | oler | riechen | においをかぐ |
| 6312. smelling salts - (n) | sels volatils | sali da fiuto | sales aromáticas | Riechsalz | 嗅塩、嗅薬 |
| 6313. smiling - (n) | sourire | sorriso | sonrisa | Lächeln | 微笑 |
| 6314. smoke - (n) | fumée | fumo | humo | Rauch | 喫煙 |
| 6315. smoke - (v) | fumer | fumare | fumar | rauchen | 喫煙する |
| 6316. smoke inhalation - (n) | inhalation de fumée | inalazione di fumo | inhalación de humo | Rauchinhalation | 煙の吸入 |
| 6317. smokeless tobacco - (n) | tabac sans fumée | tabacco senza fumo | tabaco que no se fuma | Kau- oder Schnupftabak | 噛みたばこ |
| 6318. smoking - (n) | habitude de fumer; fumage | il fumare; fumo | que fuma; fumando | Rauchen | 喫煙すること |
| 6319. smooth - (a) | lisse; poli | liscio | suave; liso | glatt | なめらかな |
| 6320. smooth muscle - (n) | muscle lisse | muscolo liscio | músculo liso | glatter Muskel | 平滑筋 |
| 6321. snake venom - (n) | venin de serpent | veleno di serpente | veneno de víbora | Schlangengift | 毒へどの毒液 |
| 6322. snare - (n) | anse | ansa | asa | Schlinge | わな、スネア |
| 6323. sneeze - (n) | éternuement | starnuto | estornudo | Niesen | くしゃみ |
| 6324. sneeze - (v) | éternuer | starnutire | estornudar | niesen | くしゃみをする |
| 6325. sneezing - (n) | éternuement | lo starnutire | estornutación | Niesen | くしゃみをすること |
| 6326. sniff - (n) | reniflement | fiutata | sorbo | Schnüffeln | においをかぐこと |
| 6327. sniff - (v) | renifler | annusare | sorber | schnüffeln | においをかぐ |
| 6328. snore - (n) | ronflement | il russare | ronquido | Schnarchen | いびき |
| 6329. snore - (v) | ronfler | russare | roncar | schnarchen | いびきをかく |
| 6330. soap - (n) | savon | sapone | jabón | Seife | 石けん |

324

| English/American | French/Français | Italian/Italiano | Spanish/Español | German/Deutsch | Japanese/日本語 |
|---|---|---|---|---|---|
| 6331. sob - (n) | sanglot | singulto | sollozo | Schluchzen | 嗚り泣き |
| 6332. sob - (v) | sangloter | piangere; singhiozzare | sollozar | schluchzen | 嗚り泣く |
| 6333. social - (a) | social | sociale | social | sozial | 社会的な |
| 6334. social class - (n) | classe sociale | classe sociale | clase social | gesellschaftliche Stellung; Klasse | 社会階級 |
| 6335. social security - (n) | sécurité sociale | sicurezza sociale | seguridad social | Sozialhilfe; Sozialversicherung | 社会保障 |
| 6336. socialization - (n) | socialisation | socializzazione | socialización | Sozialisierung | 社会化 |
| 6337. society - (n) | société | società | sociedad | Gesellschaft | 社会 |
| 6338. socioeconomic factor - (n) | facteur socioéconomique | fattore socioeconomico | factor socioeconómico | sozialwirtschaftlicher Faktor | 社会経済的因子 |
| 6339. sociology - (n) | sociologie | sociologia | sociología | Soziologie | 社会学 |
| 6340. socket - (n) | cavité; trou | cavità; incavo | cavidad | Höhle; Fassung | 槽、窩、ソケット |
| 6341. soda - (n) | soda; soude | soda; carbonato di sodio | soda; bicarbonato sódico | Soda; Natron | ソーダ |
| 6342. sodium - (n) | sodium; de soude | sodio | sodio | Natrium | ナトリウム |
| 6343. soft - (a) | moelleux; mou | soffice; molle | blando; flojo | weich | 柔らかい |
| 6344. soft endpoint - (n) | sous-objectif faible; objectif spécifique faible | variabile non facilmente misurabile | punto final flojo | nicht signifikanter Endpunkt | あいまいな終点 |
| 6345. soft outcome - (n) | résultat faible; issue faible | risultato non facilmente misurabile | resultado flojo | nicht signifikantes Ergebnis | あいまいな結果 |
| 6346. soft palate - (n) | palais mou | palato molle | paladar blando | weicher Gaumen | 軟口蓋 |
| 6347. soft tissue - (n) | tissu mou | tessuto molle | tejido blando | Bindegewebe | 軟部組織 |
| 6348. software - (n) | logiciel | software; programma per computer | software | Software | ソフトウェア |
| 6349. soil - (v) | salir; contaminer | sporcare; contaminare | ensuciar; contaminar | beschmutzen | 汚す |
| 6350. solar plexus - (n) | plexus solaire | plesso solare | plexo solar | Solarplexus | 腹腔神経叢 |
| 6351. sole - (n) | plante du pied | pianta | suela de pie | Fußsohle | 足底 |
| 6352. solid - (a) | solide | solido | sólido | solide; fest | 固形の |
| 6353. solubility - (n) | solubilité | solubilità | solubilidad | Löslichkeit | 溶解度 |

| English/American | French/Français | Italian/Italiano | Spanish/Español | German/Deutsch | Japanese/日本語 |
|---|---|---|---|---|---|
| 6354. solution - (n) | solution | soluzione | solución | Lösung | 溶液 |
| 6355. solvent - (n) | solvant | solvente | solvente | Solvens; Lösungsmittel | 溶媒、溶剤 |
| 6356. soma - (n) | soma | soma | soma | Soma; Körper | 体、体幹 |
| 6357. somatic - (a) | somatique | somatico | somático | somatisch; körperlich | 身体の |
| 6358. somatoform disorder - (n) | désordre somatoforme | disordine somatoformo | trastorno somatofórico | somatische Störung | 体性障害、心身症 |
| 6359. somato-sensory - (a) | somatosensitif | somatosensorio | somatosensorial | somatosensibe; somatosensorisch | 身体の、体幹の |
| 6360. somnolence - (n) | somnolence | sonnolenza | somnolencia | Somnolenz | 傾眠 |
| 6361. sonogram - (n) | sonogramme | sonogramma | sonograma | Sonogramm | ソノグラム、音波検査図 |
| 6362. soothing - (a) | calmant | calmante | calmante | beruhigend; schmerzlindernd | 鎮静させる |
| 6363. sophisticated analysis - (n) | analyse sophistiquée | analisi sofisticata | análisis sofisticado | anspruchsvolle Analyse; verfeinerte Analyse | 高度な分析 |
| 6364. sore - (n) | blessure; plaie | ferita; piaga | llaga | Geschwür; umschriebene Hautläsion | びらん、痛み |
| 6365. sore throat - (n) | mal de gorge | mal di gola | dolor de garganta | Angina; Halsentzündung | 咽頭炎、咽頭痛 |
| 6366. sorrow - (n) | peine; tristesse | dolore | pena; tristeza | Kummer; Sorge | 悲痛 |
| 6367. sound - (n) | son; bruit | suono | sonido | Geräusch; Ton | 音 |
| 6368. sound - (v) | sonner; ausculter | esplorare con una sonda; sonare | sonar; auscultar | sondieren | ゾンデにより体腔を検査または測定する |
| 6369. source data - (n) | données d'origine | dati originari | fuente de datos | Ursprungsdaten | 原地のデータ |
| 6370. source data verification - (n) | vérification des données d'origine | verifica dei dati originali | verificación de la fuente de datos | Ursprungsdaten-bestätigung | 原地のデータ確認 |
| 6371. source document - (n) | document d'origine | documento originario | documento fuente | Ursprungsdokument | 元の文献 |
| 6372. southern blot - (n) | analyse Southern blot | analisi di Southern blot | análisis Southern blot | Southern-Blot | サザンブロット |
| 6373. space - (n) | espace | spazio | espacio | Raum | 空間 |

326

| English/American | French/Français | Italian/Italiano | Spanish/Español | German/Deutsch | Japanese/日本語 |
|---|---|---|---|---|---|
| 6374. space flight - (n) | voyage spatial | volo spaziale | vuelo espacial | Weltraumflug | 宇宙飛行 |
| 6375. sparing effect - (n) | effet épargnant | effetto di evitamento | efecto moderador | aussparender Effekt | 回避効果 |
| 6376. spasm - (n) | spasme | spasmo | espasmo | Spasmus; Zuckung | 痙攣、痙縮 |
| 6377. spastic - (a) | spastique | spastico | espástico | spastisch; spasmodisch | 緊張過度の |
| 6378. spastic colon - (n) | côlon spastique | colite spastica | colon espástico | irritables Kolon; spastiches Kolon | 刺激結腸 |
| 6379. spatial behavior - (n) | comportement spatial | comportamento spaziale | conducta espacial | räumliches Verhalten | 空間行動 |
| 6380. spatial relationship - (n) | relation spatiale | relazione spaziale | relación espacial | räumliche Beziehung | 空間関係 |
| 6381. speak - (v) | parler | parlare | hablar | sprechen | 話す |
| 6382. special education - (n) | education spécialisée | educazione speciale | educación especial | Sonderschule | 特殊教育 |
| 6383. special patient population - (n) | population de malades spéciaux | popolazione di pazienti speciali | población de pacientes especiales | spezielle Patientenpopulation | 特殊患者母集団 |
| 6384. special senses - (n) | sens spéciaux | sensi speciali | sentidos especiales | die fünf Sinne | 特殊感覚 |
| 6385. specialism - (n) | spécialisation; spécialité | specializzazione | especialismo | Spezialisierung; Spezialfach | 専攻 |
| 6386. specialist - (n) | spécialiste | specialista | especialista | Spezialist; Facharzt | 専門家、専門医 |
| 6387. specialized study - (n) | étude spécialisée | studio specializzato | estudio especializado | spezialisierte Studie | 専門研究 |
| 6388. specialty - (n) | spécialité | specialità | especialidad | Spezialität; Fachgebiet | 専門 |
| 6389. specialty board - (n) | conseil de spécialité | consiglio di specialità | consejo de especialidad | Fachgebietsausschuß | 専門委員会 |
| 6390. species - (n) | espèces | specie | especies | Spezies; Art | 種 |
| 6391. specific - (a) | spécifique | specifico | específico | spezifisch; bestimmt | 種の、特異[的]な |
| 6392. specific gravity - (n) | poids spécifique | peso specifico | peso específico | spezifisches Gewicht | 比重 |

| English/American | French/Français | Italian/Italiano | Spanish/Español | German/Deutsch | Japanese/日本語 |
|---|---|---|---|---|---|
| 6393. specific pathogen free organism - (n) | organisme sans pathogènes | organismo senza patogeni | organismo sin patógenos | Krankheitserregerfreier Organismus | 特異病原体のない生物 |
| 6394. specificity - (n) | spécificité | specificità | especificidad | spezifische Wirksamkeit | 特異性 |
| 6395. specimen - (n) | spécimen; échantillon | campione | espécimen | Probe; Untersuchungsmaterial | 標本、検体 |
| 6396. specimen collection - (n) | accumulation de spécimens | raccolta campione | colección de espécimenes | Probensammlung | 標本収集 |
| 6397. specimen handling - (n) | manutention des spécimens | manipolazione del campione | manejo de espécimenes | Probenhandhabung | 標本の取り扱い |
| 6398. speck - (n) | point; petite tache | macchiolina; granello | pequeña mancha; punto | Fleck | 小斑点 |
| 6399. spectacles - (n) | lunettes | occhiali | gafas | Brille | 眼鏡 |
| 6400. spectral measurement - (n) | mesure spectrale | misura spettroscopica | medición espectral | Spektralmessung | スペクトル測定 |
| 6401. spectrometry - (n) | spectrométrie | spettrometria | espectrometría | Sepktrometrie | 分光［光度］法、スペクトロメトリ |
| 6402. spectroscopy - (n) | spectroscopie | spettroscopia | espectroscopia | Spektroskopie | 分光学 |
| 6403. spectrum, (pl.) spectra - (n) | spectre | spettro | espectro | Spektrum | スペクトル |
| 6404. speculum - (n) | spéculum | specolo | espéculo | Spekulum; Spiegel | 鏡 |
| 6405. speech - (n) | discours; parole | parola; linguaggio | habla | Sprache | 言語、会話 |
| 6406. speech therapy - (n) | traitement orthophonique | cura dei disturbi del linguaggio | terapia lingüística | Sprachtherapie | 言語療法 |
| 6407. sperm - (n) | sperme | sperma | esperma | Sperma | 精子、精液 |
| 6408. spermatic cord - (n) | cordon spermatique | cordone spermatico | cordón espermático | Funiculus spermaticus; Samenstrang | 精索 |
| 6409. spermatocidal agent - (n) | agent spermicide | agente spermicida | agente espermatocida | Spermizid | 殺精子剤 |

328

| English/American | French/Français | Italian/Italiano | Spanish/Español | German/Deutsch | Japanese/日本語 |
|---|---|---|---|---|---|
| 6410. spermato-genesis - (n) | spermatogénèse | spermatogenesi | espermatogénesis | Spermatogenese | 精子形成 |
| 6411. spermatozo-on - (n) | spermatozoïde | spermatozoo | espermatozoide; espermatozoo | Spermatozoon | 精子、精虫 |
| 6412. sperm-ovum interaction - (n) | interaction sperme-ovule | interazione uovo-sperma | interacción esperma/óvulo | Spermien-Ei-Interaktion | 精子と卵子の相互作用 |
| 6413. spheroid - (n) | sphéroïde | sferoide | esferoide | kugelförmige Struktur | 球状体 |
| 6414. spheroid - (a) | sphéroïdal | sferoidale | esferoidal | Sphäroid-; kugelartig | 球状の |
| 6415. sphincter - (n) | sphincter | sfintere | esfínter | Sphinkter | 括約筋 |
| 6416. sphygmomanome-ter - (n) | sphygmomanomètre | sfigmomanometro | esfigmomanómetro | Sphygmomanometer; Blutdruckmeßgerät | 血圧計 |
| 6417. spike - (n) | pointe | punta | punta; espiga | Spitzen; Stacheln | 棘波、スパイク |
| 6418. spike and wave - (n) | pointe-onde | punta e onda | puntas y ondas; espigas y ondas | Spitzen und Wogen; 'spike and wave' | 脳波 |
| 6419. spin - (n) | rotation | rotazione; spin | vuelta | Drehung | 回転、スピン |
| 6420. spin - (v) | tournoyer; centrifuger | ruotare; centrifugare | girar; centrifugar | rotieren; drehen | 回す |
| 6421. spin label - (n) | étiquette de centrifuger | etichetta di centrifugazione | etiqueta de centrifugar | Spinmarker; Spinmarkierung | スピンラベル |
| 6422. spinal - (a) | spinal | spinale | espinal | spinal | 棘の、脊柱の |
| 6423. spinal column - (n) | colonne vertébrale | colonna vertebrale | columna vertebral | Wirbelsäule | 脊柱 |
| 6424. spinal cord - (n) | moelle épinière | midollo spinale | médula espinal | Rückenmark | 脊髄 |
| 6425. spinal fluid - (n) | liquide céphalo-rachidien | liquido cefalorachidiano | líquido cefalorraquídeo | spinaler Liquor | 髄液 |
| 6426. spinal tap - (n) | ponction spinale; ponction lombaire | puntura lombare | punción lumbar | Lumbalpunktion | 脊椎穿刺 |
| 6427. spine - (n) | épine; colonne vertébrale | colonna vertebrale | espina | Rückgrat; Spina | 棘、脊柱、脊椎 |
| 6428. spiral - (n) | spirale; hélice | spirale | espiral | Spirale | らせん体 |
| 6429. spiral - (a) | spiroïdal; spiral | spirale | espiral | spiralförmig | らせん形の |

329

| English/American | French/Français | Italian/Italiano | Spanish/Español | German/Deutsch | Japanese日本語 |
|---|---|---|---|---|---|
| 6430. spirit - (n) | esprit | spirito | espíritu | Geist; Seele | 蒸留酒、蒸留された液体、酒精剤 |
| 6431. spirochete - (n) | spirochète | spirocheta | espiroqueta | Spirochäte | スピロヘータ |
| 6432. spirometry - (n) | spirométrie | spirometria | espirometría | Spirometrie | 肺活量測定 [法] |
| 6433. spit - (n) | salive | sputo | saliva; esputo | Speichel | 唾液 |
| 6434. spit - (v) | cracher; expectorer | sputare | escupir | spucken | 吐く |
| 6435. splanchnic - (a) | splanchnique | splancnico | esplácnico | Splanchniko-; viszeral- | 内臓の |
| 6436. spleen - (n) | rate | milza | bazo | Milz | 脾臓、脾 |
| 6437. splenic - (a) | splénique | splenico | esplénico | Milz-; lienal | 脾 [性] の |
| 6438. splenomegaly - (n) | splénomégalie | splenomegalia | esplenomegalia | Splenomegalie | 巨脾腫 [症] |
| 6439. splicing - (n) | épissage | splicing; rottura e risaldatura | empalme | Spleißen | スプライシング |
| 6440. splint - (n) | attelle; éclisse | stecca | férula | Schiene | 副木、腓骨 |
| 6441. splinter - (n) | esquille | scheggia | esquiria | Splitter | 破（骨）片 |
| 6442. splinter hemorrhage - (n) | hémorragie sous-unguéale | emorragia subungueale | hemorragia subungueal | Splitterblutung | 線状出血 |
| 6443. spoil - (v) | décomposer; gâter | rovinare; andare a male | deterioro; descomponer | verderben | 腐敗する |
| 6444. sponge - (n) | éponge | spugna | esponja | Schwamm; Tupfer | 海綿、スポンジ |
| 6445. sponsor - (n) | garant; répondant | garante; sponsor | patrocinador | Förderer; Sponsor | 保証人 |
| 6446. sponsoring agency - (n) | agence qui assure le patronage | agenzia garante; ditta sponsorizzatrice | agencia patrocinadora | fördernde (geldgebende) Gesellschaft | 後援機関 |
| 6447. spontaneous - (a) | spontané | spontaneo | espontáneo | spontan | 自発性の |
| 6448. sporadic - (a) | sporadique | sporadico | esporádico | sporadisch | 散在 [性] の、散発 [性] の |
| 6449. spore - (n) | spore | spora | espora | Spore | 胞子、芽胞 |
| 6450. spot - (n) | tache; macule | macchia; macula | mácula; mancha | Fleck | 点、斑点、斑 |
| 6451. spot check - (n) | contrôle intermittent | controllo salutario | comprobación en el acto | Stichprobe | 抜取り検査 |
| 6452. sprain - (n) | entorse; foulure | storta | torcedura | Verrenkung; Verstauchung | 捻挫 |

| English/American | French/Français | Italian/Italiano | Spanish/Español | German/Deutsch | Japanese/日本語 |
|---|---|---|---|---|---|
| 6453. spray - (n) | pulvérisation; vaporisation | spruzzi | pulverizador | Spray; Aerosol | 噴霧、スプレー |
| 6454. spray - (v) | faire des pulvérisations; vaporiser | spruzzare | rociar | sprayen; sprühen | 吹きかける |
| 6455. spread - (n) | propagation; étendue | espansione; estensione | extensión; propagación | Ausbreitung | 普及 |
| 6456. spread - (v) | propager; étendre | espandersi | extender; propagar | ausbreiten; verteilen | 広がる |
| 6457. spring back - (v) | guérir; recouvrer | recuperare; ristabilirsi | recobrar; restablecerse | genesen | はね返る、もどる |
| 6458. sprout - (n) | pousse; germe | germoglio | brote | Sproß; Ableger | 新芽 |
| 6459. sprout - (v) | pousser; germer | germogliare | brotar; echar | keimen; sprießen | 芽を出す |
| 6460. sprue - (n) | sprue | sprue | esprue | Sprue | スプルー |
| 6461. spur - (n) | éperon; ergot | traccia | espuela; aguijón | Sporn; Knochenzacke | [骨] 棘、葉突起 |
| 6462. spurious - (a) | faux; falsifié | spurio | espurio | falsch; Pseudo- | 偽の、(偽性の) |
| 6463. sputum - (n) | crachat; expectoration | sputo | esputo | Sputum; Auswurf | 痰 |
| 6464. squamous cell - (n) | cellule squameuse | cellula squamosa | célula escamosa | Schuppenzelle | 扁平上皮細胞 |
| 6465. square root - (n) | racine carrée | radice quadrata | raíz cuadrada | Quadratwurzel | 平方根 |
| 6466. squeeze - (v) | serrer; comprimer | spremere | comprimir; compresar | zusammendrücken; quetschen | 圧迫する |
| 6467. squint - (n) | strabisme | strabismo | estrabismo | Schielen; Strabismus | 斜視 |
| 6468. stab - (n) | coup | trafittura; puntura | puñalada | Stich | 刺し傷、刺創 |
| 6469. stab - (v) | poignarder; donner un coup | puntare; accoltellare | apuñalar | stechen | 刺す |
| 6470. stability - (n) | stabilité | stabilità | estabilidad | Stabilität; Festigkeit | 安定性、安定度 |
| 6471. stabilization - (n) | stabilisation | stabilizzazione | estabilización | Stabilisierung | 安定化 |
| 6472. stable - (a) | stable | stabile | estable | stabil; beständig | 安定した |
| 6473. staff - (n) | personnel | staff; personale | personal | Personal | スタッフ、職員 |
| 6474. staffing - (n) | personnel | personale | empleo de personal | Stellenbesetzung; Pesonalbesetzung | 職員配置 |
| 6475. stage - (n) | stade; phase | fase; stadio | estado; fase | Stadium; Phase | 病期、載物台、段階 |

331

| English/American | French/Français | Italian/Italiano | Spanish/Español | German/Deutsch | Japanese/日本語 |
|---|---|---|---|---|---|
| 6476. staging - (n) | établissement du stade | stadiazione | establecimiento del estado | Stadieneinteilung | 病期分類 |
| 6477. staging neoplasm - (n) | établissement du stade d'une néoplasie | stadiazione di una neoplasia | establecimiento del estado de una neoplasma | Stadieneinteilung des Neoplasmas | 癌の病期分類 |
| 6478. stagnation - (n) | stagnation; stase | stasi | estancamiento | Stagnieren | 停滞、うっ血 |
| 6479. stain - (n) | tache; colorant | macchia; miscela colorante | colorante; mancha | Farbstoff; Fleck | 変色、染色 [法] |
| 6480. stain - (v) | tacher; teindre | macchiare; dare la colorazione | manchar; colorar | färben | 変色させる、染色する |
| 6481. stainless steel - (n) | acier inoxydable | acciaio inossidabile | acero inoxidable | rostfreier Stahl | ステンレス |
| 6482. stalk - (n) | tige; pédoncule | stelo; picciolo | tallo; pedúnculo | Stengel; Stiel | 茎、柄 |
| 6483. stamina - (n) | vigueur; résistance | resistenza fisica | resistencia | Vitalität; Ausdauer | スタミナ |
| 6484. stammer - (v) | balbutier; bégayer | balbettare | tartamudear | stottern; stammeln | どもる、口ごもる |
| 6485. standard - (n) | standard; étalon | standard; modello | estándar; patrón | Standard; Norm | 標準 |
| 6486. standard - (a) | standard; normal | standard; normale | standard; normal | standard; normal | 標準の |
| 6487. standard deviation - (n) | déviation standard | deviazione standard | desviación estándar | Standardabweichung | 標準偏差 |
| 6488. standard error - (n) | erreur standard | errore standard | error estándar | Standardfehler | 標準誤差 |
| 6489. standard operating procedure - (n) | procédure d'opération standard; procédure à suivre | procedura operazionale standard | procedimiento estándar | gewöhnliche Betriebsverfahren | 標準の手術手順 |
| 6490. standardized scale - (n) | échelle standardisée; échelle normalisée | unità di misura standardizzata | escala normalizada | standardisierte Maßstab | 規格化された秤 |
| 6491. standing - (a) | sur pied; debout | in piedi; eretto | derecho | stehend | 起立している |
| 6492. staphylococcus - (n) | staphylocoque | stafilococco | estafilococo | Staphylokokkus | ブドウ球菌属 |

| English/American | French/Français | Italian/Italiano | Spanish/Español | German/Deutsch | Japanese 日本語 |
|---|---|---|---|---|---|
| 6493. starch - (n) | amidon | amido | almidón | Stärke | デンプン |
| 6494. stare - (n) | regard fixe | sguardo fisso | mirada fija | Blick; Starrblick | 凝視 |
| 6495. stare - (v) | regarder fixement | fissare | mirar fijamente | starren | 凝視する |
| 6496. startle reflex - (n) | réflexe de sursaut réflexe d'alarme | riflesso delle spavento | reflejo de sobresalto | Stellreflex | 驚愕反射. びっくり反射 |
| 6497. starvation - (n) | inanition | inedia | falta de alimento | Verhungern; Hungertod | 飢餓 |
| 6498. stasis - (n) | stase; stagnation | stasi | estasis | Stauung; Stase | 静止、うっ血、血行停止 |
| 6499. stat - (adv) | stat; d'extrême urgence | sul momento; immediatamente | inmediatamente | sofort | すぐに、直ちに |
| 6500. state - (n) | état; condition | stato | estado | Status; Zustand | 状態 |
| 6501. state of the art - (a) | dernier cri; fait de mieux | il migliore esistente; l'ultimo ritrovato | de punta; de avanzada | auf dem Stand der Technik | 最先端技術を用いた |
| 6502. static comparisons - (n) | comparaisons statiques | paragoni statici | comparaciones estáticas | statische Vergleiche | 静的比較 |
| 6503. statistical - (a) | statistique | statistico | estadístico | statistisch | 統計の |
| 6504. statistical method - (n) | méthode statistique | metodo statistico | método estadístico | statistisches Verfahren | 統計手段 |
| 6505. statistical report - (n) | rapport statistique | rapporto statistico | informe estadístico | statistischer Bericht | 統計報告 |
| 6506. statistically significant - (n) | statistiquement significant | statisticamente significativo | estadísticamente significativo | statistisch signifikant | 統計上顕著な |
| 6507. statistics - (n) | statistique | statistica | estadística | Statistik | 統計［量］ |
| 6508. stature - (n) | stature; taille | statura | estatura | Statur; Größe | 身長 |
| 6509. status - (n) | état | stato | estado | Status; Zustand | 状態 |
| 6510. status quo - (n) | status quo | status quo | status quo | Status quo | 現状 |
| 6511. steady state - (n) | état stable | stato di stabilità | estado estable | Fließgleichgewicht; stationärer Zustand | 安定状態 |
| 6512. steady-state - (a) | régime à l'état stable | in regime stazionario | estado-estabilidad | in stationärem Zustand | 安定状態の |

| English/American | French/Français | Italian/Italiano | Spanish/Español | German/Deutsch | Japanese日本語 |
|---|---|---|---|---|---|
| 6513. steal - (n) | vol | furto | robo | Diebstahl | 盗血 |
| 6514. steal - (v) | voler; dérober | rubare | robar | stehlen | 盗む |
| 6515. steam - (n) | vapeur | vapore | vapor | Dampf | 蒸気 |
| 6516. steatorrhea - (n) | stéatorrhée | steatorrea | esteatorrea | Steatorrhö | 脂肪便 |
| 6517. steel - (n) | acier | acciaio | acero | Stahl | 鉄鋼 |
| 6518. steering committee - (n) | comité de direction | comitati direttivi | comité directivo | Lenkungsausschuß; Leitung | 運営委員会 |
| 6519. stellate - (a) | stellaire; étoilé | stellato | estrellado; radiado | sternförmig; stellatus | 星状の |
| 6520. stem - (n) | tronc; tige | stelo | tallo | Stamm; Stiel | 茎、幹 |
| 6521. stem cell - (n) | cellule souche | cellula staminale | célula troncal | Stammzelle | 幹細胞 |
| 6522. stench - (n) | puanteur; odeur infecte | puzzo; fetore | hedor | Gestank | 悪臭 |
| 6523. stenosis - (n) | sténose; rétrécissement | stenosi | estenosis | Stenose | 狭窄 [症] |
| 6524. step - (n) | pas; marche | passo | paso | Schritt; Stufe | ステップ、段階 |
| 6525. stepwise approach - (n) | approche par étapes | approccio passo per passo | aproximación por incrementos sucesivos | stufenweiser Ansatz | 段階的アプローチ |
| 6526. stereoisomer - (n) | stéréoisomère | stereoisomero | estereoisómero | Stereoisomer | 立体異性体 |
| 6527. stereoselective - (a) | stéréosélectif | stereoselettivo | estereoselectivo | stereoselektiv | 立体選択的 |
| 6528. stereotaxic technique - (n) | technique stéréotaxique | tecnica stereotassica | técnica esterotáxica | stereotaxische Methode | 定位的技術 |
| 6529. stereotyped behavior - (n) | comportement | comportamento | conducta estereotipada | stereotypisches Verhalten | 常同的行動 |
| 6530. stereotyping - (n) | stéréotypé | stereotipato | estereotipia | Stereotypisierung | 常同症 |
| 6531. sterile - (a) | stéréotype | stereotipo | estéril | steril; keimfrei | 生殖不能の、無菌の |
| 6532. sterile powder - (n) | stérile; aseptique | sterile; asettico | polvo estéril | steriler Puder | 殺菌パウダー |
| 6533. sterility - (n) | poudre stérile | polvere sterile | esterilidad | Sterilität; Keimfraiheit | 生殖不能、無菌 |
| 6534. sterilization - (n) | stérilité; infécondité | sterilità | esterilización | Sterilisation; Sterilisierung | 不妊手術、殺菌 [法] |
| | stérilisation | sterilizzazione | | | |

334

| English/American | French/Français | Italian/Italiano | Spanish/Español | German/Deutsch | Japanese日本語 |
|---|---|---|---|---|---|
| 6535. sternocosto-clavicular - (a) | sternocostoclaviculaire | sternocostoclavicolare | esternocostoclavicular | sternokostoklavikular | 胸肋鎖骨の |
| 6536. sternum - (n) | sternum | sterno | esternón | Sternum | 胸骨 |
| 6537. steroid - (n) | stéroïde | steroide | esteroide | Steroid | ステロイド |
| 6538. steroidal - (a) | stéroïde; stéroïdien | steroideo | esteroidal | steroidisch | ステロイドの |
| 6539. stethoscope - (n) | stéthoscope | stetoscopio | estetoscopio | Stethoskop | 聴診器 |
| 6540. stick - (n) | bâton; morceau de bois | stecco | palo | Stock | 棒、線條剤 |
| 6541. stiff - (a) | rigide; raide | rigido | rígido | steif | 堅い |
| 6542. stifle - (v) | suffoquer; réprimer | soffocare | sofocar, suprimir | ersticken; unterdrücken | 窒息させる |
| 6543. stigma - (n) | stigmate | stigma | estigma | Stigma; Markierung | 徴候、スチグマ |
| 6544. still - (a) | immobile; tranquille | fermo; immobile | inmóvil; tranquilo | bewegungslos; still | 静かな |
| 6545. stillbirth - (n) | accouchement d'un mort-né | parto di un feto morto; nato morto | parto con niño muerto | Totgeburt | 死産 |
| 6546. stimulant - (n) | stimulant; excitant | stimolante | estimulante | Stimulans; Stimulator | 興奮薬、剌戟薬 |
| 6547. stimulate - (v) | stimuler | stimolare | estimular | stimulieren; anregen | 剌激する |
| 6548. stimulation - (n) | stimulation | stimolazione | estimulación | Stimulation; Reiz | 剌激 [作用] |
| 6549. stimulus - (n) | stimulus | stimolo | estímulo | Reiz; Stimulus | 興奮薬、剌戟薬、剌激 |
| 6550. sting - (n) | piqûre; brûlure | puntura d'insetto; pungiglione | picadura; escozor | Stich | 剌痛、剌す |
| 6551. stir - (v) | agiter | mescolare | agitar | rühren; umrühren | かきまぜる |
| 6552. stitch - (n) | point de suture | sutura | punto de sutura | Stich; Naht | 激痛、一針の縫合 [糸] |
| 6553. stitch - (v) | suturer | suturare | suturar | nähen; stechen | 縫う |
| 6554. stock [species] - (n) | lignée | colonia | linaje | Stamm | 株、血統 |
| 6555. stoma - (n) | stomate | stoma | estoma | Stoma; Rachen | 小孔 |
| 6556. stomach - (n) | estomac | stomaco | estómago | Magen; Bauch | 胃 |
| 6557. stone - (n) | calcul; pierre | calcolo | cálculo; piedra | Stein | 結石、石 |
| 6558. stool - (n) | selle | feci; defecazione | deposición; heces | Stuhl; Kot | 便通 |

335

| English/American | French/Français | Italian/Italiano | Spanish/Español | German/Deutsch | Japanese/日本語 |
|---|---|---|---|---|---|
| 6559. stool guaiac - (n) | analyse de sang fécale | ricerca di sangue occulto nelle feci | análisis de sangre fecal | Stuhltest auf okkultes Blut | 便のグアヤク試験 |
| 6560. stoop - (n) | inclination en avant; attitude voûtée | curvatura | cargazón de espaldas; andar encorvado | Gebeugtheit | 前かがみ込み |
| 6561. stoop - (v) | courber; incliner | chinarsi | encorvar | beugen | かがむ |
| 6562. stop condition - (n) | condition d'arrêt | condizione di arresto | condición de parada | Abbruchsbedingung | 停止状態 |
| 6563. stop item - (n) | article d'arrêt | articolo di arresto | artículo de parada | Abbruchskriterium | 停止項目 |
| 6564. stopping boundary - (n) | limite d'arrêt | limite di arresto | límite de parada | Abbruchsgrenze | 停止境界 |
| 6565. stopping rule - (n) | règle d'arrêt | regola di arresto | regla de parada | Abbruchsregel | 停止規則 |
| 6566. storage - (n) | entreposage; emmagasinage | immagazzinamento; stoccaggio | almacenaje | Aufbewahrung; Einlagerung | 貯蔵 |
| 6567. storage device - (n) | appareil d'entreposage | dispositivo di memorizzazione | dispositivo de almacenaje | Speichervorrichtung | 貯蔵装置 |
| 6568. storage disease - (n) | maladie d'accumulation; thésaurismose | tesaurismosi | enfermedad por almacenaje | Speicherkrankheit | 蓄積症 |
| 6569. strabismus - (n) | strabisme | strabismo | estrabismo | Strabismus; Schielen | 斜視 |
| 6570. straighten - (v) | redresser | raddrizzare | enderezar | geraderichten; aufrichten | まっすぐにする |
| 6571. strain - (n) | souche; entorse | distorsione; ceppo | torcedura; raza | Verstauchung; Stamm | 菌株、緊張 |
| 6572. strand - (n) | brin; fibre | filamento | hebra; filamento | Strang; Strähne | 繊維、糸状体 |
| 6573. strangle - (v) | étrangler | soffocare | estrangular | erwürgen; ersticken | 絞殺する、絞扼 |
| 6574. strangulation - (n) | étranglement | strozzamento | estrangulación | Strangulierung; Abschnürung | 絞扼、窒息、嵌頓 |
| 6575. strategy - (n) | stratégie | strategia | estrategia | Strategie | 戦略 |
| 6576. stratification - (n) | stratification | stratificazione | estratificación | Schichtung; Stratifikation | 層化 |
| 6577. stratified random allocation - (n) | allocation aléatoire stratifiée | distribuzione stratificata a caso | asignación al azar estratificada | geschichtete zufällige Zuteilung | 層化無作為割当 |

| English/American | French/Français | Italian/Italiano | Spanish/Español | German/Deutsch | Japanese/日本語 |
|---|---|---|---|---|---|
| 6578. stratified randomization - (n) | randomisation stratifiée | randomizzazione stratificata | aleatorización estratificada | geschichtete Randomisierung | 層化無作為化 |
| 6579. stratified study - (n) | étude stratifiée | studio stratificato | estudio estratificado | geschichtete Studie | 層化研究 |
| 6580. stratify - (v) | stratifier | stratificare | estratificar | schichten | 層をなす |
| 6581. stratum - (n) | stratum | strato | estrato | Schicht | 層 |
| 6582. streak - (n) | strie; raie | striscia; stria | estría | Streifen; Linie | 縞条 |
| 6583. stream - (n) | courant | flusso | corriente | Fluß; Strom | 流れ |
| 6584. strength - (n) | force; puissance | forza; concentrazione | fuerza | Kraft; Stärke | 強さ、強度 |
| 6585. streptococcus - (n) | streptocoque | streptococco | estreptococo | Streptokokke | 連鎖球菌属 |
| 6586. stress - (n) | stress; tension | stress; sforzo | estrés; tensión | Streß; Belastung | ストレス、抵抗力 |
| 6587. stress fracture - (n) | fracture de stress; fracture de tension | frattura da stress | fractura de estrés | Belastungsfraktur | 圧力骨折 |
| 6588. stress test - (n) | épreuve à l'effort | prova di stress | prueba de estrés | Belastungstest | ストレス負荷試験 |
| 6589. stretch - (n) | extension | stiramento | extensión; estirón | Strecken | 広がり、伸張 |
| 6590. stretch - (v) | distendre; étirer | stendere; stirare | extender; estirar | strecken; ausdehnen | 伸ばす |
| 6591. stria - (n) | strie; raie | stria | estría | Streifen; Stria | [線] 条 |
| 6592. striated muscle - (n) | muscle strié | muscolo striato | músculo estriado | quergestreifter Muskel; Skelettmuskel | 横紋筋 |
| 6593. stricture - (n) | stricture; rétrécissement | stenosi; restringimento | estrictura | Striktur; Verengung | 狭窄 |
| 6594. stride - (n) | grand pas; enjambée | passo | zancada; tranco | Schritt; Gang | 闊歩、歩幅 |
| 6595. stridor - (n) | stridor | stridore | estridor | Stridor | ぜん鳴、ぜん音 |
| 6596. stripe - (n) | raie; bande | striscia; banda | raya | Streifen | 縞、横紋、線 [条] |
| 6597. stroke - (n) | accident cérébro-vasculaire | colpo | ataque súbito y agudo; ataque cerebral | Anfall; Schlag | 発作、拍動 |
| 6598. stroke volume - (n) | volume systolique; volume d'éjection | gittata sistolica | volumen de eyección; volumen sistólico | Schlagvolumen | 一回拍出量、心拍血液量 |

| English/American | French/Français | Italian/Italiano | Spanish/Español | German/Deutsch | Japanese/日本語 |
|---|---|---|---|---|---|
| 6599. stroma - (n) | stroma | stroma | estroma | Stroma; interstitielles Bindegewebe | 支質 |
| 6600. stromal cell - (n) | cellule de stroma | cellula stromale | célula de estroma | Stromazelle; Bindegewebszelle | 間質細胞 |
| 6601. strontium - (n) | strontium | stronzio | estroncio | Strontium | ストロンチウム |
| 6602. structural - (a) | structural | strutturale; di struttura | estructural | strukturell; Struktur- | 構造の |
| 6603. structure - (n) | structure | struttura | estructura | Struktur | 構造 |
| 6604. structure activity relationship - (n) | relation structure - activité | relazione struttura-attività | relación estructura-actividad | Struktur-Wirkungs-Verhältnis | 構造活性関係 |
| 6605. student - (n) | étudiant | studente | estudiante | Student | 学生 |
| 6606. study - (n) | étude | studio | estudio | Studie; Versuch | 研究 |
| 6607. study arm - (n) | bras de l'étude | ramo di uno studio | rama del estudio | Versuchszweig | 研究中の腕 |
| 6608. study conduct - (n) | conduite de l'étude | condotta di studio | conducta de estudio | Studienleitung | 研究経営 |
| 6609. study coordinator - (n) | coordinateur de l'étude | coordinatore dello studio | coordinador del estudio | Studienkoordinator | 研究コーディネーター |
| 6610. study design - (n) | plan de l'étude | disegno dello studio | diseño del estudio | Studienplanung | 研究設計 |
| 6611. stunt - (v) | retarder la croissance | arrestare la crescita | atrofiar; impedir el crecimiento | hemmen; verkrüppeln | 発育を妨げる |
| 6612. stupor - (n) | stupeur | stupore | estupor | Betäubung; Stupor | 昏迷 |
| 6613. stutter - (v) | bégayer | balbettare | tartamudear | stottern | どもる |
| 6614. stuttering - (n) | bégaiement | balbettamento | tartamudez | Stottern | どもり、吃、構音障害 |
| 6615. sty - (n) | orgelet | orzaiolo | orzuelo | Gerstenkorn; -ordeolum | 麦粒腫、ものもらい |
| 6616. subacute - (a) | subaigu | subacuto | subagudo | subakut | 亜急性の |
| 6617. subarachnoid - (a) | sous-arachnoïdien | subaracnoidea | subaracnoideo | Subarachnoid | クモ膜下の |
| 6618. subcellular - (a) | sous-cellulaire | subcellulare | subcelular | subzellulär | 非細胞の |
| 6619. subchronic - (a) | subchronique | subcronico | subcrónico | subchronisch; überwiegend chronisch | 亜慢性の |
| 6620. subclavian - (a) | sous-clavière | succlavia | subclavio; subclavicular | Subklavia- | 鎖骨下の |

338

| English/American | French/Français | Italian/Italiano | Spanish/Español | German/Deutsch | Japanese/日本語 |
|---|---|---|---|---|---|
| 6621. subclinical - (a) | subclinique | subclinico | subclínico | subklinisch | 無症状の、準臨床的の |
| 6622. subconscious - (a) | subconscient | subcosciente | subconsciente | unterbewußt | 潜在意識の |
| 6623. subcutaneous - (a) | sous-cutané | sottocutaneo | subcutáneo | subkutan | 皮下の |
| 6624. subdivide - (v) | subdiviser | suddividere | subdividir | unterteilen | 細分する |
| 6625. subdural - (a) | sous-dural | subdurale; sottodurale | subdural | subdural | 硬膜下の |
| 6626. subdural hematoma - (n) | hématome sous-dural | ematoma subdurale | hematoma subdural | Subduralhämatom | 硬膜下血腫 |
| 6627. subgroup - (n) | sous-groupe | sottogruppo | subgrupo | Untergruppe | 亜群 |
| 6628. subgroup analysis - (n) | analyse de sous-groupe | analisi del sottogruppo | análisis del subgrupo | Untergruppenanalyse | 亜群分析 |
| 6629. subgroup of patients - (n) | sous-groupe des patients | sottogruppo di pazienti | subgrupo de los pacientes | Patientenuntergruppe | 患者亜群 |
| 6630. subject - (n) | sujet; patient | soggetto; paziente | sujeto; paciente | Subjekt; Proband | 被検（被験）者 |
| 6631. subject heading - (n) | rubrique | titolo del soggetto | encabezamiento del tema | Überschrift; Rubrik | 件名標目 |
| 6632. subjective - (a) | subjectif | soggettivo | subjetivo | subjektiv | 主観の |
| 6633. subjective data - (n) | données subjectives | dati soggettivi | datos subjetivos | subjektive Daten | 主観的データ |
| 6634. subjective response - (n) | réponse subjective; réaction subjective | risposta soggettiva | respuesta subjetiva | subjektive Reaktion | 主観的反応 |
| 6635. sublimation - (n) | sublimation | sublimazione | sublimación | Sublimierung; Sublimation | 昇華 |
| 6636. subliminal - (a) | subliminal | subliminale | subliminal | unterschwellig | いき値下の |
| 6637. sublingual - (a) | sublingual | sottolinguale | sublingual | sublingual | 舌下の |
| 6638. submandibular gland - (n) | glande sous-mandibulaire | ghiandola sottomandibolare | glándula submandibular | Glandula submandibularis; Unterkieferdrüse | 顎下腺 |

| English/American | French/Français | Italian/Italiano | Spanish/Español | German/Deutsch | Japanese/日本語 |
|---|---|---|---|---|---|
| 6639. submicroscopic - (a) | sous-microscopique | submicroscopico | submicroscópico | ultramikroskopisch | 超顕微鏡的な、限外顕微鏡的な |
| 6640. submitochondrial particle - (n) | particule sous-mitochondriale | particella submitocondriale | partícula submitocondrial | submitochondriales Teilchen | 亜ミトコンドリアの粒子 |
| 6641. subnormal - (a) | sous-normal | subnormale | subnormal | subnormal | 正常以下の |
| 6642. subside - (v) | tomber; s'apaiser | diminuire; ridursi | bajar; alejarse | sich absetzen; sich niederschlagen | 静まる |
| 6643. subsidiary - (a) | subsidiaire | sussidiario | subsidiario | subsidiär; Hilfs- | 補助の |
| 6644. subsidiary - (n) | filiale | sussidiario | sucursal; filial | Tochtergesellschaft | 付加物 |
| 6645. subsistence - (n) | subsistance; existence | mezzi di sussistenza | subsistencia | Lebensunterhalt Existenz | 生活、食糧 |
| 6646. substance - (n) | substance | sostanza | sustancia | Substanz | 物質 |
| 6647. substance abuse - (n) | abus de substance | abuso di sostanza | abuso de sustancia | Stoffabhängigket | 物質乱用 |
| 6648. substandard - (a) | de qualité inférieure | sotto la norma | inferior al nivel normal | minderwertig | 標準以下の |
| 6649. substantia nigra - (n) | substantia nigra; substance noire | substantia nigra; sostanza nera | substancia negra | Substantia nigra | 黒質 |
| 6650. substantial - (a) | substantiel | considerevole | sustancial; sustancioso | kräftig; beträchtlich | 本質的な |
| 6651. substitute - (n) | substitut | sostituto | sustituto | Ersatz | 代理［人］ |
| 6652. substitute - (v) | substituer | sostituire | sustituir | ersetzen | 置換する、代用する |
| 6653. substrate specificity - (n) | spécificité du substrat | specificità del substrato | especificidad del substrato | Substratspezifität | 基質特異性 |
| 6654. subtherapeutic - (a) | sous-thérapeutique | subterapeutico | subterapéutico | subtherapeutisch | （低すぎて）効果の出ない、薬のレベルの |
| 6655. subtotal - (n) | sous-total | subtotale | subtotal | Zwischensumme | 小計 |
| 6656. subtraction technique - (n) | technique de soustraction | tecnica di sottrazione | técnica de sustracción | Subtraktionsverfahren | 減算法 |
| 6657. suburban - (a) | suburbain; de banlieue | suburbano | suburbano | vorstädtisch | 郊外の |

| English/American | French/Français | Italian/Italiano | Spanish/Español | German/Deutsch | Japanese/日本語 |
|---|---|---|---|---|---|
| 6658. succession - (n) | succession; suite | successione | sucesión | Reihenfolge; Aufeinanderfolge | 連続 |
| 6659. sucking - (n) | succion; aspiration | suzione; aspirazione | succión; aspiración | Saugen; Lutschen | 吸うこと、乳を飲む |
| 6660. suckle - (v) | allaiter | allattare | amamantar | säugen | 哺乳する、乳児に |
| 6661. suckling - (n) | allaitement; nourrisson | lattante | mamón; amamantar | Säugen; Säugling | 哺乳、乳児 |
| 6662. suction - (n) | succion; aspiration | suzione | succión | Saugen | 吸引［法］、吸込み |
| 6663. sudden cardiac death - (n) | mort subite cardiaque | morte cardiaca improvvisa | muerte súbita cardiaca | plötzlicher Herztod | 心臓病による突然死 |
| 6664. sudden death - (n) | mort subite | morte improvvisa | muerte súbita | plötzlicher Tod | 突然死 |
| 6665. sudden infant death (cot death) [abbr] SID - (n) | mort subite du nourrisson | morte neonatale improvvisa | muerte súbita infantil; muerte en cuna | plötzlicher Kindestod | 乳児の突然死 |
| 6666. sudden onset - (n) | attaque soudaine | inizio improvviso | ataque súbito | plötzlicher Ausbruch | 突然の開始 |
| 6667. suffer - (v) | souffrir; subir | soffrire | sufrir | erleiden; leiden | 苦しむ |
| 6668. suffocate - (v) | suffoquer | soffocare | sofocar | ersticken | 窒息する、窒息させる |
| 6669. suffuse - (v) | se répandre sur; envahir | colorire | bañar; difundir | erfüllen | 覆う |
| 6670. sugar - (n) | sucre | zucchero | azúcar | Zucker | 砂糖 |
| 6671. suggestion - (n) | suggestion | suggestione | sugerencia; sugestión | Anregung; Vorschlag | 暗示 |
| 6672. suicidal - (a) | suicidaire | che tende al suicidio | suicida | suizidal; selbstmörderisch | 自滅的な |
| 6673. suicide - (n) | suicide | suicidio | suicidio | Suizid; Selbstmord | 自殺、自殺者 |
| 6674. suitable - (a) | convenable; approprié | adatto; appropriato | conveniente; apropiado | passend; geeignet | 適切な |
| 6675. sulfonamides - (n) | sulfonamides | sulfonamidi; sulfamidici | sulfonamidas | Sulfonamide | スルホンアミド |
| 6676. sulfur - (n) | soufre | zolfo | azufre | Schwefel | 硫黄 |
| 6677. summary - (n) | sommaire; résumé | riassunto | resumen | Zusammenfassung; Abriß | 概要 |
| 6678. sunburn - (n) | coup de soleil; érythème solaire | eritema solare | quemadura del sol | Sonnenbrand | 日焼け |
| 6679. sunlight - (n) | lumière du soleil | luce solare | luz del sol | Sonnenlicht | 日光 |

341

| English/American | French/Français | Italian/Italiano | Spanish/Español | German/Deutsch | Japanese/日本語 |
|---|---|---|---|---|---|
| 6680. sunscreen - (n) | lotion de soleil; protection du soleil | sostanza antisolare | protección contra el sol | Sonnenöl | 遮光剤 |
| 6681. sunstroke - (n) | insolation; coup de chaleur | colpo di sole | insolación | Sonnenstich | 日射病 |
| 6682. superego - (n) | surmoi | super-io; super-ego | superego | Über-Ich | 超自我 |
| 6683. superficial - (a) | superficiel | superficiale | superficial | oberflächlich | 皮相の |
| 6684. super-imposed - (a) | surimposé | sovrapposto | sobrepuesto | überlagert | 二重焼き付けの |
| 6685. super-infection - (n) | super-infection; surinfection | superinfezione | superinfección | Superinfektion | 重［複］感染 |
| 6686. superior - (a) | supérieur | superiore | superior | oberer; überlegen | 上の、上方を向いた |
| 6687. supernatant - (a) | surnageant | supernatante | sobrenadante | auf der Oberfläche schwimmend | 上澄み［液］ |
| 6688. supervisor - (n) | surveillant; directeur | supervisore | supervisor | Leiter; Aufseher | 監督者 |
| 6689. supinate - (v) | mettre en supination | supinare | supinar | supinieren; in Rückenlage bringen | 回外運動を行なう |
| 6690. supine - (a) | en supination; couché sur le dos | supino | supino | in Rückenlage | 仰臥の |
| 6691. supplement - (n) | supplément | supplemento | suplemento | Ergänzung; Zusatz | 補足 |
| 6692. supplies - (n) | approvisionnement | provvista | suministro; abastecimiento | Vorräte | 供給品 |
| 6693. support - (n) | soutien; appui | il sostenere | sostén; apoyo | Unterstützung; Abstützung | 支持、支持器 |
| 6694. support system - (n) | système de soutien; système d'appui | sistema sopportanti | sistema de apoyo | Unterstützungssystem | 支援システム |
| 6695. supportive results - (n) | résultats à l'appui | risultati di supporto | resultados respaldadores | unterstützende Ergebnisse | 支援的結果 |
| 6696. suppository - (n) | suppositoire | supposta; suppositore | supositorio | Suppositorium; Zäpfchen | 坐剤 |

342

| English/American | French/Français | Italian/Italiano | Spanish/Español | German/Deutsch | Japanese/日本語 |
|---|---|---|---|---|---|
| 6697. suppress - (v) | supprimer | arrestare; sedare | suprimir | unterdrücken; supprimieren | 抑圧する、印制する |
| 6698. suppression - (n) | suppression | soppressione | supresión | Verdrängung; Unterdrückung | 抑圧、抑制 |
| 6699. suppressor - (n) | suppresseur | soppressore | supresor | Suppressor | 抑圧剤 |
| 6700. suppurant - (a) | suppuratif | suppurante | supurante | eiterbildend | 化膿性の |
| 6701. suppuration - (n) | suppuration | suppurazione | supuración | Eiterung | 化膿 |
| 6702. suprapubic - (a) | suprapubien | suprapubico | suprapúbico | suprapubisch | 恥骨上の |
| 6703. suprarenal - (a) | supra-rénal | surrenale | suprarrenal | suprarenal; Nebennieren- | 腎上の、副腎の |
| 6704. supraventricular - (a) | supra-ventriculaire | sopraventricolare | supraventricular | supraventrikulär | 上室 [性] の |
| 6705. sural - (a) | sural | surale | sural | Waden- | ふくらはぎの、腓腹の |
| 6706. surface - (n) | surface | superficie | superficie | Oberfläche | 表面 |
| 6707. surface antigen - (n) | antigène de surface | antigene di superficie | antígeno de superficie | Oberflächenantigen | 細胞表面抗原 |
| 6708. surface properties - (n) | propriétés de surface | proprietà di superficie | propiedades de superficie | Oberflächen-eigenschaften | 表面の特性 |
| 6709. surface-active - (a) | actif en surface | tensioattivo | activo en la superficie | oberflächenaktiv | 表面活性で |
| 6710. surgeon - (n) | chirurgien | chirurgo | cirujano | Chirurg | 外科医 |
| 6711. surgery - (n) | chirurgie | chirurgia | cirugía | Chirurgie; Operation | 外科 |
| 6712. surgical - (a) | chirurgical | chirurgico | quirúrgico | chirurgisch | 外科の |
| 6713. surgical ablation - (n) | ablation chirurgicale | asportazione chirurgica | ablación quirúrgica | operative Ablation | 外科切断 |
| 6714. surgical flaps - (n) | lambeaux chirurgicaux | lembo chirurgico | colgajos quirúrgicos | Gewebelappen | (外科の) 皮弁 |
| 6715. surgical instrument - (n) | instrument chirurgical | strumento chirurgico | instrumento quirúrgico | chirurgisches Instrument | 手術用具 |

343

| English/American | French/Français | Italian/Italiano | Spanish/Español | German/Deutsch | Japanese/日本語 |
|---|---|---|---|---|---|
| 6716. surgical operation - (n) | opération chirurgicale | operazione chirurgica | operación quirúrgica | Operation; Operieren | 外科手術 |
| 6717. surgical specialty - (n) | spécialité chirurgicale | specialità chirurgica | especialidad quirúrgica | chirurgisches Spezialgebiet | 外科専門 |
| 6718. surgical stapler - (n) | agrafeuse chirurgicale | cucitrice chirurgica | abrochador quirúrgico | chirurgischer Klammerapparat | 外科のホチキス |
| 6719. surrogate - (n) | substitut; succédané | sostituto | sustituto; suplente | Ersatz; Surrogat | 代理［人］ |
| 6720. surrogate - (a) | substitut | sostitutivo | sucedáneo; suplente | Ersatz-; Leih- | 代理の |
| 6721. surrogate endpoint - (n) | point final substitut | punto finale sostitutivo | punto final de sustitución | Ersatzzielpunkt | 代理の終点 |
| 6722. surrogate outcome - (n) | résultat substitut | risultate sostitutivo | resultado sucedáneo | Ersatzergebnis | 代理結果 |
| 6723. surrounded - (a) | entouré | circondato | rodeado | umgeben | 囲まれた |
| 6724. surveillance - (n) | surveillance | vigilanza; supervisione | vigilancia | Überwachung | 監視 |
| 6725. survey - (n) | enquête | ispezione; indagine | inspección; encuesta | Überblick; Befragung | 調査 |
| 6726. survival - (n) | survie | sopravvivenza | supervivencia | Überleben | 生存、生残り |
| 6727. survivor - (n) | survivant | superstite; sopravvissuto | superviviente | Überlebende(r) | 生存者 |
| 6728. susceptibility - (n) | susceptibilité; prédisposition | predisposizione | susceptibilidad | Empfindlichkeit; Anfälligkeit | 感受性 |
| 6729. suspend - (v) | suspendre; surseoir | sospendere | suspender | ausschwemmen; suspendieren | 中止する、中断する |
| 6730. suspension - (n) | suspension | sospensione | suspensión | Aufschwemmung; Suspension | 一時的停止 |
| 6731. sustain - (v) | soutenir; maintenir | sostenere | sostener | erhalten; erleiden | 持続する |
| 6732. sustained release - (n) | libération soutenue; libération continue | rilascio continuo | liberación sostenida; liberación constante | anhaltende gleichmäßige Freisetzung | 徐放 |
| 6733. suture - (n) | suture | sutura | sutura | Naht; Nahtmaterial | 縫合［術］、縫合糸 |
| 6734. suture - (v) | suturer; coudre | suturare | suturar; coser | nähen | 縫い合わせる |
| 6735. swab - (n) | tampon | tampone | escobillón | Abstrich; Tupfer | 綿棒、スワブ |

344

| English/American | French/Français | Italian/Italiano | Spanish/Español | German/Deutsch | Japanese/日本語 |
|---|---|---|---|---|---|
| 6736. swab - (v) | tamponner | usare un tampone | limpiar | betupfen; abtupfen | 綿棒で拭く |
| 6737. swallow - (v) | avaler | inghiottire | tragar | schlucken | 飲み込む、嚥下する |
| 6738. sweat - (n) | sueur | sudore; traspirazione | sudor; transpiración | Schweiß | 汗 |
| 6739. sweat - (v) | suer; transpirer | sudare; traspirare | sudar | schwitzen | 発汗する |
| 6740. sweat gland - (n) | glande sudoripare | ghiandola sudoripara | glándula sudorípara | Schweißdrüse | 汗腺 |
| 6741. swelling - (n) | renflement; gonflement | gonfiore; edema | tumefacción; hinchazón | Schwellung | 腫脹 |
| 6742. swimming - (n) | natation | nuoto | natación | Schwimmen | 水泳 |
| 6743. swollen - (a) | gonflé; enflé | gonfio | hinchado | geschwollen | はれた |
| 6744. syllogism - (n) | syllogisme | sillogismo | silogismo | Syllogismus | 演繹法 |
| 6745. symbiosis - (n) | symbiose | simbiosi | simbiosis | Symbiose | 共生 |
| 6746. symbol - (n) | symbole | simbolo | símbolo | Symbol; Zeichen | 象徴、定式記号 |
| 6747. symbolism - (n) | symbolisme | simbolismo | simbolismo | Symbolik | 象徴性、象徴主義 |
| 6748. symmetrical - (a) | symétrique | simmetrico | simétrico | symmetrisch | 対称的な |
| 6749. sympathecto- my - (n) | sympathectomie | simpatectomia | simpatectomía | Sympathektomie | 交感神経切除 [術]、交感神経節摘出 [術] |
| 6750. sympathetic - (a) | sympathique | simpatico | simpático | sympathisch | 同情的の、交感神経 [性] の |
| 6751. sympathetic nervous system - (n) | système nerveux sympathique | sistema nervoso simpatico | sistema nervioso simpático | sympathisches Nervensystem | 交感神経系 |
| 6752. sympatholytic - (a) | sympatholytique | simpaticolitico | simpaticolítico | sympatholytisch | 交感神経遮断 [性] の |
| 6753. sympathomimet- ic - (a) | sympathomimétique; sympathicomimétique | simpaticomimetico | simpaticomimético | sympathomimetisch | 交感神経 [様] 作用の |
| 6754. symphysis - (n) | symphyse | sinfisi | sínfisis | Symphyse | [繊維軟骨] 結合、癒着の癒合 |
| 6755. symposium - (n) | symposium | simposio | simposio | Symposium | シンポジウム |
| 6756. symptom - (n) | symptôme | sintomo | síntoma | Symptom | 症状 |
| 6757. symptomatic - (a) | symptomatique | sintomatico | sintomático | symptomatisch | 症候性の |

345

| English/American | French/Français | Italian/Italiano | Spanish/Español | German/Deutsch | Japanese/日本語 |
|---|---|---|---|---|---|
| 6758. symptomatic treatment - (n) | traitement symptomatique | trattamento sintomatico | tratamiento sintomático | symptomatische Behandlung | 対症療法 |
| 6759. symptomatology - (n) | symptomatologie; séméiologie | semeiotica; sintomatologia | sintomatología | Symptomatologie | 症候学 |
| 6760. synapse - (n) | synapse | sinapsi | sinapsis | Synapse | シナプス、接合部、接合 |
| 6761. synaptic membrane - (n) | membrane synaptique | membrana sinaptica | membrana sináptica | synaptische Membran | シナプス膜 |
| 6762. synaptic receptor - (n) | récepteur synaptique | recettore sinaptico | receptor sináptico | synaptischer Rezeptor | シナプスレセプター |
| 6763. synaptosome - (n) | synaptosome | sinaptosoma | sinaptosoma | Synaptosom | シナプトゾーム |
| 6764. syncopal episode - (n) | syncope; épisode syncopal | episodio sincopatico | síncope | synkopale Episode | 失神 |
| 6765. syncope - (n) | syncope | sincope | síncope | Synkope | 失神 |
| 6766. syndrome - (n) | syndrome | sindrome | síndrome | Syndrom | 症候群 |
| 6767. synergism - (n) | synergie; synergisme | sinergismo | sinergismo | Synergismus | 共力（協力）作用、相乗作用 |
| 6768. synovia - (n) | synovie | sinovia | sinovia | Synovia; Gelenkschmiere | 滑液 |
| 6769. synovial - (a) | synovial | sinoviale | sinovial | synovial | 滑液の、滑膜の |
| 6770. synovial fluid - (n) | synovie; liquide synovial | liquido sinoviale | fluido sinovial | Synovia | 滑液 |
| 6771. synovial joint - (n) | articulation synoviale | giuntura sinoviale | articulación sinovial | Synovialgelenk | 滑膜性の連結 |
| 6772. synovial membrane - (n) | membrane synoviale | membrana sinoviale | membrana sinovial | Synovialmembran | 滑膜 |
| 6773. synthesis - (n) | synthèse | sintesi | síntesis | Synthese | 合成 |
| 6774. synthetic - (a) | synthétique | sintetico | sintético | synthetisch | 合成の |
| 6775. synthetic chemistry - (n) | chimie synthétique | chimica sintetica | química sintética | synthetische Chemie | 合成化学 |
| 6776. syringe - (n) | seringue | siringa | jeringa | Spritze | 注射器 |
| 6777. syrup - (n) | sirop | sciroppo | jarabe | Sirup | シロップ、シロップ剤 |

| English/American | French/Français | Italian/Italiano | Spanish/Español | German/Deutsch | Japanese/日本語 |
|---|---|---|---|---|---|
| 6778. system - (n) | système | sistema | sistema | System | 系[統]、体系 |
| 6779. systematic error - (n) | erreur systématique | errore sistematico | error sistemático | systematischer Fehler | 系統誤差 |
| 6780. systemic - (a) | systémique | sistemico | sistémico | systemisch | 全身性の、全身系の |
| 6781. systemic effect - (n) | effet systémique | effetto sistemico | efecto sistémico | systemische Wirkung | 全身効果 |
| 6782. systemic infection - (n) | infection systémique | infezione sistemica | infección sistémica | systemische Infektion | 全身感染 |
| 6783. systemic vascular resistance - (n) | résistance vasculaire systémique | resistenza vascolare sistemica | resistencia vascular sistémica | systemischer Gefäßwiderstand | 全身血管抵抗 |
| 6784. systems analysis - (n) | analyse de systèmes | analisi dei sistemi | análisis de sistemas | Systemanalyse | システム分析 |
| 6785. systole - (n) | systole | sistole | sístole | Systole | [心] 収縮 [期] |
| 6786. systolic blood pressure - (n) | pression sanguine systolique | pressione sanguigna sistolica | presión sanguínea sistólica | systolischer Blutdruck | 収縮期血圧 |
| 6787. systolic murmur - (n) | souffle systolique | soffio sistolico | soplo sistólico | systolisches Geräusch; Systolikum | 収縮期雑音 |

| English/American | French/Français | Italian/Italiano | Spanish/Español | German/Deutsch | Japanese/日本語 |
|---|---|---|---|---|---|
| 6788. T cell leukemia - (n) | leucémie à cellules T | leucemia a T-linfociti | leucemia de células T | T-Zellen-Leukämie | T細胞白血病 |
| 6789. T lymphocyte - (n) | lymphocyte T | linfocito T | linfocito T | T-Lymphozyt | Tリンパ球 |
| 6790. table - (n) | table | tabella | tabla | Tisch; Tabelle | 骨板、表、台 |
| 6791. table format - (n) | format de table | tipo di tabella | formato de tabla | Tabellenformat | 表形式 |
| 6792. table of contents - (n) | table des matières | elenco del contenuto | índice | Inhaltsverzeichnis | 目次 |
| 6793. tablet - (n) | tablette; comprimé | compressa; pastiglia | tableta; comprimido | Tablette | 錠 [剤] |
| 6794. tachycardia - (n) | tachycardie | tachicardia | taquicardia | Tachykardie | [心] 頻拍、頻脈 |
| 6795. tachyphylaxis - (n) | tachyphylaxie | tachiflassi | taquifilaxia | Tachyphylaxie | タキフィラキシー |
| 6796. tachypnea - (n) | tachypnée | tachipnea | taquipnea | Tachypnoe | 頻呼吸、呼吸頻数 |
| 6797. tactics - (n) | tactiques | tattica | tácticas | Taktik | 策略 |
| 6798. tactile - (a) | tactile | tattile | táctil | taktil; fühlbar | 触覚の、接触の |
| 6799. tactile fremitus - (n) | frémissement tactile | fremito tattile | frémito táctil | tastbarer Fremitus | 触覚振とう音 |
| 6800. tail - (n) | queue; fin | coda | cola; rabo | Schwanz; Ende | 尾、尾部、尾状物 |
| 6801. taint - (n) | infection; corruption | traccia | mancha; contaminación | Fleck; Makel | 病毒 |
| 6802. talc - (n) | talc | talco | talco | Talkum | 滑石、タルク |
| 6803. talk - (n) | conversation; discussion | conversazione; conferenza | conversación; conferencia | Rede | 話 |
| 6804. talk - (v) | parler; discuter | parlare | hablar; conversar | sprechen | 話す |
| 6805. tamper resistant - (a) | résistant aux intempéries | resistente alle manomissione | resistente a fractura | gegen Entnahme und nachträgliche Einfüllung gesichert | 干渉を防止する |
| 6806. tamper with - (v) | altérer; falsifier | immischiarsi; adulterare | sobornar; estropear | verfälschen; verpfuschen | 不正をする |
| 6807. tampon - (n) | tampon | tampone | tampón | Tampon | タンポン、綿球 |
| 6808. tamponade - (n) | tamponnade | tamponatura | taponamiento | Tamponade | タンポン挿入 [法]、タンポナーデ |

348

| English/American | French/Français | Italian/Italiano | Spanish/Español | German/Deutsch | Japanese/日本語 |
|---|---|---|---|---|---|
| 6809. tangent - (n) | tangente | tangente | tangente | Tangente | タンジェント |
| 6810. tantrum - (n) | accès de colère; crise de colère | accesso d'ira | rabieta; berrinche | Raptus | 立腹、かんしゃく |
| 6811. tap - (n) | ponction; robinet; petit coup | punctura; robinetto; colpetto | punción; llave; palmadita | Punktion; Perkussion | 軽くたたくこと、栓林熱、、タップ |
| 6812. tap - (v) | ponctionner; faire une ponction; frapper doucement | percuotere (leggermente) | hacer una puntura; golpear suavemente | perkutieren; punktieren | 打診する、穿刺する |
| 6813. tape recording - (n) | enregistrement sur bande | registrazione | grabación | Tonbandaufnahme | 録音 |
| 6814. tardive dyskinesia - (n) | dyscinésie tardive | discinesia tardiva | discinesia tardia | Dyskinesia tardive | 晩発性ジスキネジー |
| 6815. target - (n) | objectif; cible | bersaglio | objeto; anticátodo | Ziel | 標的、ターゲット、視標 |
| 6816. target lesion - (n) | lésion-cible | lesione bersaglio | lesión-blanco | ringförmige Läsion | 標的の病巣 |
| 6817. target organ - (n) | organe-cible | organo bersaglio | órgano-blanco | Zielorgan | 標的の臓器 |
| 6818. task force - (n) | corps de travail | unità operativa | grupo de trabajo | Arbeitsgemeinschaft | 特別調査団、対策委員会 |
| 6819. task performance - (n) | exécution d'une tâche | adempimento dell'incarico | realización de una tarea | Durchführung einer Tätigkeit | 任務遂成度 |
| 6820. taste - (n) | goût; saveur | gusto | sabor; gusto | Geschmack | 味 |
| 6821. taste - (v) | goûter; déguster | assaggiare | probar; saborear | schmecken | 味覚する |
| 6822. taste bud - (n) | papille gustative | papilla gustativa | papila gustativa | Geschmacksknospe | 味蕾、味覚芽 |
| 6823. taste panel - (n) | groupe de dégustation | pannello di degustatori | equipo de degustación | Gruppe von Geschmacksprüfern | 味覚検査グループ |
| 6824. taste test - (n) | épreuve de dégustation | test del gusto | prueba del gusto | Geschmackstest | 味覚検査 |
| 6825. tattooing - (n) | tatouage | tatuaggio | tatuaje | Tätowierung | 入れ墨すること |
| 6826. taxonomy - (n) | taxinomie; taxonomie | tassonomia | taxonomía | Taxonomie | 分類学 |
| 6827. teacher - (n) | professeur | insegnante; docente | profesor; maestro | Lehrer | 教師 |
| 6828. teaching - (n) | enseignement; instruction | insegnamento | enseñanza | Unterricht; Erziehung | 教授すること |

349

| English/American | French/Français | Italian/Italiano | Spanish/Español | German/Deutsch | Japanese/日本語 |
|---|---|---|---|---|---|
| 6829. teaching hospital - (n) | hôpital d'enseignement | clinica universitaria | hospital para enseñanza de la medicina | Lehrkrankenhaus | 教育研究病院 |
| 6830. team - (n) | équipe; groupe | gruppo di lavoro; team | equipo; grupo | Team; Gruppe | チーム |
| 6831. team player - (n) | travailleur coopératif | partecipante al gruppo di lavoro | trabajador cooperativo | Team-Spieler | 協力的な人 |
| 6832. tear - (n) | larme; déchirure | lacrime; lacerazione | lágrima; rasgón | Träne; Riß | 涙、断裂 |
| 6833. tease - (v) | débrouiller | garzare | escarmenar | zerzupfen | 掻き裂く |
| 6834. teat - (n) | tétine; mamelon | capezzolo | teta; pezón | Brustwarze; Mamille | 乳頭、乳首、乳房 |
| 6835. technician - (n) | technicien | tecnico | técnico | Techniker | 技術者 |
| 6836. technique - (n) | technique | tecnica | técnica | Verfahren; Methode | 技術 |
| 6837. technology - (n) | technologie | tecnologia | tecnología | Technologie; Technik | テクノロジー |
| 6838. technology transfer - (n) | transfert de technologie | trasferimento di tecnologia | transferencia de tecnología | Technologieübertragung | 技術移転 |
| 6839. tegument - (n) | tégument | tegumento | tegumento | Tegmentum | 外皮 |
| 6840. tegumentary - (a) | tégumentaire | tegumentale | tegumentario | Decke-; Haut- | 外皮の |
| 6841. telangiectasis - (n) | télangiectasie | telangectasia | telangiectasis | Teleangiektasie | 毛細管拡張症 |
| 6842. telencephalon - (n) | télencéphale | telencefalo | telencéfalo | Telencephalon; Telenzephalon | 終脳 |
| 6843. telepathy - (n) | télépathie | telepatia | telepatía | Telepathie; Gedankenlesen | テレパシー |
| 6844. telephone conversation report - (n) | rapport des conversations téléphoniques | rapporto dei conversazioni telefonici | informe de las conversaciones telefónicas | Telefongesprächsbericht | 電話会話報告 |
| 6845. telephone interview - (n) | entrevue téléphonique | colloquio telefonico | entrevista telefónica | telefonische Befragung | 電話でのインタビュー |
| 6846. temperament - (n) | tempérament | temperamento | temperamento | Temperament | 気質 |
| 6847. temperature - (n) | température; fièvre | temperatura; febbre | temperatura; fiebre | Temperatur; Fieber | 温度、体温 |
| 6848. template - (n) | modèle; moule | stampo; modello | plantilla; patrón | Schablone | テンプレート |

350

| English/American | French/Français | Italian/Italiano | Spanish/Español | German/Deutsch | Japanese/日本語 |
|---|---|---|---|---|---|
| 6849. temple - (n) | tempe | tempia | sien | Schläfe; Tempus | 側頭、こめかみ |
| 6850. temporal - (a) | temporal | temporale | temporal | temporal | 側頭の、こめかみの |
| 6851. temporary - (a) | temporaire; provisoire | temporaneo | temporario; provisional | vorübergehend;befristet | 時間の、一時性の |
| 6852. temporomandibular joint - (n) | articulation temporo-mandibulaire | articolazione temporomandibolare | articulación temporo-mandibular | Articulatio temporomandibularis | 側頭下顎関節 |
| 6853. tendency - (n) | tendance | tendenza | tendencia | Tendenz; Neigung | 傾向 |
| 6854. tender - (a) | tendre; sensible au toucher | dolorabile | delicado; dolorido | empfindlich | 敏感な、圧痛のある |
| 6855. tenderness - (n) | douleur à la pression | sensibilità; dolorabilità | dolor a la presión | Empfindlichkeit | 圧痛 |
| 6856. tendinitis - (n) | tendinite | tendinite | tendinitis | Tendinitis | 腱炎 |
| 6857. tendon - (n) | tendon | tendine | tendón | Sehne | 腱 |
| 6858. tendon sheath - (n) | gaine tendineuse | guaina tendinea | vaina tendinosa | Sehnenscheide | 腱鞘 |
| 6859. tenesmus - (n) | ténesme | tenesmo | tenesmo | Tenesmus | しぶり、テネスムス |
| 6860. tensile strength - (n) | résistance à la tension | resistenza alla rottura | resistencia a la tensión | Zugfestigkeit; Reißfestigkeit | 引張強度 |
| 6861. tension - (n) | tension | tensione | tensión | Spannung; Dehnung | 張力、伸圧 |
| 6862. tenuous - (a) | ténu; subtil | tenue; sottile | tenue; sutil | dünn; schwach | 希薄な |
| 6863. teratogen - (a) | tératogène | teratogeno | teratógeno | Teratogen | 催奇形物質 |
| 6864. teratogenic drugs - (n) | drogues tératogènes | farmaci teratogeni | drogas teratogénicas | teratogene Arzneimittel | 催奇形珍品 |
| 6865. teratogenic effect - (n) | effet tératogène | effetto teratogeno | efecto teratogénico | teratogene Wirkung | 催奇形性効果 |
| 6866. teratology - (n) | tératologie | teratologia | teratología | Teratologie | 奇形学 |
| 6867. teratoma - (n) | tératome | teratoma | teratoma | Teratom | 奇形腫 |
| 6868. term - (n) | terme; période | termine; periodo | término; periodo | Zeitraum; Fachausdruck | 期間、用語 |
| 6869. terminal - (n) | terminal | terminale | terminal | Endigung; Terminal | ターミナル |
| 6870. terminal - (a) | terminal | terminale | terminal | unheilbar; terminal | 終末の |

| English/American | French/Français | Italian/Italiano | Spanish/Español | German/Deutsch | Japanese/日本語 |
|---|---|---|---|---|---|
| 6871. terminal care - (n) | soins terminaux | assistenza a malati terminali | cuidados terminales | Sterbebegleitung | 終末看護 |
| 6872. terminal half life - (n) | période de demi-vie terminale | emivita terminale | vida media terminal | terminale Halbwertszeit | 終末半減期 |
| 6873. terminal illness - (n) | maladie terminale | malattia terminale | enfermedad terminal | terminale Erkrankung | 命とりの病気 |
| 6874. termination - (n) | terminaison; conclusion | fine; conclusione | terminación | Beendigung | 終末、終了 |
| 6875. terminology - (n) | terminologie | terminologia | terminología | Terminologie | 術語学 |
| 6876. tertiary care - (n) | soins tertiaires | cura terziaria | atención terciaria | tertiäre Pflege | 三次医療 |
| 6877. tertiary care center - (n) | centre de soins tertiaires | centro cura terziario | centro de atención terciario | Zentrum für tertiäre Pflege | 三次医療センター |
| 6878. test - (n) | épreuve; essai | prova; esperimento; test | prueba; análisis | Test; Untersuchung | 検査、試験 |
| 6879. test - (v) | mettre à l'épreuve; essayer | esaminare; analizzare | probar; hacer un análisis | testen; untersuchen | 検査する、試験する |
| 6880. testicular feminization - (n) | féminisation testiculaire | femminilizzazione testicolare | feminización testicular | testikuläre Feminisierung | 精巣性女性化 |
| 6881. testis - (n) | testicule | testicolo | testículo | Hoden; Testis | 精巣、睾丸 |
| 6882. tetany - (n) | tétanie | tetano | tétano | Tetanie | テタニー、強直 |
| 6883. text - (n) | texte | testo | texto | Text | テキスト |
| 6884. textbook - (n) | texte; manuel | libro di testo; manuale | libro de texto | Lehrbuch | 教科書 |
| 6885. textural - (a) | relatif à la texture | di tessitura | relativo a la textura | strukturell; Gewebe- | 組織構造上の |
| 6886. thalamic - (a) | thalamique | talamico | talámico | thalamisch | 視床の |
| 6887. thalamus - (n) | thalamus | talamo | tálamo | Thalamus | 視床 |
| 6888. theoretical - (a) | théorique | teorico | teórico | theoretisch | 理論の |
| 6889. theoretical limit - (n) | limite théorique | limite teoretico | límite teórico | theoretische Grenze | 理論の限界 |
| 6890. theory - (n) | théorie | teoria | teoría | Theorie | 理論、［学］説 |
| 6891. therapeutic - (a) | thérapeutique | terapeutico | terapéutico | therapeutisch | 治療の |

352

| English/American | French/Français | Italian/Italiano | Spanish/Español | German/Deutsch | Japanese/日本語 |
|---|---|---|---|---|---|
| 6892. therapeutic area - (n) | zone thérapeutique | area terapeutica | área terapéutica | therapeutischer Bereich | 治療部位 |
| 6893. therapeutic index - (n) | index thérapeutique | indice terapeutico | índice terapéutico | therapeutischer Index; therapeutische Breite | 治療指標 |
| 6894. therapeutic substitution - (n) | substitution thérapeutique | sostituzione terapeutica | sustitución terapéutica | therapeutische Substitution | 有効な薬の交換 |
| 6895. therapeutic window - (n) | fenêtre thérapeutique | apertura terapeutica | ventana terapéutica | therapeutisches Fenster | 有効な薬の期間 |
| 6896. therapeutics - (n) | thérapeutique | terapeutica | terapéutica | Therapeutik | 治療学 |
| 6897. therapy - (n) | thérapie | terapia | terapia | Therapie | 療法、治療 |
| 6898. thermal - (a) | thermique | termico | térmico | thermisch | 熱[性]の |
| 6899. thermal conductivity - (n) | conductibilité thermique | conducibilità termica | conductivicad térmica | Wärmeleitfähigkeit | 熱伝導度 |
| 6900. thermodilution - (n) | thermodilution | diluizione termica | termodilución | Thermodilution | 熱希釈 |
| 6901. thermodynamics - (n) | thermodynamique | termodinamica | termodinámica | Thermodynamik | 熱力学 |
| 6902. thermogram - (n) | thermogramme | termogramma | termograma | Thermogramm | 温度記録 [図] |
| 6903. thermography - (n) | thermographie | termografia | termografía | Thermographie | 温度記録 [法] |
| 6904. thermometer - (n) | thermomètre | termometro | termómetro | Thermometer | 温度計、体温計 |
| 6905. thigh - (n) | cuisse | coscia | muslo | Oberschenkel | 大腿 |
| 6906. thin layer chromatography - (n) | chromatographie sur couche mince | cromatografia su strato sottile | cromatografía de capa delgada | Dünnschicht-chromatographie | 薄層クロマトグラフィ |
| 6907. thinness - (n) | maigreur; fluidité | sottigliezza | delgadez; flaqueza | Dünne; Dünnheit | 薄さ |
| 6908. third-degree burn - (n) | brûlure du troisième degré | ustione di terzo grado | quemadura de tercer grado | Verbrennung III. Grades | 第三度の火傷 |
| 6909. third party payer - (n) | payeur de tierce personne | la terza persona paga | tercer pagador | dritte bezahlende Organisation | 第三者の支払人 |

353

| English/American | French/Français | Italian/Italiano | Spanish/Español | German/Deutsch | Japanese/日本語 |
|---|---|---|---|---|---|
| 6910. third stage labor - (n) | troisième stade du travail | doglie di terzo stadio | tercer estadio del parto | Wehen im dritten Stadium | 第三段階の労働 |
| 6911. thirst - (n) | soif | sete | sed | Durst | 渇、渇き |
| 6912. thoracentesis - (n) | thoracentèse | toracentesi | toracentesis | Thorakozentese Pleurapunktion | 胸腔穿刺 [術] |
| 6913. thoracic - (a) | thoracique | toracico | torácico | thorakal | 胸の |
| 6914. thoracic duct - (n) | canal thoracique | dotto toracico | conducto torácico | Ductus thoracicus | 胸管 |
| 6915. thorax - (n) | thorax; cage thoracique | torace | tórax | Brustkorb; Thorax | 胸郭 |
| 6916. thought leader - (n) | faiseur de pensée | formatore dell'idea | creador de pensamiento | Gedankenbildner | 思想の指導者 |
| 6917. three dimensional - (a) | à trois dimensions | tridimensionale | tridimensional | dreidimensional | 三次元の |
| 6918. three times a day - (adv) | trois fois par jour | tre volte al giorno | tres veces al día | dreimal täglich | 一日三回 |
| 6919. threshold - (n) | seuil | soglia | umbral | Schwelle | いき値 |
| 6920. thrill - (n) | vibration; frémissement | fremito; vibrazione | temblor | Schwirren; Schnurren | 振せん |
| 6921. throat - (n) | gorge | gola | garganta | Hals; Kehle | 咽喉 |
| 6922. throb - (n) | pulsation; battement | battito; pulsazione | pulsación; latido | Pulsschlag; Klopfen | 拍動 |
| 6923. thrombocyte - (n) | thrombocyte; plaquette | trombocito; piastrina | trombocito; plaqueta | Thrombozyt; Blutplättchen | 血小板 |
| 6924. thrombocyto-penia - (n) | thrombocytopénie; thrombopénie | trombocitopenia | trombocitopenia | Thrombozytopenie | 血小板減少症 |
| 6925. thrombo-cytosis - (n) | thrombocytose | trombocitosi | trombocitosis | Thrombozytose Thrombozytärmie | 血小板増加症 |
| 6926. thromboembo-lism - (n) | thrombo-embolie | tromboembolia | tromboembolia | Thrombembolie Thromboembolie | 血栓塞栓症 |
| 6927. thrombolysis - (n) | thrombolyse | trombolisi | trombólisis | Thrombolyse | 血栓前壊 |
| 6928. thrombolytic therapy - (n) | thérapie thrombolytique | terapia trombolitica | terapia trombolítica | thrombolytische Therapie | 血栓前壊療法 |

| English/American | French/Français | Italian/Italiano | Spanish/Español | German/Deutsch | Japanese/日本語 |
|---|---|---|---|---|---|
| 6929. thrombophlebitis - (n) | thrombo-phlébite | tromboflebite | tromboflebitis | Thrombophlebitis | 血栓 [性; 静脈炎 |
| 6930. thromboplastin time - (n) | temps de thromboplastine | tempo di tromboplastina | tiempo de tromboplastina | Thromboplastinzeit | トロンボプラスチン時間 |
| 6931. thrombosis - (n) | thrombose | trombosi | trombosis | Thrombose | 血栓症 |
| 6932. thrombotic - (a) | thrombotique | trombotico | trombótico | thrombotisch | 血栓の |
| 6933. thrombus - (n) | thrombus | trombo | trombo | Thrombus | 血栓 |
| 6934. thrombus formation - (n) | formation du thrombus | formazione del trombo | formación del trombo | Thrombusbildung | 血栓の形成 |
| 6935. thumb - (n) | pouce | pollice | pulgar | Daumen | 母指 |
| 6936. thymus gland - (n) | thymus | timo | timo; glándula timo | Thymus | 胸腺 |
| 6937. thyroid - (n) | thyroïde | tiroide | tiroides | Thyroidea; Schilddrüse | 甲状腺 |
| 6938. thyroid gland - (n) | glande thyroïdienne | tiroide | glándula tiroides | Thyreoidea; Schilddrüse | 甲状腺 |
| 6939. thyroid hormone receptor - (n) | récepteur aux hormones thyroïdiennes | recettore dell' ormone tiroideo | receptor de hormonas tiroides | Schilddrüsenhormonrezeptor | 甲状腺ホルモンレセプター |
| 6940. tibia - (n) | tibia | tibia | tibia | Tibia | 脛骨 |
| 6941. tibial - (a) | tibial | tibiale | tibial | tibial | 脛骨の |
| 6942. tic - (n) | tic; spasme | tic | tic | Tic(k); Zuckung | チック |
| 6943. tick - (n) | tique | zecca | garrapata; ácaro | Zecke | マダニ |
| 6944. tick borne encephalitis - (n) | encéphalite transmise par une tique | encefalite trasmessa dalla zecca | encefalitis transmitida por garrapata | durch Zecken übertragene Enzephalitis | ダニ媒介脳炎 |
| 6945. ticklishness - (n) | sensibilité au chatouillement | sensibilità al solletico | tener cosquillas; ser cosquilloso | Kitzligkeit | くすぐったさ |
| 6946. tidal volume - (n) | volume courant; air courant | volume corrente | volumen corriente | Atemzugvolumen | 一回換気量 |
| 6947. time - (n) | temps | tempo | tiempo | Zeit | 時間 |
| 6948. time-concentration - (n) | concentration temporelle | concentrazione nel tempo | tiempo/concentración | Konzentration zu einem bestimmten Zeitpunkt | 時間における薬の血中濃度 |

355

| English/American | French/Français | Italian/Italiano | Spanish/Español | German/Deutsch | Japanese/日本語 |
|---|---|---|---|---|---|
| 6949. time and events - (n) | temps et événements | tempo ed eventi | tiempo y eventos | Zeit und Ereignisse | 時と出来事 |
| 6950. time course - (n) | cours de temps | corso del tempo | curso del tiempo | zeitlicher Verlauf | タイムコース |
| 6951. time factor - (n) | facteur de temps | fattore tempo | factor de tiempo | Zeitfaktor | 時間要素 |
| 6952. time frame - (n) | intervalle du temps | intervallo di tempo | intervalo de tiempo | Zeitraum | 時間の枠 |
| 6953. time point - (n) | point dans le temps; moment dans le temps | punto temporale | momento del tiempo; punto del tiempo | Zeitpunkt | 時点 |
| 6954. time to maximal effect - (n) | temps jusqu'à l'effet maximal | tempo per raggiungere l'effetto massimo | tiempo hasta el efecto máximo | Zeit bis zur maximalen Wirkung | 最大効果までの時間 |
| 6955. time to onset of effect - (n) | temps jusqu'au début de l'effet | tempo per l'inizio dell'effetto | tiempo para inicio del efecto | Zeit bis zum Einsetzen der Wirkung | 効果出現までの時間 |
| 6956. time to peak effect - (n) | temps jusqu'à l'effet maximal | tempo per raggiungere l'effetto ottimale | tiempo hasta efecto máximo | Zeit bis zum 'peak' | 効果の最高時までの時間 |
| 6957. time to recovery - (n) | temps jusqu'à la récupération | tempo per la guarigione | tiempo hasta la recuperación | Zeit bis zur Erholung | 回復までの時間 |
| 6958. time to relapse - (n) | temps jusqu'à la rechute | tempo di ricaduta | tiempo hasta relapso | Zeit bis zum Rückfall | 再発までの時間 |
| 6959. time window - (n) | limite de temps | apertura temporale | límite de tiempo | Zeitfenster | 期間 |
| 6960. timeline - (n) | ligne de temps | linea tempo | línea de tiempo | Zeitkurve | タイムライン |
| 6961. timetable - (n) | horaire | orario | horario | Stundenplan; Zettabelle | 時間予定表 |
| 6962. tincture - (n) | teinture | tintura | tintura | Tinktur; Auszug | チンキ [剤] |
| 6963. tinea - (n) | tinea; teigne | tigna | tinea; tiña | Tinea; Dermatophytose | 白癬 |
| 6964. tingling - (n) | picotement; fourmillement | formicolio | escozor; hormigueo | Prickelgefühl; Kizeln | 刺痛 |
| 6965. tinnitus - (n) | tinnitus; tintement d'oreilles | scampanellio | zumbido | Tinnitus; Ohrgeräusch | 耳鳴 |
| 6966. tissue - (n) | tissu | tessuto | tejido | Gewebe | 組織 |
| 6967. tissue distribution - (n) | distribution tissulaire | distribuzione del tessuto | distribución de tejido | Verteilung im Gewebe | 組織分布 |

356

| English/American | French/Français | Italian/Italiano | Spanish/Español | German/Deutsch | Japanese/日本語 |
|---|---|---|---|---|---|
| 6968. tissue perfusion - (n) | perfusion tissulaire | perfusione del tessuto | perfusión de tejido | Gewebedurchblutung | 組織灌流 |
| 6969. titer (titre) - (n) | titre | titolo | título | Titer | [力] 値 |
| 6970. title - (n) | titre | titolo | título | Titel | 表題 |
| 6971. titrate - (v) | titrer | titolare | titular | titrieren | 滴定する |
| 6972. titration schedule - (n) | programme de titrage | programa di titolazione | programa de titulación | Titrierungszeitplan | 滴定スケジュール |
| 6973. tobacco - (n) | tabac | tabacco | tabaco | Tabak | タバコ |
| 6974. toe - (n) | orteil | dito del piede | dedo del pie | Zehe | 足指 |
| 6975. toilet - (n) | toilette | toletta | baño | Toilette | 清拭 |
| 6976. tolerability - (n) | tolérance | tollerabilità | ser tolerable; poder soportar | Erträglichkeit; Annehmbarkeit | 許容度 |
| 6977. tolerance - (n) | tolérance | tolleranza | tolerancia | Toleranz; Verträglichkeit | 耐性 |
| 6978. tolerate - (v) | tolérer | tollerare | tolerar | tolerieren | 我慢する |
| 6979. tomography - (n) | tomographie | tomografia | tomografía | Tomographie | 断層撮影法 |
| 6980. tone - (n) | ton | tono | tono | Ton; Tonus | 音、緊張 |
| 6981. tongue - (n) | langue | lingua | lengua | Zunge | 舌 |
| 6982. tongue depressor - (n) | abaisse-langue | abbassalingua | abatelengua | Zungenspatel | 舌圧子 |
| 6983. tonic - (n) | tonique | tonico | tónico | Tonikum | 強壮薬 |
| 6984. tonic - (a) | tonique | tonico | tónico | tonisch | 持続性の、強直性の |
| 6985. tonic-clonic seizure - (n) | convulsion tonico-clonique | crisi convulsiva tonico-clonica | epilepsia tónico-clónica | tonisch-klonischer Anfall | 強直間代性てんかん |
| 6986. tonicity - (n) | tonicité; tonus | tonicità; tono | tonicidad | Tonus; Spannungszustand | 緊張 [性]、強度 |
| 6987. tonometer - (n) | tonomètre | tonometro | tonómetro | Tonometer | 圧力計 |
| 6988. tonometry - (n) | tonométrie | tonometria | tonometría | Tonometrie | 圧力測定 [法] |
| 6989. tonsil - (n) | amygdale | tonsilla | amígdala | Tonsille; Mandel | 扁桃 |

357

| English/American | French/Français | Italian/Italiano | Spanish/Español | German/Deutsch | Japanese/日本語 |
|---|---|---|---|---|---|
| 6990. tonus - (n) | tonus; tonicité | tono; tonicità | tono; tonicidad | Tonus | 緊張、張力 |
| 6991. tooth - (n) | dent | dente | diente; muela | Zahn | 歯 |
| 6992. toothache - (n) | mal de dents; odontalgie | mal di denti; odontalgia | dolor de muelas | Zahnschmerz | 歯痛 |
| 6993. toothbrushing - (n) | brossage des dents | lavaggio dei denti | lavarse los dientes con un cepillo dental | Zähnebürsten | 歯磨き |
| 6994. toothpaste - (n) | pâte dentifrice | pasta dentifricia | pasta de dientes | Zahnpasta; Zahncreme | 歯磨き粉 |
| 6995. tophus - (n) | tophus; calcul tophacé | tofo; calcolo salivare | tofo | Tophus | 痛風結節 |
| 6996. topical - (a) | topique; local | topico; locale | tópico | topisch; lokal | 局所[性]の |
| 6997. torpor - (n) | torpeur | torpore | torpor | Torpidität; Torpor | 遅鈍、鈍麻 |
| 6998. torsion - (n) | torsion | torsione | torsión | Torsion; Verwindung | 捻転、回転 |
| 6999. torso - (n) | torse | torso; tronco | torso | Rumpf; Torso | 胴、トルソ |
| 7000. torticollis - (n) | torticolis | torcicollo | torticolis | Tortikollis; Schiefhals | 斜頸 |
| 7001. tortuous - (a) | tortueux | tortuoso | tortuoso | gewunden | 蛇行[性]の |
| 7002. torture - (n) | torture | tortura | tortura | Folterung; Marter | 苦痛 |
| 7003. total - (n) | total; tout | totale; somma | total | Gesamtheit | 総計、全体 |
| 7004. total - (a) | total | totale | total | gesamt | 合計の、全体の |
| 7005. total daily dose - (n) | dose quotidienne totale | dose totale giornaliera | dosis diaria total | Gesamttagesdosis | 一日の全服用量 |
| 7006. touch - (n) | toucher | tatto; sensibilità tattile | toque; tacto | Berührung; Tastgefühl | 触診 |
| 7007. touch - (v) | toucher | toccare | tocar; tentar | berühren | 触診する |
| 7008. tourniquet - (n) | tourniquet; garrot | tourniquet; laccio emostatico | torniquete | Tourniquet; Stauschlauch | 止血帯、駆血帯 |
| 7009. toxemia - (n) | toxémie | tossiemia | toxemia | Toxämie | 毒血症 |
| 7010. toxic - (a) | toxique | tossico | tóxico | toxisch; giftig | 毒性の |
| 7011. toxicity - (n) | toxicité | tossicità | toxicidad | Toxizität | 毒性 |
| 7012. toxicology - (n) | toxicologie | tossicologia | toxicología | Toxikologie | 毒物学 |
| 7013. toxin - (n) | toxine | tossina | toxina | Toxin | 毒素 |
| 7014. trabeculation - (n) | trabéculation | trabecolazione | trabeculación | Trabekelbildung | 肉柱形成 |

| English/American | French/Français | Italian/Italiano | Spanish/Español | German/Deutsch | Japanese/日本語 |
|---|---|---|---|---|---|
| 7015. trace - (n) | trace | traccia | tracto | Spur | 痕跡 |
| 7016. trace - (v) | tracer; suivre | seguire | seguir; investigar | aufspüren; aufzeichnen | 跡をたどる |
| 7017. trace element - (n) | oligo-élément | oligoelemento | oligoelemento | Spurenelement | 極微量の元素 |
| 7018. trachea - (n) | trachée | trachea | tráquea | Luftröhre; Trachea | 気管 |
| 7019. tracheal - (a) | trachéal | tracheale | traqueal | tracheal | 気管の |
| 7020. tracheo-esophageal - (a) | trachéo-oesophagien | tracheo-esofageo | traqueoesofágico | tracheoosophageal | 気管食道の |
| 7021. tracking - (n) | dépistage | inseguimento | seguimiento | Verfolgen | 追跡すること |
| 7022. tract - (n) | appareil; système | apparato; sistema | tracto; fascículo | Trakt; Tractus | 路、道 |
| 7023. traction - (n) | traction | trazione | tracción | Traktion; Zug | 牽引 |
| 7024. trade name - (n) | nom commercial; marque | marca; nome depositato | nombre comercial | Handelsname | 商品名 |
| 7025. trademark - (n) | marque déposée | marchio | marca de fábrica | Warenzeichen | 商標 |
| 7026. traditional medicine - (n) | médecine traditionnelle | medicina tradizionale | medicina tradicional | traditionelle Medizin | 伝統的医薬 |
| 7027. training - (n) | entraînement; éducation | istruzione; educazione | instrucción; entrenamiento | Training; Schulung | 訓練、トレーニング |
| 7028. training effect - (n) | effet d'entraînement | effetto di addestramento | efecto de entrenamiento | Trainingseffekt; Übungseffekt | 訓練効果 |
| 7029. training support - (n) | support d'entraînement | supporto per l'educazione | apoyo de entrenamiento | Übungshilfe | 訓練支援 |
| 7030. trait - (n) | trait; caractère | tratto | rasgo; característica | Eigenschaft; Charakterzug | 特性、体質 |
| 7031. trance - (n) | trance | catalessi | trance; catalepsia | Trance; Dämmerzustand | 昏睡状態、トランス状態 |
| 7032. tranquilizer - (n) | tranquillisant | tranquillante | tranquilizante | Beruhigungsmittel | トランキライザ |
| 7033. tranquilizing agent - (n) | tranquillisant | agente tranquillante | agente tranquilizante | Beruhigungsmittel | 精神安定薬 |
| 7034. transactional analysis - (n) | analyse transactionnelle | analisi transazionale | análisis transaccional | Transaktionsanalyse | 相互作用分析 |

359

| English/American | French/Français | Italian/Italiano | Spanish/Español | German/Deutsch | Japanese/日本語 |
|---|---|---|---|---|---|
| 7035. transcription - (n) | transcription | trascrizione | transcripción | Transkription | 転写 |
| 7036. transcultural - (a) | transculturel | interculturale | transcultural | interkulturell | いろいろな文化を通して共通な |
| 7037. transdermal - (a) | transdermique | transdermico | transdermal | transdermal | 経皮性の |
| 7038. transdermal patch - (n) | pièce transdermique; disque transdermique | cerotto transdermico | parche transdérmico | transdermaler Lappen | 経皮性パッチ |
| 7039. transducer - (n) | transducteur | trasduttore | transductor | Transducer; Umwandler | 変換器 |
| 7040. transduction - (n) | transduction | trasduzione | transducción | Transduktion | [形質] 導入、エネルギー変換 |
| 7041. transect - (v) | sectionner transversalement | tagliare trasversalmente | cortar transversalmente | quer durchschneiden | 離断する、横に切開する |
| 7042. transfection - (n) | transfection | transfezione | transfección | Transfektion | トランスフェクション |
| 7043. transfer - (n) | transfert | trasferimento | transferencia | Übertragung; Transfer | 移動 |
| 7044. transfer - (v) | transférer | trasferire | transferir | übertragen | 転移する |
| 7045. transfer price - (n) | prix d'un transfert | prezzo del trasferimento | precio de la transferencia | Übernahmekurs | 為替価格 |
| 7046. transfer RNA - (n) | ARN de transfert | ARN di trasporto | ARN de transferencia | Transfer-RNS | 転移RNA |
| 7047. transference - (n) | transfert | trasferimento; transfert | transferencia | Übertragung | 移転、移動、転移 |
| 7048. transference psychology - (n) | psychologie transférentielle | psicologia di transfert | psicología de transferencia | Übertragungspsychologie | 転移心理学 |
| 7049. transformation - (n) | transformation | trasformazione | transformación | Transformation; Umwandlung | 変態、[形質] 転換 |
| 7050. transformed value - (n) | valeur transformée | valore trasformato | valor transformado | transformierter Wert | 変換値 |
| 7051. transforming growth factor - (n) | facteur de croissance transformant | fattore di crescita trasformante | factor de crecimiento transformado | transformierender Wachstumsfaktor | 形質転換成長因子 |
| 7052. transfuse - (v) | transfuser | trasfondere | transfundir | transfundieren; übertragen | 輸液する |

| English/American | French/Français | Italian/Italiano | Spanish/Español | German/Deutsch | Japanese/日本語 |
|---|---|---|---|---|---|
| 7053. transfusion - (n) | transfusion | trasfusione | transfusión | Transfusion; Bluttransfusion | 輸血、輸血液 |
| 7054. transgenic - (a) | transgénique | transgenico | transgénico | transgen | トランスジェニックの |
| 7055. transient - (a) | transitoire | transitorio | transitorio | vorübergehend; transitorisch | 短命な |
| 7056. transient fall - (n) | chute transitoire | caduta transitoria | caída transitoria | transitorische Abnahme | 一時的な低下 |
| 7057. transillumination - (n) | transillumination; diaphanoscopie | transilluminazione | transiluminación | Transillumination; Diaphonoskopie | 透視 [法] |
| 7058. transitional cell - (n) | cellule transitionrelle | cellula transizionale | célula transicional | Übergangsepithelzelle | 移行細胞 |
| 7059. translation - (n) | traduction | traduzione | traducción | Übersetzung | 翻訳、トランスレーション |
| 7060. translocation - (n) | translocation | traslocazione | translocación | Translokation | 転座 |
| 7061. translucent - (a) | translucide | traslucido | translúcido | strahlendurchlässig; durchsichtig | 半透明の |
| 7062. transmission - (n) | transmission | trasmissione | transmisión | Übertragung | 伝達、広番 |
| 7063. transmitter - (n) | transmetteur | trasmettitore | transmisor | Überträger | 伝播伝物 |
| 7064. transparent - (a) | transparent | trasparente | transparente | durchsichtig | 透明な |
| 7065. transplant - (n) | greffon; greffe | organo trapiantato; trapianto | trasplante | Transplantat; Transplantation | 移植、移植組織 |
| 7066. transplant - (v) | transplanter; greffer | trapiantare | trasplantar | transplantieren | 移植する |
| 7067. transplantation - (n) | transplantation; greffe | trapianto | trasplante; trasplantación | Transplantation | 移植 [術] |
| 7068. transport - (v) | transporter | trasportare | transportar | transportieren | 移送する |
| 7069. transport pathway - (n) | voie de transport | via di trasporto | vía de transporte | Transportweg | 移送経路 |
| 7070. transportation - (n) | transportation; transport | trasporto | transporte | Transport | 移送 |
| 7071. transudate - (n) | transsudat | trasudato | transudado | Transsudat | 漏出液 |
| 7072. transverse - (a) | transverse; transversal | trasverso | transverso | transversal; quer | 横径の |

361

| English/American | French/Français | Italian/Italiano | Spanish/Español | German/Deutsch | Japanese日本語 |
|---|---|---|---|---|---|
| 7073. trauma - (n) | trauma; traumatisme | trauma; traumatismo | trauma; traumatismo | Trauma; Verletzung | 外傷 |
| 7074. trauma center - (n) | centre de traumatologie | centro di traumatologia | centro traumatológico | traumatologisches Zentrum | 外傷センター |
| 7075. traumatology - (n) | traumatologie | traumatologia | traumatología | Traumatologie | 外傷学 |
| 7076. treatment - (n) | traitement; soins | trattamento; cura | tratamiento | Behandlung; Therapie | 治療、療法 |
| 7077. treatment failure - (n) | échec du traitement | fallimento del trattamento | falla del tratamiento | Behandlungsmißerfolg | 治療の失敗 |
| 7078. treatment outcome - (n) | résultat du traitement | risultato del trattamento | resultado del tratamiento | Behandlungsergebnis | 治療結果 |
| 7079. tremble - (v) | trembler | tremare | temblar | zittern | 震える |
| 7080. tremor - (n) | tremblement | tremore | temblor | Tremor | 振せん |
| 7081. trend - (n) | tendance | tendenza | tendencia | Trend; Neigung | 傾向 |
| 7082. trend adjusted score - (n) | score ajusté à la tendance | punteggio riflettente la tendenza | puntaje ajustado a la tendencia | schwankungsbereinigte Punktzahl | 傾向に調節されたスコア |
| 7083. trephine - (n) | tréphine; trépan | trapano | trépano; trefina | Trephine | トレパン、穿孔器 |
| 7084. trephine - (v) | trépaner | trapanare | trepanar | trepanieren | 穿孔する |
| 7085. trepidation - (n) | trépidation | trepidazione | trepidación | Trepidation; Ängstlichkeit | 振せん運動、戦慄 |
| 7086. triad - (n) | triade | triade | tríada | Triade; Trias | 三つ組、三構造 |
| 7087. triage - (n) | triage | selezione; screening | triage | Triage | 三角 |
| 7088. trial - (n) | essai | prova; studio; sperimentazione clinica | ensayo; prueba | Studie, Probe | 試験 |
| 7089. trial and error - (n) | essai et erreur | prova per tentativi | prueba y error | Ausprobieren; empirische Methode | 試行錯誤 |
| 7090. trial audit - (n) | vérification de l'essai | verifica dello studio | inspección del ensayo | Studienüberprüfung | 試験監査 |
| 7091. trial design - (n) | plan de l'essai | disegno della prova | diseño del ensayo | Studienentwurf | 試験設計 |
| 7092. trial master file - (n) | fiche maîtresse de l'essai | filza principale dello studio | archivo maestro del ensayo | Stammdatei der Studie | 試験主要ファイル |

| English/American | French/Français | Italian/Italiano | Spanish/Español | German/Deutsch | Japanese 日本語 |
|---|---|---|---|---|---|
| 7093. trial monitor - (n) | moniteur de l'essai | monitoraggio dello studio | monitor del ensayo | Studienüberwacher | 試験監視 |
| 7094. trial registry - (n) | registre de l'essai | registro dello studio | registro del ensayo | Studienregister | 試験登録 |
| 7095. trial termination - (n) | terminaison de l'essai | termine dello studio | terminación del ensayo | Studienabschluß | 試験の中止 |
| 7096. trialist - (n) | participant à l'essai | paziente incluso in uno studio | sujeto que participa en el ensayo | Versuchsdurchführer | 試験実行者 |
| 7097. tricuspid valve - (n) | valvule tricuspide | valvola tricuspidale | válvula tricúspide | Trikuspidalklappe | 三尖弁 |
| 7098. trigeminal neuralgia - (n) | névralgie du trijumeau | nevralgia del trigemino | neuralgia del trigémino | Trigeminusneuralgie | 三叉神経痛 |
| 7099. trigone - (n) | trigone | trigono | trígono | Trigonum; Dreieck | 三角 |
| 7100. trimester - (n) | trimestre | trimestre | trimestre | Trimester | トリメスター |
| 7101. triple-blind - (a) | à triple aveugle | triplo-ciego | por triple ciego | dreifachblind | 三重盲検の |
| 7102. triplet - (n) | triplet | bambino trigemino | trillizo | Drilling | 三胎 |
| 7103. trismus - (n) | trismus | trisma | trismo | Trismus | 開口障害 |
| 7104. trisomy - (n) | trisomie | trisomia | trisomía | Trisomie | 三染色体性、トリソミー |
| 7105. tritium - (n) | tritium | tritio | tritio | Tritium | トリチウム |
| 7106. trivial name - (n) | nom commun | nome non ufficiale | nombre común | Trivialname | 通称 |
| 7107. troche - (n) | troche; troque | pastiglia; discoide | trocisco | Hustenbonbon; Pastille | トローチ [剤] |
| 7108. trophic change - (n) | changement trophique | cambiamento trofico | cambio trófico | trophische Veränderung | 栄養の変化 |
| 7109. trophoblast - (n) | trophoblaste | trofoblasto | trofoblasto | Trophoblast | 栄養膜、トロホブラスト |
| 7110. tropical - (a) | tropique | tropicale | tropical | tropisch | 熱帯の |
| 7111. trough - (n) | dépression; creux | depressione; solco | depresión; cuba | Rinne; Sulcus | 溝 |
| 7112. trunk - (n) | tronc | tronco | tronco | Stamm; Truncus | 体幹 |
| 7113. tubal - (a) | tubaire | tubarico | tubárico; tubario | tubar; Tuben- | 管（の） |
| 7114. tubal ligation - (n) | ligature tubaire | legatura delle tube | ligación tubárica | Tubenligatur | 卵管結紮 |
| 7115. tubal pregnancy - (n) | grossesse tubaire | gravidanza tubarica | embarazo tubárico | Eileiterschwangerschaft | 卵管妊娠 |

363

| English/American | French/Français | Italian/Italiano | Spanish/Español | German/Deutsch | Japanese/日本語 |
|---|---|---|---|---|---|
| 7116. tubal sterilization - (n) | stérilisation tubaire | sterilizzazione tubarica | esterilización tubárica | tubare Sterilisation | 管不妊手術 |
| 7117. tube - (n) | tube; trompe | tubo; salpinge | tubo; trompa | Sonde; Röhre | 管 |
| 7118. tuberculin test - (n) | épreuve à la tuberculine | prova della tubercolina | prueba a la tuberculina | Tuberkulintest | ツベルクリン試験 |
| 7119. tuberculosis - (n) | tuberculose | tubercolosi | tuberculosis | Tuberkulose | 結核 [症] |
| 7120. tubule - (n) | tubule | tubulo | túbulo | Röhrchen; Tubulus | 細管 |
| 7121. tumescence - (n) | tumescence | tumescenza | tumescencia | Tumeszenz; Intumeszenz | 腫脹 |
| 7122. tumor - (n) | tumeur | tumore | tumor | Tumor; Herd | 腫瘍 |
| 7123. tunnel vision - (n) | vision en tunnel; rétrécissement du champ visuel | visione a tunnel; visione tubulare | visión en túnel | röhrenförmiges Gesichtsfeld | トンネル視 |
| 7124. turbidimetry - (n) | turbimétrie | turbidimetria | turbidimetría | Trübungsmessung | 混度測定 |
| 7125. turbinate - (n) | os turbiné; cornet | turbinato | turbinado | Nasenmuschel | 鼻甲介 |
| 7126. turgor - (n) | turgor; turgescence | turgore | turgor | Turgor; Schwellung | トルゴール |
| 7127. twice a day - (adv) | deux fois par jour | due volte al giorno | dos veces al día | zweimal täglich | 一日二回 |
| 7128. twin - (n) | jumeau | gemello | gemelo; mellizo | Zwilling | 双生児, 双胎 |
| 7129. twitch - (n) | tic; saccade | spasmo | tirón; sacudida | Zuckung | 単収縮 |
| 7130. two-compartment model - (n) | modèle à deux compartiments | modello a due compartimenti | modelo de dos compartimientos | Modell mit zwei Kompartimenten | 二区画模型 |
| 7131. two-part study - (n) | étude à deux parties | studio in due parti | estudio de dos partes | zweiteilige Studie | 二次元の |
| 7132. two dimensional - (a) | à deux dimensions | bidimensionale | de dos dimensiones | zweidimensional | 二部構成の研究 |
| 7133. two physician method - (n) | méthode à deux médecins | metodo a due dottori | método de dos médicos | "Zwei-Ärzte"-Methode | 医師二人による方法 |
| 7134. two sided test - (n) | épreuve bilatérale | prova bilaterale | prueba bilateral | zweiseitiger Test | 両側検定 |

| English/American | French/Français | Italian/Italiano | Spanish/Español | German/Deutsch | Japanese/日本語 |
|---|---|---|---|---|---|
| 7135. two tailed test - (n) | épreuve bilatérale | prova bilaterale | prueba bilateral | zweiseitiger Test | 両側検定 |
| 7136. tympanic membrane - (n) | membrane du tympan | membrana timpanica | membrana del tímpano | Trommelfell | 鼓膜 |
| 7137. tympany - (n) | tympanisme | timpano | resonancia timpánica | Tympanie | 鼓脹 |
| 7138. type - (n) | type | tipo | tipo | Typ; Typus | 型 |
| 7139. type I error - (n) | erreur de type I | errore di tipo I | error tipo I | Typ-I-Fehler | エラー I 型 |
| 7140. type II error - (n) | erreur de type II | errore di tipo II | error tipo II | Typ-II-Fehler | エラー II 型 |

| English/American | French/Français | Italian/Italiano | Spanish/Español | German/Deutsch | Japanese 日本語 |
|---|---|---|---|---|---|
| 7141. ulcer - (n) | ulcère | ulcera | úlcera | Ulkus; Geschwür | 潰瘍 |
| 7142. ulna - (n) | cubitus | ulna; cubito | ulna; cúbito | Ulna; Elle | 尺骨 |
| 7143. ultracentrifugation - (n) | ultracentrifugation | ultracentrifugazione | ultracentrifugación | Ultrazentrifugation | 超遠心 |
| 7144. ultrafiltration - (n) | ultrafiltration | ultrafiltrazione | ultrafiltración | Ultrafiltration | 限外濾過 [法] |
| 7145. ultrasonic - (a) | ultrasonique | ultrasonico | ultrasónico; ultrasonoro | Ultraschall- | 超音波の |
| 7146. ultrasonography - (n) | ultrasonographie | ultrasonografia | ultrasonografía | Ultraschallsonographie | 超音波検査法 |
| 7147. ultrasound - (n) | ultrason | ultrasuono | ultrasonido | Ultraschall | 超音波 |
| 7148. ultrastructure - (n) | ultrastructure | ultrastruttura | ultra estructura | Ultrastruktur; Feinstruktur | 超微 [細] 構造 |
| 7149. ultraviolet - (a) | ultra-violet | ultravioletto | ultravioleta | ultraviolett | 紫外線の |
| 7150. umbilical cord - (n) | cordon ombilical | cordone ombelicale | cordón umbilical | Nabelschnur | 臍帯 |
| 7151. umbilical vein - (n) | veine ombilicale | vena ombelicale | vena umbilical | Nabelvene | 臍静脈 |
| 7152. unapproved indication - (n) | indication non approuvée | indicazione non approvata | indicación no aprobada | falsche Indikation | 不認可 (薬の) 使用法 |
| 7153. unborn - (a) | pas encore né | non ancora nato | aún no nacido | ungeboren | 未出生の |
| 7154. unbound fraction - (n) | fraction non liée | frazione non legata | fracción no unida | ungebundene Fraktion | 非結合部分 |
| 7155. uncle - (n) | oncle | zio | tío | Onkel | おじ |
| 7156. uncomplicated - (a) | non compliqué; simple | senza complicazioni | sin complicaciones; sencillo | unkompliziert; einfach | 複雑でない |
| 7157. unconjugated - (a) | non conjugué | non coniugato | no conjugado | unkonjugiert; nicht konjugiert | 接合していない |
| 7158. unconscious - (n) | inconscient | inconscio | inconsciente | Unbewußtsein | 無意識 |
| 7159. unconscious - (a) | inconscient | inconscio | inconsciente | bewußtlos; unbewußt | 無意識の |
| 7160. unconscious psychology - (n) | psychologie de l'inconscient | psicologia dell'inconscio | psicología del inconsciente | Psychologie der unbewußten Vorgänge | 無意識心理学 |

| English/American | French/Français | Italian/Italiano | Spanish/Español | German/Deutsch | Japanese日本語 |
|---|---|---|---|---|---|
| 7161. unconsciousness - (n) | évanouissement; perte de connaissance | inconscio | insensibilidad | Bewußtlosigkeit | 意識消失 |
| 7162. uncontrolled - (a) | non contrôlé | incontrollato | incontrolado | unkontrolliert | 無統制[の] |
| 7163. underlying disease - (n) | maladie sous-jacente | malattia alla base di | enfermedad primaria | Grundkrankheit | 潜在疾病 |
| 7164. underreporting - (n) | sous-rapportage | reportage incompleto | reportaje insuficiente | untertriebene Anzahl von Fällen melden | 過小報告 |
| 7165. underweight - (n) | poids insuffisant | sottopeso | bajo peso | Untergewicht | 重量不足 |
| 7166. unemployment - (n) | manque de travail; chômage | disoccupazione | desempleo | Arbeitslosigkeit | 失業 |
| 7167. unequal - (a) | inégal | ineguale | desigual | ungleich | 等しくない |
| 7168. unexpected adverse event - (n) | événement défavorable inattendu | evento avverso inaspettato | evento desfavorable no esperado | unerwartetes schädliches Ereignis | 予期されていない悪い出来事 |
| 7169. unhealthy - (a) | malsain; maladif | malato; malsano | enfermizo; malsano | ungesund; gesundheitsschädigend | 不健康な |
| 7170. unicellular - (a) | unicellulaire | unicellulare | unicelular | einzellig | 単細胞の |
| 7171. uniform - (a) | uniforme | uniforme | uniforme | einheitlich; gleichmäßig | 一様な |
| 7172. uniformity - (n) | uniformité | uniformità | uniformidad | Einheitlichkeit; Gleichmäßigkeit | 画一性 |
| 7173. unilateral - (a) | unilatéral | unilaterale | unilateral | unilateral; einseitig | 一側[性]の |
| 7174. unintentional injuries - (n) | blessures involontaires | ferite non intenzionali | lesiones involuntarias | unbeabsichtigte Schädigungen | 不慮の事故 |
| 7175. union - (n) | union | unione; consolidamento | unión | Vereinigung; Verbindung | 結合 |
| 7176. unipolar - (a) | unipolaire | unipolare | unipolar | unipolar | 一極性の |
| 7177. unit - (n) | unité | unità | unidad | Einheit | 単数、単位 |
| 7178. unit of measurement - (n) | unité de mesure | unità di misura | unidad de medición | Maßeinheit | 測定単位 |

367

| English/American | French/Français | Italian/Italiano | Spanish/Español | German/Deutsch | Japanese日本語 |
|---|---|---|---|---|---|
| 7179. universal precautions - (n) | précautions universelles | precauzioni universali | precauciones universales | allgemeine Vorsichtsmaßnahmen | 普遍的予防手段 |
| 7180. university - (n) | université | università | universidad | Universität | 大学 |
| 7181. unknown - (a) | inconnu | sconosciuto | desconocido | unbekannt | 不明の |
| 7182. unmask - (v) | démasquer | smascherare | desenmascarar | entlarven; demaskieren | 正体を現す |
| 7183. unmyelinated - (a) | amyélinique; sans myéline | amielinico | amielínico | marklos; nicht myelinisiert | 無髄の |
| 7184. unnatural - (a) | anormal; non naturel | innaturale | antinatural; no natural | unnatürlich | 不自然な |
| 7185. unsaturated - (a) | non saturé | insaturo | no saturado | ungesättigt | 不飽和の |
| 7186. unscheduled - (a) | imprévu | non messo in lista; non previsto | no programado | außerplanmäßig | 予定されていない |
| 7187. unspecified - (a) | non spécifié | imprecisato; non specificato | no especificado | nicht spezifiziert; nicht angegeben | 指定されていない |
| 7188. unstable - (a) | instable | instabile | inestable | instabil | 不安定な |
| 7189. ununited - (a) | désuni; non uni | non unito | desunido | nicht vereinigt | 結合されていない |
| 7190. upfront payment - (n) | paiement de dépôt; dépôt | pagamento anticipato | pago por adelantado | Vorschußzahlung | 前金払い |
| 7191. upper respiratory - (a) | respiratoire supérieure | delle alte vie respiratorie | respiratorio superior | obere Atmungs- | 上気道の |
| 7192. up-regulation - (n) | régulation à la hausse | regolazione ascenzionale | regulación hacia arriba | Hochregulation | アップレギュレーション |
| 7193. uptake - (n) | captage; fixation | incorporazione; captazione | captación | Aufnahme | 取り込み、摂取 |
| 7194. uptake - (v) | capter; fixer | incorporare; captare | captar | aufnehmer | 摂取する |
| 7195. urban - (a) | urbain | urbano | urbano | städtisch | 郊外の |
| 7196. urbanization - (n) | urbanisation | urbanizzazione | urbanización | Urbanisierung; Verstädterung | 郊外化 |
| 7197. urea - (n) | urée | urea | urea | Harnstoff; Carbamid | 尿素 |
| 7198. uremia - (n) | urémie | uremia | uremia | Urämie | 尿毒症 |

| English/American | French/Français | Italian/Italiano | Spanish/Español | German/Deutsch | Japanese/日本語 |
|---|---|---|---|---|---|
| 7199. ureter - (n) | uretère | uretere | uréter | Harnleiter; Ureter | 尿管 |
| 7200. urethra - (n) | urètre | uretra | uretra | Harnröhre; Urethra | 尿道 |
| 7201. urethral - (a) | urétral | uretrale | uretral | urethral; Urethra- | 尿道の |
| 7202. urgency - (n) | urgence (de miction) | urgenza (minzionale) | urgencia (de micción) | Harndrang; Dringlichkeit dringend | 緊急、尿意促進 |
| 7203. urgent - (a) | urgent | urgente | urgente | | 緊急の |
| 7204. uric acid - (n) | acide urique | acido urico | ácido úrico | Harnsäure | 尿酸 |
| 7205. urinalysis - (n) | analyse d'urine | analisi dell'urina | urinálisis | Urinuntersuchung; Urinstatus | 尿検査、検尿 |
| 7206. urinary - (a) | urinaire | urinario | urinario | Harn-; Urin- | 尿の |
| 7207. urinary tract - (n) | voie urinaire | tratto urinario | vías urinarias | Harntrakt | 尿管 |
| 7208. urination - (n) | excrétion d'urine; miction | minzione | micción | Miktion; Wasserlassen | 排尿、放尿 |
| 7209. urine - (n) | urine | urina | orina | Urin; Harn | 尿 |
| 7210. urine recovery - (n) | récupération d'urine | recupero urina | recuperación de orina | Urinausscheidungsrate | 尿回復 |
| 7211. urodynamics - (n) | urodynamique | urodinamica | urodinamia | Urodynamik | 尿力学 |
| 7212. urogenital - (a) | urogénital | urogenitale | urogenital | urogenital | 尿生殖の |
| 7213. urography - (n) | urographie | urografia | urografía | Urographie | 尿路造影（撮影）［法］ |
| 7214. urologic - (a) | urologique | urologico | urológico | urologisch | 泌尿器科学の |
| 7215. urological - (a) | urologique | urologico | urológico | urologisch | 泌尿器科学の |
| 7216. urology - (n) | urologie | urologia | urología | Urologie | 泌尿器科学 |
| 7217. urticaria - (n) | urticaire | orticaria | urticaria | Urtikaria; Nesselsucht | じんま疹 |
| 7218. use patent - (n) | droit d'usage; brevet d'utilisation | brevetto per l'uso | licencia para el uso | Anwendungspatent | 使用特許 |
| 7219. uterine contraction - (n) | contraction utérine | contrazione uterina | contracción uterina | Uteruskontraktion; Wehen | 子宮収縮 |
| 7220. uterus - (n) | utérus | utero | útero | Uterus; Gebärmutter | 子宮 |
| 7221. utilization - (n) | utilisation | utilizzazione | uso | Verwendung; Verwertung | 利用 |

369

| English/American | French/Français | Italian/Italiano | Spanish/Español | German/Deutsch | Japanese/日本語 |
|---|---|---|---|---|---|
| 7222. utricle - (n) | utricule | otricolo; utricolo | utrículo | Utriculus | 卵形嚢 |
| 7223. uvea - (n) | uvée | uvea | úvea | Uvea | ブドウ膜 |
| 7224. uvula - (n) | uvula | ugola | úvula | Zäpfchen; Uvula | 口蓋垂 |

| English/American | French/Français | Italian/Italiano | Spanish/Español | German/Deutsch | Japanese/日本語 |
|---|---|---|---|---|---|
| 7225. vaccination - (n) | vaccination | vaccinazione | vacunación | Impfung | ワクチン接種 |
| 7226. vaccine - (n) | vaccin | vaccino | vacuna | Impfstoff | ワクチン |
| 7227. vacillate - (v) | vaciller | ondeggiare; oscillare | vacilar | schwanken | 動揺する |
| 7228. vacuole - (n) | vacuole | vacuolo | vacuola | Vakuole | 小胞 |
| 7229. vacuum - (n) | vacuum | vuoto | vacío | Vakuum | 真空 |
| 7230. vagal - (a) | vagal | vagale | vagal | vagal | 迷走神経 [性] の |
| 7231. vagina - (n) | vagin | vagina | vagina | Scheide; Vagina | 鞘，腟 |
| 7232. vaginal - (a) | vaginal | vaginale | vaginal | vaginal | 鞘の，腟の |
| 7233. vaginal discharge - (n) | perte vaginale | secrezione vaginale | secreción vaginal | Scheidenausfluß | 腟分泌物 |
| 7234. vaginal smear - (n) | frottis vaginal | striscio vaginale | frote vaginal | Scheidenabstrich | 腟スミア |
| 7235. vagotomy - (n) | vagotomie | vagotomia | vagotomía | Vagotomie | 迷走神経切断 [術] |
| 7236. vague - (a) | vague; imprécis | vago; impreciso | vago | undeutlich; vage | あいまいな |
| 7237. vagus nerve - (n) | nerf pneumogastrique | nervo vago | nervio neumogástrico | (Nervus) Vagus | 迷走神経 |
| 7238. validation - (n) | validation | convalidazione | validación | Validierung | 確証，確認 |
| 7239. validity - (n) | validité | validità | validez | Validität; Gültigkeit | 妥当性 |
| 7240. value - (n) | valeur | valore | valor | Wert; Nutzen | 値，価値 |
| 7241. valve - (n) | valvule; valve | valvola | válvula | Klappe; Ventil | 弁，ひだ |
| 7242. valve stenosis - (n) | sténose valvulaire | stenosi valvolare | estenosis valvular | Klappenstenose | 弁狭窄 |
| 7243. vapor - (n) | vapeur | vapore | vapor | Dampf | 蒸気 |
| 7244. variability - (n) | variabilité | variabilità | variabilidad | Variabilität; Unbeständigkeit | 変動性 |
| 7245. variable - (n) | variable | variabile | variable | Variable | 変数，変量 |
| 7246. variable - (a) | variable | variabile | variable | variabel; veränderlich | 変異の |
| 7247. variance - (n) | variance; dispersion | varianza | dispersión | Varianz; Veränderung | 分散 |
| 7248. variant - (n) | variante | variante; variato | variante | Variante; Mutante | 変異体 |

371

| English/American | French/Français | Italian/Italiano | Spanish/Español | German/Deutsch | Japanese/日本語 |
|---|---|---|---|---|---|
| 7249. variation - (n) | variation | variazione | variación | Variation | 変動、変異 |
| 7250. varicocele - (n) | varicocèle | varicocele | varicocele | Varikozelle; Krampfaderbruch | 精索静脈瘤 |
| 7251. varicose - (a) | variqueux | varicoso | varicoso | varikös | 静脈瘤の |
| 7252. varicose veins - (n) | varices | vena varicosa | venas varicosas | Krampfadern | 拡張蛇行静脈 |
| 7253. varix - (n) | varice | varice | várice | Varize | 静脈瘤 |
| 7254. vas - (a) | vaisseau; canal | vaso; dotto | vas | Vaso- | [脈]管 |
| 7255. vas deferens - (n) | canal déférent | vaso deferente; dotto deferente | vas deferens; conducto deferente | Samenleiter; Ductus deferens | 精管 |
| 7256. vascular - (a) | vasculaire | vascolare | vascular | vaskular; Gefäß- | 脈管の、血管の |
| 7257. vascular dementia - (n) | démence vasculaire | demenza vascolare | demencia vascular | Multiinfarktdemenz | 血管性痴呆 |
| 7258. vascular resistance - (n) | résistance vasculaire | resistenza vascolare | resistencia vascular | Gefäßwiderstand | 血管抵抗 |
| 7259. vasculitis - (n) | vasculite | vasculite | vasculitis | Vaskulitis | 脈管炎 |
| 7260. vasectomy - (n) | vasectomie | vasectomia | vasectomía | Vasektomie | 精管切除 [術] |
| 7261. vasoconstriction - (n) | vasoconstriction | vasocostrizione | vasoconstricción | Vasokonstriktion | 血管収縮、血管狭窄 |
| 7262. vasoconstrictor - (n) | vasoconstricteur | vasocostrittore | vasoconstrictor | Vasokonstriktor | 血管収縮薬、血管収縮神経 |
| 7263. vasodepressor - (n) | vaso-dépresseur | vasodepressore | vasodepresor | Vasodepressor | 血管抑制薬 |
| 7264. vasodilatation - (n) | vasodilatation | vasodilatazione | vasodilatación | Vasodilatation | 血管拡張 |
| 7265. vasodilation - (n) | vasodilatation | vasodilatazione | vasodilatación | Vasodilatation | 血管拡張 |
| 7266. vasodilator - (n) | vasodilatateur | vasodilatatore | vasodilatador | Vasodilatator | 血管拡張薬、血管拡張神経 |
| 7267. vasomotor - (n) | vaso-moteur | vasomotore | vasomotor | Vasomotor | 血管運動神経 |
| 7268. vasomotor - (a) | vaso-moteur | vasomotore | vasomotor | vasomotorisch | 血管運動神経の |

| English/American | French/Français | Italian/Italiano | Spanish/Español | German/Deutsch | Japanese 日本語 |
|---|---|---|---|---|---|
| 7269. vasopressor - (n) | vaso-presseur | vasopressorio | vasopresor | Vasopressor; vasopressorische Substanz | 血管収縮薬、昇圧薬 |
| 7270. vasospasm - (n) | vasospasme; spasme vasculaire | vasospasmo | vasoespasmo | Vasospasmus; Gefäßkrampf | 血管痙攣 |
| 7271. vector - (n) | vecteur | vettore | vector | Vektor; Träger | ベクトル |
| 7272. vector analysis - (n) | analyse vectorielle | analisi vettoriale | análisis de vector | Vektoranalyse | ベクトル分析 |
| 7273. vectorcardiography - (n) | vectocardiographie | vettocardiografia | vectocardiografía | Vektorkardiographie | ベクトル心電図 [記録] 法 |
| 7274. vegetable - (n) | végétal; légume | vegetale | vegetal | Gemüse | 野菜 |
| 7275. vegetarian - (n) | végétarien | vegetariano | vegetariano | Vegetarier | 菜食主義者 |
| 7276. vegetarian - (a) | végétarien | vegetariano | vegetariano | vegetarisch | 菜食の |
| 7277. vehicle - (n) | véhicule | veicolo | vehículo; medio | Vehikel; Träger | 賦形剤、媒介物 |
| 7278. vein - (n) | veine | vena | vena | Vene | 静脈 |
| 7279. vena cava - (n) | veine cave | vena cava | vena cava | Vena cava | 大静脈 |
| 7280. vendor - (n) | vendeur | venditore | vendedor | Verkäufer | 売り主 |
| 7281. venereal disease - (n) | maladie vénérienne | malattia venerea | enfermedad venérea | Geschlechtskrankheit | 性病 |
| 7282. venipuncture - (n) | ponction veineuse | venopuntura | venipuntura | Venenpunktion | 静脈穿刺 |
| 7283. Venn diagram - (n) | diagramme de Venn | diagramma di Venn | diagrama de Venn | Vennsches Diagramm | ベン図 (式) |
| 7284. venom - (n) | venin | veleno | veneno | tierisches Gift | 毒物、毒液 |
| 7285. venous - (a) | veineux | venoso | venenoso | venös | 静脈 [性] の |
| 7286. venous pressure - (n) | pression veineuse | pressione venosa | presión venosa | venöser Blutdruck | 静脈圧 |
| 7287. ventilation - (n) | ventilation | ventilazione; ossigenazione | ventilación; oxigenación | Lüftung; Ventilation | 換気、通気 |

| English/American | French/Français | Italian/Italiano | Spanish/Español | German/Deutsch | Japanese/日本語 |
|---|---|---|---|---|---|
| 7288. ventilation perfusion ratio - (n) | rapport ventilation/ perfusion | rapporto ventilazione-perfusione | relación ventilación-perfusión | Verhältnis zwischen Ventilation und Perfusion | 換気血流比 |
| 7289. ventilator - (n) | ventilateur; respirateur | ventilatore | ventilador; respirador | Respirator; Beatmungsgerät | 換気器 |
| 7290. ventilator weaning - (n) | sevrage du respirateur | eliminazione graduale del ventilatore | destete del respirador | Entwöhnung von der künstlichen Beatmung | 換気器離脱 |
| 7291. ventral - (a) | ventral; abdominal | ventrale; addominale | ventral; abdominal | ventral | 腹の |
| 7292. ventricle - (n) | ventricule | ventricolo | ventrículo | Ventrikel; Kammer | 室、心室、脳室 |
| 7293. ventricular - (a) | ventriculaire | ventricolare | ventricular | ventrikulär | 心室の、脳室の |
| 7294. ventricular fibrillation - (n) | fibrillation ventriculaire | fibrillazione ventricolare | fibrilación ventricular | Kammerflimmern | 心室［性］細動 |
| 7295. ventricular tachycardia - (n) | tachycardie ventriculaire | tachicardia ventricolare | taquicardia ventricular | Kammertachykardie | 心室［性］頻拍（頻脈） |
| 7296. ventriculogra-phy - (n) | ventriculographie | ventricolografia | ventriculografía | Ventrikulographie | 脳室造影（撮影）［法］ |
| 7297. venule - (n) | veinule | venula | vénula | Venole; Venula | 細静脈、小静脈 |
| 7298. verbal - (a) | verbal | verbale | verbal | verbal; Wort- | 言葉の |
| 7299. verbatim - (a) | mot à mot | alla lettera | palabra por palabra | wörtlich | 言葉どおりの |
| 7300. verification - (n) | vérification | verificazione | verificación | Verifikation; Bestätigung | 立証 |
| 7301. verify - (v) | vérifier; confirmer | verificare | verificar; comprobar | bestätigen; verifizieren | 立証する |
| 7302. vermiform - (a) | vermiforme | vermiforme | vermiforme | wurmförmig | 虫状の |
| 7303. vermin - (n) | vermine; parasites | parassiti | parásitos; alimañas | Ungeziefer; Schädling | 外客生虫、寄生動物 |
| 7304. verruca - (n) | verrue | verruca | verruga | Warze; Verruca | ゆうぜい、いぼ |
| 7305. vertebra - (n) | vertèbre | vertebra | vértebra | Wirbel | 椎骨 |
| 7306. vertebral - (a) | vertébral | vertebrale | vertebral | vertebral; Wirbel- | ［脊］椎骨の |
| 7307. vertebral column - (n) | colonne vertébrale | colonna vertebrale | columna vertebral | Wirbelsäule | 脊柱 |

374

| English/American | French/Français | Italian/Italiano | Spanish/Español | German/Deutsch | Japanese 日本語 |
|---|---|---|---|---|---|
| 7308. vertebrate - (n) | vertébré | vertebrato | vertebrado | Wirbeltier; Vertebrat | 脊椎動物 |
| 7309. vertex - (n) | vertex | vertice | vértice | Scheitel; Vertex | 頂，頭頂 |
| 7310. vertical - (a) | vertical | verticale | vertical; del vértice | vertikal; senkrecht | 頂の，垂直の |
| 7311. vertical integration - (n) | intégration verticale | integrazione verticale | integración vertical | vertikale Integrierung | 垂直的統合 |
| 7312. vertigo - (n) | vertige | vertigine | vértigo | Schwindel; Vertigo | めまい |
| 7313. vesicle - (n) | vésicule | vescicola; vescichetta | vesícula | Bläschen; Vesikel | 小胞 |
| 7314. vesicular - (a) | vésiculaire | vescicolare; vescicoso | vesicular | vesikulär; blasenförmig | 小胞の |
| 7315. vessel - (n) | vaisseau | vaso | vaso | Gefäß | [脈] 管 |
| 7316. vestibular - (a) | vestibulaire | vestibolare | vestibular | vestibulär; Gleichgewichts- | 前庭の |
| 7317. vestibular toxicity - (n) | toxicité vestibulaire | tossicità vestibolare | toxicidad vestibular | toxische Wirkung auf das Gleichgewichtsorgan | 前庭毒性 |
| 7318. vestibule - (n) | vestibule | vestibolo | vestíbulo | Vorhof; Vestibulum | 前庭 |
| 7319. vestibulo-ocular reflex - (n) | réflexe oculo-vestibulaire | riflesso vestibolo-oculare | reflejo óculo-vestibular | Okulovestibularisreflex | 前庭眼球反射 |
| 7320. vestige - (n) | vestige | vestigio; rudimento | vestigio | Rudiment; rudimentärer Körperteil | 痕跡 [部] |
| 7321. veteran - (n) | vétéran | veterano | veterano | Veteran | ベテラン |
| 7322. veterinary medicine - (n) | médecine vétérinaire | medicina veterinaria | medicina veterinaria | Tiermedizin | 獣医学 |
| 7323. viable - (a) | viable | vitale | viable | lebendig; lebensfähig | 生活可能な |
| 7324. vial - (n) | fiole | fiala | frasco | Phiole; kleines Fläschchen | バイアル、小びん |
| 7325. vibration - (n) | vibration | vibrazione | vibración | Vibration; Schwingung | 振とう法，振動 |
| 7326. vibratory sensation - (n) | sensation vibratoire | sensazione vibratoria | sensibilidad vibratoria | Vibrationsempfinden | 振動感覚 |

375

| English/American | French/Français | Italian/Italiano | Spanish/Español | German/Deutsch | Japanese/日本語 |
|---|---|---|---|---|---|
| 7327. villi - (n) | villosités | villi | vellos | Zotten | 絨毛、絨毛状突起 |
| 7328. violation - (n) | violation | violazione | violación | Übertretung; Zuwiderhandlung | 違反 |
| 7329. violence - (n) | violence | violenza | violencia | Gewalt | 暴力 |
| 7330. viral - (a) | viral | virale | viral | viral | ウイルス[性]の |
| 7331. viral agent - (n) | agent viral | agente virale | agente viral | viraler Organismus | ウイルス性病原体 |
| 7332. viral culture - (n) | culture virale | coltura virali | cultivo viral | Virenkultur | ウイルス培養 |
| 7333. viral shedding - (n) | dissémination virale; effusion virale | diffusione di un virus | eliminación viral | Virenausscheidung; Virenabstoßung | ウイルスの放出 |
| 7334. viremia - (n) | virémie | viremia | viremia | Virämie | ウイルス血症 |
| 7335. virile - (a) | viril | virile | viril; varonil | männlich; maskulin | 男性の |
| 7336. virilization - (n) | virilisation | virilizzazione | virilización | Virilisierung; Vermännlichung | 男性化 |
| 7337. virion - (n) | virion | virione | virión | Virion; Viruspartikel | ビリオン |
| 7338. virology - (n) | virologie | virologia | virología | Virologie | ウイルス学 |
| 7339. virulence - (n) | virulence | virulenza | virulencia | Virulenz | ビルレンス、毒力 |
| 7340. virus - (n) | virus | virus | virus | Virus | ウイルス |
| 7341. viscera - (n) | viscères; entrailles | visceri | víscera | Viszera; Eingeweide | 内臓 |
| 7342. viscid - (a) | visqueux | viscido; gelatinoso | viscoso; glutinoso | viskös; klebrig | 粘着性の |
| 7343. viscosity - (n) | viscosité | viscosità | viscosidad | Viskosität; Zähflüssigkeit | 粘性 |
| 7344. viscus, viscous - (a) | visqueux | viscoso | viscoso | viskös; zähflüssig | 粘性の |
| 7345. vision - (n) | vision; vue | vista; visione | visión | Sehvermögen; Sehen | 視覚、視力 |
| 7346. visual - (a) | visuel | visuale | visual | visuell | 視覚の |
| 7347. visual acuity - (n) | acuité visuelle | acuità visiva | agudeza visual | Sehschärfe | 視力 |
| 7348. visual analogue scale - (n) | échelle analogue visuelle | scala analoga visiva | escala analoga visual | sichtbare Analogskala | 視覚アナログ尺度 |
| 7349. visual evoked potential - (n) | potentiel évoqué visuel | potenziale evocato visivo | potencial evocado de la visión | visuell evoziertes Potential | 視覚誘発電位 |

| English/American | French/Français | Italian/Italiano | Spanish/Español | German/Deutsch | Japanese/日本語 |
|---|---|---|---|---|---|
| 7350. visual field - (n) | champ visuel | campo visivo | campo visual | Sehfeld; Gesichtsfeld | 視野 |
| 7351. visual impairment - (n) | trouble visuel | diminuzione dell'acuità visiva | daño visual | Verschlechterung des Sehvermögens | 視覚障害 |
| 7352. visualization - (n) | visualisation | visualizzazione | visualización | Visualisierung; Sichtbarmachung | 心像 |
| 7353. vital capacity - (n) | capacité vitale | capacità vitale | capacidad vital | Vitalkapzität | 肺活量 |
| 7354. vital signs - (n) | signes vitaux | segni vitali | signos vitales | Lebenszeichen | 生きている兆候 |
| 7355. vital statistics - (n) | statistiques démographiques | statistica demografica | estadísticas demográficas | Biostatistik | 動態統計［学］ |
| 7356. vitamin - (n) | vitamine | vitamina | vitamina | Vitamin | ビタミン |
| 7357. vitreous - (a) | vitré | vitreo | vítreo | gläsern; glasig | ガラス状の |
| 7358. vitreous body - (n) | corps vitré | corpo vitreo | cuerpo vítreo | Glaskörper | 硝子体 |
| 7359. vitreous humor - (n) | humeur vitrée | umore vitreo | humor vítreo | Glaskörperflüssigkeit | 硝子体液 |
| 7360. vivisect - (v) | pratiquer la vivisection | vivisezionare | hacer la vivisección de | vivisezieren | 生体解剖を行なう |
| 7361. vocabulary - (n) | vocabulaire | vocabolario | vocabulario | Wortschatz; Vokabular | 語彙 |
| 7362. vocal cords - (n) | cordes vocales | corde vocali | cuerdas vocales | Stimmbänder | 声帯 |
| 7363. vocational - (a) | professionnel | professionale | vocacional; profesional | beruflich | 職業の |
| 7364. voice - (n) | voix | voce | voz | Stimme | 音声、声 |
| 7365. void - (n) | vide | vuoto | vacío | Hohlraum; Lücke | 空虚 |
| 7366. void - (v) | vider; évacuer | evacuare; vuotare | vaciar; evacuar | evakuieren; leeren | 排出する |
| 7367. volatile - (a) | volatil | volatile | volátil | ätherisch; gasförmig | 揮発性の |
| 7368. volatile oil - (n) | huile volatile | olio volatile | aceite volátil | ätherisches Öl | 揮発油 |
| 7369. volume - (n) | volume | volume | volumen | Volumen; Lautstärke | 音量、容積 |
| 7370. volume of distribution - (n) | volume de la distribution | volume di distribuzione | volumen de la distribución | Verteilungsvolumen | 分布の容量 |
| 7371. voluntary - (a) | volontaire | volontario | voluntario | freiwillig | 随意の、任意の |
| 7372. voluntary muscle - (n) | muscle volontaire | muscolo volontario | músculo voluntario | Willkürmuskulatur | 随意筋 |

| English/American | French/Français | Italian/Italiano | Spanish/Español | German/Deutsch | Japanese/日本語 |
|---|---|---|---|---|---|
| 7373. voluntary worker - (n) | travailleur volontaire | lavoratore volontario | trabajador voluntario | freiwilliger Arbeiter | ボランティア労働者 |
| 7374. volunteer - (n) | volontaire | volontario | voluntario | Freiwillige(r) | ボランティア |
| 7375. volunteer - (v) | offrir volontairement | offrirsi volontariamente | ofrecer(se) | etwas freiwillig tun | 志願する |
| 7376. vomiting - (n) | vomissement | vomito | vómito | Erbrechen | 嘔吐 |
| 7377. vulnerable - (a) | vulnérable | vulnerabile | vulnerable | verletzlich | 傷を受けやすい |
| 7378. vulva - (n) | vulve | vulva | vulva | Vulva | 外陰 [部] |
| 7379. vulvar - (a) | vulvaire | vulvare | vulvar | vulvar | 外陰 [部] の |

378

| English/American | French/Français | Italian/Italiano | Spanish/Español | German/Deutsch | Japanese/日本語 |
|---|---|---|---|---|---|
| 7380. waddling gait - (n) | démarche en canard; démarche dandinante | andatura ondeggiante | andar como un pato | Watschelgang | 動揺性歩行 |
| 7381. waist - (n) | taille; ceinture | vita; cintola | talle; cintura | Taille | 腰 |
| 7382. waiting list - (n) | liste d'attente | lista d'attesa | lista de espera | Warteliste | 補欠人名簿 |
| 7383. waiver - (n) | renonciation; désistement | rinuncia | renuncia; desistimiento | Verzicht; Verzichtserklärung | 権利放棄 |
| 7384. wake - (v) | réveiller | svegliarsi; svegliare | despertar | aufwachen; (auf)wecken | 覚醒させる |
| 7385. wakefulness - (n) | insomnie | mancanza di sonno; insonnia | insomnio | Schlaflosigkeit | 不眠症 |
| 7386. waking hours - (a) | heures de veille | ore di veglia | horas de vela | von früh bis spät | めざめている時間 |
| 7387. walk - (n) | démarche; promenade | passo; passeggiata | marcha; paseo | Gang; Spaziergang | 歩行 |
| 7388. walk - (v) | marcher; se promener | camminare; deambulare | andar, caminar | gehen | 歩く |
| 7389. walking chromosome - (n) | chromosome ambulant | cromosoma ambulante | cromosoma ambulante | wandernder Chromosom | クロモソーマル ウォーキング |
| 7390. wall - (n) | mur; paroi | muro | pared | Wand | 壁 |
| 7391. wane - (v) | diminuer; décliner | declinare | menguar; decaer | schwinden; abnehmen | 衰える |
| 7392. ward - (n) | salle d'hôpital | corsia | sala de hospital | Abteilung; Krankensaal | 病棟 |
| 7393. warm - (v) | chauffer | riscaldare | calentar | erwärmen; aufwärmen | 暖める |
| 7394. warm - (a) | chaud | caldo | tibio; caliente | warm | 暖かい |
| 7395. warning - (n) | avertissement; avis | avvertimento | advertencia; aviso | Warnung | 前兆 |
| 7396. wart - (n) | verrue | verruca | verruga | Warze | いぼ |
| 7397. wash - (n) | lavage; lotion | lavata; lozione | lavado; loción | Spülung; Lotion | 洗浄、洗浄液 |
| 7398. wash - (v) | laver | lavare; lavarsi | lavar | waschen; spülen | 洗浄する |
| 7399. washout - (n) | lavage; désastre | enterolisi isoperistaltica; insuccesso | lavado; desastre | Auswaschung; Mißerfolg | 流出、失敗 |
| 7400. waste - (n) | perte; gaspillage; déchets | spreco; residuo; deperimento | superfluo; desecho; desperdicios | Verschwendung; Abfall | 老廃物、浪費 |
| 7401. waste - (v) | perdre; gaspiller | deperire | derrochar; perder | verschwenden | むだにする |

| English/American | French/Français | Italian/Italiano | Spanish/Español | German/Deutsch | Japanese/日本語 |
|---|---|---|---|---|---|
| 7402. wasting - (n) | émaciation | emaciazione | emaciación | Schwund; Auszehrung | るいそう |
| 7403. water - (n) | eau | acqua | agua | Wasser | 水 |
| 7404. water deprivation - (n) | privation d'eau | privazione di acqua | privación de agua | Wasserverlust | 水分欠乏 |
| 7405. water solubility - (n) | solubilité dans l'eau | solubilità in acqua | solubilidad en agua | Wasserlöslichkeit | 水溶性 |
| 7406. water-soluble - (a) | soluble dans l'eau; hydrosoluble | solubile in acqua; idrosolubile | soluble en agua; hidrosoluble | wasserlöslich | 水溶性の |
| 7407. watery stools - (n) | stelles liquides | feci acquosi | heces acuosas | waßrige Stühle | 水様便 |
| 7408. waveform - (n) | forme d'onde | forma d'onda | forma de onda | Wellenform | 波形 |
| 7409. wavelike motion - (n) | mouvement ondulatoire | movimento ondoso | movimiento ondulado | wellenförmige Bewegung | 波形動作 |
| 7410. wax - (n) | cire | cera | cera | Wachs | ろう |
| 7411. weak - (a) | faible | debole | débil; flojo | schwach | 虚弱な |
| 7412. weakness - (n) | faiblesse | debolezza | debilidad; flojedad | Schwäche; Debilität | 腕弱 |
| 7413. wean - (v) | sevrer | svezzare | destetar | abstillen; entwöhnen | 離乳させる |
| 7414. weariness - (n) | lassitude; fatigue | stanchezza | cansancio; fatiga | Ermüdung | 疲労 |
| 7415. webbed neck - (n) | cou palmé | pterigio congenito | cuello membranoso | Pterygium colli | 翼状頸 |
| 7416. wedge shaped - (a) | en coin; en forme de coin | a forma di cuneo | en forma de cuña | keilformig | くさび形 |
| 7417. week - (n) | semaine | settimana | semana | Woche | 週 |
| 7418. weeping - (n) | pleurs; exsudation | piangente; essudazione | lágrimas; supurante | Weinen; Exsudation | 泣くこと |
| 7419. weight - (n) | poids | peso | peso | Gewicht | 重量 |
| 7420. weight bearing - (a) | soutenant poids | carico | cargando peso | gewichtstragend | 重量支持 |
| 7421. weight gain - (n) | augmentation de poids | aumento di peso | subido de peso | Gewichtszunahme | 体重の増加 |
| 7422. weight lifting - (n) | haltérophilie | pesistica | halterofilia | Gewichtheben | 重量上げ |
| 7423. weight loss - (n) | perte pondérale; perte de poids | perdita di peso; dimagramento | perdida de peso | Gewichtsverlust | 体重の減少 |

| English/American | French/Français | Italian/Italiano | Spanish/Español | German/Deutsch | Japanese/日本語 |
|---|---|---|---|---|---|
| 7424. weighted value - (n) | valeur pondérée | valore soppesato | valor ponderado | gewogener Wert | 加重値 |
| 7425. weightless-ness - (n) | apesanteur | assenza di peso | ingravidez | Schwerelosigkeit | 無重量感 |
| 7426. welding - (n) | soudure; soudage | saldatura | soldadura | Schweißen | 溶接 |
| 7427. well-being - (n) | bien-être | benessere | bienestar | Wohl; Wohlfahrt | 福祉 |
| 7428. Western blot - (n) | analyse Western bot | analisi di Western blot | análisis Western blot | Western-Blot | ウエスタンブロット |
| 7429. wet - (a) | mouillé | bagnato | mojado | feucht; naß | 湿気のある |
| 7430. wheal - (n) | pustule; urticaire | pustola; nodulo | roncha; grano | Quaddel | 膨疹 |
| 7431. wheal and flare reaction- (n) | réaction érythémateuse-allergique | reazione papulo-eritematosa | reacción de roncha y brote | Quaddel-Erythem-Reaktion | 膨疹と発赤 |
| 7432. wheelchair - (n) | chaise roulante | sedia a rotelle | silla de ruedas | Rollstuhl | 車椅子 |
| 7433. wheeze - (v) | respirer bruyamment | avere il respiro affannoso | resollar; respirar con dificultad | keuchen; schnaufen | 喘鳴する |
| 7434. whiplash - (n) | syndrome cervical traumatique | colpo di frusta cervicale | desnucamiento | Peitschenschlag-verletzung | むち打ち |
| 7435. whisper - (n) | chuchotement | sussurro | cuchicheo; susurro | Geflüster | ささやき |
| 7436. whisper - (v) | chuchoter | sussurrare | cuchichear; susurrar | flüstern | ささやく |
| 7437. white - (a) | blanc | bianco | blanco | weiß | 白、白色 |
| 7438. white blood cell - (n) | globule blanc; leucocyte | globulo bianco; leucocito | glóbulo blanco | Leukozyt | 白血球 |
| 7439. white cell count - (n) | décompte leucocytaire | conta leucocitaria | conteo de glóbulos blancos | Leukozytenzahl; Leukozytenzählung | 白血球数 |
| 7440. white matter - (n) | substance blanche | sostanza bianca | materia blanca | weiße Substanz | 白質 |
| 7441. whole - (a) | entier; tout | tutto; completo; intero | entero; todo | voll; ganz | 全ての |
| 7442. whole blood - (n) | sang total; sang complet | sangue intero | sangre total | Vollblut | 全血 |
| 7443. whole blood exchange transfusion - (n) | exsanguino-trans-usion de sang complet | exsanguino-trasfusione di sangue intero | exanguinotransfusión de sangre total | Vollblutaustausch-transfusion | 全血交換輸血 |

| English/American | French/Français | Italian/Italiano | Spanish/Español | German/Deutsch | Japanese/日本語 |
|---|---|---|---|---|---|
| 7444. whole body plethysmography - (n) | pléthysmographie pancorporelle | pletismografia dell'intero corpo | pletismografía del cuerpo entero | Ganzkörperplethysmographie | 全身プレチスモグラフィ |
| 7445. wholesaler - (n) | grossiste; marchand en gros | grossista | comerciante al por mayor | Großhändler | 卸売り業者 |
| 7446. widening - (n) | élargissement | allargamento; slargamento | ampliación; extensión | Verbreiterung | 広くすること |
| 7447. will - (n) | volonté; testament | volontà; testamento | voluntad; testamento | Wille; Testament | 意志、遺言書 |
| 7448. will power - (n) | volonté | forza di volontà | fuerza de voluntad | Willenskraft | 自制心、意志力 |
| 7449. wing - (n) | aile | ala | aleta; ala | Flügel | 翼 |
| 7450. wipe - (v) | essuyer | pulire; strofinare | enjugar; limpiar | wischen | 拭う |
| 7451. witch doctor - (n) | sorcier | stregone | hechicero | Medizinmann | 妖術師 |
| 7452. withdrawal - (n) | abstinence; sevrage | sospensione; astinenza | eliminación; abstinencia | Entnahme; Entzug | 離脱、停止 |
| 7453. withdrawal delirium - (n) | délire d'abstinence; délire de sevrage | delirio da privazione | delirio por abstinencia | Entzugsdelir | 離脱せん妄 |
| 7454. withdrawal symptom - (n) | symptôme d'abstinence; symptôme de sevrage | sindrome di astinenza | síntoma de abstinencia | Entzugssymptom | 離脱症状 |
| 7455. wither - (v) | atrophier; dessécher | avvizzire | consumir; debilitar | verdorren; austrocknen | 萎える |
| 7456. witnessed verbal consent - (n) | consentement verbal devant témoin | consenso verbale con testimoni | consentimiento verbal atestiguado | bezeugte mündliche Einwilligung | 証人のある口頭での同意 |
| 7457. woman - (n) | femme | donna | mujer | Frau | 女性 |
| 7458. womb - (n) | utérus | utero | útero | Gebärmutter; Uterus | 子宮 |
| 7459. work - (n) | travail | lavoro | trabajo | Arbeit | 労働 |
| 7460. work capacity - (n) | capacité de travail | capacità di lavoro | capacidad de trabajo | Arbeitskapazität | 労働量 |
| 7461. work force - (n) | main d'oeuvre | forza lavoro | mano de obra | gesamte Arbeitskraft | 労働力 |
| 7462. workaholic - (n) | bourreau de travail | stacanovista del lavoro | trabajador obsesivo | Arbeitswütige(r) | 働きすぎ |
| 7463. workers' compensation - (n) | assurance contre accidents de travail | assicurazione contro infortuni professionali | compensación por accidente de trabajo | Arbeitsunfallversicherung | 労働者の報酬 |

382

| English/American | French/Français | Italian/Italiano | Spanish/Español | German/Deutsch | Japanese/日本語 |
|---|---|---|---|---|---|
| 7464. workload - (n) | charge de travail | carico di lavoro | cantidad de trabajo | Arbeitslast | 作業負荷 |
| 7465. workshop - (n) | séminaire; conférence | corso pratico | seminario | Seminar; Arbeitstagung | ワークショップ |
| 7466. World Health Organization [abbr] WHO - (n) | Organisation Mondiale de la Santé OMS | Organizzazione Mondiale della Sanità, OMS | Organización Mundial de la Salud, OMS | Weltgesundheits-organisation | 世界保健機関 |
| 7467. worldwide - (a) | mondial; universel | universale | mundial | weltweit; global | 世界的な |
| 7468. worldwide development - (n) | développement mondial | sviluppo universale | desarrollo mundial | weltweite Entwicklung | 世界的発展 |
| 7469. worm - (n) | ver | verme | lombriz | Wurm | 虫様構造 |
| 7470. worsening - (n) | aggravation; détérioration | peggioramento | agravación | Verschlechterung | 悪化すること |
| 7471. worst case - (n) | le pire cas | caso peggiore | peor de los casos | schlechtester Fall | 最悪例 |
| 7472. wound - (n) | blessure; plaie | ferita | herida | Wunde | 創傷 |
| 7473. wound - (v) | blesser | ferire | herir | verwunden | 傷つける |
| 7474. wounded - (a) | blessé | ferito | herido | verwundet | 傷ついた |
| 7475. wrinkle - (n) | ride | ruga; plega | arruga | Hautfältchen | しわ、ひだ |
| 7476. wrist - (n) | carpe; poignet | polso | muñeca | Handgelenk | 手根 |
| 7477. write - (v) | écrire | scrivere | escribir | schreiben | 書く |
| 7478. written informed consent - (n) | consentement éclairé | consenso informato scritto | consentimiento escrito | Einverständniserklärung schriftliche Bestellung; | 文書告知同意書 |
| 7479. written order - (n) | ordre écrit | ordine scritto | orden escrita | schriftlicher Befehl | 文書での命令 |

383

| English/American | French/Français | Italian/Italiano | Spanish/Español | German/Deutsch | Japanese/日本語 |
|---|---|---|---|---|---|
| 7480. X chromosome - (n) | chromosome X | cromosoma X | cromosoma X | X-Chromosom | X染色体 |
| 7481. xanthomatous nodule - (n) | nodule xanthomateux | nodulo xantomatoso | nódulo xantomatoso | xanthomatöser Knoten | 黄色腫［性］小結節 |
| 7482. x-axis - (n) | axe des abscisses; axe des x | asse delle x; ascissa | abscisa | X-Achse; Abscisse | X軸 |
| 7483. xenobiotic - (n) | xénobiotique | xenobiotico | xenobiótico | Fremdstoff | 生体異物 |
| 7484. xiphoid process - (n) | appendice xiphoïde | processo xifoide | apófisis; xifoides | Processus xiphoideus | 剣状突起 |
| 7485. X-ray - (n) | rayon X; radiographie | raggio X; radiografia | rayo x; radiografía | Röntgenstrahl; Röntgenaufnahme | X線、X線写真 |
| 7486. X-ray - (v) | radiographier | radiografare | radiografiar | röntgen | X線撮影する |
| 7487. X-ray computed tomography - (n) | tomographie par ordinateur | tomografia computerizzata | tomografía computada | Röntgencomputertomographie | X線コンピューター連動断層撮影［法］ |
| 7488. X-ray densitometry - (n) | densitométrie par rayons X | densitometria a raggi X | densitometría con rayos x | Röntgendensitometrie | X線デンシトメトリー |
| 7489. X-ray film - (n) | film à rayon X; film radiologique | pellicola per raggi X | película de rayos x | Röntgenfilm | X線フィルム |

384

| English/American | French/Français | Italian/Italiano | Spanish/Español | German/Deutsch | Japaaese/日本語 |
|---|---|---|---|---|---|
| 7490. Y chromosome - (n) | chromosome Y | cromosoma Y | cromosoma Y | Y-Chromosom | Y染色体 |
| 7491. yawn - (v) | bâiller | sbadigliare | bostezar | gähnen | あくびする |
| 7492. y-axis - (n) | axe des y; axe des ordonnées | asse delle y; ordinata | ordenada | Y-Achse; Ordinate | Y軸 |
| 7493. year - (n) | an; année | anno; annata | año | Jahr | 年 |
| 7494. years of survival - (n) | années de survie | anni di sopravvivenza | años de supervivencia | Überlebensjahre | 生存年月 |
| 7495. yeast - (n) | levure | lievito | levadura | Hefe | 酵母、イースト |
| 7496. yellow card system - (n) | système de carte jaune | sistema di catelle gialle | sistema de tarjeta amarilla | 'gelbes-Karten-System' | イエローカードシステム |
| 7497. yellow vision - (n) | xanthopsie | xantopsia | visión amarilla; xantopsia | Gelbsehen; Xanthoposie | 黄 [色. 視 [症] |
| 7498. yoke - (n) | joug | giogo | yugo | Jugum | ヨーク、隆起 |
| 7499. yolk - (n) | jaune d'œuf; vitellus | vitello; tuorlo | yema; vitelo | Dotter; Eigelb | 卵黄 |
| 7500. young - (a) | jeune | giovane | joven | jung | 若い |
| 7501. youth - (n) | jeunesse; jeune | gioventù | juventud; joven | Jugend | 青年 |

| English/American | French/Français | Italian/Italiano | Spanish/Español | German/Deutsch | Japanese/日本語 |
| --- | --- | --- | --- | --- | --- |
| 7502. z-axis - (n) | axe des z; axe des cotes | asse z | eje de las z | Z-Achse | Z軸 |
| 7503. zero order infusion rate - (n) | taux d'infusion de l'ordre zéro | velocità d'infusione di ordine zero | velocidad de infusión de orden cero | Infusionsrate nullter Ordnung | 零次点滴速度 |
| 7504. zero order kinetics - (n) | cinétique d'ordre zéro | cinetica di ordine zero | cinética de orden cero | Kinetik nullter Ordnung | 零次関数速動 |
| 7505. zona glomerulosa - (n) | zona glomerulosa; zone glomérulaire | zona glomerulosa | zona glomerulosa | Zona glomerulosa | 球状帯 |
| 7506. zonal centrifugation - (n) | centrifugation zonale | centrifugazione zonale | centrifugación zonal | Zonalzentrifugation | ゾーナル遠心法 |
| 7507. zone - (n) | zone | zona | zona | Zone | 帯 |
| 7508. zoonosis - (n) | zoonose | zoonosi | zoonosis | Zoonose | 人獣共通伝染病、ゾーノージス |
| 7509. zoster - (n) | zoster; zona | herpes zoster | zona | Zoster | 帯状疱疹 |
| 7510. z-test - (n) | épreuve z | test z | prueba z | Z-Test | Z検査 |

cours 1552
cours clinique 1196
cours de temps 6950
court 6214
coussin graisseux 2525
coût 1531
coût de service direct 1914
coût-utilité 1534
coûts indirects 3378
coûts intangibles 3503
coutume 1629
couverture 1555
couverture 4012
couveuse 3364
covalent 1553
covariance 1554
coeliaque 1027
coeur 2985
coeur-poumon artificiel 3000
crachat 6463
cracher 6434
craindre 2533
crainte 2532
crampe 1558
crâne 1561
crâne 6285
crânien 1559
craquer 1557
créatinine 1563
crépitation 1565
crépitation articulaire 3663
crête 5934
crête du tibia 6209
crête iliaque 3268
crétinisme 1566
creux 7111
crevasse 1567
crime 1569
crise 1571
crise 6104

crise blastique 734
crise cardiaque 2987
crise d'épilepsie 2320
crise de colère 6810
crise intermenstruelle 4251
cristal 1604
cristallin 1605
cristallin 1606
cristallin 3768
cristallisation 1607
critère 1573
critères d'admissibilité 2211
critères d'éligibilité 2211
critères d'entrée 2294
critères d'exclusion 2404
critères d'inclusion 3349
croisement 1580
croisement entre races 4227
croisement génétique 2820
croissance 2924
croupe 1594
croupion 1594
croûte 1598
croûte 6031
croûte 6302
cryochirurgie 1603
cryopréservation 1601
cryoprotecteur 1602
cubitus 7142
cuir chevelu 6036
cuisse 6905
cultiver 1611
culture 1610
culture cellulaire 1031
culture de la société 1324
culture et sensibilité 1612
culture médiatique 4064
culture sanguine 762
culture virale 7332
culturel 1609

cumulatif 1615
curatif 5785
cure 1620
curette 1623
curriculum vitae 1625
cuspide 1628
cutané 1630
cutané 1824
cyanose 1634
cybernétique 1635
cycle 1636
cycle de dosage 2021
cycle menstruel 4124
cycles par seconde 1637
cylindre hyalin 3163
cyphose 3160
cyphose 3694
cystadénocarcinome 1640
cystectomie 1641
cystite 1643
cystoscopie 1644
cytogénétique 1645
cytologie 1647
cytométrie de flux 2635
cytoplasme 1648
cytoprotecteur 1649
cytosol 1651
cytosquelette 1650
cytotoxicité 1652
cytotoxine 1653
d'âge moyen 4198
d'avoir des enfants 1114
d'éducation 2151
d'extrême urgence 6499
d'opération 4671
d'un certain âge 4198
daltonien 1297
dans le sens des aiguilles d'une montre 1226
date 1696
date d'admission 1697

date d'expiration 1698
date d'expiration 2439
de banlieue 6657
de croissance 1851
de début tardif 3729
de durée courte 6216
de haute-technologie 3082
de lot à lot 3881
de lot à lot 616
de métal 4156
de nuit 4501
de pointe 3082
de propriété 5442
de qualité inférieure 3893
de qualité inférieure 6648
de soude 6342
débat en commission 4822
débile 4298
débilité 1711
débilité 1712
débit cardiaque 948
debout 6491
déboîtement 1713
dérouiller 6833
début 4649
début graduel 2892
début lent 6304
décanter 1714
décarboxylation 1715
décentralisation 1718
décès 1708
déchets 7400
déchirement 5978
déchirure 6832
décibel 1722
décimale 1725
décimètre 1726
déclin 1731
décliner 1732
décliner 7391

décollement 1840
décoloration 1924
décoloration 735
décompensation 1733
décomposer 6443
décomposition 1734
décompression 1735
décompte d'œufs 2166
décompte des colonies microbiennes 4168
décompte leucocytaire 7439
décongestionnant 1737
décontamination 1738
découverte 1929
décubitus 1739
déduction logique 1742
défaillance 2501
défaillance cardiaque 2990
défaut 1747
défaut 2625
défaut 738
défaut de remplissage 2591
défaut du tube neural 4460
défaut enzymatique 2301
défavorable 115
défécation 1746
défectueux 1748
défense 1749
défense abdominale 6
défense involontaire 3610
déféquer 1745
défibrillateur implantable 3321
défibrillation 1752
déficience 1753
déficience en lactase 3707
déficience mentale 4130
définitif 2597
définition 1754
définition opérationnelle 4670
déformabilité 1755
déformé 4234

dégénération hépatolenticulaire 3051
dégénéré 1757
dégénéré 1759
dégénérer 1758
dégénérescence 1760
dégénérescence maculaire 3948
dégradation 1762
dégranulation 1763
degrés de liberté 1764
déguster 6821
déhiscence 1765
déjà vu 1768
délai d'une drogue 2068
délais 6952
délétère 1772
délétion 1773
délétion chromosomique 1147
délire 1774
délire d'abstinence 7453
délire de sevrage 7453
délire 5669
delirium tremens 1775
délivrance 1115
délivre 136
demande d'édition 2146
démangeaison 3652
démangeaison 3654
démarche 215
démarche 2761
démarche 7387
démarche dandinante 7380
démarche en canard 7380
démarche propulsive 5448
démasquer 7182
démence 1782
démence 3467
démence 3912
démence par infarcissements multiples 4335
démence présénile 5335
démence sénile 6131

démence vasculaire 7257
dément 3465
dément 3466
demi-ton 2943
demi-vie 2942
demi-vie d'élimination 2215
démographie 1784
démographie 1785
démyélinisation 1786
dénaturation 1787
dénaturation protéique 5460
dénaturation protidique 5460
dendrite 1788
dénervation 1790
densité 1792
densité optique 4684
densitométrie 1791
densitométrie par rayons X 7488
dent 6991
dent de lait 1724
dent permanente 5010
dentaire 1794
dentelé 6172
dentelure 3367
dentier 1805
dentier 5169
dentifrice 1799
dentine 800
dentiste 1801
dentisterie 802
dentition 1803
dentition complète 1351
dentition primaire 5363
dents fausses 2512
déodorant 1806
déontologie médicale 1259
département 1607
département médical 4073
dépendance physique 5094
dépendant 1809

dépendant des anticorps 325
dépense 2428
dépense 2429
dépilation 2318
dépistage 1841
dépistage 7021
dépistage aléatoire 5640
dépistage de masse 4017
déplacement 1946
déplacement vers l'arrière 570
dépolarisation 1814
déposer 1816
dépôt 7190
dépôt 1815
dépôt 1817
dépôt cutané 6279
dépôt osseux 815
dépouille 6302
dépression 1819
dépression 7111
dépression nerveuse 4454
dépression respiratoire 5851
dépriman: 1818
dérivation 6221
dérivé 1822
dermatite 1825
dermatite de contact 1452
dermatologie 1826
dermatose 1827
dermite 1825
dernier cr 6501
dérober 6514
derrière 5976
des voies respiratoires inférieures 3898
désastre 7399
descendant 1828
descendant 4630
description 1830
désensibilisation 1832
déséquilibre 1935

# French/Français

déséquilibre 3277
déshydratation 1767
déshydrater 1766
désinfecter 1836
désintégration 1716
désintégration 1937
désistement 7383
desmosome 1838
désordre 1941
désordre affectif 128
désordre affectif bipolaire 708
désordre affectif psychotique 5512
désordre convulsif 1506
désordre cutané 1631
désordre d'anxiété 367
désordre de coagulation 1240
désordre de l'appétit 2126
désordre de personnalité marginal 819
désordre du comportement 636
désordre du mouvement 4324
désordre électrolytique 2189
désordre émotionnel 2237
désordre foetal 2560
désordre inflammatoire 3417
désordre maniaque 3990
désordre mental 4131
désordre métabolique 4149
désordre nutritionnel 4580
désordre obsédant 4601
désordre phobique 5074
désordre post-combat 1304
désordre psychotique 5513
désordre somatoforme 6358
désordres factices 2492
désorganisé 1942
désorientation 1943
desséchant 1834
dessécher 1835
dessécher 7455
dessiccatif 1833

dessiccation 1836
dessin 1837
dessin 2042
dessin 4939
dessin d'entrecroisement 1592
dessin factoriel 2495
dessin médicamenteux 2062
dessins par ordinateur 1373
désuni 7189
détection 1841
détection radioimmunologique 5617
détergent 1843
détérioration 1845
détérioration 3314
détérioration 7470
détérioration clinique 1197
détérioration cognitive 1267
détérioré 3313
détériorer 1844
détermination de l'étendue des doses 2015
deuil 646
deutérium 1848
deux fois par jour 7127
développement 1850
développement 2387
développement analytique 252
développement chimique 1094
développement clinique 1198
développement commun 3664
développement de médicament 2063
développement de produit 5399
développement en médecine 4093
développement global 2859
développement mondial 7468
déviant 1852
déviation 1853
déviation 9
déviation au protocole 5470
déviation septale 6145
déviation standard 6487

dextro-isomère 1855
diabète 1856
diabète mellitus 1857
diabète sucré 1857
diabétique 1858
diabétique 1859
diagnostic 1861
diagnostic 1862
diagnostic différentiel 1889
diagnostic oral 4694
diagnostique 1863
diagramme 1869
diagramme circulaire 5117
diagramme de Venn 7283
dialyse 1870
diaphanoscopie 7057
diaphorèse 1872
diaphragme 1873
diapositive 6295
diarrhée 1874
diastéréo-isomère 1876
diastole 1877
diathèse 1880
diathèse hémorragique 3042
dictionnaire des réactions indésirables 117
diencéphale 1881
diète 1882
diète athérogénique 480
diète restrictive 5866
diète sans sel 6004
diététicien 1886
diététique 1884
diététique 1885
différenciation 1890
différenciation de produit 5400
difforme 4234
difformité 13
difformité 1756
diffus 1892
diffuser 1891

diffusion 1893
diffusion de l'innovation 1894
digérer 1896
digestion 1897
dilatation 1903
dilatation 1905
dilatation capillaire 922
dilatation par ballonnet 589
dilater 3418
diLuer 1906
dimension 6274
dimensions 1907
diminué 3313
diminuer 7391
diminution 1908
diminution progressive de la dose 2019
dioptrie 1909
dioxyde de carbone 929
dipeptide 1910
diplocoque 1911
diploïdie 1912
diplopie 1913
directeur 1916
directeur 6688
directeur médical 4075
direction 3742
directives 3491
directives aux auteurs 3492
discours 6405
discussion 6803
discuter 6804
dislocation 1940
disloquer 1939
dispensaire 1944
dispersion 7247
dispersion graphique 6048
disposer en groupes 2921
dispositif anti-conceptionel intra-uterin 3578
disposition 1951
disqualificateur 1952

# French/Français

droit d'usage 7218
droitier 5937
du côlon 1290
du comportement 635
du métier 4614
duodénal 2090
duodénum 2092
duperie 1719
dure-mère 2093
durée 2094
durée de conservation 6207
durée du séjour 3766
durillon 1512
durillon 909
dysarthrie 2102
dyscinésie 2106
dyscinésie tardive 6814
dyscrasie 2103
dysenterie 2104
dysfonction 2105
dysfonction sexuelle 6187
dysfonctionnement du sommeil 6291
dyskinésie 2106
dyslexie 2107
dyslexique 2108
dyslexique 2109
dysménorrhée 2110
dyspepsie 2111
dysphagie 2112
dysphasie 2113
dysphorie 2114
dysplasie 2115
dysplasie bronchopulmonaire 869
dysplasie ectodermique 2138
dyspnée 2116
dyspnée d'effort 2412
dyspnée nocturne paroxystique 4877
dyspnéique 6215
dysrythmie 2117
dystonie 2118

dystrophie 2119
dysurie 2120
eau 7403
eau corporelle 800
eau distillée 1965
eau douce 2732
eau fraîche 2732
eaux d'égout 6180
écaille 6034
écailleux 6038
ecchymose 2127
échange 2397
échange fœto-maternel 4035
échantillon 1585
échantillon 6008
échantillon 6395
échantillon aléatoire 5639
échantillonnage 6012
échappement 2415
écharpe 6297
échauder 6033
échaudure 6032
échec 2501
échec de bon développement 2502
échec du traitement 7077
échelle 6034
échelle analogique visuelle 7348
échelle arithmétique 413
échelle d'anxiété manifeste 3991
échelle d'état psychiatrique 5492
échelle d'évaluation 5662
échelle de sévérité de la blessure 3450
échelle graduée 2894
échelle logarithmique 3861
échelle normalisée 6490
échelle standardisée 6490
échocardiographie 2128
échocardiographie Doppler 1998
échocardiographie 2129
échoencéphalographie 2130

écholalie 2131
éclampsie 2132
éclater 891
éclisse 6440
école 6059
écologie 2133
économe de maison 3147
économie 2136
économique 2136
écorcher 16
écorchure 17
écoulement 2632
écoulement de mucus 4333
écoulement nauséabond 2708
écran 6070
écrire 7477
ectoderme 2137
ectopie 2140
eczéma 2141
éditeur 2148
édition 2147
édition 3650
éditorial 2149
éducatif 2151
éducation spécialisée 6382
éducation 2150
éducation 7027
éducation de santé 2973
éducation de troisième cycle 2883
effectif 2153
effectuer un caryotype 3675
efférent 2155
effet 2152
effet d'entraînement 7028
effet de cohorte 1271
effet de premier passage 2609
effet de reste 980
effet épargnant 6375
effet placebo 5151
effet plafond 1026

effet réversible 5904
effet secondaire 6228
effet systémique 6781
effet tératogène 6865
efficace 2153
efficacité 2154
efficacité 2158
efficacité 2162
efficacité clinique 1199
efficacité-coût 1533
effluent 2163
effondrement 1284
effort 2411
effusion 2164
effusion pleurale 5181
effusion virale 7333
égalité 4872
égratigner 6069
égratignure 6068
éjaculation 2168
élaboration diagnostique 1868
élargissement 7446
élasticité 1354
élasticité 2172
élasticité 5836
élastique 2171
électrique 2176
électro-oculographie 2199
électro-encéphalogramme 2185
électro-encéphalographie 2186
électrocardiogramme, ECG 2178
électrocardiographie 2180
électrochimie 2181
électrochirurgie 2204
électrochoc 2203
électrocoagulation 2182
électroconvulsif 2183
électrode 2184
électrode implantée 3322
électrodes d'électrocardiogramme 2179

# French/Français

essai central 5148
essai clinique 1222
essai clinique ouvert 4659
essai contrôlé 1498
essai contrôlé avec placebo 5150
essai contrôlé et randomisé 5646
essai d'ensemencement 6099
essai d'équivalence 2332
essai d'étiquette ouverte 4661
essai dans un seul centre 6256
essai de confirmation 1411
essai de prévention primaire 5368
essai et erreur 7089
essai immunologique 5616
essai interprocessus 3463
essai médicamenteux multidose 4338
essai multicentrique 4337
essai pilote 5130
essai sur les êtres humains 3155
essai transversal 1586
essayer 6879
essence 2624
essentiel 2356
essuyer 7450
estérification 2357
estimation 2358
estimation 463
estimer 2359
estomac 6556
établir la priorité 5374
établissement d'un programme 6051
établissement du stade 6476
établissement du stade d'une néoplasie 6477
étalon 6485
étalon argent 6248
étalonnage 906
étancher 5586
étape clinique 1216
état 1395
état 6500

état 6509
état acide-base 51
état clinique 1217
état de décérébration 1720
état de santé 2979
état fonctionnel 2748
état matrimonial 4001
état mental 4137
état nutrionnel 4581
état po teur 978
état stable 6511
étendre 6456
étendu 5453
étendu 5691
étendu 5710
étendue 6455
étendue de mouvement 5648
étendue des doses 2014
éternuement 6323
éternuement 6325
éternuer 6324
éther 2362
éthique 2366
éthologie 2370
étiologie 2371
étiquetage du matériel clinique 3698
étiquetage restrictif 5868
étiquette 3696
étiquette d'affinité 135
étiquette de centrifuger 6421
étirer 3590
étoilé 6519
étourderie 2694
étrange 4622
étranger 2687
étrangement 1443
étrangement 6574
étranger 6573
être en incubation 3361
étude 6606

étude à deux parties 7131
étude clinique 1219
étude clinique 2588
étude comparative 1327
étude contrôlée 1498
étude d'observation 4595
étude dans une communauté 1321
étude de cas 988
étude de cas témoin 983
étude de cohorte 1272
étude de commission 4823
étude de comparabilité 1326
étude de compatibilité 1335
étude de conduction nerveuse 4448
étude de diffusion 1895
étude de première phase 5065
étude de reproduction 5818
étude de suivi 2669
étude diagnostique 1866
étude équilibrée 585
étude ouverte 4662
étude pharmacocinétique 5050
étude prospective 5450
étude rétrospective 5896
étude spécialisée 6387
étude stratifiée 6579
étude transversale 1587
étude vite faite 5588
études de prix 5359
étudiant 6605
étudier 3599
eugénique 2372
euphorie 2373
euthanasie 2375
évacuer 2376
évacuer 4693
évacuer 7366
évaluable 2377
évaluation 2378
évaluation 463

évaluation Apgar 375
évaluation clinique globale 2854
évaluation commune 3665
évaluation d'invalidité 1919
évaluation de l'exécution 4981
évaluation de sécurité 5991
évaluation du rendement 4981
évaluation globale 2860
évaluation psychométrique 5500
évanouissement 7161
évanouissement 728
éveil 417
événement adverse grave 616C
événement clinique 1201
événement défavorable inattendu 7168
événement primaire 5364
événement secondaire 6085
événements modifiant la vie 3737
éventrer 891
éversion 2381
évidence 2384
éviscération 2385
évolution 2387
évulsion 2388
exacerbation 2389
exactitude 40
examen 2390
examen 2391
examen 5906
examen à microscope 4182
examen avec une lampe à fente 6301
examen de base 608
examen de contrôle 2667
examen de la littérature 5908
examen des systèmes 5909
examen du patient 4927
examen et interrogatoire 6072
examen gastroscopique 2793
examen médical 1087
examen paramétrique 4845

French/Français

examen pelvien bimanuel 673
examen physique 5095
examen rectal 5708
examiner 3599
examiner 5907
exanthémateux 2393
exanthème 2392
exanthème 5656
excellent 2394
excentricité 5591
excès de reportage 4771
excessif 2396
excipient 2399
exciser 2400
excision 2401
excitabilité 2402
excitant 6546
excitation (sexuelle) 417
excitation 2403
exclure 5975
excoriation 6068
excorier 6069
excrément 2405
excrément 799
excrétion 2406
excrétion biliaire 669
excrétion d'urine 7208
exécution 4980
exécution d'une tâche 6819
exercer 2408
exercice 2407
exercice physique 5096
exercice respiratoire 852
exfoliation 2413
exhalation 2414
exhiber 2416
exigence 5821
exigence de la taille d'un échantillon 6011
exigences d'autorisation 3791
existence 6645

exocrine 2417
exocytose 2419
exogène 2420
exon 2421
exophtalmie 2422
exotoxine 2423
expansion 2424
expectant 2425
expectorant 2427
expectoration 6463
expectorer 6434
expérience 2430
expérience 2432
expérience clinique 1202
expérience d'entrecroisement 1593
expérimental 2434
expérimenter 2433
expert 2436
expiration 2438
expiratoire 2440
exploration 2441
exposer à grands traits 4758
exposition antérieure 568
exposition 2442
expression 2443
expulser 2470
expulsion 2445
exsanguiner 2446
exsanguino-transfusion 2398
exsanguino-transfusion de sang complet 7443
exsudat 2472
exsudation 7418
extenseur 2450
extension 2448
extension 6589
extension de ligne 3822
extérieur 2687
extérieur 4629
externe 2451
extirpation 2452

extra-corporel 2454
extracellulaire 2453
extraction 2457
extraction 555
extraction de cataracte 998
extrahépatique 2458
extraire 2456
extrait 2455
extrait 25
extrapolation 2461
extrapolation de données 1675
extrapolation des données 2462
extrasystole 2464
extrasystole 5317
extravasation 2465
extravasculaire 2466
extrémité 2468
extrémité 3815
extrinsèque 2469
extubation 2471
fabricant à contrat 1477
fabricant forfaitaire 1477
fabrication 3998
fabrication 5397
fabrication 5405
facial 2484
faciès d'allure masquée 4013
faciès lunaire 4287
facilitation 2488
facilité 2489
facteur 2493
facteur d'activation 63
facteur de confusion 1416
facteur de croissance 2925
facteur de croissance transformant 7051
facteur de relaxation 5779
facteur de risque 5945
facteur de temps 6951
facteur environnemental 2299
facteur natriurétique 4412

facteur non-spécifique 4526
facteur sanguin 764
facteur socioéconomique 6338
faculté 2497
faculté de médecine 4082
fade 731
Fahrenheit 2499
faible 2085
faible 2716
faible 7411
faiblesse 1712
faiblesse 2504
faiblesse 7412
faim 3161
faire des plans 5423
faire des pulvérisations 6454
faire la moyenne de 550
faire mauvais usage 4238
faire une conférence 3752
faire une incision 6300
faire une incision dans 3345
faire une ponction 6812
faire une scanographie 6040
faisabilité 2534
faisceau de His 885
faiseur d'opinion 4679
faiseur de pensée 6916
fait 2491
fait de mieux 6501
falsification 1548
falsifié 6462
falsifier 6806
familial 2513
famille 2514
fantasme 1781
fascia 2518
fasciculation 2520
fatal 2526
fatigue 2527
fatigue 7414

406

407

# French/Français

411

ingrédient 3431
ingrédient actif 67
inguérissable 3365
inguinal 3432
inhalant 3434
inhalation 3435
inhalation de fumée 6316
inhaler 3436
inhérent 3437
inhibiteur 3441
inhibition 3440
initiales 3444
initialisation d'une session 3863
initiation 3445
injecté de sang 783
injecter 3446
injection 3448
injection intraveineuse continue 1468
inné 3340
inné 3452
innerver 3454
innocent 3455
innovation 3457
inoculer 3458
inoffensif 3456
inopérable 3459
inotrope 3460
inquiétude 5862
inscription 2286
inscription 5743
insecte 3468
insecticide 3469
insémination 3470
insémination artificielle 447
insensible 3472
inséré 3474
insertion 3473
insidieux 3475
insolation 6681
insoluble 3476

insomnie 3477
insomnie 6294
insomnie 7385
inspection 3478
inspiration 3479
inspiratoire 3480
inspirer 3481
instabilité 3482
instable 7188
installation 2489
installation de production 5406
installation de santé 2974
instillation 3483
instinct 2049
instinct 3484
institut 3485
institution 3486
institution mère 4864
institutionnalisation 3490
institutionnel 3487
instruction 3748
instruction 6828
instructions 3491
instrument 3493
instrument chirurgical 6715
instrument de recherche 5826
instrumentation 3494
insuffisance 2501
insuffisance 3495
insuffisance cardiaque 2990
insuffisance cardiaque congestive 1423
insuffisance hépatique 3852
insuffisance mitrale 4248
insuffisance rénale 5793
insuffisance ventriculaire gauche 3757
insuffler 3497
insuline 3498
insulino-dépendant 3499
intégration 3504
intégration verticale 7311

intégrité 3505
intellect 3507
intelligence 3508
intelligence artificielle 448
intelligence épidémiologique 2310
intempérance 3512
intensif 3514
intensification 3359
intensification de dose 2011
intensifier 3360
intensité de la réaction 3513
interaction 3519
interaction alimentaire 2674
interaction médicamenteuse 2067
interaction sperme-ovule 6412
intercostal 3522
interculturel 578
interdisciplinaire 3524
interface par ordinateur 1375
interféron 3525
intérim 3526
intérimaire 3527
intermittent 3529
interna 3539
interna 5832
international 3535
interne 3442
interne 3614
internes 3146
interneurone 3537
interniste 3538
interphase 3540
interprétation 3541
interprétation de données 1680
interprétation erronée de données 1682
interréaction 583
interréactivité 1584
interréagir 1582
interrompu 1927
interruption 1926

interruption de l'axe 843
interruption de la méthode en aveugle 844
interstice 3542
interstitiel 3543
intertolérance 1589
intervalle 3544
intervalle de confiance 1406
intervalle de dose 2012
interva le du temps 6952
interva les de naissance 715
interven-tion 3546
intervention de crise 1572
interventriculaire 3548
interventi 3597
interview 3550
interviewer 3551
intestin 2933
intestin 3556
intestin 824
intestin grêle 6307
intestinal 3552
intima 3557
intolérance 3558
intolérance à la chaleur 3005
intolérance alimentaire 2675
intolérance au froid 1277
intolérant 3559
intoxication 3560
intoxication à la caféine 897
intoxication alimentaire 2676
intoxication au mercure 4140
intoxication aux métaux lourds 3010
intra-artériel 3561
intra-articulaire 3562
intra-oculaire 3571
intracellulaire 3563
intradermique 3565
intrahépatique 3566
intralésionnel 3567
intramural 3568

| | | | |
|---|---|---|---|
| lubrifiant 3900 | macule 3949 | maladie d'origine inconnue 1933 | maniaque-dépressif 3989 |
| lucide 3901 | macule 6450 | maladie de Crohn 5740 | manie 3988 |
| lumbago 3885 | maculo-papule 3950 | maladie de la paupière 2480 | manifestation 1947 |
| lumière 3810 | magnésium 3952 | maladie de spécialité 1934 | manifestation 3992 |
| lumière 3908 | maigre 3747 | maladie dégénérative 1761 | manifeste 390 |
| lumière du soleil 6679 | maigre 5220 | maladie disséminée 1955 | manifester 1948 |
| luminescence 3910 | maigreur 6907 | maladie du sérum 6176 | manipulation 2949 |
| luminescence chimique 1099 | main 2947 | maladie fibrokystique 2579 | manomètre 3993 |
| lunettes 2477 | main-d'oeuvre 3995 | maladie héréditaire 3439 | manométrie 3994 |
| lunettes 2854 | main d'oeuvre 7461 | maladie infectieuse 3405 | manoeuvre 3986 |
| lunettes 6399 | maintenir 6731 | maladie mentale 4135 | manoeuvrer 3987 |
| lutéinisation 3919 | maintien 3956 | maladie pulmonaire obstructive chronique 1151 | manquant 20 |
| luxation 1940 | maison 3110 | maladie rare 5655 | manquant 4235 |
| lymphadénopathie 3925 | maison de soins infirmiers 4575 | maladie sous-jacente 7163 | manque de mémoire 2694 |
| lymphadénopathie régionale 5741 | mal 3960 | maladie terminale 6873 | manque de travail 7166 |
| lymphatique 3926 | mal 6226 | maladie transmise sexuellement, MTS 6194 | manuel 3996 |
| lymphe 3922 | mal de dents 6992 | maladie transmissible 1318 | manuel 6884 |
| lymphocytaire 3930 | mal de dos 566 | maladie vénérienne 7281 | manuel d'utilisation 3997 |
| lymphocyte 3928 | mal de gorge 6365 | maladif 7169 | manufacture 3998 |
| lymphocyte B 562 | mal de tête 2965 | malaise 1925 | manutention des spécimens 6397 |
| lymphocyte T 6789 | mal des caissons 640 | malaise 2504 | marchand en gros 7445 |
| lymphocytose 3931 | mal des transports 4312 | malaise 3965 | marche 6524 |
| lymphoïde 3932 | malabsorption 3961 | mâle 5582 | marché 4004 |
| lymphome 3933 | malacie 3962 | mâle 3966 | marcher 7388 |
| lymphoprolifératif 3934 | malade 3588 | mâle 3967 | marge (sur)élevée 2208 |
| lyophilisation 2724 | malade 3589 | malformation 13 | marge 817 |
| lyophilisation 3935 | malade 4920 | malformation 3969 | mariage 4008 |
| lyophilisé 2725 | malade en consultation externe 4759 | malin 3970 | marketing 4006 |
| lyse 3937 | maladie 1344 | malin 3971 | marque 7024 |
| lyser 3936 | maladie 1932 | malnutrition 3974 | marque brevetée 5444 |
| lysogénie 3938 | maladie 3272 | malocclusion 3975 | marque d'affinité 135 |
| lysosome 3939 | maladie 3964 | malsain 7169 | marque de fabrication 842 |
| lytique 3940 | maladie 6226 | mamelon 4496 | marque déposée 7025 |
| macération 3941 | maladie cardiaque 2989 | mamelon 6834 | marqué radioactivement 5619 |
| mâchoire 3656 | maladie cardiovasculaire 963 | mammaire 3979 | marques d'hachures 2958 |
| macrocéphalie 3943 | maladie chronique 1150 | mammifère 3978 | marqueur 4003 |
| macrocyte 3944 | maladie coexistante 1264 | mammogramme 3980 | marqueur physiologique 5109 |
| macroglobuline 3945 | maladie concomitante 1392 | mammographie 3981 | masculin 4010 |
| macrophage 3946 | maladie cyclique 1638 | mandibule 3984 | masochisme 4014 |
| macula 3949 | maladie d'accumulation 6568 | manger 2125 | masque 4011 |

416

French/Français

métaphore 4160
métastase 4161
métastatique 4162
méthémoglobine 4164
méthode 4165
méthode à deux médecins 7133
méthode en aveugle 742
méthode séro-épidémiologique 6162
méthode statistique 6504
méthodes multivariées 4348
méthylation 4166
mètre 4163
mettre à l'épreuve 6879
mettre bas 3850
mettre en abduction 8
mettre en adduction 80
mettre en quarantaine 5585
mettre en supination 6689
mettre un bandage sur 591
micro-électrode 4176
micro-onde 4192
micro-ordinateur 4175
micro-organisme 4180
micro-injection 4178
microbe 4167
microbiologie 4171
microbiologiste 4170
microcéphale 4173
microchirurgie 4187
microcirculation 4174
microfiche 4177
micron 4179
microscope 4181
microscope électronique 2193
microscope électronique de balayage 6042
microscope optique 3812
microscopie 4184
microscopie électronique 2194
microsome 4185
microsphère 4186

microtome 4188
microtubule 4189
microvasculaire 4190
microvilli 4191
miction 7208
midi 4532
migraine 4202
migrateur 4203
migration 4204
migratoire 4205
milieu 4094
milieu 4210
milieu de culture 1613
militaire 4211
milligramme 4213
millimètre 4214
minéral 4216
minéral 4217
minéralocorticoïde 4218
miniaturisation 4219
minimum 4220
misanthropie 4225
miscible 4228
mise en code 1260
mise en commun de données 1686
mise en mémoire de données 1692
misogamie 4231
misogynie 4232
mission 4236
mite 4239
mitochondrial 4241
mitochondrie 4240
mitogène 4242
mitose 4244
mitotique 4245
mitral 4247
mobilité 4256
modalité 4257
mode 4258
mode d'administration de drogue 2061

modelage par ordinateur 1376
modèle 4259
modèle 4939
modèle 6848
modèle à deux compartiment 7130
modèle à un compartiment 4645
modèle animal 288
modèle de prescription 5331
modèle de réponse 4940
modèle linéaire 3826
modèle linéaire logarithmique 3869
modèle logistique 3867
modèle mathématique 4038
modéré 4262
modérer 4261
modification de protocole 5469
modifié 4263
moelle épinière 6424
moelle 4009
moelle osseuse 812
moelleux 6343
mois 4286
moisissure 4267
molaire 4266
môle 4268
môle 4268
moléculaire 4269
molécule 4272
moment dans le temps 6953
moment de calme 3902
mondial 7467
moniliase 4273
moniteur 4274
moniteur clinique 1208
moniteur clinique 2586
moniteur de clinique 1190
moniteur de données 1684
moniteur de Holter 3109
moniteur de l'essai 7093
moniteur fœtal 2562

monitorage 4276
monoamine biogénique 690
monoclonal 4279
monocyte 4281
monoinsaturé 4284
monomanie 4282
monothérapie 4283
monoxyde de carbone 930
monozygote 4285
montrer 1948
moral 4288
moral 4289
morbide 4290
morbidité 4292
morceau 2714
morceau de bois 6540
mordre 724
morgue 4294
moribond 4295
morose 4299
morphogénèse 4300
morphologie 4301
morsure 723
mort 1704
mort 1708
mort 2100
mort cérébrale 835
mort subite 6664
mort subite cardiaque 6663
mort subite du nourrisson 1540
mort subite du nourrisson 1568
mort subite du nourrisson 6665
mortalité 4303
mortalité par cause spécifique 1019
mortel 2526
mortel 3771
mortel 4302
mosaïque 4306
mosaïsme 4307
mot à mot 7299

418

neuropathie 4472
neuroscience 4473
neurosécrétoire 4474
neurotoxine 4479
neurotransmetteur 4480
neutralisation 4482
neutraliser 1546
neutre 4481
neutron 4484
neutropénie 4485
neutrophile 4486
névralgie 4461
névralgie du trijumeau 7098
névrome 4467
névrose 4475
névrose obsessionnelle 4601
névrotique 4477
névrotique 4478
nez 4545
niveau 3782
niveau d'anesthésie 3784
niveau de conscience 3785
niveau macroscopique 3942
niveau plasmatique 5161
niveau plasmatique maximal 4944
niveau sanguin 767
nocicepteur 4499
nociception 4498
nocif 4553
nocturne 4501
nodule 4505
nodule osseux 816
nodule xanthomateux 7481
nom 4394
nom chimique 1095
nom commercial 7024
nom commun 7106
nom générique 4765
nombre du lot 3880
nombres aléatoires 5638

nombril 4422
nomenclature 4508
nominal 4509
nomogramme 4511
non compliqué 7156
non conjugué 7157
non contrôlé 7162
non miscible 3284
non naturel 7184
non saturé 7185
non spécifié 7187
non uni 7189
non-aléatoire 4524
non-estérifié 4516
non-évaluable 4517
non-insulinodépendant 4518
non-médicament 4515
non-pénétrant 4522
non-répondeur 4525
non-stéroïdien 4527
non-union 4529
non-viable 4531
noradrénaline 4533
noradrénergique 4534
norépinéphrine 4535
normal 4536
normal 6486
norme de référence 5722
norme éthique 2365
normochrome 4541
normocytaire 4542
normotensif 4543
nosocomial 4547
nosologie 4549
note de progrès 5418
note en bas de la page 2679
notification 4550
nourri au biberon 821
nourri au sein 846
nourrisson 6661

nourriture 2672
nourriture 4577
nouveau-né 3398
nouveau-né 4489
nouvelle approche 4552
nouvelle entité chimique 4488
noyau caudé 1015
noyau cyclique 5941
nœud 4503
nœud auriculo-ventriculaire 497
nœud sino-auriculaire 6261
nœud sinusal 6261
nu 4562
nucléaire 4555
nucléole 4559
nucléosome 4560
nucléus 4561
nuisible 1772
nuisible 4553
nuit 4491
nuit 4495
numération cellulaire du sang 757
numération des globules rouges 5715
numération différentielle 1888
numéro 4566
numéro d'identification 3258
numéro d'identification du patient 4928
numéro de patient 4929
numéro de protocole 5471
numéro du lot 615
nutrition 4578
nutritionnel 4579
nutritionniste 4582
nycturie 4500
nylon 4584
nystagmus 4585
obèse 4586
obèse 4773
obésité 4587
obésité morbide 4291

obésité pathologique 4291
objectif 158
objectif 2875
objectif 4588
objectif 6815
objectif clinique 1200
objectif primaire 5366
objectif secondaire 6087
objectif social 1520
objectif spécifique faible 6344
objectif spécifique majeur 2955
obligations des investigateurs 4590
obligations des répondants 4591
oblique 4592
oblique 6276
observateur 4598
observation 4593
observation anecdotique 265
observation répétée 5802
obsession 4599
obsessionnel 4600
obstétrical 4602
obstétrique 4603
obstructif 4605
obstruction 4604
obturation 752
obturation 3451
obturation 4606
occipital 4607
occiput 4608
occlusion 4609
occlusion 723
occlusion fécale 2536
occlusif 4610
occulte 4611
occupation 4613
occupation des lits 626
oculaire 4618
oculaire 4619
oculomoteur 4621

423

phase 1 5064
phase 4992
phase 5063
phase 6475
phase après l'étude 5254
phase de repos 5860
phase lutéale 3918
phases de sommeil 6292
phénomène 5067
phénomène de la roue dentée 1268
phénomène secondaire 6151
phénotype 5068
phéromone 5069
phlébite 5070
phlébotomie 5071
phobie 5073
phonation 5075
phonétique 5076
phonocardiographie 5077
phosphore 5078
photochimie 5080
photocopie 5081
photocopier 5082
photographie 5083
photographier 5084
photophobie 5085
photosensibilité 5087
photosensible 3814
photosensible 5086
photothérapie 5089
phrénique 5090
phrénologie 5091
physiologie 5111
physiologique 5108
physionomie 5106
physiothérapie 5102
physiothérapie 5112
physique 5092
physique 5105
pic 4942

pica 5114
picacisme 5114
picogramme 5115
picotement 6964
pie-mère 5113
pièce transdermique 7038
pied 2677
pied tombant 2678
piège 5141
pierre 6557
pigment 5119
pigment sanguin 768
pigmentation 5120
pile 619
pile de globules rouges 5964
pilomoteur 5127
pilule 5123
pilule anticonceptionnelle 713
pilulier 5124
pince hémostatique 1171
pincer 1172
pinéal 5132
pipette 5138
piqûre 6550
placebo 5149
placebo apparié 4033
placenta 5152
plaie 6364
plaie 7472
plan 1837
plan 4757
plan 6050
plan aponéurotique 2519
plan carré latin 3733
plan d'urgence 1461
plan de l'essai 7091
plan de l'étude 6610
plan de la facilité 2490
plan du fascia 2519
plan séquentiel 6156

planificateur 5155
planification de santé 2977
planisme familiale 2516
plantaire 5157
plante 5156
plante comestible 2144
plante du pied 6351
plante médicinale 4091
plaque 5158
plaque 5169
plaque de croissance 2927
plaque épiphysaire 2322
plaque osseuse 813
plaque terminale 2252
plaquette 5170
plaquette 6923
plaquette 746
plaquette sanguine 769
plasma 5159
plasmaphérèse 5162
plasmide 5163
plasmine 5164
plasticité 5168
plastique 5165
plastique 5166
plat 3783
platine 5174
plâtre 989
pléthore 5177
pléthysmographie 5178
pléthysmographie pancorporelle 7444
pleur 1600
pleurer 4319
pleurésie 5182
pleurs 7418
plèvre 5179
plexus 5183
plexus choroïdien 1144
plexus lombo-sacré 3907
plexus solaire 6350

pl 2659
plier 2660
plomb 3741
pneumocoque 5184
pneumonie 5185
pneumonie d'aspiration 460
pneumonie lobaire 3855
pneumonite 5186
pneumothorax 5187
poche 5188
poche 5275
poche 5980
podologie 5189
pods 7419
pods à la naissance 718
pods corporel 801
pods insuffisant 7165
pods moléculaire 4271
pods spécifique 6392
poignarder 6469
poignet 7476
poïkilocytose 5190
poil 2938
poils corporels 793
point 2026
point 6398
point dans le temps 6953
point de décision 1728
point de repère 1685
point de suture 6552
point final 2277
point final substitut 6721
pointage brut 5671
pointe 6417
pointe-onde 6418
poison 5194
poitrine 845
poli 6319
politique 5198
politique 5201

424

politique publique 5521
pollen 5202
polluant 5203
pollution 5204
poly-insaturé 5217
polyamine biogénique 691
polyarthrite 5205
polycystique 5206
polycythémie 5207
polydipsie 5208
polygraphe 5209
polymère 5210
polymorphisme génétique 2823
polymyosite 5211
polynévrite 5212
polype 5213
polyphagie 5214
polypharmacie 5215
polyploïdie 5216
polyurie 5218
pommade 4632
pompe 5544
pompe à l'infusion 3429
pompe à proton 5475
pompe ionique 3619
pomper 5545
ponction 5547
ponction 6811
ponction lombaire 3906
ponction lombaire 6426
ponction spinale 6426
ponction veineuse 7282
ponctionner 6812
pont 5219
pontage 894
pontage artériel 433
pontage cardiopulmonaire 956
pontage coronaire 1518
pontage coronarien 1518
poplité 5221

population 5222
population de malades spéciaux 6383
population générale 2810
pore 5223
poreux 5224
porphyrine 5225
porte 5226
portée 3849
portée moyenne 4200
portefeuille 5229
portafolio 5229
porteur 976
positif 5232
position 508
position 5230
positionner 5231
posologie 5234
possédant le pouvoir rotatoire 1122
possibilité 1076
post mortem 5247
post-natal 5249
post partum 5251
post-anesthésie 5236
post-coït 5237
post-convulsion 5243
post-dose 5233
post-essai 5258
post-essai 5259
post-ganglionnaire 5241
post-ménopausique 5246
post-mise en marché 5244
post-nasal 5248
post-traitement 5256
post-traitement 5257
postérieur 5240
postérieur 5976
posthume 5242
postmarketing 5244
postopératoire 5250
postprandial 5252

postpubère 5253
postsynaptique 5255
postulat 5260
postuler 5261
postural 5262
posture 5265
posture assise 6270
potable 5266
potassium 5267
potentiation 5272
potentiel 5270
potentiel 5271
potentiel d'abus 27
potentiel d'action 61
potentiel de membrane 4109
potentiel évoqué 2386
potentiel évoqué visuel 7349
potentiométrie 5273
potion 5274
pou 3884
pouce 6935
poudre 5278
poudre stérile 6532
pouls 5540
pouls artériel 424
pouls bigéminé 663
pouls paradoxal 4837
poumon 3913
pour cent 4966
pourcentage 4966
pourcentage 4970
pourcentage cumulatif 1617
pourcentage de la réponse maximale 4968
pourcentage du changement 4967
pourcentage du total 4969
pourrir 1717
poursuite pour négligence professionnelle 3977
pousse 6458
pousser 6459
poussière 2095

pratique 5282
pratique dentaire 1798
pratique facultaire 2498
pratique médicale 4078
pratique privée 5378
pratique professionnelle 5409
pratiquer la vivisection 7360
pré-éclampsie 5303
préanesthésique 5286
précancéreux 5287
précaution 5288
précautions universelles 7179
précédent 5289
précédent 5373
préceptorat 5290
précipitant 5291
précipitation 5292
précision 40
précision 5293
préclinique 5294
précoce 5295
précurseur 5298
prédiabétique 5299
prédictif 5301
prédiction 5300
prédisposé 5434
prédisposition 5302
prédisposition 6728
préexistant 5357
préganglionnaire 5305
préimplantation 5310
préinfusion 5311
préinjection 5312
préjudice 5313
préjugé 655
prélèvement d'échantillons sanguins 775
prémarketing 5315
prématuré 5316
prématurité 5320
prémédication 5321

428

risque de base 609
risque de dépendance 1808
risque excessif 2395
risque relatif 4623
risque relatif 5774
risquer 5943
robinet 6811
robotique 5950
robustesse 5951
Roentgen 5954
ronchis 5927
ronflement 6328
ronfler 6329
rongeur 5952
rongeur 5953
Röntgen 5954
rotation 5960
rotation 6419
rotation d'inventaire 3593
rotation optique 4686
rotule 4902
rougir 2649
rouleau 5964
roulement de personnel 5020
route 5967
routine 5970
routinier 5971
rubicond 6015
rubrique 6631
rudimentaire 5974
rupture 5978
rural 5979
rythme 5928
rythme alpha 201
rythme cardiaque 949
rythme circadien 1164
rythme de galop 2766
rythme nodal 4502
s'affaisser 1285
s'affoler 4825

s'apaiser 6642
s'effondrer 1285
s'enflammer 2621
s'étrangler 1127
s'évanouir 2503
sac 5980
sac amniotique 583
saccade 5981
saccade 7129
sacro-iliaque 5983
sacro-lombaire 5984
sacrum 5985
sadisme 5986
sado-masochisme 5987
sage-femme 4201
sagittal 5996
saigrée 782
saignement de nez 4546
sain 2980
sain 6014
saiscnnier 6078
salin 5998
salin hypertonique 3212
salir 6349
salivaire 6001
salive 6000
salive 6433
salle d'hôpital 7392
salle d'opération 4668
salle d'urgence 2229
salutaire 6005
sanatorium 6013
sang 753
sang autologue 533
sang complet 7442
sang occulte 4612
sang total 7442
sanglant 784

sanglot 6331
sangloter 6332
sangsue 3753
sanguin 6015
sanitaire 6016
sans abris 3112
sans assurance médicale 4085
sans douleur 4797
sans failles 2500
sans myéline 7183
sans ordonnance 4523
santé 2968
santé d'esprit 6020
santé générale 4766
santé globale 4766
santé holistique 3108
santé mentale 4132
santé professionnelle 4615
santé publique 5520
sarcome 6021
satiété 6026
satiété 6027
satisfaction 6029
satisfaction de la vie 3799
saturation d'oxygène artériel 423
saturé 6030
sauvetage 5822
saveur 2623
saveur 6820
savon 6330
scalpel 6037
scan par tomographie d'émission positronique 5028
scanographie 6039
scanographie 6041
scansion 6043
scatologie 6047
scellé thermocontractile 3008
schéma 6052
schéma 6054

schématique 6053
schizoïde 6055
schizophrène 6057
schizophrénie 6056
sciatique 6060
science 6061
scientifique 6062
scientifique 6064
sclérotique 6065
scoliose 6066
score ajusté à la tendance 7082
score d'efficacité 2160
score de changement 1080
score de comportement 633
scotome 6067
scrotum 6075
se flétrir 6219
se gangrener 4305
se gargariser 2779
se gélifier 2801
se mettre en contact 1451
se mouvoir soudainement 3651
se pencher en arrière 638
se pencher en avant 639
se promener 7388
se ratatiner 6219
se remettre 5711
se répandre sur 6669
se rétablir 5711
séance 5270
secondaire 6083
secours 5822
sécréter 6089
sécrétion 1921
sécrétion 3650
sécrétion 6090
sécrétion biliaire 668
secteur privé 5379
secteur publique 5523

431

stat 6499
statistique 6503
statistique 6507
statistique de Bayes 620
statistiquement signifiant 6506
statistiques démographiques 7355
statistiques descriptives 1831
stature 6508
status quo 6510
stéatorrhée 6516
stellaire 6519
stelles liquides 7407
sténose 6523
sténose mitrale 4249
sténose valvulaire 7242
stéréoisomère 6526
stéréosélectif 6527
stéréotype 6530
stérie 3407
stérile 6531
stérilisation 6534
stérilisation tubaire 7116
stérilisé 455
stérilité 6533
sternocostoclaviculaire 6535
sternum 6536
stéroïde 6537
stéroïde 6538
stéroïdes anabolisants 237
stéroïdien 6538
stéthoscope 6539
stigmate 6543
stimulant 6546
stimulateur cardiaque 4788
stimulation 1074
stimulation 6548
stimulation photique 5079
stimulation répétée 5689
stimuler 6547
stimulus 6549

stomate 6555
stomatite aphteuse 379
strabisme 6467
strabisme 6569
strate 3739
stratégie 6575
stratégie clinique 1218
stratification 6576
stratifier 6580
stratum 6581
streptocoque 6585
stress 6586
stricture 6593
stridor 6595
strie 6582
strie 6591
stroma 6599
strontium 6601
structural 6602
structure 2718
structure 6603
structure chimique 1097
structure organisationnelle 4710
structure protéique 5461
stupeur 6612
style de vie 3800
style en paires appariées 4032
subaigu 6616
subchronique 6619
subclinique 6621
subconscient 6622
subdiviser 6624
subir 6667
subir une mutation 4363
subjectif 6632
sublimation 6635
subliminal 6636
sublingual 6637
subordonné 263
subsidiaire 6643

subsistance 6645
substance 4041
substance 6646
substance blanche 7440
substance cancérigène 935
substance cancérogène 935
substance chimique 1091
substance dangereuse 2961
substance grise 2912
substance noire 6649
substance nutritive 4576
substances biocompatibles 685
substantia nigra 6649
substantiel 6650
substituer 6652
substitut 6651
substitut 6719
substitut 6720
substitution thérapeutique 6884
subtil 6862
suburbain 6657
subvention 2902
suc gastrique 2787
succédané 6719
succession 6658
succion 6659
succion 6662
sucre 6670
suer 6739
sueur 6738
sueur nocturne 4493
suffocant 2783
suffoquer 6542
suffoquer 6668
suggestion 6671
suicidaire 6672
suicide 6673
suintant 4654
suintement infect 2708
suite 6150

suite 6152
suite 6658
suivre 7016
suivre de près 2664
suivre un régime 1883
su et 6630
su fonamides 6675
su per-infection 6685
su percherie 2720
su perficiel 6683
su périeur 6686
su pplément 6691
su pport d'entraînement 7029
su ppositoire 6696
su ppresseur 6699
su ppression 6698
su ppression génétique 2825
su pprimer 6697
su ppuratif 6700
su ppuration 2557
su ppuration 6701
su ppurer 2558
su pra-ventriculaire 6704
su pra-rénal 6703
su pra-rénal 6703
su prapubien 6702
su r pied 6491
su r place 4650
su ral 6705
su rcharge 4770
su rdité 1707
su rdose 4767
su rdose intentionnelle 3518
su rdoser 4768
su rface 6706
su rface articulaire 443
su rface corporelle 797
su ractant pulmonaire 5533
su rimposé 6684
su rinfection 1581
su rinfection 6685

434

# French/Français

technique bactériologique 577
technique cytologique 1646
technique de dilution avec indicateur 3375
technique de relaxation 5778
technique de soustraction 6656
technique Delphi 1778
technique stéréotaxique 6528
technologie 6837
technologie d'information 3423
technologie de libération contrôlée 1497
tégument 3506
tégument 6839
tégumentaire 6840
teigne 6963
teindre 2099
teindre 6480
teint 1353
teinture 2098
teinture 6962
télangiectasie 6841
télencéphale 6842
télépathie 6843
témoin historique 3103
tempe 6849
tempérament 6846
température 6847
température corporelle 798
temporaire 6851
temporal 6850
temps 6947
temps d'acceptation 400
temps de circulation 1167
temps de coagulation 1241
temps de coagulation 1249
temps de prothrombine 5466
temps de saignement 737
temps de thromboplastine 6930
temps de thromboplastine partiel 4882
temps et événements 6949
temps jusqu'à l'effet maximal 6954

temps jusqu'à l'effet maximal 6956
temps jusqu'à la rechute 6958
temps jusqu'à la récupération 6957
temps jusqu'au début de l'effet 6955
tendance 6853
tendance 7081
tendance future 2759
tendances passées 4899
tendinite 6856
tendon 6252
tendon 6857
tendre 6854
ténesme 6859
tension 6586
tension 6861
tentative de suicide 503
ténu 6862
tératogène 6863
tératologie 6866
tératome 6867
terme 6868
terme préféré 5304
termes anatomiques 260
terminaison 6874
terminaison de l'essai 7095
terminaison nerveuse 4449
terminal 6869
terminal 6870
terminal d'ordinateur 1378
terminal intelligent 3511
terminal muet 2088
termination 1234
terminologie 6875
terne 2085
testament 7447
testicule 6881
tétanie 6882
tête 2962
téine 6834
texte 6883

texte 6884
thalamique 6886
thalamus 6887
théorie 6890
théorie décisionnelle 1729
théorie 6888
thérapeutique 6891
thérapeutique 6896
thérapie 6897
thérapie comportementale 634
thérapie d'aversion 552
thérapie de chélation 1090
thérapie de deuxième ligne 6080
thérapie de première ligne 2607
thérapie de remplacement 5806
thérapie de sauvetage 6006
thérapie maritale 4002
thérapie occupationnelle 4617
thérapie orthomoléculaire 4720
thérapie physique 5102
thérapie thrombolytique 6928
thermique 6898
thermodilution 6900
thermodynamique 6901
thermogramme 6902
thermographie 6903
thermomètre 6904
thésaurismose 6568
thoracentèse 6912
thoracique 6913
thorax 1106
thorax 6915
thorax en tonneau 597
thrombo-embolie 6926
thrombo-phlébite 6929
thrombocyte 6923
thrombocytopénie 6924
thrombocytose 6925
thrombolyse 6927
thrombopénie 6924

thrombose 6931
thrombose veineuse profonde 1744
thrombotique 6932
thrombus 6933
thymus 6936
thyroïde 6937
tibia 6940
tibial 6941
tic 6942
tic 7129
tige 6482
tige 6520
tir ea 6963
tir nitus 6965
tintement d'oreilles 6965
ticue 6943
tissu 6966
tissu calleux 3132
tissu conjonctif 1430
tissu germinal 2843
tissu mou 6347
tittage biologique 693
titre 6969
titre 6970
titre d'anticorps 324
titrer 6971
toilette 6975
tolérance 6976
tolérance 6977
tolérance à l'exercice 2410
tolérer 6978
tomber 6642
tomographie 6979
tomographie assistée par ordinateur 1379
tomographie axiale par ordinateur 1372
tomographie cérébrale 836
tomographie d'émission par ordinateur 2234
tomographie par ordinateur 1369
tomographie par ordinateur 7487
ton 6980

| | | | |
|---|---|---|---|
| tonicité 6986 | toxicomanie 2059 | transculturel 7036 | transversal 7072 |
| tonicité 6990 | toxicomanie 77 | transdermique 7037 | transverse 7072 |
| tonique 6983 | toxire 7013 | transducteur 7039 | trappe 5141 |
| tonique 6984 | toxine bactérienne 575 | transducteur de pression 5349 | trauma 7073 |
| tonomètre 6987 | toxines marines 4000 | transduction 7040 | trauma cérébral 834 |
| tonométrie 6988 | toxique 7010 | transduction génétique 2827 | traumatisme 7073 |
| tonus 6986 | trabeculation 7014 | transfection 7042 | traumatisme crânien 2964 |
| tonus 6990 | trace 7015 | transférer 7044 | traumatologie 7075 |
| tonus postural 5264 | tracé à boites 827 | transfert 7043 | travail 2244 |
| tophus 6995 | tracer 7016 | transfert 7047 | travail 3701 |
| topique 6996 | tracés sériées 6157 | transfert de technologie 6838 | travail 7459 |
| torpeur 6997 | traceur radioactif 5609 | transfert passif 4897 | travail induit 3385 |
| torse 6999 | trachéal 7019 | transformation 5390 | travail prématuré 5318 |
| torsion 6998 | trachée 7018 | transformation 7049 | travail provoqué 3385 |
| torticolis 7000 | trachéo-oesophagien 7020 | transformation cellulaire néoplasique 4438 | travailleur coopératif 6831 |
| tortueux 7001 | traction 7023 | transformation de données 1693 | travailleur volontaire 7373 |
| torture 7002 | tractus gastro-intestinal 2792 | transformer métaboliquement 4153 | trématode 2644 |
| total 21 | traduction 7059 | transfuser 7052 | tremblant 6212 |
| total 7003 | trait 7030 | transfusion 7053 | tremblement 5592 |
| total 7004 | trait mendélien 4114 | transfusion sanguine 776 | tremblement 7080 |
| toubib 5573 | traitement 5390 | transgénique 7054 | tremblement fin 2602 |
| toucher 7006 | traitement 7076 | transillumination 7057 | trembler 6197 |
| toucher 7007 | traitement assigné 464 | transitoire 7055 | trembler 6211 |
| tourner 5911 | traitement concomitant 1390 | translocation 7060 | trembler 7079 |
| tourniquet 5959 | traitement curatif 1619 | translucide 7061 | trépan 7083 |
| tourniquet 7008 | traitement de contrôle 1495 | transmetteur 7063 | trépaner 7084 |
| tournoyer 6420 | traitement de données 1688 | transmission 7062 | tréphine 7083 |
| tous les deux jours 2383 | traitement des données automatique 537 | transparent 7064 | trépidation 7085 |
| tous les jours 2382 | traitement orthophonique 6406 | transpiration 5021 | triade 7086 |
| tousser 1542 | traitement postopératoire 137 | transpirer 6739 | triage 7087 |
| tout 7003 | traitement symptomatique 6758 | transplantation 7067 | trigone 7099 |
| tout 7441 | traitement témoin 1495 | transplantation cardiaque 2996 | trimestre 7100 |
| toux 1541 | trance 7031 | transplantation coeur-poumon 3301 | triplet 7102 |
| toxémie 7009 | tranquille 5590 | transplanter 7066 | trismus 7103 |
| toxicité 7011 | tranquille 6544 | transport 7070 | trisomie 7104 |
| toxicité foetale 2563 | tranquillisant 7032 | transport actif 68 | tristesse 6366 |
| toxicité limitant la dose 2013 | tranquillisant 7033 | transport d'électrons 2195 | tritium 7105 |
| toxicité vestibulaire 7317 | transcriptase de réversion 5903 | transportation 7070 | troche 7107 |
| toxicologie 7012 | transcription 7055 | transporter 7068 | trois fois par jour 6918 |
| toxicomane 76 | transcription génétique 2826 | transsudat 7071 | troisième stade du travail 6917 |

# French/Français

## Italian/Italiano

# Italian/Italiano

agente sensibilizzante alle radiazioni 5602
agente spermicida 6409
agente tranquillante 7033
agente virale 7331
agenzia 143
agenzia garante 6446
agenzia governativa 2890
agenzia sponsorizzatrice 2751
aggiuntivo 78
aggiuntivo 90
aggiustamento 92
aggiustare 91
agglutinazione 146
agglutinina 147
aggravare 148
aggregazione 149
aggregazione piastrinica 5172
aggressione 150
agire contro 1546
agitare 6197
agitazione 152
ago 4429
ago da biopsia 702
agonista 153
agonista parziale 4880
agopuntura 73
agranulocitosi 155
aiuto sanitario 2969
ala 7449
albero bronchiale 861
albero di decisioni 1730
albero genealogico 2808
albero genealogico 4950
albinismo 168
albumina 169
albuminuria 170
alcali 181
alcaloide 182
alcalosi 183
alcalosi respiratoria 5850

alcolismo 2045
alcool 171
alcool di acido grasso 2529
alcoolico 172
alcoolismo 174
algoritmo 176
alienazione 177
alienazione mentale 3912
alimentare 178
alimentazione 1882
alimentazione 2543
alimentazione mediante sonda gastrica 2797
alimento 2672
aliquota 5594
alitosi 2944
alitosi 581
alla lettera 7299
allacciare 3807
allacciatura 3808
allacciatura 3809
allargamento 2285
allargamento 7446
allargato 2284
allattamento 3708
allattamento artificiale 822
allattare 6660
allattato al seno 846
allattato artificialmente 821
allele 185
allenamento fisiologico 5110
allergene 186
allergia 189
allergia alimentare 2673
allergico 187
allevamento 854
alleviare 190
alloggio 3148
allucinazione 2945
alluminio 206
allungamento 3767

allungare 1906
alogeno 2946
alopecia 198
alta frequenza 3077
alta pressione 3078
alta tecnologia 3081
altamente tecnologico 3082
alterato 3313
alterazione 3314
alterazione cognitiva 1267
alternativa 203
alternativo 204
alternato 202
alterno 202
altezza 3012
alto rischio 3079
altro 202
altruismo 205
alveolare 207
alveolo 208
alveolo polmonare 160
alzare 3804
amalgama 209
amaro 725
ambidestro 210
ambientale 2298
ambiente 2297
ambiente 4210
ambiente 567
ambiente della società 1324
ambiente domestico 1992
ambiguità 211
ambivalenza 212
ambliopia 213
ambulanza 214
ambulatorio 216
ambulatorio cura cancro 916
ambulatorio sanitario 2974
ameba 218
amebiasi 219

amenorrea 221
amianto 449
amido 6493
amielinico 7183
amilasi 234
amiloide 235
amiloidosi 236
amina 222
aminoacido 223
aminoaciduria 224
ammiccamento 744
amministratore 2887
amministratore 96
amministrazione 3983
amministrazione 95
ammissione ospedaliera 3136
ammoniaca 225
amnesia 226
amniocentesi 227
amorfo 229
ampiezza 5647
amplificatore 231
amplificazione 230
amplificazione genica 2806
ampolla 232
amputazione 233
anabolismo 238
anaerobico 240
anaerobio 239
anafase 254
anafilassi 256
anale 241
analettico 243
analgesia 244
analgesico 245
analisi 249
analisi a coppie contrapposte 4031
analisi attuariale 71
analisi chimica 1092
analisi costo-beneficio 1532

442

444

Italian/Italiano

assaggiare 6821
assaggio 461
asse 558
asse delle x 7482
asse delle y 7492
asse destro 5936
asse fratturato 858
asse rotto 858
asse sinistro 3754
asse z 7502
assegnazione 191
assegnazione casuale 5637
assegnazione dosaggio 2004
assente 20
assenza di peso 7425
assicurazione 3500
assicurazione contro infortuni professionali 7463
assicurazione per la salute 2975
assistenza a malati terminali 6871
assistenza ambulatoriale 217
assistenza domiciliare 3111
assistenza in ospizio 3134
assistenza medica completa 1361
assistenza primaria 5362
assistenza sanitaria 2970
assistenza socio-psicologica 1543
assistito 465
assistito dall' elaboratore 1371
associato 466
associato ricerca clinica 1212
associazione 467
assoluto 21
assone 559
assorbente 110
assorbente igienico 6017
assorbimento 111
assorbimento 24
assorbimento intestinale 3553
assorbire 109
assorbire 23

assorbire 786
assunzione clinica 1193
astenia 469
asterisco 468
astigmatismo 471
astinenza 7452
astringente 472
astrocitoma 473
atassia 3358
atassia 478
atelettasia 479
atenoma 481
ateriosclerosi 482
atebsi 483
atipco 509
atecico 484
atlo-assiale 485
atmosfera 486
atmosferico 487
atomizzatore 4424
atonia 489
atonico 490
atopia 491
atresia 492
atriale 493
atrio 498
atrofia 500
atrofico 499
attaccatura 501
attacco 2612
attacco 502
attacco 6104
attacco cardiaco 2987
attentpato 2174
attendibilità 5730
attenuato 506
attenuazione 1
attenuazione 507
attenzione 504
attenzione 965

attesa di vita 3798
attitudine 402
attitudine 508
attivazione 62
attività 70
attività del tempo libero 3765
attività farmacologica 5052
attività fisica 5093
attività intrinseca 3583
attività locomotoria 3860
attività quotidiana 69
attivo 64
attuale 5336
audiometria 510
aumentare 3360
aumento 3359
aumento del dosaggio 2010
aumento di peso 7421
aumento proporzionale 6035
aura 515
auricola 517
auricolare 493
auricolare 516
ausiliario 263
ausiliario 548
autismo 521
autistico 522
autoanalisi 523
autoanalizzatore 524
autoanticorpo 525
autoantigene 526
autobiografia 527
autoclave 528
autocontrollo biologico 689
autodistruzione 6112
autoesame 6113
autoimmune 530
autoimmunità 531
autoinnesto 529
autoipnosi 6114

autolimitante 6115
autolisi 534
autologo 532
automaticità 538
automazione 539
automedicamento 6116
autonomo 540
autopsia 542
autoradiografia 543
autore 520
autorità 519
autorità che concede licenze 3792
autorizzazione 1182
autorizzazione 37
autosoma 546
autosomministrazione 6108
autostimolazione 6118
autosuggestione 547
autosupervisione 6117
autotrapianto 529
autovalutazione 6109
avambraccio 2684
aver paura 2533
avere il respiro affannoso 7433
avere un collasso 1285
avere un colloquio 3551
avitaminosi 553
avulsione 555
avvelenamento de metallo pesante 3010
avvelenamento 5197
avvelenare 5195
avverso 115
avvertimento 7395
avvincente 1336
avvizzire 7455
azienda a contratto 1475
azione legale per negligenza 3977
azione tardiva 138
azotemia 560
azoto 4497

Italian/Italiano

dormire 6290
dorsale 2000
dorsalgia 565
dorso 564
dorsolaterale 2002
dosaggio 2003
dosaggio consentito 195
dosaggio in forma parenterale 4866
dosare 2009
dose 2008
dose accumulata 1616
dose alta 3076
dose bolo 804
dose di induzione 3854
dose di mantenimento 3957
dose di mezzogiorno 4195
dose di rovesciamento 5902
dose eccessiva 4767
dose-effetto 2016
dose giornaliera 1855
dose iniziale 3443
dose letale 3772
dose ottimale 4689
dose permissibile 195
dose prima di andare a letto 630
dose serale 2379
dose totale giornaliera 7005
dose-limite per la tossicità 2013
dosimetro 2020
dossaggio biologico 681
dossaggio biologico 693
dossier 2025
dossier ospedaliero 3137
dossier regolatorio 5754
dotto 2082
dotto 7254
dotto arterioso pervio 4906
dotto biliare 667
dotto deferente 7255
dotto ghiandolare 2083

dotto toracico 6814
dottore 1987
drenaggio 2041
droga 2056
due volte al giorno 7127
duodenale 2080
duodeno 2092
dura madre 2093
durata 2094
durata della degenza 3766
durata di immagazzinamento 6207
durata di uno studio 4993
ebbro 2078
eccellente 2394
eccentrico 726
eccessivo 2396
ecchimosi 2127
ecipiente 2399
eccitabilità 2402
eccitamento 417
eccitazione 2403
eclampsia 2132
ecocardiografia 2129
ecocardiografia Doppler 1998
ecocardiogramma 2128
ecoencefalografia 2130
ecofrasia 2131
ecolalia 2131
ecologia 2133
economia 2136
ectoderma 2137
ectopia 2140
eczema 2141
eczema puntiforme 5546
edema 2142
edema 6741
edema della caviglia 296
edema depressibile 5143
edema facciale 2486
edema pedale 4947

edificio 2489
editazione 2147
editoria 5525
editoriale 2149
edizione 3650
educativo 2151
educazione 2150
educazione 7027
educazione continua 1465
educazione sanitaria 2973
educazione speciale 6382
efelide 2721
efferente 2155
effetto 2152
effetto carry-over 980
effetto collaterale 6228
effetto coorte 1271
effetto di addestramento 7028
effetto di evitamento 6375
effetto indesiderato 116
effetto limite massimo 1026
effetto placebo 5151
effetto primo passo 2609
effetto reversibile 5904
effetto rimanenza 980
effetto sistemico 6781
effetto teratogeno 6865
efficace 2153
efficacia 2154
efficacia 2158
efficacia 5279
efficacia clinica 1199
efficienza 2154
efficienza 2162
effluente 2163
effusione 2164
effusione pericardica 4986
eiaculazione 2168
elaboratore 1370
elaboratore dati automatizzato 537

elaborazione 5390
elaborazione di dati 1688
elaborazione diagnostica 1868
elasticità 2172
elastico 5836
elastico 2171
elastiscità 1354
eleggibilità del paziente 4925
elementi di consenso 2206
elemento 2205
elemento di dati 1681
elemento sanguigno 763
elenco del contenuto 6792
elenco farmaci restituiti 5900
elettrico 2176
elettrocardiografia 2180
elettrocardiogramma, ECG 2178
elettrochimica 2181
elettrochirurgia 2204
elettrocoagulazione 2182
elettroconvulsivante 2183
elettrodo 2184
elettrodo impiantato 3322
elettroencefalografia 2186
elettroencefalogramma 2185
elettrofisiologia 2201
elettroforesi 2200
elettrolisi 2187
elettroliti sierici chi 6175
elettrolito 2188
elettromiografia 2191
elettrone 2192
elettronico 2196
elettronistagmografia 2198
elettrooculografia 2199
elettroretinografia 2202
elettroshock 2177
elettroshock 2203
elevatore 3781
elevazione 2209

456

Italian/Italiano

eliminazione 2214
eliminazione graduale del ventilatore 7290
elio 3013
elisir 2216
elminte 3014
emaciamento 2217
emaciazione 7402
emangioma 3016
emartrosi 3017
ematemesi 3018
ematocrito 3019
ematologia 3021
ematologico 3020
ematoma 3022
ematoma subdurale 6626
ematuria 3025
ematuria microscopica 4183
emboli cerebrali 1061
embolia gassosa 161
embolia grassosa 2524
embolismo 2221
embolizzazione 2222
embolo 2223
embolo 759
embriologia 2225
embrionale 2226
embrione 2224
emendamento del protocollo 5469
emergenza 2227
emesi 2230
emetico 2231
emialgia 3026
emicrania 4202
emigrazione 2232
eminenza mediana 4067
emiplegia 3028
emisfero 3029
emissione 2233
emivita 2942
emivita d'eliminazione 2215

emivita terminale 6872
emoagglutinazione 3015
emocitometria 761
emocoltura 762
emocralisi 3030
emocinamica 3031
emofilia 3039
emoglobina 3032
emoglobinopatia 3033
emoglobinuria 3034
emogruppo 766
emolisi 3035
emolitico 3036
emolliente 2235
emoperfusione 3038
emopoiesi 3023
emorragia 3041
emorragia 736
emorragia intestinale 3554
emorragia nasale 4546
emorragia subugueale 6442
emorroide 3044
emorroidi 5122
emostasi 3045
emotivo 2239
emotisi 3040
emozione 126
emozione 2236
empatia 2240
empiema 2245
empirico 2242
emulsione 2246
enantiomero 2248
enartrosi 588
encefalite 2249
encefalite trasmessa dalla zecca 6944
encefalo 831
endarterectomia 2253
endemica 2254
endocardio 2256

endocarcite 2255
endocitosi 2260
endocrino 2257
endocrinologia 2259
endodontico 2261
endogeno 2262
endolinfa 2264
endometriale 2265
endometrio 2267
endometriosi 2266
endorfina 269
endoscopia 2272
endoscopico 2271
endoscopio 2270
endoteliale 2274
endotelio 2275
endotossina 2276
energia 2231
enfisema 2241
enterale 2287
enterico 2288
enterite 2290
enterocolite pseudomembranosa 5487
enterolisi isoperistaltica 7399
enterotossina 2292
entrata 2293
entrata 3351
entrata dati 1674
entrata di dati distribuzione 1970
entrata di dati doppi 2029
enucleare 2295
enucleazione dell'occhio 2473
enuresi 2296
enuresi 631
enzima 2302
enzimologia 2303
eosinofilia 2305
eosinofilo 2304
eparina a bassa dose 3890
epatico 3048

epatite 3049
epatologia 3052
epatoma 3053
epatomegalia 3054
epicardio 2306
epidemia 2307
epidemico 2308
epidemiologia 2311
epidemiologico 2309
epidermico 2312
epidermide 2313
epididimo 2314
epidurale 2315
epifisi 2323
epifisi 5133
epigastrico 2316
epiglottide 2317
epilessia 2319
epinefrina 2321
epiploon 4639
episiotomia 2324
episodio 2325
episodio sincopatico 6764
epistassi 2326
epistassi 4546
epiteliale 2327
epitelio 2329
equilibrio 2330
equilibrio 584
equilibrio acido-base 50
equilibrio fluido-elettroliti 2639
equivalente 2333
equivalente 2334
equo 2505
erba 2910
erba 3055
erbicida 3057
ereditarietà 3438
eredità 3059
eredità 3438

461

| | | | |
|---|---|---|---|
| geriatrico 2839 | giovanile 3672 | gocciolare 2048 | granello 6398 |
| germe 2840 | gioventù 7501 | gola 6921 | granulazione 2903 |
| germinale 2842 | girare 5911 | gomito 2173 | granulo 2904 |
| germogliare 6459 | gittata cardiaca 948 | gomma 2932 | granulocità 2905 |
| germoglio 6458 | gittata sistolica 6598 | gonade 2881 | granuloma 2906 |
| gerontologia 2844 | giudizio 3667 | gonfiare 1963 | granulomatoso 2907 |
| gesso 990 | giudizio clinico 1207 | gonfiare 3418 | grasso 2522 |
| gestazionale 2846 | giugulare 3668 | gonfio 6743 | grasso 2523 |
| gestazione 2845 | giuntura 444 | gonfio 747 | grasso bruno 873 |
| gestione 3983 | giuntura sinoviale 6771 | gonfiore 6741 | graza 2913 |
| gestione della professione 5284 | giunzione 3671 | governante 2887 | grave 6159 |
| gettare nel panico 4825 | giunzione intercellulare 3521 | governo 2889 | grave 6178 |
| ghiandola 2851 | giunzione neuromuscolare 4469 | governo della casa 3147 | gravida 5309 |
| ghiandola endocrina 2084 | giustapporre 3673 | governo federale 2540 | gravidanza 1113 |
| ghiandola endocrina 2258 | giusto 2505 | gozzo 2876 | gravidanza 5306 |
| ghiandola esocrina 2418 | glande 2852 | gozzo nodulare 4504 | gravidanza ectopica 2139 |
| ghiandola linfatica 3923 | glaucoma 2855 | gradazione 6195 | gravidanza interrotta 4226 |
| ghiandola paratiroide 4861 | glaucoma ad angolo aperto 4658 | gradevole al palato 4800 | gravidanza tubarica 7115 |
| ghiandola parotide 4874 | glicogeno 2873 | gradi di libertà 1764 | gravido 2911 |
| ghiandola pituitaria 5146 | glicoside cardiaco 945 | gradiente di densità 1793 | gravità 6179 |
| ghiandola salivare 6002 | glicosidi digitalici 1902 | grado delle stato psichiatrico 5492 | griglia 2913 |
| ghiandola sebacea 6079 | glicosuria 2874 | graffiare 6069 | grossista 7445 |
| ghiandola sottomandibolare 6638 | glioblastoma 2856 | graffio 6068 | grucce 1599 |
| ghiandola sudoripara 6740 | glioma 2857 | grafica computerizzata 1374 | gruppo 2920 |
| già visto 1768 | globina 2862 | grafici 2909 | gruppo a basso rischio 3895 |
| gibbo di bufalo 880 | globo oculare 2475 | grafici puntiformi 5191 | gruppo a rischio 5947 |
| gigantismo 2849 | globulina 2863 | grafico a settori 5118 | gruppo bersaglio 2658 |
| ginecologia 2934 | globulo 756 | grafico a valori sparsi 6048 | gruppo consumatori 1449 |
| ginecomastia 2935 | globulo bianco 7438 | grafico lineare 3823 | gruppo di confronto 1330 |
| ginocchio 3691 | globulo rosso 5714 | grafico rettangolo 827 | gruppo di controllo 1493 |
| giocare 5176 | glomerulonefrite 2865 | grafico sopravvivenza 3802 | gruppo di lavoro 6830 |
| giogo 7498 | glottide 2867 | gram-negativo 2899 | gruppo di osservazione 4596 |
| giornale delle valutazioni dei pazienti 4936 | glucocorticoide 2868 | gram-positivo 2900 | gruppo di pressione 5347 |
| giornale di bordo 3862 | gluconeogenesi 2869 | grammo 2898 | gruppo etnico 2369 |
| giornale di visite di controllo 4278 | glucosio 2870 | grammomolecola 4268 | gruppo in prima fase 5066 |
| giornaliero 1654 | glucoso 2870 | gran forame occipitale 2681 | gruppo medico 967 |
| giornata 1700 | gluteo 2872 | grande cellula 3717 | gruppo sanguigno 766 |
| giornate senza farmaco 2065 | gobba di bufalo 880 | grande male 2901 | gruppo senza trattamento 4551 |
| giorno 1700 | goccia 2047 | grandezza 3954 | gua na 6204 |
| giovane 7500 | gocciolamento 2047 | grandezza 6274 | gua na mielinica 4374 |

| | | | |
|---|---|---|---|
| guaina tendinea 6858 | idrocele 3171 | imbecille 4298 | immunosoppressivo 3309 |
| guancia 1088 | idrofilo 3176 | imbiancamento 735 | immunosoppressore 3307 |
| guarigione 2967 | idrofobico 3177 | imbianchimento 735 | immunosorbente 3306 |
| guarigione 5700 | idrofobo 3177 | imbrogliare 1085 | immunoterapia 3310 |
| guarire 1621 | idrofobo 5595 | imbroglione 5573 | immunotossina 3311 |
| guarire 2966 | idrogeno 3173 | imene 3180 | imparare a discriminare 1931 |
| guarire 5711 | idrogeno pesante 1848 | immagazzinamento 6566 | impari 561 |
| guida 2928 | idrolisi 3175 | immagine 3275 | impedenza 3315 |
| guida 3742 | idrope 2054 | immagine corporea 794 | impedimento 1846 |
| guidare 2929 | idrosolubile 7406 | immaturo 3280 | imperforato 3316 |
| guscio 6208 | idrossilazione 3178 | immediatamente 3282 | impermeabile 3317 |
| gusto 2623 | igiene 3179 | immediatamente 6499 | impiantabile 3320 |
| gusto 6820 | igiene 6018 | immediato 328? | impiantare 3319 |
| gusto residuo 139 | igienico 6016 | immigrazione 3283 | impianti per la produzione 5406 |
| habitus 2937 | igienista dentale 1797 | immischiarsi 6606 | impianto 3318 |
| hardware 2957 | il bere 2045 | immiscibile 3264 | impianto dentale endosseo 2273 |
| herpes labiale 1278 | il fumare 6318 | immissione dati 1674 | impianto di silicone 6246 |
| herpes zoster 7509 | il margiare 2125 | immobile 3285 | impiegato 2243 |
| hertz 1637 | il migliore esistente 6501 | immobile 6544 | impiego 2244 |
| hertz 3065 | il nutre 2543 | immobilizzato 2287 | impilamento dei globuli rossi 5964 |
| hiatus 3073 | il pensare laterale 3731 | immobilizzazione 3286 | implosivo 3323 |
| high-tech 3081 | il percere 6205 | immune 3288 | importante 6242 |
| high-tech 3082 | il russare 6328 | immunità 3290 | importanza 6241 |
| hotline 3145 | il sostenere 6693 | immunità acquisita dalla madre 4036 | importanza clinica 1203 |
| iatrogeno 3251 | ileale 3263 | immunità attiva 66 | impotenza 3324 |
| ibridazione 3167 | ileo 3266 | immunità naturale 4416 | imprecisato 7187 |
| ibridizzazione 1580 | ileo 3267 | immunità passiva 4896 | impreciso 7236 |
| ibrido 3165 | ileo-colite granulomatosa 5740 | immunizzazione 3291 | impregnazione 3325 |
| ibrido 3166 | ileodigiunale 3658 | immunochimica 3293 | impressione diagnostica 186? |
| ibridoma 3168 | ileostomia 3265 | immunocompetenza 3294 | impronta 3326 |
| ideazione 3254 | iio 3269 | immunoeficierza 3296 | impronta digitale 2605 |
| identificazione 3256 | illuminare 3627 | immunodiffusio ne 3297 | impulso 2049 |
| identità sessuale 2804 | illusione 3273 | immunoelettroforesi 3298 | impulso 3328 |
| idiopatico 3259 | illustrazione 2589 | immunofenotipo 3304 | impulso apicale 381 |
| idiosincrasia 3260 | illustrazione 3274 | immunogenetica 3299 | impulso nervoso 4451 |
| idiota 3261 | ilo 3083 | immunoglobulir e, Ig 3300 | impurezza 3330 |
| idiota erudito 3262 | imballaggio 4789 | immunoistochinica 3301 | impurità 3330 |
| idratato 3169 | imba samazione 2219 | immunologia 3303 | imputazione 3331 |
| idrocarburo 3170 | imba co 6210 | immunologica 3302 | in attesa 2425 |
| idrocefalo 3172 | imbecille 3278 | immunosoppressione 3308 | in buona salute 2980 |

Italian/Italiano

inghiottire 6737
ingrandimento 2285
ingrandito 2284
ingrediente 3431
ingrediente attivo 67
ingresso 2293
ingresso 97
ingresso di dati a distanza 5790
inguaribile 3365
inguinale 3432
inguine 2917
ingurgitato 2283
inibire 5586
inibitore 3441
inibizione 3440
iniettare 3446
iniezione 3448
iniziali 3444
iniziazione 3445
inizio improvviso 6666
inizio lento 6304
inizio tardivo 3729
innato 3340
innato 3437
innato 3452
innaturale 7184
innervare 3454
innestabile 3320
innestare 2896
innestare 3319
innesto 2895
innesto 3318
innesto di cute 6281
innesto endocavitario 3451
innesto omologo 3119
innesto osseo 811
innocente 3455
innocuo 3456
innovazione 3457
inoculare 3458

inoperabile 3459
inotropo 3460
inporta digitale ADN 1984
inquiramento 5204
insanguinato 784
insan·a 3467
insat·ro 7185
inseg namento 6828
insegnante 6827
insegdimento 7021
inseminazione 3470
inseminazione artificiale 447
insensibile 2085
insersibile 3472
inseribile 3474
inserire la parola d'ordine in un computer per attivare 3863
inserviente 4701
inserzione 3473
inserzione 501
inseticida 3469
inseto 3468
insidoso 3475
insolto 4622
insolubile 3476
insonnia 3477
insonnia 6294
insonnia 7385
insongenza 4649
insorgenza graduale 2892
inspirare 3481
inspiratorio 3480
inspirazione 3479
instabile 7188
instabilità 3482
instillazione 3483
insuccesso 7399
insufficiente 5220
insufficiente sollievo 3496
insufficienza 2501

insufficienza 3495
insufficienza cardiaca 2990
insufficienza cardiaca congestizia 1423
insufficienza epatica 3852
insufficienza mitralica 4248
insufficienza renale 5793
insufficienza ventricolare sinistra 3757
insufflare 3497
insulina 3498
insulino dipendente 3499
intarsio 3451
integrazione 3504
integrazione verticale 7311
integrità 3505
intelletto 3507
intelligenza 3508
intelligenza artificiale 448
intelligenza epidemiologica 2310
intemperanza 3512
intensità della razione 3513
intensivo 3514
interazione 35·9
interazione alimentare 2674
interazione farmaci 2067
interazione uovo-sperma 8412
intercostale 3522
interculturale 1578
interculturale 7036
interdisciplinare 3524
interfaccia corr puterizzata 1375
interfase 3540
interferone 3525
interim 3526
intermittente 3529
internato 1186
internato 3539
internazionale 3535
interneurone 3537
intervista 3538
interno 3614

interno all'azienda 3442
interno 7441
interpretazione 3541
interpretazione di dati 1680
interpretazione errata 4230
interruzione 1926
interruzione di studio cieco 844
interscarmbio genetico 1591
interstiziale 3543
intervalle tra dosi 2012
intervallo 3526
intervallo 3544
intervallo di sicurezza 1406
intervallo di tempo 6952
intervallo tra nascite 715
intervento 3546
intervento di crisi 1572
interventricolare 3548
intervista 3550
intervistare 3551
intestinale 3552
intestino 2933
intestino 3556
intestino 824
intestino crasso 3718
intestino tenue 6307
intima 3557
intirizzimento 4567
intirizzire 4564
intirizzito 4565
intollerante 3559
intolleranza 3558
intolleranza al caldo 3005
intolleranza al freddo 1277
intolleranza alimentare 2675
intorpidimento 4567
intorpidire 4564
intorpidire 4565
intossicazione 3392
intossicazione 3560

# Italian/Italiano

orecchio medio 4197
organello 4705
organi genitali 2830
organi sessuali 6190
organi sessuali femminili 2549
organi sessuali maschili 3968
organico 4706
organismo 4708
organismo patogeno 4910
organismo senza patogeni 6393
organizzazione 4709
organizzazione a contratto 1479
organizzazione di ricerca a contratto 1481
organizzazione mantenimento sanitario 2976
organizzazione per la ricerca medica 4081
Organizzazione Mondiale della Sanità, OMS 7466
organo 4704
organo bersaglio 6817
organo di senso 6135
organo riproduttore 5819
organo trapiantato 7065
organulo 4705
orgasmo 4711
orgoglioso 5481
orientale 4712
orientamento 4713
orifizio 373
orifizio 4714
orinare 4193
orizzontale 3127
ormone 3129
ormone adrenocorticotropo, ACTH 108
ormone luteinizzante 3920
ormone pituitario 5147
ormone sessuale 6183
ormonodipendente 3130
ormonoterapia 3131
oro 2877
orofaringe 4716

orofaringeo 4715
orologico biologico 694
orticaria 3106
orticaria 7217
ortodontia 4719
ortodonzia correttiva 1522
ortognatodonzia 4719
ortopedico 4721
ortopnea 4722
ortostasi 4723
orzaiolo 6615
oscillare 7227
oscillografo 4726
oscilloscopio 4727
osmolalità 4728
osmolarità 4730
ospedale 3135
ospedale 3413
ospedaliero 4547
ospedalizzazione 3139
ospite 3140
ospite immunocompromesso 3295
ospizio 3133
ossa del carpo 975
ossa della faccia 2485
osseo 4732
osservatore 4598
osservazione 4593
osservazione aneddotica 265
osservazione ripetuta 5802
ossessione 4599
ossessivo 4600
ossicino dell'orecchio 2122
ossidante 4778
ossidazione 4779
ossidoriduzione 4780
ossiemoglobina 4786
ossificazione 4733
ossigenare 4784
ossigenazione 4785

ossigenazione 7287
ossigeno 4782
ossigeno iperbarico 3187
ossimetria 4781
osso 807
osso del pube 5517
osteite 4734
osteoartrite 4735
osteoartropatia 4736
osteoblasto 4737
osteoclasto 4738
osteoma 4739
osteomielite 4740
osteopatia 4742
osteoporosi 4743
osteosarcoma 4744
osteotomia 4745
ostetrica 4201
ostetricia 4603
ostetrico 4602
ostilità 3142
ostomia 4746
ostruttivo 4605
ostruzione 4604
ostruzione 752
otico 4747
otite 4748
otite esterna 4749
otite media 4750
otorinolaringoiatria 4751
otoscopio 4752
otricolo 7222
ottenuto per mezzo di coltura 1609
ottica 4688
ottica delle fibre 2570
ottico 4673
ottico 4682
ottico 4683
ottico 4687
otturatore 4606

otturazione 4606
ottusità 2086
ottuso 2085
ovaia 4763
ovarico 4762
ovariectomia 4653
ovario 4763
ovidotto 4774
ovocita 4651
ovogenesi 4652
ovulare 4775
ovulazione 4776
ozono 4787
p-value 5561
pacchetto trasparente 746
pacemaker 4788
padiglione auricolare 517
paese 1551
paese in via di sviluppo 1849
paese membro 4106
pagamento 4941
pagamento anticipato 7190
palato 4801
palato leporino 1185
palato molle 6346
palatoschisi 1185
palliare 4802
palliativo 4803
palliativo 4804
pallore 4805
palma 4806
palpabile 4809
palpazione 4810
palpebra 2479
palpebrale 4811
palpitare 4812
palpitazione 4813
panacea 1622
panacea 4815
pancitopenia 4818

percento del totale 4969
percentuale 4966
percentuale 4970
percentuale accumulata 1617
percentuale di cambio 4967
percentuale di risposta massima 4968
percettivo 4973
percezione 4972
percezione dei rumori 3883
percezione del timbro 5140
percezione di moto 4311
percezione in profondità 1821
percuotere (leggermente) 6812
percuotere 4974
percussione 4975
perdere 3744
perdere i sensi 2503
perdita 3745
perdita 3875
perdita 646
perdita d'acqua insensibile 3471
perdita dei capelli 2941
perdita della memoria 4112
perdita di calore 3006
perdita di coscienza 3876
perdita di fluidi 2641
perdita di peso 3877
perdita di peso 7423
perdita uditiva 2983
perdite di bit 2052
perenne 4977
perforazione 4979
perforazione manuale 3683
perfusione 4983
perfusione del tessuto 6968
periapicale 4984
pericardio 4985
pericardio 4987
periferico 5001
perimetro 4988

perinatale 4989
perineale 4990
perineo 4991
periodicità 4996
periodico 3666
periodico 4994
periodico 4995
periodo 4992
periodo 6868
periodo de screening 6074
periodo di controllo 2668
periodo di follow-up 2668
periodo di incubazione 3363
periodo di latenza 3728
periodo di osservazione 4594
periodo di reclutamento 5706
periodontale 4997
periodonzia 4998
periorbitale 4999
periostio 5000
peristalsi 5004
peritoneale 5007
peritoneo 5008
peritonite 5009
permeabile 5012
permeabilità 5011
permeabilità capillare 924
permeabilità della membrana 4108
pernicioso 5013
perone 2584
perorale 5014
perossido 5015
persona 5016
personale 5017
personale 5019
personale 6473
personale 6474
personalità 5018
personalità schizotipica 6058
perspirazione 5021

perversione 5023
pervertito 5024
pervietà 4904
pesistica 7422
peso 7419
peso alla nascita 718
peso del corpo 801
peso eccessivo 4773
peso molecolare 4271
peso specifico 6392
pessario 5025
peste 5027
peste 5153
pesticida 5026
pestilenza 5027
Pet scan 5028
petecchia 5029
petrolato 5031
petto 845
pettorale 4946
pezzo 2714
pia madre 5113
pia meninge 5113
piaga 6364
piaga da decubito 1740
piangente 7418
piangere 6332
pianificazione familiare 2516
pianificazione sanitaria 2977
piano 3783
piano 5422
piano contingente 1461
piano di crescita 2927
piano fasciale 2519
pianta 5156
pianta 6351
pianta commestibile 2144
pianta medicinale 4091
pianto 1600
piastra 5169

piastrina 5170
piastrina 6923
piastrina 769
piazzare 5231
pica 5114
picacismo 5114
picciolo 6482
picco 4942
piccolo 6214
piccolo male 5030
picogrammo 5115
pidocchio 3884
piede 2677
piega 2659
piega 7475
piegare 2660
piegarsi all'indietro 638
piegarsi in avanti 639
pielonefrite 5562
piemia 5563
pietra miliare 4208
pigmentazione 5120
pigmento 5119
pigmento sanguigno 768
pigro 3740
pia 619
pillola 5123
pillola anticoncezionale 713
pillola ricoperta 1252
pilomotore 5127
piloro 5565
pineale 5132
pinza 2683
pinza chirurgica 1171
pinza emostatica 3046
pinza emostatica rotante 5959
pinzare 1172
piogenico 5566
piogeno 5566
piombo 3741

Italian/Italiano

precisione 40
precisione 5293
preclinico 5294
precoce 5295
preconcetto 5313
precursore 5298
prediabetico 5299
predisposizione 5302
predisposizione 6728
predittivo 5301
predizione 5300
pregangliare 5305
pregiudizio 5313
pregiudizio 655
pregno 2911
preimpianto 5310
preinfusione 5311
preiniezione 5312
premarketing 5315
prematurità 5320
prematuro 5316
premedicazione 5321
premorto 310
prenatale 311
prenatale 5322
preoperatorio 5323
preparato 5325
preparto 312
prepuberale 5326
prepuzio 2693
presbiopia 5328
presbitismo 5328
prescrizione 5332
prescrizione multipla 5215
preselezionare 6071
preselezione 5334
preselezione casuale 5640
presentante 5338
presentazione 5337
presentazione del medicamento 2005

presentazione di dati 1687
presentazione podalica 853
presentazione regolatoria 5755
preservativo 5340
preservativo 5341
preservazione 5339
preservazione del sangue 771
presinaptico 5350
pressare 1363
pressione 5346
pressione arteriosa 422
pressione arteriosa polmonare 5536
pressione atmosferica 488
pressione d'incuneamento polmonare 5531
pressione del sangue 772
pressione del sangue bassa 3886
pressione diastolica 1878
pressione ematica 772
pressione intracranica 3564
pressione intraoculare 3573
pressione osmotica 4731
pressione pulsatoria 5542
pressione sanguigna sistolica 6786
pressione venosa 7286
pressione venosa centrale 1048
pressione ventricolare sinistra di fine diastole
  3756
pressorecettore 5345
pressorio 5344
prestazione 4980
pretese farmaco 2060
pretrattamento 5351
pretrial 5352
prevalenza 5353
preventivo 5355
prevenzione 5354
prevenzione primaria 5367
prezzo del trasferimento 7045
prigioniero 5376
prima fase 5064

primario 5360
primario 5361
primate 5369
primipara 5370
primitivo 5360
principio 5372
principio informatore 2879
priorità 5375
prioritizzazione 5374
privato 5377
privazione 646
privazione di acqua 7404
privo di assicurazione medica 4085
proaritmico 5380
probabile 5449
probabilità 5381
probabilmente correlato al farmaco 5382
problema 5385
problema di redazione testo 2146
problema etico 2364
problema linea di condotta 5199
procedura 5388
procedura di una operazione 4667
procedura invasiva 3590
procedura non invadente 4519
procedura operazionale standard 6489
procedura simulata 6200
processo 3847
processo 4165
processo 5389
processo decisionale 1727
processo mastoideo 4027
processo xifoide 7484
proconvulsivante 5391
procreazione 5392
proctoscopio 5393
prodotti farmaceutici 5042
prodotto 5398
prodotto caseario 1657
prodotto chimico 1091

prodotto competitivo 1343
prodotto naturale 4418
prodromo 5395
produttore 5397
produzione 3998
produzione 4761
produzione 5405
produzione in grande scala 2744
produzione in scala ridotta 5129
profarmaco 5396
profase 5437
professionale 4614
professionale 5408
professionale 7363
professione 4613
professione 5282
professione infermiera 4574
professore 5410
professore universitario 2497
profilassi 5440
profilattico 5438
profilattico 5439
profilo cinetico 3689
profilo di sicurezza 5994
profilo efficacia 2159
profilo farmaco 2070
profondità del respiro 5852
progenitore 262
progestativo 5411
progestinico 5412
progetto 1837
progetto 5422
progetto a coppie contrapposte 4032
progetto pilota 5128
prognosi 5413
prognostica 5414
programma di titolazione 6972
programma 5415
programma 6050
programma di studi 1624

478

Italian/Italiano

programma per computer 6348
programma per la salute nazionale 4409
programmare 5416
programmare 6051
programmatore 5155
progressivo 5419
proibito 5420
proibizione 5421
proiettore 5425
proiezione 5424
prolasso 5426
proliferazione 5427
prolungamento 2448
prolungamento 5429
prolungare 5428
prominenza 5430
promotore 5431
promozione 5432
pronazione 5433
pronto soccorso 2606
propagare 5435
propensione di dipendenza 1808
proporzione sopravvivente 5441
proprietà 5436
proprietà di superficie 6708
propriocezione 5445
proptosi 5446
propulsione 5447
prosencefalo 2685
prospettico 5449
prospettiva del paziente 4938
prossimale 5485
prostata 5451
prostrato 5434
prostrato 5453
prostrazione 5454
proteasi 5455
proteina 5458
proteina chimerica 1120
proteina del sangue 773

proteina vettrice 977
proteinasi 5462
proteinuria 5463
proteolisi 5464
protesi 5452
protesi acustica 2982
pretezione 5456
protezione addominale 6
protezione brevetto 4907
protezione involontaria 3610
proto-oncogene 5467
protocollo 5468
protocollo aggiuntivo 2449
protocollo comune 1316
protocollo di continuità 1463
protocollo di eccezione per compassione 1332
protocollo umanitario 3156
protone 5474
protoplasma 5476
protozoa 5477
protozoario 5478
protozoi 5477
protrombina 5465
protrusione 5480
prova 2384
prova 461
prova 6878
prova 7088
prova a unico ramo 4647
prova aggiuntiva 79
prova bilaterale 7134
prova bilaterale 7135
prova controllata con placebo 5150
prova dell'esercizio 2409
prova della realtà 5679
prova della tubercolina 7118
prova di fissazione del complemento 1347
prova di ipotesi unilaterale 4646
prova di stress 6588
prova equivalenza 2332

prova fatta in comunità 1321
prova immunoenzimatica 3292
prova in cross-over 1593
prova interprocesso 3463
prova multicentrica 4337
prova per tentativi 7089
prova pilota 5130
provare 2431
provincia 5482
provitamina 5483
provocato 3384
provocazione 1074
provvisorio 3527
provvista 6692
prudere 3653
prurito 3652
prurito 3654
prurito 5-86
pseudo- 5483
psicanalisi 5495
psicanalitco 5496
psiche 5489
psichedelico 5490
psichiatria 5493
psichiatrico 5491
psichico 5494
psicochirurgia 5509
psicofarmacologia 5504
psicologia 5499
psicologia criminale 1570
psicologia dell'inconscio 7160
psicologia di condizionamento 1400
psicologia di transfert 7048
psicologico 5497
psicometria 5501
psicomotorio 5502
psicopatologia 5503
psicosessuale 5505
psicosi 5506
psicosi alcoolica 173

psicosociale 5507
psicosomatico 5508
psicoterapia 5510
psicotico 5511
psicotropico 5514
pterigio congenito 7415
ptosi 5515
ptosi palpebrale 3795
pubblicazione 5524
pubblicità diretta al consumatore 1915
pubblico 5519
pube 5518
pubertà 5516
pubertà precoce 5296
pudendo 5526
puerile 5527
puerperale 5528
puerperio 1410
puerperio 3921
pulire 2649
pulire 7450
pulsare 5541
pulsazione 5539
pulsazione 6922
punctua 6811
pungiglione 6550
punizione 5548
punta 6417
punta e onda 6418
puntare 6469
punteggio comportamentale 633
punteggio della severità della lesione 3450
punteggio di Apgar 375
punteggio di cambio 1080
punteggio efficacia 2160
punteggio originale 5671
punteggio riflettente la tendenza 7082
punto 2026
punto cardinale 953
punto cieco 741

Italian/Italiano

punto dati 1685
punto decisivo 1728
punto finale 2277
punto finale ben definibile 2955
punto finale sostitutivo 6721
punto temporale 6953
puntura 5547
puntura 6468
puntura 723
puntura d'insetto 6550
puntura lombare 3906
puntura lombare 6426
pupilla 5549
pupille dilatate 1904
purezza 5554
purga 5551
purgante 5551
purgativo 5552
purulento 5556
pus 5557
pustola 5131
pustola 5558
pustola 7430
putrefazione 5559
putrido 5560
puzzo 6522
quadrante 5574
quadrato latino 3732
quadriplegia 5575
qualità 5577
qualità commerciale 1310
qualità della vita 5581
qualitativo 5576
quantitativo 5583
quarantena 5584
quarantinizado 2289
questionario 5587
questionario finale di uno studio controllato 2251
quieto 5590
quorum 5593

quota pazienti 4932
quotidiano 1654
quotidiano 2382
quoziente d'intelligenza, QI 3509
rabbia 275
rabbia 5632
rabbico 5595
rabbrividire 6211
rabdomiosarcoma 5915
racchiuso 2250
raccolta campione 6396
raccolta campione ematico 775
raccolta di dati 1669
raccolta di dati 1686
raccolta fondi 2749
raddrizzare 6570
radiante 5598
radiazione 5600
radiazione ionizzante 3621
radicale 5604
radicale 5605
radicale libero 2722
radice 5956
radice nervosa 4452
radice quadrata 6465
radio 5630
radioattivo 5608
radiobiologia 5611
radiochirurgia 5628
radiografare 7486
radiografia 5613
radiografia 5615
radiografia 7485
radiografia d'intervento 3547
radiografia panoramica 4827
radiografico 5614
radioimmunoassay 5616
radioisotopo 5618
radioligando 5620
radiologia 5622

radiologo 5621
radiomarcato 5619
radiometria 5623
radionuclide 5624
radioonda 5607
radiopaco 5625
radiosensibile 5626
radiosensibilizzatore 5627
radioterapia 5603
radioterapia 5629
radon 5631
raffreddore 1275
raffreddore comune 1315
ragazzo 828
raggi gamma 2771
raggi infrarossi 3426
raggio 5630
raggio X 7485
raggiungere un massimo 4943
raggrinzarsi 6219
raggruppamento 1244
raggruppamento di dati 1667
raggruppare 2921
ragione fondamentale 5666
ramo 3758
ramo 414
ramo di trattamento 3759
ramo di trattamento 415
ramo di uno studio 6607
randomizzare 5645
randomizzazione 5641
randomizzazione a blocchi 750
randomizzazione stratificata 6578
rango 5649
rantoli 5634
rantoli grossi 1250
rantoli umidi 4264
rapporto 1429
rapporto 3523
rapporto 5663

rapporto 5809
rapporto beneficio/rischio 643
rapporto costo-beneficio 1537
rapporto dei conversazioni telefonici 6844
rapporto di dati da campo 2587
rapporto di previsione 4623
rapporto dose-risposta 2018
rapporto medico 4080
rapporto medico finale 2598
rapporto medico-paziente 5104
rapporto rischio-beneficio 5944
rapporto sessuale 6189
rapporto statistico 6505
rapporto statistico finale 2599
rapporto tra sessi 6184
rapporto ventilazione-perfusione 7288
rappresentante 5997
rappresentante marketing 4007
rappresentativo 5812
raschiamento 17
raschiatoio 1623
rash 5656
rata di secrezione 6091
ratto 5657
raucedine 3107
razionale 5665
razionale clinico 1210
razionalizzazione 5667
razionamento 5668
razione 5664
razza 5596
reagente 5678
realizzazione 45
reattività crociata 1584
reattivo 5675
reattivo 5678
reattore nucleare 4557
reazione 5673
reazione 5857
reazione alla sofferenza 2915

480

reazione allergica 188
reazione anafilattica 255
reazione chimica 1096
reazione crociata 1583
reazione papulo-eritematosa 7431
rebound 5682
recensione 5906
recensire 5907
recessivo 5688
recessivo autosomico 545
recesso 5687
recettore 5686
recettore adrenergico 107
recettore alpha 200
recettore beta 650
recettore colinergico 1134
recettore de complemento 1348
recettore dell' ormone tiroideo 6939
recettore delta 1780
recettore di fattore crescita 2926
recettore farmaco 2071
recettore gamma 2772
recettore mitogeno 4243
recettore mu 4326
recettore per l'homing dei linfociti 3929
recettore purinergico 5553
recettore sensoriale 6139
recettore sinaptico 6762
recettore sostanza endogena 2263
recidiva 5764
recipiente 1455
reclamo assicurazione 3501
reclinato 5710
reclutamento 5704
recrudescenza 5703
reclutamento di pazienti 4933
recuperare 6457
recupero urina 7210
redattore 2148
redazione 2147

redazione dati 1673
redito 3351
referenza 5720
refrattario 5731
regime 5736
regime a bassa dose 3891
regime di dosaggio 2006
regionale 5738
regione 410
regione 5737
regstrare 5697
registrazione 2286
registrazione 5743
registrazione 5744
registrazione 6813
registrazione del paziente 4926
registrazione dosaggio 2023
registrazione elettrica 2197
registro dei pazienti 4934
registro dello studio 7094
regola dell' interruzione anticipata 2124
regola di arresto 6565
regolamento a losterico 193
regolare 5750
regolare 91
regolatore 5753
regolazione 5751
regolazione 92
regolazione abbassa 2037
regolazione ascenzionale 7192
regredire 5745
regredire 5891
regredire 5893
regressione 5746
regressione alla media 5749
reidratazione 3758
reinfarto 5760
reinfezione 5761
relativo 5770
relazione 5811

relazione con il paziente 4935
relazione dose-risposta 2018
relazione esperta 2437
relazione lineare 3827
relazione medica 986
relazione non lineare 4520
relazione sessuale 6193
relazione spaziale 6380
relazione struttura-attività 6604
relazioni csplite-parassite 3143
relazioni pubbliche 5522
religione 5782
remineralizzazione 5787
remissione 1
remissione 5788
remittente 5789
renale 5792
rendere igienico 6019
rendere inattivo 3336
rendimento 2162
rendimento 4980
rene 3684
reologia 5916
reparto cure intensiva 3516
reparto di pronto soccorso 2229
reparto ospedaliero 1189
reparto terapia intensiva 3517
reperimento 5888
replicazione 5807
reportage eccessiva 4771
reportage incompleto 7164
repressione 5814
reprimere 5813
repulsivo 5820
requisiti di licenza 3791
requis.to 5821
requis.to per il dimensione di campione 6011
resecabile 5828
resecare 5827
resezione 5829

residenza 5831
residenziale 5833
residuo 5834
residuo 5835
residuo farmaco 2072
resilienza 5836
resina 5837
resistente alle manomissione 6805
resistenza 2279
resistenza 5838
resistenza alla rottura 6860
resistenza dell'ospite 3141
resistenza delle vie aere 165
resistenza fisica 6483
resistenza polmonare vascolare 5535
resistenza vascolare 7258
resistenza vascolare sistemica 6783
resoconto di posti 6269
respiratore 5846
respiratorio 5847
respirazione 5845
respirazione a pressione positiva 5233
respirazione bocca a bocca 4322
respirazione debole 6198
respiro 849
respiro 851
respiro affannoso 2783
respiro corto 6215
respiro di Kussmaul 162
responsabilità 36
responsabilità 3787
responsabilità dose farmaco 2058
resto 5784
restringimento 4401
restringimento 6593
restrizione 5867
restrizione fluidi 2642
rete 4457
rete neurale di computer 4459
reticolare 5878

481

riposarsi 5859
riposo 5858
riproducibile 5816
riproducibilità 5815
riproduttivo 1114
riproduzione 5817
riprovocazione 5689
ripulsivo 5820
risata 3734
risata 3736
riscaldamento 3009
riscaldare 3003
riscaldare 7393
rischiare 5943
rischio 2960
rischio 5942
rischio della salute professionale 4616
rischio di base 609
rischio eccessivo 2395
rischio relativo 5774
riscontro interno 3532
risecare 5827
riserva 5830
riso 3736
risoluzione 5839
risolvere 5840
risolversi 5840
risonanza 5841
risonanza magnetica nucleare 4556
risonanza magnetica per imagini 3953
risorsa 5843
risorse naturale 4419
rispondente parziale 4881
risposta 5857
risposta accumulata 1618
risposta anamnestica 253
risposta clinica 1213
risposta di sazietà 6028
risposta galvanica cutanea 2768
risposta massimale 4945

risposta ritardata 1770
risposta soggettiva 6634
rista alirsi 6457
risultate sostitutivo 6722
risultati di supporto 6695
risultati equivoci 2335
risultati inconclusivi 3356
risultati non favorevoli 4528
risultato 4754
risultato 5398
risultato 5869
risultato ben definibile 2956
risultato del trattamento 7078
risultato di paziente 4930
risultato non facilmente misurabile 6345
risultato numerico 4570
risultato secondario 6088
risuscitare 5910
risveglio 417
ritarcato 1769
ritarcato 5874
ritarco 5873
ritarco di un farmaco 2068
ritarco mentale 4130
ritarco mentale 4136
ritegno 1456
ritenzione 5877
ritenzione denti 1804
ritenzione fecale 2536
ritiro 2052
ritiro 5886
ritmc 5928
ritmc alfa 201
ritmc cardiaco 949
ritmc circadiano 1164
ritmc di galoppo 2766
ritmc nodale 4502
riuniene 4096
rivalutazione 5719

rivascolarizzazione 5901
rivelazione 1923
robinetto 6811
robotica 5950
robustezza 5951
roditore 5852
roditore 5853
rombencefalo 3084
rompere 1557
ronchi grossi 1251
ronco 5927
röntgen 5954
rosso d'uovo 2187
rossore 2620
rossore 2648
rossore 2651
rotare 5911
rotazione 5960
rotazione 6419
rotazione ottica 4686
rotazioni dell'inventario 3593
rotto 1927
rottura 1556
rottura 5978
rottura e risaldatura 6439
rottura nell'asse 843
rotula 4902
routine 5970
rovinare 6443
rubare 6514
rubricazione 3372
rudimentale 5974
rudimento 7320
ruga 7475
rumore 4506
rumore 875
rumore cardiaco 2995
rumore di sfregamento 2736
rumore respiratorio 850
rumori intestinali 826

rumori peristaltici 5005
ruotare 5420
rurale 5979
russare 6329
rutto 637
sacca 5188
sacca 5980
sacco 5188
sacco amniotico 583
sacro 5985
sacroiliaco 5983
sacrolombare 5984
sadismo 5986
sadomasochismo 5987
sagittale 5996
sala di recupero 5701
sala neonati 4573
sala operatoria 4668
salasso 782
saldatura 7426
sale 6003
sali da fiuto 6312
saliva 6000
salivare 6001
salpinge 7117
salutare 6005
salute 2914
salute 2968
salute fisica 5097
salute mentale 4132
salute ol stica 3108
salute professionale 4615
salvataggio 5822
salvezza 5989
sanare 2966
sanatorio 6013
sangue 753
sangue autologo 533
sangue intero 7442
sangue occulto 4612

seno paranasale 4846
sensazione 6132
sensazione da puntura di spillo 5135
sensazione vibratoria 7326
sensi speciali 6384
sensibile 6136
sensibilità 2544
sensibilità 6137
sensibilità 6855
sensibilità al solletico 6945
sensibilità alla percussione 4976
sensibilità tattile 7006
sensibilizzazione crociata 1588
senso 6133
senso comune 1317
senso di nausea 5582
sensorio 6138
sentimento 2544
sentire 2431
sentire 6134
sentire odore di 6311
senza casa 3112
senza complicazioni 7156
separato 6141
separazione 1840
separazione 6142
sepsi 6143
sequela 6151
sequenza 6152
sequenza ADN automatizzata 536
sequenza di basi 605
sequenza segnale 6239
sequenziale 6154
serie di casi 987
serio 6159
serotoninergico 6168
servizi a contratto 1482
servizio informazioni 3422
servizio sanità mentale 4134
servizio sanitario 2978

sessione 6177
sessione sosttutiva 3959
sesso 2803
sesso 6181
sessuale 6186
sete 6911
setticemia 6148
setticemia 770
settico 6146
settimana 7417
setto 6149
setto nasale 4404
settore privato 5379
settore pubblico 5523
severo 6178
sezionare 1953
sezionare 6093
sezione 6092
sezione congelata 2741
sezione istologica 3098
sezione trasversale 1585
sferoidale 6414
sferoide 6413
sfigmomanometro 6416
sfintere 6415
sfintere anale 242
sfondo etnico 2368
sforzo 2411
sforzo 2527
sforzo 6586
sfregio 6287
sguardo fisso 6494
shock 6213
shock cardiogeno 954
shock da calore 3007
shock elettrico 2177
shock emorragico 3043
shock settico 6147
shunt 6221
shunt cardiaco 950

sicurezza 1067
sicurezza 5989
sicurezza del prodotto 5403
sicurezza sociale 6335
sicuro 5888
sicuro da guasti 2500
SIDA 156
siero 6173
sieroalbumina 6174
sierodiagnosi 6161
sierologia 6163
sieropositività 6165
sieropositivo 6164
sieroprevalenza 6166
sieropurulento 6167
sifiloma primario 1077
sigaretto 1158
sigari 1159
sigmoideo 6231
sigmoidoscopia 6234
sigmoidoscopio 6233
significamente differente 6243
significato 6241
significato clinico 1214
silente 6245
silenzicso 5590
silogismo 6744
simbiosi 6745
simbolismo 6747
simbolo 6746
simbolo di codificazione 1261
simmetrico 6743
simpatectomia 6749
simpatico 6750
simpaticolitico 6752
simpaticomimetico 6753
simposio 6755
simulare 6250
simulare una malattia 3972
simulazione computerizzata 1377

simulazione di una malattia 3973
simultaneo 6251
sinapsi 6760
sinaptosoma 6763
sincope 6765
sindrome 6766
sindrome da immunodeficienza acquisita, SIDA 58
sindrome delle gambe irrequiete 5861
sindrome di astinenza 7454
sindrome di Down 2038
sindrome di Ekbom 5861
sindrome dolore miofasciale 4386
sindrome mielodisplastica 4377
sindrome postgastrectomia 2089
sinergismo 6767
sinergismo tra farmaci 2074
sinfisi 6754
singhiozzare 6332
singhiozzo 3074
singolo 3382
singolo 6254
singulto 6331
sinistro 6260
sinovia 6768
sinoviale 6769
sintesi 6773
sintesi chimica 1098
sintetico 6774
sintomatico 6757
sintomatologia 6759
sintomi affettivi 129
sintomi di raffreddamento 1280
sintomi fisici 5101
sintomo 6235
sintomo 6756
sintomo clinico 1220
sintomo evidente 4772
sintomo soggettivo 1344
sinusite 6263

siringa 6776
siringa ipodermica 3226
sistema 6778
sistema 7022
sistema cardiovascolare 964
sistema del secondo messaggero 6081
sistema di accecamento 742
sistema di catetle gialle 7496
sistema di sopravvivenza 3801
sistema ematico 3027
sistema immunitario 3289
sistema in linea 4648
sistema ipofisi-surrenale 5145
sistema ipotalamo ipofisario 3237
sistema limbico 3816
sistema linfatico 3927
sistema motorio 4317
sistema muscolare 4356
sistema nervoso 4455
sistema nervoso autonomo 541
sistema nervoso centrale 1047
sistema nervoso parasimpatico 4856
sistema nervoso simpatico 6751
sistema portale 5227
sistema sopportanti 6694
sistemazione dei pazienti 192
sistemico 6780
sistole 6785
sito allosterico 194
sito di legame 678
sito investigativo 3603
sito satellite 6025
situs 6272
slargamento 7446
smaltimento dei rifiuti 1950
smalto 2247
smascherare 7182
smemoratezza 2694
sociale 6333
socializzazione 6336

società 1323
società 6337
società multinazionale 4344
sociologia 6339
soda 6341
soddisfatto 5481
soddisfazione 6029
soddisfazione nel livello di vita 3799
sodio 6342
sofferenza 1968
sofferenza 2914
sofferenza fetale 2561
soffice 6343
soffio 4352
soffio 875
soffio cardiaco 2992
soffio diastolico 1879
soffio sistolico 6787
soffocare 1127
soffocare 6542
soffocare 6573
soffocare 6668
soffrire 6667
software 6348
soggettivo 6632
soggetto 6630
soglia 6919
soglia del dolore 4795
soglia sensoriale 6140
sognare a occhi aperti 1703
sogno 2043
solco 2610
solco 2918
solco 7111
solido 6352
solitario 3871
sollievo 5781
solo 3871
solo 6254
solubile in acqua 7406

solubilità 6353
solubilità in acqua 7405
soluzione 6354
soluzione del problema 5386
soluzione ipertonica 3213
soluzione salina 5998
soluzione salina ipertonica 3212
solvente 6355
soma 6356
somatico 6357
somatosensorio 6359
somma 7003
somministrare una dose 2009
somministrazione 95
somministrazione orale 4692
somministrazione orale 4695
sonare 6368
sonda 5383
sonda ADN 1986
sondare 5384
sonnambulismo 6293
sonno 6289
sonno REM 5783
sonnolenza 2055
sonnolenza 6360
sonogramma 6361
soporifero 4677
sopporti 829
soppressione 6698
soppressione genetica 2825
soppressore 6699
sopracciglia 872
sopracciglio 2476
sopradossaggio intenzionale 3518
sopraventricolare 6704
sopravvissuto 6727
sopravvivenza 6726
sorcio 4320
sordità 1707
sordo 1705

sordo 2085
sordomuto 1706
sorriso 6313
sorveglianza di un prodotto 5404
sorveglianza farmacologica 2073
sorveglianza successiva al marketing 5245
sospendere 6729
sospensione 1926
sospensione 6730
sospensione 7452
sospensione prematura 5319
sospeso 1927
sospiro 6229
sostanza 4041
sostanza 6646
sostanza antisolare 6680
sostanza bianca 7440
sostanza chimica 1091
sostanza con alta affinità plasmatica 3080
sostanza grigia 2912
sostanza inquinante 5203
sostanza nera 6649
sostanza nutriente 4576
sostanza pericolosa 2961
sostanza ricca di fibre 5963
sostenere 6731
sostituire 6652
sostitutivo 6720
sostituto 6651
sostituto 6719
sostituzione 5805
sostituzione terapeutica 6894
sottigliezza 6907
sottile 6862
sotto la norma 6648
sottocutaneo 6623
sottodurale 6625
sottogruppo 6627
sottogruppo di pazienti 6629
sottolinguale 6637

Italian/Italiano

sottopeso 7165
sottrazione digitale 1901
sovradosare 4768
sovrapposizione 4770
sovrapposto 6684
spalla 6218
spargimento dati 1672
spartire 1979
spasmo 6376
spasmo 7129
spasmo bronchiale 860
spasmolitico 5776
spastico 6377
spazio 6373
spazio intermedio 3542
spazio vuoto 732
specialista 6386
specialità 6388
specialità chirurgica 6717
specialità clinica 4083
specializzazione 6385
specializzazione malattia 1934
specie 2695
specie 6390
specificità 6394
specificità del substrato 6653
specifico 6391
specolo 6404
speculazione 2769
spedizione 6210
sperimentale 2434
sperimentare 2433
sperimentazione clinica 7088
sperimentazione controllata 1498
sperimentazione randomizzata controllata 5646
sperma 6407
spermatogenesi 6410
spermatozoo 6411
sperone 5934
sperone di calcio 904

spesa 2428
spesa 2429
spessore dello strato sottocutaneo 6284
spettro 6403
spettro infrarosso 3427
spettrofotometria di Raman 5635
spettrometria 6401
spettroscopia 6402
spigolo 2143
spin 6419
spira sacrale 5982
spirale 6422
spirale 6428
spirale 6429
spirito 4289
spirito 6430
spirocheta 6431
spirometria 6432
splancnico 6435
splenico 6437
splenomegalia 6438
splicing 6439
splicing dell'ARN 5949
spondilite anchilosante 298
spoisor 6445
spostaneo 6447
spoia 6449
spo adico 6448
spo care 6349
spo ozoito 733
spossatezza 2415
spostamento 1946
spostamento all'indietro 570
spreco 7400
spremere 6466
spremitura 2443
spri e 6460
sprizzare 6454
spriizzi 6453
spugna 6444

spurio 6462
sputare 6434
sputo 6433
sputo 6463
squalificante 1952
squama 6034
squamoso 6038
squilibrio 1935
squilibrio 3277
squilibrio elettrolitico 2189
stabile 6472
stabilità 6470
stabilità fisica 5100
stabilizzazione 6471
stacanovista del lavoro 7462
stadi del sonno 6292
stadiazione 6476
stadiazione di una neoplasia 6477
stadio 6475
stadio clinico 1216
stadio di riposo 5860
stadio di un medico interno 5832
staff 6473
staff paramedico 4843
staff permanente 3146
stafilococco 6492
stagionale 6078
stagione 6077
stampelle 1599
stampo 4267
stampo 6848
stampo 989
stampo 990
stanchezza 3726
stanchezza 7414
standard 6485
standard 6486
standard di argento 6248
standard di riferimento 2878
standard di riferimento 5722

standard di riferimento 6244
standard etica 2365
stare a dieta 1883
starnutire 6324
starnuto 6323
stasi 6478
stasi 6498
statistica 6507
statistica demografica 7355
statistica descrittiva 1831
statistica di Bayes 620
statisticamente significativo 3506
statistico 6503
stato 6500
stato 6509
stato acido base 51
stato clinico 1217
stato decerebrato 1720
stato di allerta 175
stato di famiglia 4001
stato di portatore 978
stato di stabilità 6511
stato funzionale 2748
stato generale delle salute £766
stato mentale 4137
stato nutritivo 4581
statura 6508
status quo 6510
steatorrea 2531
steatorrea 6516
stecca 6440
stecco 6540
stellato 6519
stelo 6520
stendere 6590
stenosi 6523
stenosi 6593
stenosi mitralica 4249
stenosi valvolare 7242
stereoisomero 6526

487

terapia comportamentale 634
terapia della coppia 4002
terapia di avversione 552
terapia di inalazione ossigeno 4783
terapia di prima linea 2607
terapia di recupero 6006
terapia di seconda linea 6080
terapia occupazionale 4617
terapia ormonale 3131
terapia ortomolecolare 4720
terapia sostitutiva 5806
terapia trombolitica 6928
teratogeno 6863
teratologia 6866
teratoma 6867
termico 6898
terminale 6869
terminale 6870
terminale computer 1378
terminale intelligente 3511
terminale muto 2088
terminazione nervosa 4449
termine 1235
termine 6868
termine dello studio 7095
termine preferito 5304
termini anatomici 260
terminologia 6875
termodinamica 6901
termografia 6903
termogramma 6902
termometro 6904
tesaurismosi 6568
tesi 1957
tessuto 6966
tessuto connettivo 1430
tessuto corneo 3132
tessuto germinale 2843
tessuto molle 6347
test 6878

test campione 1586
test cutaneo 6282
test d'intelligenza 3510
test dei segni 6237
test del chi quadrato 1125
test del gusto 6824
test della funzione uditiva 2984
test delle colture linfocitarie miste 4253
test di compatibilità 1335
test di complementazione 1349
test di conferma 1411
test di fertilità 2555
test di funzionalità polmonare 5532
test di germinazione: test di inseminazione 6099
test di gravidanza 5307
test di prestazione 4982
test di sensibilità microbica 4169
test di tolleranza al glucosio 2871
test epicutaneo 4901
test intra-trattamento 653
test intradermico 4901
test mutagenetico 4360
test non parametrico 4521
test parametrico 4845
test provocatorio 5484
test radioimmunologico 5616
test su animali 290
test sul corpo umano 3155
test unità formanti colonie 1295
test z 7510
testa 2962
testamento 7447
testicolo 6881
testo 6883
tetano 6882
tetro 4299
tibia 6940
tibiale 6941
tic 6942
tigna 6963

timo 6936
timore 2532
timpano 2077
timpano 2123
timpano 7137
tingere 2099
tintura 2098
tintura 6962
tipizzazione immunologica 3304
tipo 7138
tipo di tabella 6791
tipo sanguigno 777
tiroide 6937
tiroide 6938
titolare 6971
titolo 6969
titolo 6970
titolo anticorpale 324
titolo del soggetto 6631
toccare 7007
tofo 6995
toletta 6975
tollerabilità 6976
tolleranza 6977
tolleranza all'esercizio 2410
tolleranza crociata 1589
tollerare 6978
tomografia 6979
tomografia ad emissione di positroni 5028
tomografia assiale computerizzata 1372
tomografia computerizzata 1369
tomografia computerizzata 1379
tomografia computerizzata 7487
tomografia computerizzata d'emissione 2234
tomografia dell'encefalo 836
tonicità 6986
tonicità 6990
tonico 6983
tonico 6984
tono 6980

tono 6986
tono 6990
tono cardiaco 2995
tono posturale 5264
tonometria 6988
tonometro 6987
tonsilla 6989
topico 6996
tipo 4320
torace 1106
torace 6915
torace a botte 597
toracentesi 6912
toracico 6913
torbido 1242
torcicollo 7000
torpore 2055
torpore 6997
torsione 6998
torso 6999
tortuoso 7001
tortura 7002
tosse 1541
tossicità 7011
tossicità fetale 2563
tossicità vestibolare 7317
tossico 7010
tossicologia 7012
tossicomane 76
tossicomania 2059
tossicomania 77
tossiemia 7009
tossina 7013
tossina batterica 575
tossine marine 4000
tossire 1542
totale 21
totale 7003
totale 7004
tourniquet 7008

Italian/Italiano

ulcera da decubito 5348
ulcera da decubito 628
ulcera duodenale 2091
ulcera peptica 4962
ulcerazione 918
ulna 7142
ultimo 2597
ultracentrifugazione 7143
ultrafiltrazione 7144
ultrasonico 7145
ultrasonografia 7146
ultrastruttura 7148
ultrasuono 7147
ultravioletto 7149
umano 3150
umidità 3158
umidità 4265
umidità relativa 5772
umorale 3159
umore acqueo 405
umore vitreo 7359
una volta al giorno 4640
unghia 2604
unghia 4393
unguento 4632
unguento 6007
unicellulare 7170
uniforme 7171
uniformità 7172
uniformità contenuto 1459
unilaterale 7173
unione 7175
unipolare 7176
unità 7177
unità di cura coronaria 1519
unità di misura 7178
unità di misura standardizzata 6490
unità internazionale 3536
unità operativa 6818
universale 7467

università 7180
universitario 6059
uomo 3982
uomo singolo 3381
uovo 2165
uovo 4777
urbanizzazione 7196
urbano 7195
urea 7197
uremia 7198
uretere 7199
uretra 7200
uretrale 7201
urgente 7203
urgenza (minzionale) 7202
urgenza 2227
urina 7209
urinare 4193
urinario 7206
urodinamica 7211
urogenitale 2833
urogenitale 7212
urografia 7213
urologia 7216
urologico 7214
urologico 7215
usare impropriamente 4238
usare un tampone 6736
uscito dallo studio 3878
uso 396
uso improprio 4237
uso per compassione 1333
ustione 887
ustione chimica 1093
ustione di terzo grado 6908
utero 7220
utero 7458
utilizzazione 7221
utricolo 7222
uvea 7223

vaccinare 3458
vaccinazione 7225
vaccino 7226
vacuolo 7228
vagale 7230
vagina 7231
vaginale 7232
vago 7236
vagotomia 7235
validazione dati 1694
validità 7239
validità contenuto 1460
validità interna 3534
valore 7240
valore basale 606
valore critico 1577
valore di controllo 1496
valore di riferimento 5723
valore erratico 4756
valore medio 549
valore metabolico basale 600
valore normalizzato 4540
valore nutritivo 4583
valore p 5561
valore rettificato 1521
valore soppesato 7424
valore stimato 2358
valore trasformato 7050
valori seriali 6158
valutabile 2377
valutazione 2378
valutazione 463
valutazione clinica globale 2858
valutazione congiunta 3665
valutazione della disabilità 1919
valutazione delle prestazioni 4981
valutazione di sicurezza 5991
valutazione globale 2860
valutazione psicometrica 5500
valvola 7241

valvola aortica 371
valvola cardiaca 2997
valvola ileocecale 3264
valvola mitrale 4250
valvola polmonare 5534
valvola tricuspidale 7097
vampata di calore 3144
vantaggio 641
vapore 6515
vapore 7243
variabile 7245
variabile 7246
variabile confondente 1417
variabile di sicurezza 5995
variabile dipendente 1810
variabile efficacia 2161
variabile indipendente 3369
variabile non facilmente misurabile 6344
variabilità 7244
variabilità binaria 674
variabilità tra pazienti 652
variante 7248
varianza 7247
variato 7248
variazione 1078
variazione 7249
varice 7253
varicocele 7250
varicoso 7251
variegato 4318
vasca a sedile 6273
vascolare 7256
vasculite 7259
vasectomia 7260
vaso 7254
vaso 7315
vasc deferente 7255
vaso sanguigno 779
vasocostrittore 7262
vasocostrizione 7261

# Italian/Italiano

amiloide 235
amiloidosis 236
amina 222
aminoácido 223
aminoaciduria 224
amnesia 226
amniocentesis 227
amoníaco 225
amontonamiento 1614
amontonamiento dentario 1595
amorfo 229
ampliación 7446
amplificación 230
amplificación de genes 2806
amplificador 231
amplio espectro 856
ampolla 232
ampolla de múltiples dosis 4339
amputación 233
anabolismo 238
anaeróbico 240
anaerobio 239
anafase 254
anafilaxia 256
anal 241
analéptico 243
analgesia 244
analgésico 245
análisis 249
análisis 6878
análisis actuarial 71
análisis costes-ventajas 1532
análisis de agrupamiento 1245
análisis de datos 1861
análisis de espectro de Raman 5635
análisis de la varianza 250
análisis de los factores de riesgo 5946
análisis de mutaciones de ADN 1985
análisis de pares correlacionados 4031
análisis de regresión 5747

análisis de sangre 758
análisis de sangre fecal 6559
análisis de sistemas 6784
análisis de vector 7272
análisis del punto final 2278
análisis del subgrupo 6628
análisis discriminante 1930
análisis económico 2134
análisis factorial 2494
análisis interno 3528
análisis mínimo-cuadrático 3750
análisis multivariante 4347
análisis Northern blot 4544
análisis numérico 4568
análisis planimétrico 5154
análisis por espectrografía de masas 4018
análisis químico 1092
análisis secuencial 6155
análisis secuencial de grupo 2923
análisis sofisticado 6363
análisis Southern blot 6372
análisis transaccional 7034
análisis Western blot 7428
analito 251
analogía 248
análogo 247
anamnesis 3104
anamnesis 3105
anamnesis 984
anamnesis natural de enfermedades 4415
anasarca 257
anastomosis 258
anastomosis 6221
anastomosis 894
anastomosis arteriovenosa 430
anatomía 261
anatómica 259
andar 7388
andar como un pato 7380
andar encorvado 6560

andrógeno 264
anemia 266
anemia aplástica 383
anemia hemolítica 3037
anemia megaloblástica 4067
anencefalia 267
anestesia 268
anestesia a circuito cerrado 1233
anestesiar 4564
anestésico 270
anestésico 271
anestesiología 269
anestesista 272
aneuploidía 273
aneurisma 274
anexos 98
angina 276
angina pectoris 277
angiocardiograma 278
angiografía 280
angioma 281
angioneurótico 282
angiopatía 283
angioplastia 284
ángulo 285
angustia 366
anillo 301
anillo 5941
animación 291
animal 286
anión 292
anisocitosis 294
anisocoria 293
ano 365
anomalía 302
anorexia nerviosa 303
anormal 12
anormalidad 13
anosmia 304
anovulación 305

anoxemia 306
anoxia 307
anquilosis 299
ansiedad 366
ansiolítico 368
antagonista 309
antagonista competitivo 1341
antagonista del calcio 902
antagonista no competitivo 4512
antebrazo 2684
antebrazo 2690
antecedentes 567
anteojos 2854
antepasado 262
anterior 313
anterior 5289
antes de la muerte 310
antes del parto 312
anti- 317
antiácido 308
antianginal 318
antiarrítmico 319
antiarrítmico 320
antibacteriano 321
antibiótico 322
antibiótico de amplio espectro 857
anticátodo 6815
anticoagulante 327
anticolinérgico 326
anticonceptivo 1471
anticonceptivo 1472
anticonceptivo hormonal 3128
anticonvulsivante 328
anticuerpo 323
anticuerpo monoclonal 4288
anticuerpo neutralizante 4463
anticuerpos de fijación del complemento 1350
antidepresivo 329
antidiarreico 330
antidiurético 331

Spanish/Español

antídoto 332
antiemético 333
antiepiléptico 334
antifibrinolítico 335
antifúngico 336
antígeno 337
antígeno carcinoembrionario 934
antígeno de superficie 6707
antihelmíntico 315
antihemorrágico 338
antihipertensivo 340
antihistamínico 339
antiinfeccioso 341
antiinflamatorio 342
antilipémico 343
antimalárico 344
antimetabolito 345
antimicrobiano 346
antinatural 7184
antineoplásico 347
antinuclear 348
antioxidante 349
antipatía 350
antipirético 352
antipsicótico 351
antiséptico 354
antisuero 355
antitoxina 357
antitrombina 356
antituberculoso 358
antitumoral 359
antitusivo 360
antiviral 361
antro 362
antro pilórico 5564
antropología 316
anual 300
anulus 301
anuresis 363
anuria 364

año 7493
año de vida ajustado a la calidad 5578
año-gente 4960
años de supervivencia 7494
aorta 369
aórtico 370
apagar 5586
aparato 1854
aparato acústico 2982
aparato cardiovascular 984
aparato de Golgi 2880
aparato de ortodoncia 4718
aparato del uso mitótico 4246
aparato digestivo 1898
aparato ortótico 4725
aparatos odontológicos 829
aparatos ortopédicos 829
apareamiento 4799
aparente 390
apariencia 392
apatía 372
apéndice 393
apéndice 394
apéndice 89
apertura 373
apetito 395
apetitoso 4800
apilamiento de los glóbulos rojos 5964
aplásico 382
aplástico 382
aplicación 396
apnea 384
apocrino 385
apoenzima 386
apófisis mastoidea 4027
apolipoproteína 387
aponeurosis 2518
apoplejía 388
apoproteína 389
aportación 3502

apódisis 7484
apoyo 6693
apoyo de entrenamiento 7029
apraxia 401
aprendizaje de discriminación 1931
aprendizaje de evasión 554
aprensión 399
aprobación ética 2363
apropiado 6674
aptitud 402
apuesta 2769
apuñalar 6469
arácnido 406
aracnoide 407
árbol bronquial 861
árbol de decisiones 1730
árbol genealógico 2808
archivamiento de datos 1662
archivo 2590
archivo 409
archivo de datos 1677
archivo del investigador 3606
archivo limpio 1180
archivo maestro de drogas 2069
archivo maestro del ensayo 7092
arco 408
arco reflejo 5727
área 410
área bajo una curva 411
área con atención médica insuficiente 4084
área terapéutica 6892
aréola 412
ARN antisenso 353
ARN de doble cadena 2033
ARN de transferencia 7046
ARN mensajero 4146
arriesgar 5943
arritmia 418
arruga 5934

arruga 7475
arrugar 6219
arte 420
artefacto 445
arteria 432
arteria carótida 972
arteria coronaria 1517
arterial 421
arteriograma 425
arteriola 426
arteriosclerosis 427
arteriovenoso 429
arteritis 431
articulación 3662
articulación 444
articulación de la cadera 3087
articulación esférica y hueca 588
articulación mandibular 3985
articulación sinovial 6771
articulación temporomandibular 6852
articular 440
artículo 439
artículo de parada 6563
artificial 446
artralgia 434
artritis 435
artritis reumatoide 5921
artrografía 436
artroplastia 437
artroscopia 438
asa 6322
asbesto 449
ascendente 450
ascitis 451
asepsia 453
aséptico 454
aséptico 455
asexual 457
asfixia 458
asignación 191

cálculo biliar 2767
cálculo del tamaño de la muestra 6010
cálculo dental 1795
cálculo renal 3685
calefacción 3009
calentar 3003
calentar 7393
calibración 906
calidad 5577
calidad de vida 5581
caliente 7394
calistenia 908
callado 5590
callo 1512
callo 909
calmante 6362
calmar 190
calmar 3803
calor 3002
caloría 911
calórico 910
calorimetría 912
calvicie 587
calvo 586
cama 624
camada 3849
cámara 1075
cámara 913
cámara anterior 314
camas ocupadas 626
cambio 1078
cambio 2397
cambio de personal 5020
cambio porcentual 4967
cambio trófico 7108
cambios patológicos 4915
caminar 7388
camino crítico 1576
campo 2585
campo de datos 1676

campo electromagnético 2190
campo pulmonar 3915
campo visual 7350
campo visual periférico 5003
canal 1081
canal 2918
canal 914
canal de potasio 5268
canal del parto 710
canal inguinal 3433
canal iónico 3617
canales semicirculares 6121
cáncer 915
candidato de reserva 569
canino 917
cansancio 7414
cantidad de camas 625
cantidad de trabajo 7464
cánula 920
cañería 5137
capa 3739
capa externa 6208
capacidad 10
capacidad 2614
capacidad de trabajo 7460
capacidad de unión 677
capacidad vital 7353
capilar 921
cápsula 926
cápsula bacteriana 573
cápsula de gelatina 2802
cápsula rellenada a mano 2948
captación 7193
captación radioactiva 5610
captar 7194
caquexia 885
cara 2481
carácter 1083
carácter de la droga 2064
característica 1084

característica 7030
carbohidrato 927
carbono 928
carboxihemoglobina 932
carbunclo 933
carcinogénesis 936
carcinogenicidad 936
carcinogénico 937
carcinógeno 935
carcinoma 939
cardíaco 940
card aco 941
cardiología 955
cardiopatía reumática 5919
cardiospasmo 958
cardiotónico 959
cardiotónico 960
cardiotoxicidad 961
cardiovascular 862
cargando peso 7420
cargazón de espaldas 6560
cariarse 1717
carie 968
caries 1716
cariotipaje 3676
cariot pear 3675
cariotipo 3674
carnal 969
carne 2626
carne 4555
caroteno 970
carótida 971
carpeta 5229
carpeta reguladora 5754
carpiano 974
carta médica 4072
cartel 5239
cartera 5229
cartílago 981
cartílago articular 441

cartílago hialino 3162
casa 3110
caso 982
caso avanzado 113
caso base 603
casc índice 3371
caso modelo 4260
casos correlacionados 4029
caspa 1658
castigo 5548
castración 2218
castrar 991
casualidad 1076
catabolismo 992
catalepsia 7031
catalepsia 993
catálisis 994
catalítico 995
cataplexia 996
catarata 997
catarro 1275
catarro 1315
catarro 999
catarsis 1007
catártico 1008
catatonía 1000
catatónico 1001
catecolamina 1002
categoría 1005
categorías de investigación 6076
categorización 1004
catéter 1009
cateterismo 1010
cateterismo cardiaco 944
catgut 1006
catión 1011
catión divalente 1975
caucásico 1012
caucásico 1013
caudal 1014

causa de la muerte 1018
causa y efecto 1017
causalidad 1016
cáustico 1020
cáustico 1021
cauterizar 1022
cavidad 1024
cavidad 5188
cavidad 6340
cavidad aérea 160
cavidad corporal 789
cavidad pleural 5180
cavitación 1023
cefalea 2965
cegar 739
ceguera 743
ceguera nocturna 4492
ceja 2476
ceja 872
celdas mastoideas 4026
celiaco 1027
célula 1028
célula aérea 160
célula blástica 733
célula de estroma 6600
célula de la granulosa 2908
célula de las islas de Langerhans 3638
célula dendrítica 1789
célula enterocromafina 2291
célula epitelial 2328
célula escamosa 6464
célula germinal 2841
célula gigante 2847
célula grande 3717
célula killer 3687
célula natural killer 4417
célula nerviosa 4447
célula plasmática 5160
célula progenitora eritroide 2349
célula progenitora hematopoyética 3024

célula progenitora humana 3154
célula transicional 7058
célula troncal 6521
celular 1036
celulitis 1038
celulosa 1039
cemento 1041
centígrado 1043
central 1044
central 4196
centralización 1049
centralizado 1050
centrifugación 1051
centrifugación zonal 7506
centrifugar 1053
centrifugar 6420
centrífugo 1052
centrífugo 2155
centro 1042
centro 2656
centro coordinador 1508
centro de atención terciario 6877
centro de coordinador de datos 1670
centro de datos 1666
centro de la salud mental 4133
centro de toxicología 5196
centro médico 2972
centro para el tratamiento del cáncer 916
centro satélite 6023
centro traumatológico 7074
centrómero 1054
centros combinados 1308
cepa bacteriana 574
cera 7410
cercado 2250
cerebelo 1056
cerebeloso 1055
cerebral 1057
cerebro 1066
cerebro 831

cerebroespinal 1064
cerebrovascular 1065
cerrado 2250
cerrar 1231
certeza 1067
certificación 1068
certificado de nacimiento 711
cerumen 1069
cervical 1070
ceto-acidosis 3680
cetoacidosis diabética 1860
cetona 3681
cetosis 3682
chamuscar 6253
chancro 1077
chasquido de apertura 4664
chequeo 1087
choque 6213
choque cardiogénico 954
choque eléctrico 2177
choque hemorrágico 3043
choque por calor 3007
choque séptico 6147
cianosis 1634
ciática 6060
cibernética 1635
cicatriz 6045
cicatrizar 6046
ciclo 1636
ciclo de dosis 2021
ciclo menstrual 4124
ciclos por segundo 1637
ciego 1025
ciego 740
ciego simple 6255
ciencia 6061
científico 6062
científico 6064
cierre 1235
cifosis 3160

cifosis 3694
cira 2589
cigarrillos 1158
cigarros 1159
cilindro hialino 3163
cilio 1161
cilium 1161
c·ma 374
c·neangiografía 1162
c·nerradiografía 1163
cinética 3690
cinética de orden cero 7504
cinética de primer orden 2608
cinética de segundo orden 6082
cintura 7381
circulación 1166
circulación colateral 1287
círculo 1165
circunsición 1168
cirrosis 1169
cirugía 6711
cirugía con láser 3725
cirugía electiva 2175
cirugía estética 1530
cirugía plástica 5167
cirujano 6710
cistectomía 1641
cístico 1642
cistitis 1643
cistoadenocarcinoma 1640
cistoscopia 1644
cita 398
citoesqueleto 1650
citogenética 1645
citología 1647
citometría de flujo 2635
citoplasma 1648
citoprotector 1649
citosol 1651
citotoxicidad 1652

502

degenerado 1757
degenerado 1759
degenerar 1717
degenerar 1758
degenerar 5891
degradación 1762
dehisencia 1765
dejo 139
del vértice 7310
del yeyuno 3657
deleción 1773
deleción cromosómica 1147
deletéreo 1772
delgadez 6907
delgado 3747
delicado 6854
delirar 5669
delirio 1774
delirio por abstinencia 7453
delirium tremens 1775
delito 1569
delusión 1781
demanda de edición 2146
demencia 1782
demencia 3467
demencia por múltiples infartos 4335
demencia presenil 5335
demencia senil 6131
demencia vascular 7257
demente 3466
demografía 1784
demografía 1785
demora farmacológica 2068
dendrita 1788
denegación 5733
densidad 1792
densidad óptica 4684
densitometría 1791
densitometría con rayos x 7488
dentadura completa 1351

dentaduras 1805
dental 1794
dentición 1803
dentición primaria 5363
dentífrico 1799
dentina 1800
dentista 1801
dentistería 1802
departamento 1807
departamento de medicina 4073
dependencia física 5094
dependiente 1809
dependiente de hormonas 3130
dependiente de los anticuerpos 325
depilación 2318
depilar 1811
depleción 1813
depositar 1816
depósito 1815
depósito 1817
depósito en la piel 6279
depósito óseo 815
depresión 1819
depresión 7111
depresión respiratoria 5851
depresor 1818
deprivación 1820
depuración 1182
depuración de la creatinina 1564
derecho 6491
derivativo 1822
dermatitis 1825
dermatitis de contacto 1452
dermatología 1826
dermatosis 1827
dérmico 1824
derramamiento 6205
derramar 3744
derrame 2164

derrame 2632
derrame pericárdico 4986
derrame pleural 5181
derrame seroso 6170
derrochar 7401
desangrar 2446
desarregó 1941
desarrollo 1552
desarrollo 1850
desarrollo 2387
desarrollo analítico 252
desarrollo clínico 1198
desarrollo conjunto 3664
desarrollo de drogas 2063
desarrollo de la medicina 4093
desarrollo del producto 5398
desarrollo global 2859
desarrollo mundial 7468
desarrollo químico 1094
desastre 7399
desastre de la naturaleza 4414
desbridamiento 1713
descalificador 1952
descansar 5975
descar 5975
descarboxilación 1715
descartar 5975
descendente 1828
descendiendo 1828
descendiente 4630
descentralización 1718
descoloramiento 1924
descompensación 1733
descompone 6443
descomposición 1734
descompresión 1735
descongestionante 1737
desconocido 7181
descontaminación 1738
descoyuntar 1939
descripción 1830

descripción de la droga 2070
descripción de la eficacia 2159
descubrimiento 1841
descubrimiento 1929
desecación 1836
desecante 1833
desecante 1834
desecar 1835
desechable 1949
desecho 7400
desempleo 7168
desenmascarar 7182
desensibilización 1832
deseo vehemente 1562
desequilibrio 1935
desequilibrio 3277
desequilibrio de electrólitos 2189
desestímulo 1721
desfibrilación 1752
desfibrilador implantable 3321
desgranulación 1763
deshidratación 1767
deshidratar 1766
desigual 7167
desinfectar 1936
desintegración 1937
desintegrado 3938
desintegrar 3936
desistimiento 7383
desmayarse 2503
desmayo 2504
desmayo 728
desmielinación 1786
desmielinización 1786
desmosoma 1838
desnaturalización 1787
desnaturalización de proteínas 5460
desnervación 1790
desnucamiento 7434
desnudo 4562

507

508

encía 2932
encinta 2425
encorvar 6561
encuesta 6725
endarterectomía 2253
endémico 2254
enderezar 6570
endocardio 2256
endocarditis 2255
endocitosis 2280
endocrino 2257
endocrinología 2259
endodoncia 2261
endógeno 2262
endolinfa 2284
endometrial 2265
endometrio 2267
endometriosis 2266
endofina 2269
endoscopia 2272
endoscópico 2271
endoscopio 2270
endotelial 2274
endotelio 2275
endotoxina 2276
enema 2280
enema de bario 596
energía 2281
enfermedad 1344
enfermedad 1932
enfermedad 3272
enfermedad 3414
enfermedad 3964
enfermedad 6226
enfermedad cardíaca 2989
enfermedad cardiovascular 963
enfermedad cíclica 1638
enfermedad coexistente 1264
enfermedad concurrente 1392
enfermedad contagiosa 1318

enfermedad crónica 1150
enfermedad de Crohn 5740
enfermedad de especialidad 1934
enfermedad de los buzos 640
enfermedad de origen desconocido 1933
enfermedad de Quincke 279
enfermedad de transmisión sexual 6194
enfermedad degenerativa 1761
enfermedad del párpado 2480
enfermedad del suero 6176
enfermedad diseminada 1955
enfermedad fibroquística 2579
enfermedad hereditaria 3439
enfermedad infecciosa 3405
enfermedad mental 4135
enfermedad poco común 5655
enfermedad por almacenaje 6568
enfermedad primaria 7163
enfermedad pulmonar obstructiva crónica 1151
enfermedad terminal 6873
enfermedad venérea 7281
enfermera 4571
enfermera diplomada 5742
enfermería 3413
enfermería 4574
enfermizo 3412
enfermizo 7169
enfermo 3412
enfisema 2241
enfocar 2657
enfoque isoeléctrico 3641
engaño 1719
enjugar 7450
enlace de hidrógeno 3174
enlace de los registros 5698
enmascaramiento 4012
enmienda al protocolo 5469
enojado 3624
enrojecer 2621
enrojecimiento 2648

enrojecimiento 2651
ensangrentado 784
ensayo 461
ensayo 7088
ensayo biológico 693
ensayo clínico abierto 4659
ensayo con animales 290
ensayo de compatibilidad 1335
ensayo de equivalencia 2332
ensayo de etiqueta abierta 4661
ensayo de siembra 6099
ensayo doble ciego 2028
ensayo en una comunidad 1321
ensayo interprocesal 3463
ensayos sobre seres humanos 3155
enseñanza 6828
ensuciar 6349
ensueño 1703
enteral 2287
entérico 2238
enteritis 2290
entero 7441
enterocolitis seudomembranosa 5487
enterotoxina 2292
entrada 2293
entrada de datos 1674
entrada de datos distribuida 1970
entrada de datos dobles 2029
entrada remota de datos 5790
entrenamiento 7027
entrenamiento fisiológico 5110
entrevista 3550
entrevista psicológica 5498
entrevista telefónica 6845
entrevistar 3551
enucleación del ojo 2473
enuclear 2295
enuresis 2296
enuresis nocturna 631
envasado 4789

envase a prueba de niños 1112
envejecimiento 151
envejecimiento 6129
envenenamiento 5197
envenenamiento alimentario 2676
envenenamiento por mercurio 4140
envenenamiento por metales pesados 3010
envenenamiento sanguíneo 770
envenenar 5195
enyesado 990
enzima 2302
enzimología 2303
eosinofilia 2305
eosirófilo 2304
epicardio 2306
epidemia 2307
epidemia 4753
epidémico 2308
epidemiología 2311
epidemiológico 2309
epidémico 2312
epidermis 2313
epidídimo 2314
epidural 2315
epifisis 2323
epigástrico 2316
epiglotis 2317
epilación 2318
epilepsia 2319
epilepsia gran mal 2901
epilepsia tónico-clónica 6985
epinefrina 2321
epiplón 4639
episiotomía 2324
episodio 2325
epistax's 2326
epitelial 2327
epitelio 2329
equilibrio 2330
equilibrio 584

511

equilibrio de fluidos y electrólitos 2639
equilibrio ácido-base 50
equimosis 2127
equipo 2331
equipo 6830
equipo de atención médica 967
equipo de degustación 6823
equipos 2957
equivalente 2333
equivalente 2334
erección 2338
erecto 637
eritema 2337
eritema palmar 4807
eritroblasto 2346
eritrocito 2347
eritropoyesis 2350
erosión de la piel 2339
erosión ósea 809
error 2340
error alfa 199
error beta 649
error de refracción 5730
error estándar 6488
error mínimo 4221
error sistemático 6779
error tipo I 7139
error tipo II 7140
eructo 637
erupción 2344
erupción 4753
erupción cutánea 5656
erupción de la piel 6280
erupción en forma de mariposa 892
erupción morbiliforme 4293
erupción punteada 5546
escala 6034
escala analoga visual 7348
escala aritmética 413
escala de ansiedad manifiesta 3991

escala de calificación 5662
escala del estado psiquiátrico 5492
escala graduada 2894
escala logaritmica 3861
escala normalizada 6490
escaldar 6033
escalofrío 1117
escalofrío 6220
escalpelo 6037
escama 6034
escamoso 6038
escansión 6043
escape 2415
escápula 6044
escara 6045
escarmenar 6833
escatología 6047
escayola 989
escayolado 990
escisión 2401
escisión 5829
esclerótica 6065
escobillón 6735
escoliosis 6066
escollo 5141
escotoma 6067
escozor 6550
escozor 6964
escribir 7477
escroto 6075
escuela 6059
escupir 6434
esencial 2356
esferoidal 6414
esferoide 6413
esfigmomanómetro 6416
esfinter 6415
esfínter anal 242
esfuerzo 2411

esfuerzo 5876
esmalte 2247
esófago 2353
esófago 2355
esofagoscopia 2354
espacio 6373
espacio en blanco 732
espacio sacular 5188
espalda 564
espasmo 6376
espasmo arterial 428
espasmo bronquial 860
espasmo cardiaco 958
espástico 6377
especialidad 6388
especialidad médica 4083
especialidad quirúrgica 6717
especialismo 6385
especialista 6386
especies 6390
especificidad 6394
especificidad del substrato 6653
específico 6391
espécimen 6395
espectro 6403
espectro infrarrojo 3427
espectrometría 6401
espectroscopia 6402
especulación 2769
espéculo 6404
esperma 6407
espermatogénesis 6410
espermatozoide 6411
espermatozoo 6411
espiga 6417
espigas y ondas 6418
espina 6427
espina sacra 5982
espinal 6422
espinilla 6209

espiral 6428
espiral 6429
espíritu 6430
espirometria 6432
espiroqueta 6431
esplácnico 6435
esplénico 6437
esplenomegalia 6438
espolones del calcio 904
espondilitis anquilosante 298
esponja 6444
espontáneo 6447
espora 6449
esporádico 6448
esprue 6460
espuela 6461
espurio 6462
esputo 6433
esputo 6463
esqueleto 6275
esquema 6052
esquemático 6053
esquiria 6441
esquizofrenia 6056
esquizofrénico 6057
esquizoide 6055
estabilidad 6470
estabilidad física 5100
estabilización 6471
estable 6472
establecimiento del estado 6476
establecimiento del estado de una neoplasma 6477
estación 6077
estacional 6078
estadia en el hospital 3138
estadística 6507
estadística de Bayes 620
estadística descriptiva 1831
estadísticamente significativo 6506

512

evaluación del rendimiento 4981
evaluación global 2860
evaluación psicométrica 5500
evento adverso significativo 6160
evento clínico 1201
evento desfavorable no esperado 7168
evento principal 5364
evento secundario 6085
eventos que cambian la vida 3797
eversión 2381
evidencia 2384
evisceración 2385
evolución 2387
evolución de paciente 4930
evulsión 2388
exacerbación 2389
exactitud 40
examen 1087
examen al azar 5640
examen al microscopio 4182
examen de base 608
examen de oído 2984
examen de seleccionar 6073
examen del paciente 4927
examen físico 5095
examen gastroscópico 2793
examen masivo 4017
examen masivo 6072
examen pélvico bimanual 673
examen por lámpara de hendidura 6301
examen rectal 5708
examinar 5907
exanguinotransfusión 2398
exanguinotransfusión de sangre total 7443
exantema 2392
exantematoso 2393
excelente 2394

excesivo 2396
exceso de reportaje 4771
excipiente 2399
excitabilidad 2402
excitación (sexual) 417
excitación 2403
excluir 5975
excreción 2406
excreción biliar 669
excremento 2405
excremento 799
exfoliación 2413
exhalación 2414
exhibir 2416
exigencias de licenciación 3791
éxito comercial 1311
exocitosis 2419
exocrino 2417
exoftalmos 2422
exogénico 2420
exón 2421
exotoxina 2423
expansión 2424
expansión pulmonar 3916
expectante 2425
expectativa de vida 3798
expectorante 2427
expeler 2470
experiencia 2430
experiencia clínica 1202
experimental 2434
experimentar 2431
experimentar 2433
experimento 2432
experimento clínico 1222
experto 2436
expiración 2438
expiratorio 2440
explicar en términos generales 4758
exploración 2441

explotar 891
exponer 1948
exposición 2442
exposición de fondo 568
expresión 2443
expulsión 2445
exsanguinar 2446
extender 6456
extender 6590
extensión 2448
extensión 5647
extensión 6455
extensión 6589
extensión 7446
extensión linear 3822
extensor 2450
externo 2451
extirpación 2336
extirpación 2452
extirpación 5791
extracción 2457
extracción de catarata 998
extracelular 2453
extracorporal 2454
extracto 2455
extracto 25
extraer 2456
extrahepático 2458
extraño 2887
extraño 4622
extraño 726
extrapolación 2461
extrapolación de datos 1675
extrapolación de los datos 2462
extrasístole 2464
extravasación 2465
extravascular 2466
extremidad 2468
extremidad 3815
extrínseco 2469

extubación 2471
exudado 2472
eyaculación 2168
fabricación 3998
fabricación 5405
fabricante contratado 1477
facial 2484
facies de máscara 4013
facies lunar 4287
facilidad 2489
facilidad de fabricación 5406
facilitación 2488
facilitado 465
factibilidad 2534
factor 2493
factor ambiental 2299
factor de activación 63
factor de confusión 1416
factor de crecimiento 2925
factor de crecimiento transformado 7051
factor de relajación 5779
factor de riesgo 5945
factor de tiempo 6951
factor natriurético 4412
factor sanguíneo 764
factor socioeconómico 6338
factores no específicos 4526
facultad 2497
facultad de medicina 4082
fagocito 5032
fagocito 6049
fagocitosis 5033
fagosoma 5034
Fahrenheit 2499
falange 5035
fálico 5036
falla 2501
falla del tratamiento 7077
fallo cardiaco 2990
falsificación 1548

514

# Spanish/Español

fluido pulmonar extravascular 2467
fluido sinovial 6770
fluir 2633
flujo 2632
flujo 2653
flujo de datos 1678
flujo pulsátil 5538
flujo respiratorio 5849
flujo sanguíneo regional 5739
flujo seminal 6124
flujograma 2634
flujograma 2637
fluoración 2646
fluorescencia 2645
fluorización 2846
fluoroscopia 2847
flutter 2652
flutter auricular 495
fobia 5073
foco 2656
folicular 2663
folículo 2662
folículo capilar 2940
folículos de Graaf 2891
folleto del investigador 3607
folleto del investigador clínico 1206
fonación 5075
fondo 2753
fondo 567
fondo gástrico 2786
fonética 5076
fonocardiografía 5077
fontanela 2671
foramen 2680
foramen occipital 2681
fórceps 2683
forense 2691
forma 2695
forma 6201
forma de dosis parenteral 4866

forma de onda 7408
formación 2150
formación 2699
formación de imágenes 3276
formación de pequeñas impresiones 5142
formación del concepto 1386
formación del trombo 6934
formación en roseta 5958
formal 2696
formato 2698
formato de tabla 6791
fórmula 2700
formulación 2704
formulado 2703
formulario 2701
formulario de datos 1679
fornicación 2705
fortificado 2706
fosa 2707
fosa axilar 416
fosa nasal 4403
fósforo 5078
fotocopia 5081
fotocopiar 5082
fotofobia 5085
fotografía 5083
fotografiar 5084
fotoquímica 5080
fotosensibilidad 5087
fotosensible 5086
fototerapia 5089
fóvea 5139
fracción 2710
fracción de eyección 2170
fracción ligada 823
fracción no unida 7154
fracción unida 823
fraccionamiento 2711
fractura 2712
fractura de estrés 6587

fractura expuesta 4660
fractura ósea 810
fractura patológica 4916
fractura por compresión 1365
frágil 2716
frágil 855
fragilidad 2713
fragilidad capilar 923
fragmentación 2715
fragmento 2714
fragmento de péptido 4964
frasco 7324
fraude 1719
fraude 2720
frecuencia 2730
frecuencia cardíaca 2994
frémito 2727
frémito táctil 6799
frenesí 2729
frénico 5090
frenillo 3828
frenología 5091
frente 2686
frénulo 2728
friable 2733
fricción 2735
frigidez 2737
frío 1275
frío 1278
frontal 2739
frote pericárdico 2736
frote vaginal 7234
frotis 6308
frotis de Pap 4829
frotis de sangre 774
frustración 2743
fruta 2742
fruto 2742
fuente de datos 1691
fuente de datos 6369

fuera del sitio 4629
fuerza 6584
fuerza de prehensión 2916
fuerza de voluntad 7448
fuerza designada 3697
fuerza marcada 3697
fulminante 2745
fumando 6318
fumar 6315
fumar una pipa 5136
función 2746
función cognitiva 1266
funcional 2747
funcionamiento hepático 3853
funeral 2754
fungicida 2756
fúngico 2755
furioso 3951
furúnculo 802
fusión 2758
gafas 2477
gafas 6399
galactorrea 2762
galactosemia 2763
galope 2765
gama de referencias 5721
gama normal 4539
gammaglobulina 2770
gammagrama 6039
gammagrama 6041
ganglio 2774
ganglio linfático 3923
ganglio linfático 3924
ganglioma 2773
ganglionar 2775
ganglriones basales 599
gangrena 2776
gangrena gaseosa 2781
gangrenarse 4305
garantía de calidad 5579

Spanish/Español

garganta 6921
gargarismo 2778
gargarizar 2779
garrapata 6943
garrotillo 1594
gas 2780
gas en la sangre 765
gasa 2796
gaseoso 2782
gasto 2428
gasto 2429
gasto cardiaco 948
gastos generales 4769
gastos por cabeza 925
gástrico 2784
gastroenterologia 2789
gastrointestinal, GI 2791
gastroscopia 2794
gel 2800
gemelo 7128
gemelos fraternos 2719
gemelos idénticos 3255
gemelos monocigóticos 3255
gene 2805
gene dominante 1995
genealogia 4950
general 2809
generalización 2813
generalizado 2814
genérico 2817
género 2803
género 2837
genético 2818
genital 2829
genitales 2831
genitales 2832
genitourinario 2833
genoma 2834
genotipo 2836
gerencia 3963

geriátrico 2339
germen 2840
germinal 2642
gerontologia 2844
gestación 2845
gestacional 2846
gigantismo 2849
ginecologia 2934
ginecomastia 2935
girar 5911
girar 6420
glande 2852
glándula 2851
glándula endocrina 2084
glándula endocrina 2258
glándula exocrina 2083
glándula exocrina 2418
glándula paratiroidea 4861
glándula parótida 4874
glándula pineal 5133
glándula pituitaria 5145
glándula salival 6002
glándula sebácea 6073
glándula submandibular 6638
glándula sudoripara 6740
glándula timo 6936
glándula tiroides 6938
glaucoma 2855
glaucoma de ángulo abierto 4658
glicósidos digitálicos 902
glioblastoma 2856
glioma 2857
glóbina 2862
globo ocular 2475
globulina 2863
glóbulo blanco 7438
glóbulo rojo 5714
glóbulo sanguíneo 756
glomerulonefritis 2865
glotis 2867

glucocorticoide 2868
glucógeno 2873
gluconeogénesis 2869
glucosa 2870
glucósido cardiaco 945
glucosuria 2874
glúteo 2872
glutinoso 7342
gobierno 2889
gobierno de la casa 3147
gobierno federal 2540
golpe por calor 3004
golpear suavemente 6812
goma 2932
gónada 2881
gordo 2523
gota a gota 2047
gotear 2048
grabación 6813
gradiente de densidad 1793
grados de libertad 1764
gráfica en cuadros 827
gráfico curvilíneo 1627
gráfico de barras 594
gráfico de columnas 1302
gráfico de sectores 5117
gráfico de sectores 5118
gráfico de supervivencia 3802
gráfico lineal 3823
gráficos 2909
gráficos ejecutados por computadora 1374
gráficos puntiformes 5191
gramnegativo 2899
gramo 2898
grampositivo 2900
grano 5131
grano 7430
granulación 2903
gránulo 2904
granulocito 2905

granuloma 2906
granulomatoso 2907
grasa 2522
grasa parda 873
graso 2523
grave 6159
grave 6178
gravedad 6179
grávida 2911
grávida 5309
grieta 1556
gripe 3419
grosor del pliego de la pie 6284
grupo 2920
grupo 6830
grupo a riesgo 5947
grupo de bajo riesgo 3896
grupo de comparación 1390
grupo de consumidores 1149
grupo de control 1493
grupo de enfoque 2658
grupo de presión 5347
grupo de trabajo 6818
grupo étnico 2369
grupo minoritario 4222
grupo que no recibe tratamiento 4551
grupo sanguíneo 766
grupo sanguíneo 777
guardería 1701
guardería 1702
guardería 4573
guia 2928
guiar 2929
gusto 2623
gusto 6820
gusto metálico 4157
habilidad 10
habilidad 2489
habilidad 6277
hábito 2936

hiperparatiroidismo 3202
hiperplasia 3204
hiperpotasemia 3196
hiperreactividad 3205
hiperreflexia 3206
hipersensibilidad 3208
hipersensibilidad tipo retardada 1771
hipersensible 3207
hipertensión 3209
hipertensión renovascular 5797
hipertermia 3210
hipertiroidismo 3211
hipertonicidad 3214
hipertrigliceridemia 3215
hipertrofia 3217
hipertrofia cardíaca 946
hipertrófico 3216
hiperventilación 3218
hipnosis 3219
hipnótico 3220
hipnotizar 4143
hipo 3074
hipo- 3221
hipocampo 3088
hipocondria 3222
hipocondria 3224
hipocondríaco 3223
hipocrómico 3225
hipofisectomía 3232
hipófisis 3233
hipófisis 5144
hipófisis 5146
hipofunción 3227
hipoglucémico 3228
hipolipoproteinemia 3229
hipomenorrea 3230
hiponatremia 3231
hipopituitarismo 3234
hipoplasia 3235
hipotálamo 3238

hipotensión 3236
hipotensión orostática 4724
hipotensión postural 5263
hipotermia 3239
hipótesis 3240
hipótesis nula 4563
hipotético 3241
hipotiroideo 3242
hipotiroidismo 3243
hipotonía 3244
hipotónico 3245
hipoxemia 3246
hipoxia 3247
hirsuto 3089
hispánico 3090
histamina 3061
histaminérgico 3092
histerectomía 3248
histeria 3249
histerosalpingografía 3250
histiocitosis 3093
histiocitoquímica 3095
histocompatibilidad 3094
histograma 3096
histograma de punción 4431
histograma invertido 3598
histograma piramidal 5568
histología 3100
histológico 3097
histólogo 3099
histopatología 3101
historia 3104
historia alcohólica 2046
historia clínica 984
historia de uso de drogas ilícitas 3271
historia médica 4076
historia médica 4898
historial familiar 2515
historial profesional 1625
historial sexual 6188

hito 4206
hoja 6206
hoja de comprobación 1086
hoja de datos 1690
hombre 3982
hombro 6218
homeopatía 3113
homeostasis 3114
homicidio 3115
homocigótico 3126
homocigoto 3125
homogenado 3116
homogeneidad 3117
homogéneo 3118
homoinjerto 3119
homología 3121
homología secuencial 6153
homólogo 3120
homosexual 2798
homosexual 2799
homosexual 3122
homosexual 3123
homosexualidad 3124
hongo 2757
honorarios y gastos 2545
hora de dormir 629
horario 6961
horario de dosis 2007
horario de dosis 2024
horas de vela 7386
horizontal 3127
hormigueo 6964
hormona 3129
hormona adrenocorticotrópica, ACTH 108
hormona luteinizante 3920
hormona pituitaria 5147
hormona sexual 6183
hosco 4299
hospicio 3133
hospital 3135

hospital 3413
hospital para enseñanza de la medicina 6829
hospitalario 4547
hospitalización 3139
hostilidad 3142
hueso 807
hueso púbis 5517
huesos del carpo 975
huesos faciales 2485
huésped 3140
huésped inmunocomprometido 3295
nuevo 2165
humano 3149
humano 3150
humedad 3158
humedad 4265
humedad relativa 5772
húmero 3157
humo 5314
humor acuoso 405
humor vítreo 7359
humoral 3159
iatrogénico 3251
ictericia 3655
ictérico 3253
ictiosis 3252
ideación 3254
identidad sexual 2804
identificación 3256
identificación genética de ADN 1984
idioma 3714
idiopático 3259
idiosincrasia 3260
idiota 3261
idiota sabio 3262
igual 4951
igualdad 4872
ileal 3263
ileitis regional 5740
íleo 3267

523

# Spanish/Español

maniaco-depresivo 3989
manifestación 1947
manifestación 3992
manifestar 1948
manifiesto 390
maniobra 3986
maniobrar 3987
mano 2947
mano de obra 3995
mano de obra 7461
manometría 3994
manómetro 3993
mantenimiento 3956
manual 3996
manual de utilización 3997
manufacturación 3998
mañana 4296
mapeo 3999
mapeo de genes 2807
mapeo de péptidos 4965
marca comercial 842
marca de fábrica 7025
marca de nacimiento 719
marcación del material clínico 3698
marcado radioactivamente 5619
marcador 4003
marcador de afinidad 135
marcador fisiológico 5109
marcapasos 4788
marcas de rayas cruzadas 2958
marcha 2761
marcha 7387
marcha propulsora 5448
mareado 3813
mareo 1982
mareo 4312
margen 2143
margen 817
margen elevado 2208
margen posológico 2014

marketing 4006
masa 4015
masa crítica 1575
masaje 4019
masaje cardiaco 2991
masajear 4020
máscara 4011
máscara facial 2483
mascelino 4010
maselero 4021
masoquismo 4014
mastectomía 4022
mastectomía radical 5606
masticación 1107
masticación 4023
masticdeo 4025
mastoides 4024
masturbación 4028
matai 3686
matemáticas 4039
mateia 4041
mateia blanca 7440
material de obturación 2592
materiales biocompatibles 685
mate nal 4034
mate nidad 4037
mate no 4034
maticez 2086
matrimonio 4008
matriz 4040
maxiar 4045
maxiar 4046
máxima respuesta 4945
máximo 4047
máximo 4942
mayer 2174
meao 4056
mecánico 4057
mecanismo 4059
mecanismo de acción 4060

mecanismo de defensa 1750
mecanorreceptor 4061
meconio 4062
media 4050
media de cultivo 4064
media geométrica 2838
media vida de eliminación 2215
mediador 4069
mediana 4066
mediar 4070
mediastino 4068
medicación 4088
medicación de escape 2352
medicado 4087
medicamento 4086
medicamento de uso especifico 4490
medicamento genérico 2816
medicamento preempaquetado 5324
medicamento sin receta 4764
medicar 2009
medicina 4092
medicina aeroespacial 124
medicina bajo receta 5333
medicina comparativa 1328
medicina de emergencia 2228
medicina defensiva 1751
medicina forense 2692
medicina herbaria 3056
medicina interna 3533
medicina legal 2692
medicina osteopática 4741
medicina popular 2661
medicina preventiva 5356
medicina tradicional 7026
medicina veterinaria 7322
medicinal 4089
medición del dolor 4794
medición espectral 6400
médico 1987
médico 4071

médico 5103
médico 5285
médico generalista 2811
medida 4052
medida de errores 2342
medida de prevención 1461
medida objetiva 4589
medio 4034
medio 4196
medio 551
medio 7277
medio de contraste 1489
medio de cultivo 1613
medio de radiocontraste 5612
medio tono 2943
mediodía 4532
medios 4051
medios de comunicación 4013
medios de comunicación 4063
medir 4053
médula espinal 6424
médula ósea 4009
médula ósea 812
médula suprarrenal 104
megalomania 4098
meiosis 4099
mejilla 1088
mejor caso 647
mejora de los síntomas 220
mejoram ento 3327
mejoría 3327
mejoría clínica 1204
melancolia 4100
melanina 4101
melanoc to 4102
melanoma 4103
melena 4104
mellizo 7128
membra na 4107
membra na basal 611

modelo logístico 3867
modelo matemático 4038
moderado 4262
moderar 4261
modificación por índice 3372
modificado 4263
modo 4258
modorra 2055
moho 4267
mojado 7429
mol 4268
mola 4268
molar 4266
molde 4267
molécula 4272
molecular 4269
momento del tiempo 6853
moniliasis 4273
monitor 4274
monitor clínico 1208
monitor de clínica 1190
monitor de datos 1684
monitor de Holter 3109
monitor del ensayo 7093
monitor en el campo 2586
monitor fetal 2562
monitorear 4275
monitoreo 4276
monitoreo del producto 5404
monitoreo fisiológico 5107
monoamina biogénica 690
monocigótico 4285
monocito 4281
monoclonal 4279
monoinsaturado 4284
monomania 4282
monoterapia 4283
monóxido de carbono 930
moral 4288
moral 4289

morbididad 4292
morbido 4290
mordedura 723
morder 724
morfogénesis 4300
morfología 4301
morgue 4294
moribundo 4295
morón 4298
mortal 3771
mortal 4302
mortalidad 4303
mortalidad con causa específica 1019
mosaico 4306
mosaiquismo 4307
moscas volantes 2630
mosquito 4308
motivación 4313
motor 4314
motricidades finas 2601
movilidad 4256
movilidad 4309
movimiento 4310
movimiento 4323
movimiento coreiforme 1139
movimiento corporal 796
movimiento extraocular 2460
movimiento involuntario 3611
movimiento ondulado 7409
movimiento sacádico 5981
movimientos clónicos 1230
movimientos oculares rápidos 5653
mucocutáneo 4327
mucoproteína 4328
mucosa 4329
mucosa bucal 878
mucosa friable 2734
mucoso 4330
mudo 2087
mudo 4365

muela 6991
muerte 1708
muerte 2100
muerte cerebral 835
muerte en cuna 6665
muerte en la cuna 1563
muerte infantil súbita 1540
muerte súbita 6664
muerte súbita cardíaca 6663
muerte súbita infantil 6665
muerto 704
muesca 3367
muestra 8003
muestra seleccionada al azar 5639
muestras gráficas 5116
muestras pictóricas 5116
muestreo 6012
mujer 2547
mujer 7457
muletas 1589
multicéntrico 4336
multigrávida 4341
multinacional 4342
multinacional 4343
multípara 4345
múltiple 4346
mundial 7467
municipal 4349
muñeca 7476
mural 4350
murino 4351
muscular 4354
musculatura 4356
músculo 4353
músculo cardíaco 2993
músculo contráctil 1484
músculo estriado 6592
músculo involuntario 3612
músculo liso 6320
músculo voluntario 7372

musculoesquelético 4357
muslo 6905
mutación 4364
mutación por cambio de encuadre 2717
mutación puntiforme 5192
mutagénesis 4359
mutagénesis de sitio 6266
mutágeno 4358
mutante 4361
mutante 4362
mutar 4363
mutilar 4366
n de un ensayo 4391
naciente 4406
nacimiento 709
nacionalidad 4410
nadir 4392
nalga 393
nalgas 5976
narcisismo 4396
narcolepsia 4397
narcosis 4398
narcótico 4399
narcótico 4400
nariz 4545
nasal 4402
nasofaríngeo 4408
natación 6742
natalidad 1113
natriuresis 4411
natural 4413
náusea 4421
náusea 5582
nebulizador 4424
necesidad médica 4077
necrólisis 4426
necropsia 4427
necrosis 4428
necrosis aséptica 456
necrosis focal 2654

# Spanish/Español

osteopatía 4742
osteoporosis 4743
osteosarcoma 4744
ostectomía 4745
ostomía 4746
ótico 4747
otitis 4748
otitis externa 4749
otitis media 4750
otorrinolaringología 4751
otoscopio 4752
ovárico 4762
ovario 4763
oviducto 4774
ovulación 4776
ovular 4775
óvulo 4777
oxidación 4779
oxidante 4778
oxigenación 4785
oxigenación 7287
oxigenar 4784
oxígeno 4782
oxígeno hiperbárico 3187
oxihemoglobina 4786
oximetría 4781
ozono 4787
pabellón de la oreja 517
paciente 4920
paciente 4921
paciente 6630
paciente admisible 2213
paciente ambulatorio 4759
paciente de control 1494
paciente elegible 2213
paciente interno 3461
paciente no elegible 3395
padre (madre/padre) 4862
pago 4941
pago por adelantado 7190

país 1551
país en vías de desarrollo 1849
país miembro 4106
palabra por palabra 7299
paladar 4801
paladar blando 6346
paladar fisurado 1185
paliar 4802
paliativo 4803
paliativo 4804
palidecer 730
palidez 4805
palma 4806
palmadita 6811
palo 6540
palpable 4809
palpación 4810
palpebral 4811
palpitación 4813
palpitar 4812
panacea 1622
panacea 4815
pancitopenia 4818
páncreas 4816
pancreatitis 4817
pandémico 4819
pandémico 4820
panel 4821
pánico 4824
pantalla 6070
pañal 1871
paño higiénico 6017
papel 4830
papel autocopiante sin carbón 931
papel de tornasol 3848
papila gustativa 6822
papilar 4832
papiledema 4833
papiloma 4834
pápula 4835

par 4951
par correlacionado 4030
para- 4836
para tener hijos 1114
paradigma de la dosis 2022
parafina 4838
paralelo 4840
parálisis 4814
parálisis 4841
parálisis flácida 2619
parálisis motora 4316
paralizar 4842
parámetro 4844
paranoia 4847
paranoide 4848
paraparesia 4849
paraplejía 4850
parapsicología 4851
parasimpático 4855
parasimpaticolítico 4857
parasimpaticomimético 4858
parasitario 4853
parásito 4852
parasitología 4854
parásitos 7303
paratiroideo 4859
paratiroideo 4860
parche transdérmico 7038
parcial 4879
parcialidad 5313
pared 7390
pared celular 1035
pareja 6191
parenteral 4865
parentescos 5768
paresia 4869
paresia 4890
parestesia 4870
parestesia 4985
paricárdico 4985
paridad 4872

pariente 5769
parietal 4871
parir 3850
paro cardiaco 2986
paro cardiaco 942
parótida 4873
paroxismo 4875
paroxístico 4876
párpado 2479
parte accesoria 32
partenogénesis 4878
partes de un estudio 4888
partes por... 4889
participación 4884
participante 4883
partícula submitocondrial 6640
partida de datos 1681
partida de defunción 1709
parto 1115
parto 1410
parto 1776
parto 4891
parto con niño muerto 6545
parto falso 2508
parto inducido 3385
parto prematuro 5318
parturición 4891
parturiente 4890
pasaje 4894
pasar 4893
pasatiempos 3765
paseo 7387
pasillo 4892
pasivo 4895
paso 6524
pasta de dientes 6994
pasteurización 4900
pasto 2910
pata delantera 2690
patela 4902

530

profesional 4614
profesional 5408
profesional 7363
profesor 6827
profiláctico 5438
profiláctico 5439
profilaxis 5440
profundidad respiratoria 5852
progestacional 5411
progestógeno 5412
prognosis 5413
programa 5415
programa 6050
programa de aleatorización 5643
programa de salud nacional 4409
programa de titulación 6972
programación 6051
programar 5416
progresivo 5419
prohibición 1120
prohibido 5420
prolapso 5426
proliferación 5427
prolongación 2448
prolongación 3767
prolongación 5429
prolongar 5428
promedio 4050
promedio oscilante 5955
promedio variable 4325
prominencia 5430
prominencia glútea 893
promoción 5432
promotor 5431
pronación 5433
pronóstico 5300
pronóstico 5413
pronóstico 5414
propagación 6455

propagar 5435
propagar 6456
propensión 655
propiedad 5436
propiedades de superficie 6708
propietario 5442
propiocepción 5445
proporción 5663
proporción sexual 6184
propósito 1837
propósito 5446
propulsión 5447
prosencéfalo 2885
prospectivo 5449
próstata 5451
proteasa 5455
protección 5456
protección contra el sol 6680
protección de patente 4907
proteína 5458
proteína quimérica 1120
proteína sanguínea 773
proteína transportadora 977
proteinasa 5462
proteinuria 5463
proteólisis 5464
prótesis 5452
protocolo 5468
protocolo común 1316
protocolo de continuación 1463
protocolo de extensión 2449
protocolo de utilización por compasión 1332
protocolo humanitario 3156
protón 5474
protooncogén 5467
protoplasma 5476
protozoa 5477
protozoario 5478
protrombina 5465
protrusión 5480

protuberancia 3911
protuberancia de la membrana del tímpano 882
proveedor de asistencia médica 966
provincia 5482
provisional 6851
provitamina 5483
provocación 1074
provocación repetida 5689
proximal 5485
proyección 5424
proyectar 5423
proyecto 5422
proyecto piloto 5128
proyector 5425
prueba 2384
prueba 461
prueba 6878
prueba 7088
prueba a la tuberculina 7118
prueba añadida 79
prueba bilateral 7134
prueba bilateral 7135
prueba chi-cuadrado 1125
prueba con animales 290
prueba cutánea 6282
prueba de complementación 1349
prueba de corte transversal 1586
prueba de cultivo mixto linfocitario 4253
prueba de ejercicio 2409
prueba de estrés 6588
prueba de fertilidad 2555
prueba de fijación del complemento 1347
prueba de función pulmonar 5532
prueba de hipótesis unilateral 4646
prueba de inteligencia 3510
prueba de intercambio de genes 1593
prueba de mutagenicidad 4360
prueba de parche 4901
prueba de plana 4790
prueba de prevención primaria 5368

prueba de provocación 5484
prueba de rendimiento 4982
prueba de sensibilidad microbiana 4169
prueba de signos 6237
prueba de tolerancia a la glucosa 2871
prueba de una rama 4647
prueba de unidades formadoras de colonias 1295
prueba del embarazo 5307
prueba del gusto 6824
prueba diagnóstica 1867
prueba en multi-centros 4337
prueba entre tratamientos 653
prueba medicamentosa de múltiples dosis 4338
prueba no paramétrica 4521
prueba Pap 4829
prueba para confirmar resultados 1411
prueba paramétrica 4845
prueba piloto 5130
prueba t en pares 4798
prueba y error 7089
prueba z 7510
prurito 5486
psicoanálisis 5495
psicoanalítico 5496
psicocirugía 5509
psicodélico 5490
psicofarmacología 5504
psicología 5499
psicología criminal 1570
psicología de condicionamiento 1400
psicología de transferencia 7048
psicología del inconsciente 7160
psicológico 5497
psicometría 5501
psicomotor 5502
psicopatología 5503
psicosexual 5505
psicosis 5506
psicosis alcohólica 173

| | | | |
|---|---|---|---|
| psicosocial 5507 | punción 6811 | que fuma 6318 | quiral 1122 |
| psicosomático 5508 | punción lumbar 3906 | que no penetra 4522 | quirófano 4668 |
| psicoterapia 5510 | punción lumbar 6426 | que no responde 4525 | quiropráctica 1123 |
| psicódico 5511 | punta 6417 | que responde parcialmente 4881 | quiropraxia 1123 |
| psicotrópico 5514 | puntaje ajustado a la tendencia 7082 | que vuelve a infartarse 5760 | quirúrgico 6712 |
| psique 5489 | puntaje de Apgar 375 | quebradizo 2716 | quiste 1639 |
| psiquiatría 5493 | puntaje de cambio 1080 | quebradizo 855 | quórum 5593 |
| psiquiátrico 5491 | puntaje de eficacia 2160 | quelato 1089 | rabdomiosarcoma 5915 |
| psíquico 5494 | puntaje de severidad de la lesión 3450 | queloide 3677 | rabia 5632 |
| ptosis 5515 | puntaje en bruto 5671 | quemadura 887 | rabieta 6810 |
| pubertad 5516 | puntas y ondas 6418 | quemadura de tercer grado 6908 | rabiosc 5595 |
| pubertad precoz 5296 | punto 2026 | quemadura del sol 6678 | rabo 6300 |
| pubis 5518 | punto 4942 | quemadura química 1093 | ración 5664 |
| publicación 5524 | punto 6398 | quemar 888 | racional 5665 |
| publicación 5525 | punto ciego 741 | quemosis 1102 | racionalización 5667 |
| publicidad orientada directamente al consumidor 1915 | punto de datos 1685 | queratina 3678 | racionamiento 5668 |
| | punto de decisión 1728 | queratinizado 2289 | radiación 5600 |
| público 5519 | punto de sutura 6552 | queratinocito 3679 | radiación ionizante 3621 |
| pudendo 5526 | punto del tiempo 6953 | queratotomía radial 5597 | radiado 6519 |
| puente 5219 | punto final 2277 | quetora 3681 | radiante 5598 |
| puente arterial 433 | punto final de sustitución 6721 | quetosis 3682 | radical 5604 |
| puente coronario 1518 | punto final definido 2955 | quiasma 1108 | radical 5605 |
| pueril 5527 | punto final flojo 6344 | quiescente 1999 | radical libre 2722 |
| puerperal 5528 | punto medio 4065 | quieto 5589 | radio 5630 |
| puerperio 3921 | punto político 5199 | quilo 1155 | radioactivo 5608 |
| puerta 5226 | puntuación de la conducta 633 | quilomicrón 1156 | radiobiología 5611 |
| pulgar 6935 | puntuación numérica 4570 | quimera 1118 | radiocirugía 5628 |
| pulimento 5200 | puñalada 6468 | quimérico 1119 | radiografía 5613 |
| pulmón 3913 | pupila 5549 | química 1100 | radiografía 5615 |
| pulmonar 5530 | pupilas dilatadas 1904 | química cerebral 833 | radiografía 7485 |
| pulpa 5537 | pureza 5554 | química clínica 1195 | radiografía intervencionista 3547 |
| pulsación 5539 | purgante 5551 | química medicinal 4090 | radiografía panorámica 4827 |
| pulsación 6922 | purgativo 5552 | química orgánica 4707 | radiografiar 7486 |
| pulsar 5541 | pú pura 5555 | química sintética 6775 | radiográfico 5614 |
| pulso 5540 | purulento 5556 | quimídisis 1101 | radioinmunoanálisis 5616 |
| pulso arterial 424 | pus 5557 | quimioluminiscencia 1099 | radioinmunodetección 561~ |
| pulso bigeminado 663 | pústula 5558 | quimidáctico 1103 | radioisótopo 5618 |
| pulso paradójico 4837 | pústula pequeña 5131 | quimictaxis 1104 | radioligando 5620 |
| pulverizador 6453 | putrefacción 5559 | quimioterapia 1105 | radiología 5622 |
| punción 5547 | pútrido 5560 | quimo 1157 | radiólogo 5621 |

# Spanish/Español

# Spanish/Español

reflujo 5728
reflujo gastroesofágico 2790
reflujo hepatoyugular 3050
reforzamiento 5762
refracción 5729
refractario 5731
regeneración 5735
regenerador 5863
régimen de dosis baja 3891
régimen 5736
régimen de dosis 2006
región 410
región 5737
regional 5738
registrar 5697
registro 3862
registro 5696
registro 5743
registro 5744
registro clínico 985
registro de dosis 2023
registro de drogas devueltas 5900
registro de exploración de pacientes 4936
registro de los problemas 5387
registro de pacientes 4934
registro de reclutamiento 5705
registro de visitas de monitoreo 4278
registro del ensayo 7094
registro electrónico 2197
registro médico 4079
regla cardinal 953
regla de interrupción precoz 2124
regla de oro 2879
regla de parada 6565
regresar 5745
regresión 5746
regresión hacia la media 5749
regulación 5751
regulación alostérica 193
regulación hacia abajo 2037

regulación hacia arriba 7192
regulador 5752
reguladora 5753
regular 5750
regurgitación 5756
rehabilitación 5757
rehicratación 5758
rehusador 5734
reinfección 5761
reír 3735
rejilla 2913
relación 5663
relación beneficio/riesgo 643
relación costo-beneficio 1537
relación de probabilidades 4623
relación dosis-respuesta 2018
relación espacial 6380
relación estructura-actividad 6604
relación huésped-parásito 3143
relación lineal 3827
relación médico-paciente 5104
relación no lineal 4520
relación riesgo-beneficio 5944
relación sexual 6193
relación ventilación-perfusión 7288
relacionado 466
relacionado con una bolsa 890
relaciones con el paciente 4935
relaciones públicas 5522
relajación 5777
relajante 5776
relajar 5775
relajsar 5765
relajso 5764
relativo 5770
relativo a la textura 6885
religión 5782
reloj biológico 694
remanente 979
remedio 5786

remedio de patente 5443
remineralización 5787
remisión 1
remisión 5720
remisión 5724
remisión 5788
remitente 5789
remodelación ósea 814
remover quirúrgicamente 2400
renal 5792
rendimiento 4960
renovación 5796
rentabilidad 1533
renuncia 7383
renuncia en caso de embarazo 5308
reología 5916
reoperación 5798
reorganización 5681
reparación 5799
repasar 5607
reperfusión 5803
repetición 5800
repetir 5801
replicación 5807
repliegue 2659
repolarización 5808
reportaje 5811
reportaje insuficiente 7164
reposar 5859
reposo 5858
reposo en cama 627
representante 5812
representante comercial 4007
representante de ventas 5997
represión 5814
reprimir 5813
reproducción 5817
reproducción 354
reproducibilidad 5815
reproducible 5816

repuesto 5805
repulsivo 5820
requisito 5821
requisito del tamaño de la muestra 6011
resabio 139
resaca 2951
resbalar 6296
rescate 5822
resecable 5828
resecar 5827
resección 5829
reservorio 5830
residencia 5831
residencial 5833
residual 5834
residuo 5784
residuo 5835
residuo de la droga 2072
resiliencia 5836
resina 5837
resistencia 2279
resistencia 5838
resistencia 6483
resistencia a la tensión 6860
resistencia de la vía respiratoria 165
resistencia del huésped 3141
resistencia vascular 7258
resistencia vascular pulmonar 5535
resistencia vascular sistémica 6783
resistente a fractura 6805
resollar 7433
resolución 5839
resolución de problema 5386
resolver 5840
resonancia 5841
resonancia magnética nuclear 4556
resonancia timpánica 7137
respiración 5845
respiración 849
respiración 851

537

supurar 2558
sural 6705
surco 2918
surfactante pulmonar 5533
susceptibilidad 6728
suspender 6729
suspensión 6730
suspiro 6229
sustancia 4041
sustancia 6646
sustancia celulósica 5963
sustancia gris 2912
sustancia peligrosa 2961
sustancia que no despolariza 4514
sustancia química 1091
sustancial 6650
sustancioso 6650
sustitución 5805
sustitución terapéutica 6894
sustituir 6652
sustituto 6651
sustituto 6719
sustracción digital 1901
susurrar 7436
susurro 7435
sutil 6862
sutura 6733
suturar 6553
suturar 6734
tabaco 6873
tabaco que no se fuma 6317
tabique nasal 4404
tabla 6790
tabla de contingencia 1462
tabla de mortalidad 3803
tabla de píldoras 5124
tableta 3899
tableta 6793
tableta bañada 1252
tacha 738

tácticas 6797
táctil 6798
tacto 7006
talámico 6886
tálamo 6887
talco 6802
talle 7381
tallo 6482
talón 6520
talón 3011
tamaño 6274
tamaño de la muestra 6009
tamaño de la muestra observada 4597
tamaño de la partícula 4886
tamaño de los bloques 751
tampón 6807
tampón 881
tangente 6809
tanque de descompresión 1736
taponamiento 6808
taponamiento cardiaco 951
taquicardia 6794
taquicardia auricular 496
taquicardia ventricular 7295
taquifilaxia 6795
taquipnea 6796
tartamudear 6484
tartamudear 6613
tartamudez 6614
tasa 5658
tasa de errores 2343
tasa de eventos 2380
tasa de filtración glomerular 2864
tasa de hospitalización 5660
tasa de inscripción 5659
tasa de metabolismo basal 600
tasa de mortalidad 1710
tasa de mortalidad 4304
tasa de natalidad 717
tasa de rendimiento descuentado 1928

tatuaje 6825
taxonomía 6828
técnica 6836
técnica bacteriológica 577
técnica citológica 1646
técnica de dilución indicadora 3375
técnica de relajación 5778
técnica de sustracción 6656
técnica Delphi 1778
técnica esterotáxica 6528
técnico 6835
tecnología 6837
tecnología de información 3423
tecnología de liberación controlada 1497
tegumentario 6840
tegumento 6839
tejido 6966
tejido adiposo 2522
tejido blando 6347
tejido conectivo 1430
tejido córneo 3132
tejido germinal 2843
telangiectasis 6841
teléfono rojo 3145
telencéfalo 6842
telepatía 6843
tema político 5199
temblando 6212
temblar 6211
temblar 7079
temblor 5592
temblor 6920
temblor 7080
temblor de enfermedad de Parkinson 5126
temblor fino 2602
temer 2533
temperamento 6846
temperatura 6847
temperatura corporal 798
temporal 6850

temporario 6851
tendencia 6853
tendencia 7081
tendencia futura 2759
tendencias pasadas 4899
tendinitis 6856
tendón 6857
tener cosquillas 6945
tener miedo 2533
tener reacción cruzada 1582
tenesmo 6859
tensión 6586
tensión 6861
tentar 7007
tenue 6862
teñir 2099
teoría 6890
teoría de la decisión 1729
técnico 6888
terapéutica 6896
terapéutico 6891
terapia 6897
terapia con hormonas 3131
terapia de aversión 552
terapia de inhalación de oxígeno 4783
terapia de la conducta 634
terapia de primera línea 2607
terapia de quelación 1090
terapia de segunda línea 6080
terapia de sustitución 5806
terapia física 5102
terapia lingüística 6406
terapia matrimonial 4002
terapia ocupacional 4617
terapia ortomolecular 4720
terapia trombolítica 6928
teratógeno 6863
teratología 6866
teratoma 6867
tercer estadio del parto 6910

# Spanish/Español

venas varicosas 7252
venda 590
vendaje 2044
vendaje 590
vendar 591
vendar 592
vendedor 7280
veneno 5194
veneno 7284
veneno de víbora 6321
venenoso 7285
venipuntura 7282
ventana terapéutica 6895
ventilación 7287
ventilación de presión positiva intermitente 3531
ventilador 7289
ventral 7291
ventricular 7293
ventrículo 7292
ventrículo cerebral 1063
ventrículo cerebral 839
ventriculografía 7296
vénula 7297
verbal 7298
verificación 7300
verificación de datos 1695
verificación de la fuente de datos 6370
verificar 7301
vermiforme 7302
verruga 7304
verruga 7309
vértebra 7305
vertebrado 7308
vertebral 7306
vertical 7310
vértice 7309
vértigo 2848
vértigo 7312
vesícula 7313
vesícula 745

vesícula biliar 2764
vesícula seminal 6125
vesicular 7314
vestibular 7316
vestíbulo 7318
vestigio 7320
vestimenta 1238
veterano 7321
vía 4919
vía 5967
vía aferente 132
vía de administración 5968
vía de aire 163
vía de aire 164
vía de eliminación 5969
vía de transporte 7069
vía eferente 2157
vía metabólica 4150
vía respiratoria 163
vía respiratoria 164
viable 7323
vías urinarias 7207
vibración 7325
vida 3796
vida diaria 1656
vida media 2942
vida media terminal 6872
vidrio 2853
viejo 4633
vientre 3
vigilancia 175
vigilancia 6724
vigilancia de posmarketing 5245
violación 5652
violación 7328
violación del protocolo 5473
violencia 7329
viral 7330
viremia 7334
viril 7335

virilización 7336
virión 7337
virología 7338
viruela 5280
virulencia 7339
virus 7340
virus sincitial respiratorio 5853
víscera 7341
viscosidad 7343
viscosidad sanguínea 780
viscoso 7342
viscoso 7344
visión 6230
visión 7345
visión amarilla 7497
visión borrosa 787
visión doble 2034
visión en colores 1298
visión en túnel 7123
visita a la clínica 1191
visita al consultorio 4627
visita al emplazamiento 6268
visita de aleatorización 5644
visita de monitoreo 4277
visita de monitoreo de rutina 5972
visita de paciente 4937
visita de seguimiento 2670
visita de supervisión 4277
visita inicial 610
visita previa a la randomización 5327
vista 6230
visual 7346
visualización 1947
visualización 7352
visualización de datos 1671
vitamina 7356
vitelo 7499
vítreo 7357
vivacidad 175
vivacidad 291

vivienda 3148
vivo 180
vocabulario 7361
vocacional 7363
volátil 7367
volumen 7369
volumen cardíaco 952
volumen corriente 6946
volumen de distribución aparente 391
volumen de eyección 6598
volumen de la distribución 7370
volumen expiratorio forzado 2682
volumen pulmonar 3917
volumen sanguíneo 781
volumen sistólico 6598
voluntad 7447
voluntario 7371
voluntario 7374
vomitar 5875
vómito 2230
vómito 7376
voz 7364
vuelo espacial 6374
vuelta 6419
vulnerable 7377
vulva 7378
vulvar 7379
xantopsia 7497
xenobiótico 7483
xifoides 7484
yema 7499
yema de huevo 2167
yeso 989
yeyunal 3657
yeyuno 3659
yeyunoileal 3658
yodo 3615
yugo 7498
yugular 3668
yuxtaponer 3673

zancada 6594
zona 7507
zona 7509
zona de servicio de salud 2971
zona enrojecida 2620
zona glomerulosa 7505
zoonosis 7508
zumbido 6965
zurdo 3755

550

bösartig 3971
botanisch 820
Boten-RNS 4146
Bradykardie 830
Bradylalie 6305
brandig machen 4305
Brandwunde 887
Brandwunde durch Chemikalien 1093
Brauch 1629
braunes Fettgewebe 873
brechen 5875
Brechmittel 2231
Brechreiz 4421
Brechungsfehler 5730
Breitband 856
Breitband-Antibiotikum 857
breites Wirkungsspektrum 856
brennen 888
Brennpunkt 2656
Brille 2477
Brille 2854
Brille 6399
bröcklig 2733
bronchial 859
Bronchialbaum 861
Bronchialspasmus 860
Bronchie 871
Bronchiektasie 862
Bronchien- 859
Bronchiole 863
Bronchiolitis 864
Bronchiolus 863
Bronchitis 865
bronchoalveolare Lavage 866
Bronchodilatator 868
Bronchokonstriktion 867
bronchopulmonale Dysplasie 869
Bronchoskopie 870
Bronchus 871
Broschüre für alle teilnehmenden Untersucher

1206
Broschüre für die Untersucher einer Studie 3607
Bruch 2710
Bruch 2712
Bruch 3061
Bruch in der Achse 843
brüchig 855
Bruchstück 2714
Brücke 5219
Brunst 2361
Brust 845
Brustkorb 1106
Brustkorb 6915
Brusttumor 847
Brustwarze 4496
Brustwarze 6834
Brutapparat 3364
Bubo 876
buccal 877
Buchprüfer 513
Buchprüfung 511
Bulbus olfactorius 4636
Bulimie 883
Bundes- 2539
Bundesregierung 2540
bursal 890
Bypass 894
Caissonkrankheit 640
Calcium 901
Carbamid 7197
Catgut 1006
Caudatum 1015
Cerebellum 1056
Cerebrum 1066
Cervix uteri 1072
Chancenverhältnis 4623
Charakter 1083
Charakter 5018
Charakteristikum 1084
Charakterzug 7030

Charge 3879
Chargennummer 3880
Chargennummer 615
Checkliste 1086
Chelat 1089
Chelatbildungstherapie 1090
Chemie 1100
Chemikalie 1091
chemische Analyse 1092
chemische Reaktion 1096
chemische Struktur 1097
chemische Synthese 1098
chemischer Name 1095
Chemolumineszenz 1099
Chemolyse 1101
Chemosis 1102
chemotaktisch 1103
Chemotaxis 1104
Chemotherapie 1105
Chi-Quadrat Test 1125
Chi-Quadrat-Verteilung 1124
Chiasma 1108
chimär 1119
Chimäre 1118
Chimären- 1119
chimäres Protein 1120
chiral 1122
Chiropraxis 1123
Chirurg 6710
Chirurgie 6711
chirurgisch 6712
chirurgischer Klammerapparat 6718
chirurgisches Instrument 6715
chirurgisches Spezialgebiet 6717
Chlorid 1126
Cholangiographie 1128
Cholelithiasis 1131
Cholesterin 1132
cholesterinarme Kost 3889
Cholesterol 1132

Cholezystektomie 1129
Cholezystitis 1130
cholinerg 1133
cholinergischer Rezeptor 1134
Chondrocalcinose 1135
Chondrodystrophie 47
Chorda 1136
Chordae tendineae 1137
Chorea 1138
choreatiforme Bewegung 1139
Chorioidea 1143
Chorion- 1141
Chorionkarzinom 1140
Chorionzotten 1142
Chromatin 1145
Chromatographie 1146
Chromosom 1148
Chromosomendeletion 1147
chronisch 1149
chronische Krankheit 1150
chronische obstruktive Lungenerkrankung 1151
Chronobiologie 1152
Chronologie 1153
chronotrop 1154
Chylomikrone 1156
Chylus 1155
Chymus 1157
Computer 1370
Computeremissionstomographie 2234
computergestützt 1371
Computergrafik 1374
Computerschnittstelle 1375
Computersimulation 1377
Computertomogramm 1372
Computertomogramm 1379
Computertomographie 1369
Computertomographie des Schädels 836
Computerzeichnungen 1373
Conjugata 1425
Corpus geniculatum 2828

Cortex cerebri 1059
Crista 5934
Crohn-Krankheit 5740
Cross-over 1591
Crowding der Zähne 1595
Damenbinde 6017
Dämmerzustand 7031
Dampf 6515
Dampf 7243
dämpfendes Mittel 1818
Dämpfung 2086
Darm 2933
Darm- 3552
Darm 3556
Darm 824
Darm- 2288
Darmbein 3269
Darmbeinkamm 3268
Darmblutung 3554
Darmgeräusche 5005
Darmgeräusche 826
Darmschmerz 3555
Darmverschluß 3267
Darreichung 95
Darreichungsform 2005
darstellen 1948
darstellend 5338
Darstellung 1947
das Becken betreffend 4953
Datei 1677
Datei 2590
Daten 1660
Daten von Tierversuchen 287
Datenanalyse 1661
Datenanzeige 1671
Datenarchivierung 1662
Datenaufbereitung 1673
Datenauswertung 1680
Datenbank 1664
Datenbank 1665

Datenblatt 1690
Datenbogen 1690
Datendarstellung 1687
Datenelement 1681
Datenerfassung 1669
Datenerfassung 1674
Datenfehlinterpretation 1682
Datenfeld 1676
Datenferneingabe 5790
Datenformular 1679
Datengruppierung 1667
Datenhochrechnung 1675
Datenhochrechnung 2462
Datenkodierung 1668
Datenkoordinierungszentrum 1670
Datenprüfung 1663
Datenprüfung 1694
Datenquelle 1691
Datenreduktion 1689
Datensammlung 1669
Datensammlung 1686
Datenspeicherung 1692
Datenstation 1378
Datenstrom 1678
Datentransformation 1693
Datenüberprüfung 1695
Datenveränderung (durch statistische Methoden) 1672
Datenverarbeitung 1688
Datenverdichtung 1689
Datenverfälschung 1683
Datenwort 1681
Datenzentrum 1666
Datum 1696
Datum 1699
Dauer- 1467
Dauer 2094
Dauerinfusion 1441
Dauersonde 3391
Daumen 6935

Debile(r) 4298
Debilität 7412
Débridement 1713
Deckblatt 1555
Decke- 6840
Decubitus 628
dedizierter Computer 1741
deduktive Logik 1742
Defäkation 1746
Defekt 1747
Defekt - 1748
defensive Medizin 1751
Defibrillation 1752
Definition 1754
Defizienz 1753
Deformität 1756
Degeneration 1760
degenerative Erkrankung 1761
degenerieren 1758
degeneriert 1759
degenerierter Mensch 1757
Degranulation 1763
Dehiszenz 1765
dehnen 1963
Dehnung 6361
Dehydratation 1767
dehydratisieren 1766
dehydrieren 1766
Dehydrierung 1767
Déjà-vu-Erlebnis 1768
Dekarboxylation 1715
Dekompensation 1733
Dekompression 1735
Dekompressionskammer 1736
Dekontamination 1738
Dekubitalgeschwür 1740
Dekubitus 5348
Dekubitus 1739
Delirium 1774
Delirium tremens 1775

Dellenbildung 5142
Delphi Verfahren 1778
Deltainfektion 1779
Deltarezeptor 1780
demaskieren 7182
Derrenz 1782
Derrographie 1784
Derrographie 1785
demographische Daten ~783
Demyelinisierung 1786
Denaturierung 1787
Dendrit 1788
dendritische Zelle 1789
Denervation 1790
Densitometrie 1791
dental 1794
Dentin 1800
Deodorant 1806
Depolarisation 1814
Depot 1817
Depression 1819
Deprivation 1820
Derivat 1822
dermal 1824
Dermatitis 1825
Dermatologie 1826
Dermatophytose 6963
Dermatose 1827
Desensibilisierung 1832
desinfizieren 1936
Desintegration 1937
deslozieren 1939
Desmosom 1838
desorganisiert 1942
Desorientierung 1943
Desorientierung 1943
Desoxyribonukleinsäure, DNS 1983
destillieren 1964
destilliertes Wasser 1965

German/Deutsch

562

gehen 7388
Gehirn 831
Gehirnchemie 833
Gehirnentzündung 2249
Gehirnerschütterung 834
Gehirnhäute 4116
Gehirnischämie 1062
Gehirnnerv 1560
Gehirnschlag 388
(Gehirnstamm 837
Gehirntumor 838
Gehirnventrikel 1063
Gehirnventrikel 839
Gehör- 514
Gehörknöchelchen 2122
Gehörmessung 510
Geist 4215
Geist 6430
Geist- 5090
Geistes Alter 4128
Geistesschwache(r) 4298
geisteskrank 3466
geisteskrank 3951
Geisteskranker 3465
Geisteskrankheit 3467
Geisteskrankheit 4135
Geistesstand 4137
Geistesstörung 4131
geistig 4127
geistig gesund 6014
geistige Behinderung 4136
geistige Gesundheit 4132
geistige Gesundheit 6020
geistige Retardierung 4130
geistige Verwirrung 4129
gekennzeichnete Stärke 3697
gekoppelt 1426
Gekröse 4142
gekühlte Lagerung 5732
Gel 2800

Gelächter 3736
Gelatinekapsel 2802
gelatinieren 2801
'gelbes-Karten-System' 7496
Gelbsehen 7497
Gelbsucht 3655
Geldbeschaffung 2749
Geldstipendium 2752
Gelenk 3662
Gelenk 444
Gelenkband 442
Gelenkentzündung 435
Gelenkfläche 443
Gelenkknorpel 441
Gelenkkrepitation 3663
Gelenkplastik 437
Gelenkschmerz 434
Gelenkschmiere 6768
Gelenkversteifung 299
gemeinsam 1314
gemeinsame Bewertung 3665
Gemeinschaft 1320
gemeinschaftliche Weiterentwicklung 3664
gemischt 4252
gemischter Lymphozyten-Kultur-Test 4253
Gemüse 7274
Gen 2805
Gen-Manipulation 2821
Gen-Zusammensetzung 2822
Genamplifikation 2806
Genauigkeit 40
Genauigkeit 5293
Genaustausch 1591
Genehmigung 1182
Genehmigung 3790
Genehmigung von ethischen Grundsätzen her 2363
generalisiert 2814
generalisierter Anfall 2815
Generalisierung 2613

generell 2809
Generikum 2816
genesen 6457
Genesung 1501
genetisch 2818
genetische Kreuzung 2820
genetische Polymorphie 2823
genetische Rekombination 2824
genetische Transduktion 2827
genetische Transkription 2826
genetische Unterdrückung 2825
genetischer Kode 2819
genießbar 4800
genital 2829
Genitalien 2831
Genitalien 2832
Genitalorgan 5819
Genkartierung 2807
Genom 2834
genomische DNS-Bank 2835
Genotyp 2836
Genus 2803
geometrisches Mittel 2838
gepaarte Fälle 4029
gepaarte Placebo 4033
gepaarte Werte 4030
geraderichten 6570
Gerät 2331
Geratologie 2844
Geräusch 4352
Geräusch 4506
Geräusch 6367
Geräusch 875
gerecht 2505
geriatrisch 2839
Gerichtsmedizin 2692
geringgradig 3893
geringgradig 4207
geringgradiger Fehler 4221
geringgradiges Fieber 3894

Gerinnung 1248
Gerinnungszeit 1241
Gerinnungszeit 1249
germinal 2842
germinativ 2842
Gerontologie 2844
Gerstenkorn 6615
Geruch 4625
Geruch 6310
Geruchssinn 6310
gesamt 7004
gesamte Arbeitskraft 7461
Gesamtheit 7003
Gesamttagesdosis 7005
Gesäß 893
gesättigt 6030
Geschäftsleitung 3983
geschichtete Randomisierung 6578
geschichtete Studie 6579
geschichtete zufällige Zuteilung 6577
Geschlecht 2803
Geschlecht 6181
geschlechtlich 2829
Geschlechts- 6186
Geschlechtschromosom 6182
geschlechtsgebunden 6185
Geschlechtshormon 6183
Geschlechtsidentität 2804
Geschlechtskrankheit 6194
Geschlechtskrankheit 7281
geschlechtslos 457
Geschlechtsorgane 2830
Geschlechtsorgane 6190
Geschlechtsverhältnis 1424
Geschlechtsverkehr 6184
Geschlechtsverkehr 6189
Geschlechtsverteilung 6184
geschlossenes Narkosesystem 1233
Geschmack 2623

Geschmack 6820
Geschmacksknospe 6822
Geschmackstest 6824
geschützt 5442
geschützter Name 5444
geschütztes Handelspräparat 5443
geschwächt 3313
Geschwisterteil 6223
geschwollen 2283
geschwollen 6743
Geschwür 18
Geschwür 6364
Geschwür 7141
Geschwür 918
Gesellschaft 1323
Gesellschaft 6337
gesellschaftliche Stellung 6334
Gesetzgebung 3762
Gesicht 2481
Gesichts- 2484
Gesichtsfarbe 1353
Gesichtsfeld 7350
Gesichtshautstraffung 2482
Gesichtsknochen 2485
Gesichtsmaske 2483
Gesichtsödem 2486
Gesichtsröte 2648
gespalten 660
gesprenkelt 4318
Gestagen 5412
Gestalt 2695
Gestank 6522
Gestation 2845
Gestations- 2846
gestillt 846
gestört 3313
gestörte Daten 4507
gesund 2980
gesunder Menschenverstand 1317
Gesundheit 2614

Gesundheit 2968
Gesundheitsbeeinträchtigung 3270
Gesundheitseinrichtung 2974
Gesundheitserhaltungsorganisation 2976
Gesundheitserziehung 2973
Gesundheitsfürsorge 2970
Gesundheitsplanung 2977
gesundheitsschädigend 7169
Gesundheitswesen 2978
Gesundheitswesen 5520
Gesundheitszentrum 2972
Gesundheitszustand 2979
getrennt 6141
Gewalt 7329
Gewebe 6963
Gewebe- 6865
Gewebedurchblutung 6968
Gewebelappen 6714
Gewicht 7419
Gewichtheben 7422
gewichtstragend 7420
Gewichtsverlust 3877
Gewichtszunahme 7421
Gewissen 1432
gewogener Wert 7424
Gewohnheit 2936
gewöhnliche Betriebsverfahren 6489
gewunden 7001
gezackt 6172
Gift 5194
giftig 7010
Gigantismus 2849
Gingiva 2850
Gipfel 374
Gips 989
Gitter 2913
Glandula submandibularis 6638
Glas 2853
gläsern 7357

glasig 7357
Glaskörper 7358
Glaskörperflüssigkeit 7359
Glaskörpertrübungen 2630
glatt 6319
glatte Muskulatur 3612
glatter Muskel 6320
Glaukom 2855
Gleiche(t) 4951
Gleichgewicht 2330
Gleichgewicht 584
Gleichgewichts- 7316
Gleichgültigkeit 372
Gleichheit des Inhalts 1459
gleichmäßig 7171
Gleichmäßigkeit 7172
Gleichrangige(r) 4951
gleichzeitig 1389
gleichzeitig 1391
gleichzeitig 6251
gleichzeitige Behandlung 1390
gleichzeitige Erkrankung 1264
gleichzeitige Krankheit 1392
gleiten 6296
Gleiten 6295
gleitender Durchschnitt 4325
Gleitmittel 3900
Gliedmaße 4105
Glioblastom 2856
Gliom 2857
global 7467
globale Auswertung 2860
globale Entwicklung 2859
globale Introspektion 2861
globale klinische Auswertung 2858
Globin 2863
Globulin 2862
Glomerulonephritis 2865
Glomerulusfiltrationsrate 2864
Glottis 2867

Glück 2954
Glücksspiel 2769
Glukkortikoid 2868
Glukoneogenese 2869
Glukose 2870
Glukosetoleranztest 2871
gluteal 2872
Glykogen 2873
Glykosurie 2874
Gold 2877
goldene Regel 2879
goldene Sittenregel 2879
Goldstandard 2878
Golgi-Apparat 2880
Gonade 2881
Graaf-Follikel 2891
Grad 3782
Grad Celsius 1043
Grad der Anästhesie 3784
Grade nteilung manifester Angst 3991
Grafik 2909
Gramm 2898
grammnegativ 2899
grampositiv 2900
Grand-mal-Epilepsie 2901
Granulation 2903
Granulom 2906
granulomatös 2907
Granulosazelle 2908
Granulozyt 2905
graphische Datenverarbeitung 1374
Gras 2910
graue Substanz 2912
gravid 2911
Greifstärke 2916
Gremium 4821
Grenz- 818
Grenze 1409
Grenzwert 1633
Grippe 3419

578

German/Deutsch

Lymphozyt 3928
lymphozytär 3930
lymphozytenlenkender Rezeptor 3929
Lymphozytose 3931
Lymphsystem 3927
Lyophilisation 3935
Lyse 3937
Lysogenie 3938
Lysosom 3939
lytisch 3940
Macht 5279
Magen- 2784
Magen 6556
Magen-Darm-Kanal 2792
Magen-Darm-Kanal 179
Magenaspirat 2785
Magenfundus 2786
Magenpförtner 5565
Magensaft 2787
Magenspülung 2788
Magenstein 654
mager 3747
Magersucht 303
Magnesium 3952
Mahlzeit 4049
Makel 6801
Makro-Ebene 3942
Makroglobulin 3945
Makropathologie 2919
Makrophage 3946
Makrophagenkolonie 3947
Makrozephalie 3943
Makrozyt 3944
Makula 3949
Makuladegeneration 3948
Mal 3960
Malabsorption 3961
Malazie 3962
Malformation 3969
maligne 3970

maligne 3971
maligne Granulozytopenie 155
Malnutrition 3974
Malokklusion 3975
Mamille 4496
Mamille 6834
mammär 3979
Mammogramm 3980
Mammographie 3981
Mandel 6989
Mandibula 3984
Mandibulargelenk 3985
Mangel 1753
Mangelernährung 3974
Manie 3988
Manifestation 3992
manisch-depressiv 3989
manische Störung 3990
Mann 3966
Mann 3982
männlich 3967
männlich 4010
männlich 7335
männliche Geschlechtsorgane 3968
Manometer 3993
Manometrie 3994
Manöver 3986
manövrieren 3987
manuelles Lochen 3683
Mapping 3999
Mark 4009
Markenname 842
Marker 4003
Marketing 4006
markhaltige Nervenfaser 4375
Markierung 6543
marklos 7183
Markt 4004
Marker 7002
Maß 4052

Maßeinheit 7178
masernähnlicher Ausschlag 4293
mäßig 4262
mäßigen 4261
Maske 4011
Maskengesicht 4013
Maskierung 4012
maskulin 4010
maskulin 7335
Maßlosigkeit 3512
Maßnahme 4052
Masochismus 4014
Massage 4019
Masse 1357
Masse 4015
Masse 4041
Massenmedien 4016
Massenscreening 4017
Massenspektrumanalyse 4018
massieren 4020
(maßstäbliches) Vergrößern 6035
Mastektomie 4022
Mastoid 4024
Mastoid- 4025
Masturbation 4028
maternal 4034
Maternität 4037
Mathematik 4039
mathematisches Modell 4038
Matrix 4040
Maturation 4042
Maus 4320
Maxilla 4045
maxillär 4046
maximal tolerierte Dosis 4048
maximale Reaktion 4945
Maximalwert 1026
Maximum 4047
Mazeration 3941
Meatus 4056

mechanisch 4057
mechanisches Gerät 4054
mechanisches Verhalten 3962
Mechanismus 4059
Mechanorezeptor 4061
Median 4065
Medianebene 4199
Mediastinum 4068
Mediator 4069
Medien 4063
Medikament 2056
Medikament 4086
Medikament mit hoher Bincungsaffinität 3080
Medikament mit spezifischer Anwendung 4490
Medikamenteigenschaften 2060
Medikamentenabhängigkei 2059
Medikamentenentwicklung 1094
Medikamentenentwicklung 2063
Medikamentenhauptverzeichnis 2069
Medikamentenpause 2065
Medikamentensynergismus 2074
Medikamentenentwicklung 4093
Medikamentenüberwachung 2073
Medikamentenverabreichungssystem 2061
Medikamentenverzeichnis 2701
medikamentös 4089
medikamentöse Behandlung 4088
Medika mentrezeptor 2071
Medikamentrückstand 2072
Medikamentverabreichung aus humanitären
Gründen 1333
Medikation 4088
Medium 4094
Medizin 4092
medizinisch 4071
medizinisch 4089
medizinische Abteilung 4070
medizinische Chemie 4090
medizinische Fakultät 4082
medizinische Forschungseinrichtung 4081

Nephropathie 4443
Nephrotoxizität 4444
Nerv 4445
Nervenblockade 4446
Nervenendigung 4449
Nervenfaser 4450
Nervenimpuls 4451
Nervensystem 4455
Nervenwurzel 4452
Nervenzelle 4447
Nervenzusammenbruch 4454
nervös 4453
Nervosität 4456
Nervus facialis 2487
(Nervus) Vagus 7237
Nesselfieber 3106
Nesselsucht 7217
Netz 4457
Netz 4639
Netzhaut 5882
Netzhaut- 5883
Netzwerk 4457
neuartiger Ansatz 4552
neue chemische Entität 4488
Neuerung 3457
neugeboren 4435
neugeboren 4489
Neugeborenenstation 4573
Neugeborenes 3398
Neuordnung 5681
neural 4458
Neuralgie 4461
Neuralrohrdefekt 4460
Neurochirurgie 4476
neurogene Blase 4462
Neuroleptikum 4463
Neurologie 4466
neurologisch 4464
neurologisch 4465
Neurom 4467

neuromuskulär 4468
neuromuskuläre Verbindung 4469
Nauron 4470
neuronal 4471
neuronales Computernetzwerk 4459
Nauropathie 4472
Naurose 4475
neurosekretorisch 4474
Neurotiker 4477
neurotisch 4478
Neurotoxin 4479
Neurotransmitter 4480
Neurowissenschaft 4473
neutral 4481
neutralisieren 1546
neutralisierender Antikörper 4483
Neutralisierung 4482
Neutron 4484
Neutropenie 4485
neutrophiler Leukozyt 4486
Neuverteilung 5680
Nexus 3832
nicht abschätzbar 4517
nicht angegeben 7187
nicht behandelte Gruppe 4551
nicht depolarisierendes Mittel 4514
nicht eindeutige Resultate 2335
nicht konjugiert 7157
nicht lebensfähig 4531
nicht mehr zur Nachuntersuchung verfügbar 3878
nicht myelinisiert 7183
nicht penetrierend 4522
nicht perforiert 3316
nicht signifikanter Endpunkt 6344
nicht signifikantes Ergebnis 6345
nicht spezifiziert 7187
nicht-steroidal 4527
nicht stützende Ergebnisse 4528
nicht systematisch getestetes Medikament 4515

nicht überzeugende Ergebnisse 3356
nicht vereinigt 7189
nicht verträglich 3352
nicht wegdrückbares Ödem 5143
nicht zufällig 4524
Nicht-Responder 4525
Nichteinhaltung 4513
nichtinvasives Verfahren 4519
nichtkompetitiver Antagonist 4512
nichtlineare Beziehung 4520
nichtprogrammierbare Datenstation 2088
Nichtvereinigung 4529
Niederkunft 1410
Niederschlag 6097
niedrig dosiertes Heparin 3890
niedriger Blutdruck 3886
Niere 3684
Nieren- 5792
Nierenbecken 4954
Nierenbecken 5794
Nierenblockade 364
Nierenstein 3685
Nierentubuli 5795
Nierenversagen 5793
niesen 6324
Niesen 6323
Niesen 6325
Niveau 3782
Nodulus 4505
Nodus 4503
Nomenklatur 4508
Nominaldaten 4510
nominell 4509
Nomogramm 4511
non-verbale Kommunikation 4530
Noradrenalin 4533
noradrenerg 4534
Norepinephrin 4535
Norm 8485
normal 4536

normal 5750
normal 6486
Normalbereich 4538
Normalbreite 4539
normaler Krankheitsverlau 4415
normalisierter Wert 4540
Normalverteilung 4537
normochrom 4541
normcton 4543
normczytär 4542
Northern-Blot 4544
nosokomial 4547
nosokomiale Infektion 4548
Nosologie 4549
Not 1968
Notfall 2227
Notfallmedizin 2228
Notiz über den Fortschritt 5418
Nozizeption 4498
Nozizeptor 4499
Nucleus 4561
Nucleus caudatus 1015
nuklear 4555
Nukleinsäure 4558
Nukleclus 4559
Nukleosom 4560
Nullhypothese 4563
numerische Analyse 4568
numerische Daten 4569
numerisches Ergebnis 4570
Nutzen 641
Nutzen 7240
Nutzen-Risikoverhältnis 643
nützen 642
Nyktalcpie 4492
Nykturie 4500
Nylon 4584
Nystagmus 4585
obdachlos 3112
Oberarm 3157

obere Atmungs- 7191
oberer 6686
Oberfläche 6706
Oberflächenaktiv 6709
oberflächenantigen 6707
Oberflächeneigenschaften 6708
oberflächlich 6683
Oberschenkel 2551
Oberschenkel 6905
Obesität 4587
Objektiv 4588
objektive Messung 4589
Objektträger 6295
Obsession 4599
Obst 2742
obstinat 5731
Obstipation 1442
obstruktiv 4605
Obturation 4606
Ödem 2142
offen 4657
offenbar 390
offene klinische Studie 4659
offene randomisierte Studie 4662
offener Bruch 4660
offener ductus arteriosus 4906
offensichtliches Symptom 4772
öffentlich 5519
öffentliche Belange 5521
öffentliche Meinungspflege 5522
öffentlicher Bereich 5523
öffentliches Interesse 5521
Öffentlichkeit 2810
Öffentlichkeitsarbeit 5522
offiziell 2696
öffnen 4656
Öffnung 373
Öffnung 4663
Öffnung 5223
ohne Krankenversicherung 4085

Ohnmachtsgefühl 2504
Ohr 2121
Ohr- 516
Ohrentrichter 4752
Ohrgeräusch 6965
-ohrig 4747
Ohrmuschel 517
Ohrspeicheldrüse 4873
Ohrspeicheldrüse 4874
Okklusion 4609
okklusiv 4610
okkult 4611
okkultes Blut 4612
Ökologie 2133
Ökonomie 2136
Okular 4618
okulär 4619
okuläre Konvergenz 4620
okulomotorisch 4621
Okulovestibularisreflex 7319
okzipital 4607
Okziput 4608
Öl 4631
olfaktorisch 4635
Oligämie 4637
Oligokardie 830
Oligurie 4638
Omentum 4639
Onanie 4028
Onkel 7155
Onkogen 4641
Onkogenese 4642
Onkologie 4644
onkologisch 4643
Online-System 4648
Oogenese 4652
Oophorektomie 4653
Oozyte 4651
opak 4655
operante Konditionierung 4666

Operation 4669
Operation 6711
Operation 6716
Operationssaal 4668
operativ 4671
operative Ablation 6713
operierbar 4665
Operieren 6716
Operon 4672
Ophthalmologie 4674
Ophthalmoskopie 4675
Opiat 4399
Opiat 4676
Opiat 4677
Opisthotonus 4680
opportunistische Infektion 4681
opthalmisch 4673
Optik 4688
Optiker 4687
Optikuspapille 4685
Optimaldosis 4689
optisch 4682
optisch 4683
optische Dichte 4684
optische Drehung 4686
optischer Festspeicher 4685
Optometrie 4690
oral 4691
oral 877
orale Pharmakotherapie 4695
orale Verabreichung 4692
orales Kontrazeptivum 4693
orbital 4698
orbitalis 4698
Orchitis 4699
ordinal 4702
Ordinate 4703
Ordinate 7492
Ordnung 4700
Ordnung nach Priorität 5374

Organ 4704
Organelle 4705
Organisation 4709
Organisationsaufbau 4710
organisch 4706
organische Chemie 4707
Organismus 4711
Orgasmus 4711
orientalisch 4712
Orientierung 4713
Orifizium 4714
oropharyngeal 4715
Oropharynx 4716
Orphan-Drug 4717
Ortauswahl 6267
Orthodontie 4719
orthomolekulare Therapie 4720
orthopädisch 4721
Orthopnoe 4722
Orthostase 4723
orthostatische Hypotonie 4724
orthostatische Hypotonie 5263
orthotisches Gerät 4725
örtlich 3857
Ortsbesichtigung 6268
Ortsbesichtigungsbericht 6269
ortsgerichtete Mutagenese 6266
Os ischii 3637
Os sacrum 5985
Osmolalität 4728
osmolare Konzentration 4729
Osmolarität 4730
osmotischer Druck 4731
ösophageal 2353
Ösophagoskopie 2354
Ösophagus 2355
osseous 4732
Ossifikation 4733
Osteoarthritis 4735
Osteoarthropathie 4736

584

German/Deutsch

Perforation 4979
Perfusion 4983
periapikal 4984
Pericardium 4987
Perikard 4987
Perikarderguß 4986
perikardial 4985
Perimeter 4988
perineal 4989
perineal 4990
Perineum 4991
Periode 5063
periodisch 4994
Periodizität 4996
periodontal 4997
Periodontologie 4998
periorbital 4999
Periost 5000
Periostenum 5000
peripher 5001
peripherer Nerv 5002
peripheres Gesichtsfeld 5003
Peristaltik 5004
peristaltische Welle 5006
peritoneal 5007
Peritoneum 5008
Peritonitis 5009
Perkussion 4975
Perkussion 6811
perkutieren 4974
perkutieren 6812
permeabel 5012
Permeabilität 5011
perniziös 5013
peroral 5014
Peroxid 5015
Person 5016
Personal 5019
Personal 6473
persönlich 5017

Persönlichkeit 1083
Persönlichkeit 5018
Perspektive des Patienten 4938
Perspiration 5021
Pert-Diagramm 5022
pervers 5024
Perversion 5023
Perzentile 4971
perzeptiv 4973
Pessar 5025
Pest 5027
Pest 5153
Pestilenz 5027
Pestizid 5026
Pet-Scan 5028
Petechie 5029
Petit mal 5030
Petrolatum 5031
Pfeifenrauchen 5136
Pfeil 419
Pflanze 3055
Pflanze 5156
Pflege 965
Pflegeanstalt für Krebserkrankte 916
Pflegegruppe 967
Pflegeheim 3110
Pfleger 966
Pflegestation 3413
Pflegestation für Koronarpatienten 1519
Pfortader 5228
Pfortadersystem 5227
Pforte 3083
Pforte 5226
Pfund 5276
Phagosom 5034
Phagozyt 5032
Phagozyt 6049
Phagozytose 5033
Phalanx 5035

phallisch 5036
Phänomen 5067
Phänotyp 5068
phantasieren 5669
Phantomglied 5037
Pharmakodynamik 5045
Pharmakoepidemiologie 5047
Pharmakogenetik 5048
Pharmakognosie 5049
Pharmakokinetik 5051
pharmakokinetische Studie 5050
Pharmakologe 5053
Pharmakologie 5054
pharmakologische Aktivität 5052
Pharmakopöe 5055
Pharmakotherapie 5056
Pharmakowirtschaft 5046
Pharmapolitik 5060
Pharmaunternehmen 5040
pharmazeutisch 5038
pharmazeutisch 5039
pharmazeutische Industrie 2066
Pharmazie 5043
Pharmazie 5058
pharyngeal 5061
Pharynx 5062
Phase 1 5064
Phase-1-Einheit 5066
Phase-1-Studie 5065
Phase 4992
Phase 5063
Phase 6475
Phase nach der Studie 5254
Pheromon 5069
Phiole 7324
Phlebitis 5070
Phlebotomie 5071
Phlegma 5072
Phobie 5073
Phobieerkrankung 5074

Phonation 5075
Phonetik 5076
Phonokardiographie 5077
Phosphor 5078
Photochemie 5080
Photophobie 5085
Photosensibilisator 5088
Photostimulation 5079
Phototherapie 5089
Phrenologie 5091
Physik 5105
physikalische Therapie 5102
Physiognomie 5106
Physiologie 5111
physiologisch 5108
physiologische Marker 5109
physiologische Überwachung 5107
physiologisches Training 5110
Physiotherapie 5112
physisch 5092
physische Stabilität 5100
Pia mater 5113
Pica 5114
Pickel 5131
Pigment 5119
Pigmentation 5120
Pigmentierung 5120
Pigmentnävus 5121
Pikazismus 5114
Pikogramm 5115
Pille 5123
Pillendrehertremor 5126
Pillentablett 5124
Pillenzahl 5125
pilomotorisch 5127
Pilotprojekt 5128
Pilotstudie 5130
Pilz- 2755
Pilz 2757
pilzartig 2755

Probe 461
Probe 6008
Probe 6395
Probe 7088
Probenentnahme 6012
Probenhandhabung 6397
Probensammlung 6396
Problem 5385
problembezogenes Protokoll 5387
Problemlösung 5386
Processus xiphoideus 7484
Prodrom 5395
Produkt 5398
Produktentwicklung 5399
Produktion 5397
Produktion 5405
Produktionsanlage 5406
Produktionscharge 5407
Produktspezialisierung 5400
Produktüberwachung 5404
Produktzulassung 5401
Produktzulassungsantrag 5402
Professor 5410
progesteronartig 5411
Prognose 5413
prognostisch 5414
Programm 5415
programmieren 5416
Programmiersprache 5417
progressiv 5419
Prohibition 5421
Projekt 5422
Projektion 5424
Projektor 5425
projizieren 5423
Proktosigmoidoskopie 5394
Proktoskop 5393
Prolaps 5426
Proliferation 5427
Promotion 5432

Pronation 5433
Prophase 5437
prophezeiend 5301
prophylaktisch 5439
prophylaktisches Mittel 5438
Prophylaxe 5354
Prophylaxe 5440
Propriozeption 5445
Propulsion 5447
propulsiver Gang 5448
Prosenzephalon 2685
prospektive Studie 5450
Prostata 5451
Prostration 5454
Protease 5455
Protein 5458
Proteinase 5455
Proteinase 5462
Proteinbindung 5459
Proteindenaturierung 5460
Proteinstruktur 5461
Proteinurie 5463
Proteolyse 5464
Prothese 5452
Prothrombin 5465
Prothrombinzeit 5466
Protokoll 3862
Protokoll 5468
Protokoll der Arztbesuche des Überwachers 4278
Protokollabweichung 5470
Protokolländerung 5469
Protokollergänzung 5469
Protokollnummer 5471
Protokollüberprüfungsausschuß 5472
Protokollübertretung 5473
Protokollverletzung 5473
Proton 5474
Protonenpumpe 5475
Protoonkogen 5467

Protoplasma 5476
Protozoen 5477
Protozoon 5478
Protrusion 5480
Provinz 5482
Provision 1312
Provitamin 5483
Provokation 1074
Provokationstest 5484
proximal 5485
Prozent 4966
Prozent der Änderung 4967
Prozent der Gesamtsumme 4969
Prozent der maximalen Reaktion 4968
Prozeß 3847
Prozeß 5389
Prüfliste 1086
Prüfpfad 512
Prüfung 2390
Prüfung 2391
Pruritus 3654
Pruritus 5486
Pseudo- 2507
Pseudo- 5488
Pseudo- 6462
Pseudogicht 1135
pseudomembranöse Enterokolitis 5487
Pseudoneurotransmitter 2510
Psyche 5489
psychedelisch 5490
Psychiatrie 5493
psychiatrisch 5491
psychisch 4127
psychisch 5494
psychisches Gesundheitswesen 4134
Psychoanalyse 5495
psychoanalytisch 5496
Psychochirurgie 5509
Psychologie 5499
Psychologie der unbewußten Vorgänge 7160

psychologisch 5497
psychologische Befragung 5498
Psychometrie 5501
psychometrische Bewertung 5500
psychomotorisch 5502
Psychopathologie 5503
Psychopharmakologie 5504
Psychose 5506
psychosexuell 5505
psychosomatisch 5508
psychosozial 5507
psychosoziale Beratung 1543
Psychotherapie 5510
psychotisch 5511
psychotische Affektstörung 5512
psychotische Störung 5513
psychotrop 5514
Pterygium colli 7415
Ptosis 5515
Pubertas praecox 5296
Pubertät 5516
Puder 5278
puerperal 5528
Puffer 881
pulmonal 5530
Pulmonalarterienverschlußdruck 5536
Pulmonalklappe 5534
Pulpa 5537
Puls 5540
Pulsation 5539
Pulsdruck 5542
pulsieren 5541
pulsierender Fluß 5538
Pulsschlag 6922
Pulsus bigeminus 663
Pulsus paradoxus 4837
Pulswelle 5543
Pulver 5278
Pumpe 5544
pumpen 5545

German/Deutsch

Rhombus 3899
Rhonchus 5927
Rhythmus 5928
Ribonukleinsäure, RNS 5930
Ribosom 5932
ribosomale DNS 5931
Richtlinie 2930
Richtlinien für die Praxis 5283
Richtlinien für die Verfasser 3492
Rickettsie 5933
riechen 6311
Riechkolben 4636
Riechsalz 6312
Riesenzelle 2847
Rift-Tal-Fieber 5935
Rigidität 5938
Rigidität 5939
Rigor 5939
Rigor mortis 5940
Rille 1081
Rinde 1526
Rinde 6208
Ring 301
Ring 5941
ringförmige Läsion 6816
Rinne 2918
Rinne 7111
Rippe 5929
Rippenfellentzündung 5182
Riß 1556
Riß 2625
Riß 5978
Riß 6632
Risiko 5942
Risikofaktor 5945
Risikofaktoranalyse 5946
Risikogruppe 5947
Risikoreduktion 5948
riskieren 5943
Risiko-Vorteil-Verhältnis 5944

RNS-Spleißen 5949
Robotertechnik 5950
Robustheit 5951
Rohdaten 5670
Röhrchen 7120
Röhre 7117
röhranförmiges Gesichtsfeld 7123
(Rohr)leitung 5137
Rohwert 5671
Rolle 5964
Rollstuhl 7432
röntgen 7486
Röntgen 5954
Röntgenaufnahme 5613
Röntgenaufnahme 7485
Röntgencomputertomographie 7487
Röntgendensitometrie 7488
Röntgenfilm 7489
Röntgenstrahl 7485
Rosettenbildung 5958
rostfreier Stahl 6481
Rotation 5960
Rotatorenmanschette 5961
rotes Auge 5134
rotieren 5911
rotieren 6420
rotierende Adepresse 5059
Roçte 5967
Routine 5970
routinemäßig 5971
routinemäßiger Überwachungsbesuch 5972
RS-Virus 5853
Rubrik 6631
Rückbildung 3613
Rückbildung 5746
Rücken 564
Rückenmark 6424
Rückenmarkshäute 4117
Rückenschmerzen 565
Rückenschmerzen 566

Rückerstattung 5759
Rückfall 5764
Rückfallsirzidenz 5766
Rückfließen 5756
Rückführung 2542
Rückgängigmachen der Provokation 1721
Rückgrat 6427
Rückkopplung 2541
Rückkopplungsschleife 2542
Rückresorption 5672
Rückstand 5784
Rückstand 5835
Rückstoß 5682
Rücktrittsklausel 2351
rückwärtige Verdrängung 570
rückwärts beugen 638
Rudiment 7320
rudimentär 5874
rudimentärer Körperteil 7320
Ruhe 5853
Ruhelosigkeit 5862
ruhen 5859
ruhend 1899
Ruhestand 5868
ruhig 5590
ruhig 6245
rühren 6551
Rülpsen 637
Rumpf 6999
runder Tisch 5966
Rundfalte 5964
Ruptur 5978
rutschen 6296
Sabbem 2050
Saccus 5980
Sack 5275
Sack 5980
Sack 889
sacrolumbal 5984
Sadismus 5986

Sadomasochismus 5987
sagittal 5996
Sakkade 5981
Sakralwirbel 5982
sakroiliakal 5983
Sakrum 5985
Salbe 4632
Salbe 6007
salinische Kontrolle 5999
Saliva 6000
Salz 6003
salzarme Kost 3896
salzarme Kost 3897
salzfreie Diät 6004
Salzlösung 5998
Samen 6120
Samenblase 6125
Samenerguß 2168
Samenflüssigkeit 6124
Samenleiter 7255
Samenstrang 6408
Sanatorium 6013
Sanierung 6018
sanitär 6016
Sanitäter 4701
Sanitation 6018
Sarkom 6021
sarkoplasmatisches Retikulum 6022
Satelliten-DNS 6024
Satellitenort 6025
Satellitenzentrum 6023
Sattheit 6027
Sättigung 6026
Sättigungsreaktion 6028
saubere Datei 1180
saubere Datenbank 1179
Sauerstoff 4782
Sauerstoffinhalationstherapie 4783
Sauerstoffmessung 4781
Sauerstoffzufuhr 4785

591

592

septisch 6146
septischer Schock 6147
Septum 6149
Septumdefekt 6144
Septumdeviation 6145
sequentiell 6154
sequentielle Analyse 6155
sequentieller Entwurf 6156
Sequenz 6152
Sequenzhomologie 6153
Serie 619
Serienaufzeichnungen 6157
Serodiagnostik 6161
seroepidemiologische Methode 6162
Serologie 6163
seropositiv 6164
Seropositivität 6165
Seroprävalenz 6166
seröser Erguß 6170
serotonerg 6168
Serotypisierung 6169
Serum 6173
Serumalbumin 6174
Serumelektrolyte 6175
Serumkrankheit 6176
seßhaft 6096
Seuche 5153
Seufzer 6229
Sexualität 6181
Sexualpartner 6191
sexuell 6186
sexuelle Funktionsstörung 6187
sexuelle Potenz 6192
sexuelle Vorgeschichte 6188
sexuelles Verhältnis 6193
sezernieren 6089
sezieren 1953
Shading 6195
Shedding 6205
Shunt 6221

Sialo- 6001
Sialographie 6222
sich absetzen 6642
sich in Verbindung setzen 1451
sich niederschlagen 6642
sich verändernder Durchschnitt 5955
sich zurückentwickeln 5893
sich zuziehen 1474
Sichelzellanämie 6225
Sichelzelle 6224
sicher 5988
Sicherheit 1067
Sicherheit 5989
Sicherheit des Produkts 5403
Sicherheitsausschuß 5990
Sicherheitsbewertung 5991
Sicherheitsindex 5992
Sicherheitsprofil 5994
Sicherheitsüberwachungsausschuß 5993
Sicherheitsvariable 5995
Sicht 6230
sichtbare Analogskala 7348
Sichtbarmachung 7352
sickernd 4654
Sigma 6232
sigmoid 6231
Sigmoid 6232
Sigmoidoskop 6233
Sigmoidoskopie 6234
Signal 6238
Signalausfall 2052
Signalsequenz 6239
Signatur 6240
signifikant verschieden 6243
Signifikanz 6241
Silberfärbung 6247
'Silberstandard' 6248
Silikonimplantat 6246
simulieren 6250
simultan 6251

Sinn 6133
Sinnesapparat 6138
Sinnesempfindung 6132
Sinnesorgan 6135
Sinus 6262
Sinusitis 6263
Sinusknoten 6261
Sirup 6777
Sitte 1629
Sitzangst 166
Sitzbad 6273
Sitzbein 3637
sitzen 2613
sitzend 6096
sitzen 6271
Sitzung 6177
Sitzung 6270
Skala 6034
Skalpell 6037
skandierende Sprache 6043
Skapula 6044
Skatologie 6047
Skelett 6275
Skelettmuskel 6592
Sklera 6065
Skoliose 6066
Skotom 6067
Skrotum 6075
Soda 6341
Sodbrennen 2999
sofort 3281
sofort 3282
sofort 6499
Software 6348
Solarplexus 6350
solide 6352
Solvens 6355
Soma 6356
somatisch 6357
somatische Störung 6358

sematosensibel 6359
sematosensorisch 6359
Sommersprosse 2721
Somnambulismus 6293
Somnolenz 6360
Sende 5383
Sende 7117
Senderschule 6382
sendieren 5384
sendieren 6368
Sendierung 5383
Sennenbrand 6678
Sennenlicht 6679
Sennenöl 6680
Sennenstich 6681
Senogramm 6361
Serge 6366
Southern-Blot 6372
sozial 6333
Sozialhilfe 6335
Sozialisierung 6336
Sozialversicherung 6335
sozialwirtschaftlicher Faktor 6338
Soziologie 6339
Spalte 1183
Spalte 1567
Spalte 6299
Spaltlampenuntersuchung 6301
Spannung 6861
Spannungszustand 6986
spasmodisch 6377
Spasmus 6376
spastiches Kolon 6378
spastisch 6377
späteinsetzend 3729
Spätwirkung 138
Spaziergang 7387
Speichel 6000
Speichel- 6001
Speichel 6433

594

Steatorrhö 6516
stechen 6469
stechen 6553
Stechmücke 4308
stehend 6491
stehlen 6514
steif 6541
Steife 5938
Steifheit mit Zahnradphänomen 1268
Stein 6557
Stein 905
Steinleiden 3845
Steiß 5976
Steißbein 1254
Steißlage 853
stellatus 6519
Stelle 6264
Stellenbesetzung 6474
Stellreflex 6496
Stellungs- 5262
Stengel 6482
Stenokardie 277
Stenose 6523
Sterbebegleitung 6871
Sterbehilfe 2375
Sterbeklinik 3133
Sterben 2100
Sterbetafel 3803
Sterbeurkunde 1709
Sterbeziffer 1710
sterblich 4302
Sterblichkeit 4303
Sterblichkeitsrate 4304
Stereoisomer 6526
stereoselektiv 6527
stereotaxische Methode 6528
stereotypisches Verhalten 6529
Stereotypisierung 6530
steril 6531
steriler Puder 6532

Sterilisation 6534
sterilisieren 6019
Sterilisierung 6534
Sterilität 6533
Sternchen 468
sternförmig 6519
sternokostoklavikulär 6535
Sternum 6536
Steroid 6537
steroidisch 6538
Stethoskop 6539
steuern 1492
Steuerung 1491
Stich 6468
Stich 6550
Stich 6552
Stichprobe 6008
Stichprobe 6451
Stichprobenerhebung 6012
Stichprobengröße 6009
Stickstoff 4497
Stiel 6482
Stiel 6520
Sternacken 880
Stiftung 2709
Stiftung 2751
Stigma 6543
still 5590
still 6544
Stille 3902
Stimmapparat 2867
Stimmbänder 7362
Stimme 7364
Stimulans 6546
Stimulation 6548
Stimulator 6546
stimulieren 6547
Stimulierung 4313
Stimulus 6549
Stipendium 2546

Stipendium 2902
Stirn 2686
Stirn- 2739
Stirn 872
Stirnbeinhöhle 2740
Stock 6540
Stoffabhängigkeit 6647
Stoffwechsel- 4148
Stoffwechsel 4151
Stoffwechselstörung 4149
Stoffwechselweg 4150
stolz 5481
Stoma 6555
Stomaanlage 4746
Störfaktor 1416
Störsignal 2051
Störung 1941
Störung 9
Störvariable 1417
stottern 6484
stottern 6613
Stottern 6614
Strabismus 6467
Strabismus 6569
Strafe 5548
Sträfling 5376
Strahlenbiologie 5611
strahlend 5598
strahlendurchlässig 7061
strahlenempfindlich 5626
strahleninduziert 5601
strahlensensibilisierendes Mittel 5602
Strahlentherapie 5603
Strahlentherapie 5629
strahlenundurchlässig 5625
Strahlung 5600
Strähne 6572
Strang 6572
Strangulierung 6574
Strategie 6575

Stratifikation 6576
strecken 6590
Strecken 6589
Streckmuskel 2450
Streichung 1773
Streifen 6582
Streifen 6591
Streifen 6596
Streptokokke 6585
Streß 6586
Streuungsdiagramm 6048
Stria 6591
Strichkodierung 593
Stridor 6595
Striktur 6593
Strom 6583
Stroma 6599
Stromazelle 6600
Strömung 2632
Strontium 6601
Struktur 2698
Struktur- 6602
Struktur- 6603
Struktur-Wirkungs-Verhältnis 6604
strukturell 6602
strukturell 6885
Struma 2876
Struma nodularis 4504
Student 6605
Studie 6606
Studie 7088
Studie der ersten Phase 5065
Studie mit enthülltem Etikett 4661
Studienabschluß 7095
Studienentwurf 7091
Studienentwurf mit gepaarten Werten 4032
Studienkoordinator 6609
Studienleitung 6608
Studienplanung 6610
Studienregister 7094

Ventrikulographie 7296
Venula 7297
verabreichend 1945
verabreichung 1776
Verabreichungssystem 1777
veränderlich 7246
Veränderung 1078
Veränderung 7247
Verantwortlichkeit 36
Verantwortung 3787
Verarbeitung 5390
Verarbeitungdiagramm 2637
verbal 7298
Verband 2044
Verband 590
Verbesserung der Symptome 220
verbinden 591
verbindlich 676
Verbindung 1357
Verbindung 1429
Verbindung 3662
Verbindung 3671
Verbindung 3832
Verbindung 7175
Verbindung von Unterlagen 5698
verborgen 4611
Verbot 5421
verboten 5420
Verbrauch 2428
verbrauchen 1447
verbrauchen 1812
Verbraucher 1448
Verbrauchergruppe 1449
Verbrechen 1569
Verbreiterung 7446
Verbreitung 1956
Verbreitung von Erneuerungen 1894
verbrennen 888
Verbrennung 6032
Verbrennung 887

Verbrennung III. Grades 6908
verbrühen 6033
Verbrühung 6032
verbunden 1307
verbunden 466
verbunden 90
verbundene Daten 1309
verbundene Zentren 1308
Verdachtsdiagnose 1864
verdauen 1896
Verdauung 1897
Verdauungsapparat 2792
Verdauungskanal 179
Verdauungsstörung 3377
Verdauungssystem 1898
Verdauungstrakt 1899
verderben 6443
Verdichtung 1394
verdorren 7455
verdrängen 5813
Verdrängung 1946
Verdrängung 6698
verdrießlich 4299
verdünnen 1906
Vereinigung 467
Vereinigung 7175
Verengung 4401
Verengung 6593
vererbte Krankheit 3439
Vererbung 3059
Vererbung 3438
Verfahren 4165
Verfahren 5388
Verfahren 5389
Verfahren 6836
Verfahrensfrage 5199
Verfahrensregeln 1259
Verfall 1731
verfallender Zahn 1724
Verfallsdatum 2439

verfälschen 6806
Verfärbung 1924
verfaulen 1717
verfaulend 5560
verfeinerte Analyse 6363
Verfolgen 7021
Verformbarkeit 1755
Verformung 1756
Verführung 6098
Vergehen 4626
Vergeßlichkeit 2694
Vergessenheit 2694
Vergewaltigung 5652
vergiften 5195
Vergiftung 3560
Vergiftung 5197
Vergiftungsberatungsstelle 5196
Vergleich 1329
Vergleichbarkeit 1325
Vergleichbarkeitsstudie 1326
Vergleichermedizin 1328
Vergleichsgruppe 1330
Vergleichsstudie 1327
vergrößert 2284
Vergrößerung 2285
Vergrößerung 230
Verhalten 632
Verhaltens- 635
Verhaltensforschung 2370
verhaltensgestört 3963
Verhaltenspunktzahl 633
Verhaltensregeln 2366
Verhaltensstörung 636
Verhaltenstherapie 634
Verhältnis 5663
Verhältnis zwischen Ventilation und Perfusion 7288
Verhandlungen 4434
Verhärtung 3389
Verhungern 6497

Verhütungsmittel 1471
Verfikation 7300
verifizieren 7301
verkalkt 899
Verkalkung 898
Verkäufer 7280
Verkehr 3523
verkrüppeln 6611
Verlagerung 1946
Verlagerung 5424
Verlangen 1562
verlängern 5428
verlängerte Standardkurve 2447
verlängertes Mark 4095
Verlängerung 2448
Verlängerung 3767
Verlängerung 5429
Verlaufs-Röntgenaufnahme 3547
Verlaufskontrolle 2665
verleihen 1404
ve-letzlich 7377
Verletzung 3449
Verletzung 7073
Verlust 3875
Vermännlichung 7336
Verminderung 1731
Verminderung 1908
vermitteln 4070
Vermögen 10
vernarben 6046
Vernebler 4424
veröffentlichen 5525
Veröffentlichung 5524
Verordnung 5332
Verpackung 4789
Verpackungsbeilage für Patienten 4931
verpaßter Untersuchungstermin 4233
verpflanzen 2896
Verpflichtungen der Sponsoren 4591
Verpflichtungen der Untersucher 4590

# German/Deutsch

verpfuschen 6806
Verrenkung 6452
Verruca 7304
Versagen 2501
Versammlung 4096
Versand- 3955
Verschattung 6196
Verschiedenheit 1977
verschlechtem 148
verschlechtem 1844
Verschlechterung 1845
Verschlechterung 7470
Verschlechterung des Sehvermögens 7351
Verschließung 4606
Verschlimmerung 2389
Verschluß 1235
Verschluß 4609
Verschmutzung 5204
Verschreiber 5330
Verschreibungsmuster 5331
verschreibungspflichtiges Medikament 5333
verschwenden 7401
Verschwendung 7400
verschwommenes Sehvermögen 787
Versicherung 3500
Versicherungsanspruch 3501
versicherungsstatistische Analyse 71
Verstädterung 7196
Verstärker 231
verstärkt 2706
Verstärkung 5762
Verstauchung 6452
Verstauchung 6571
Verstopfung 1442
Verstopfung 4604
Verstoß 4626
verstümmeln 4366
Versuch 2432
Versuch 461
Versuch 6606

Versuch mit mehreren Dosierungen 4338
Versuchsbedingungen 2435
Versuchsdurchführer 7096
Versuchsende 1232
Versuchskaninchen 2931
Versuchsprojekt 5128
Versuchsvalidierung 462
Versuchszweig 6607
Versuchung 6098
vertebral 7306
Vertebrat 7308
verteilen 6456
verteilte Datenbank 1971
verteilte Datenerfassung 1970
Verteilung 1972
Verteilung im Gewebe 6967
Verteilungskoeffizient 4887
Verteilungsvolumen 7370
Vertex 7309
Vertigo 7312
vertikal 7310
vertikale Integrierung 7311
Vertrag 1473
vertraglich festgelegte Kundendienstleistungen 1482
Verträglichkeit 1334
Verträglichkeit 6977
Vertragsbüro 1478
Vertragsfirma 1475
Vertragsforschung 1480
Vertragsforschungsorganisation 1481
Vertragshersteller 1477
Vertragslabor 1476
Vertragsorganisation 1479
Vertrauensgrenzen 1407
Vertrauensintervall 1406
Vertraulichkeit 1408
Vertreter 5997
ve:unreinigen 1457
Verunreinigung 1458

Verunreinigung 3330
Verunreinigung 5204
Verwachsung 86
Verwalter 96
Verwaltung 3983
Verwaltung der Praxis 5284
Verwaltungsbehörde 2890
Verwaltungsweg 5968
Verwander 1419
Verwander 5769
Verwandtschaft 5768
Verweiblichung 2218
Verweigerer 5734
Verweilkatheter 3391
verwelken 6219
Verwendung 7221
Verwertung 7221
Verwesung 5559
Verwindung 6998
verwirrend 1415
verwirrt 3813
Verwirrtheit 1418
Verwirrung 1418
verwunden 7473
verwundet 7474
Verzeichnis schädlicher Reaktionen 117
Verzerrung 1967
Verzicht 7383
Verzichterklärung bei Schwangerschaft 5308
Verzichtserklärung 7383
verzögert 1789
verzögerte Reaktion 1770
Verzögerung 5873
verzweigte Kette 841
Vesikel 7313
vesikular 7314
vestibulär 7316
Vestibulum 7318
Veteran 7321
Vibration 7325

Vibrationsempfinden 7326
Vieldeutigkeit 211
vielleicht medikamentös bedingt 5235
viral 7330
viraler Organismus 7331
Virämie 7334
Virenabstoßung 7333
Virenausscheidung 7333
Virenkultur 7332
Virilisierung 7336
Virion 7337
Virologie 7338
Virulerz 7339
Virus 7340
Viruspartikel 7337
viskös 7342
viskös 7344
Viskosität 7343
Visualisierung 7352
visuell 7346
visuell evoziertes Potential 7349
Viszera 7341
viszeral- 6435
Vitalität 6483
Vitalkapzität 7353
Vitamin 7356
vivisezieren 7360
Vokabular 7361
Volksgesundheit 5520
Volksgruppe 2369
Volksmedizin 2661
voll 7441
Vollblut 7442
Vollblutaustauschtransfusion 7443
Vollmondgesicht 4287
Vollprothese 1351
Volumen 7369
vom Standort entfernt 4629
von Charge zu Charge 3861
von früh bis spät 7386

weiterführend 1464
weiterführende Studie 2669
weitergeben 4893
weitsichtig 2517
Weitwinkelglaukom 4658
Wellenform 7408
wellenförmige Bewegung 7409
Weltgesundheitsorganisation 7466
Weltraumflug 6374
weltweit 7467
weltweite Entwicklung 7468
Wendung 3594
Werbung direkt zum Verbraucher 1915
Wert 7240
wesentlich 2356
Western-Blot 7428
wichtig 6242
widerlich 5820
widernatürlich 5024
widerspenstig 5731
Widerstand 5838
Widerstandsfähigkeit 5951
Wiederaufbau 5694
Wiederauffinden 5888
Wiederauftreten 5703
Wiederauftreten 5712
wiederbeleben 5870
wiederbeleben 5910
Wiederbelebung 5871
Wiederdurchblutung 5803
Wiedereinlösen eines Rezepts 5059
Wiederherstellung 5695
Wiederherstellung 5757
wiederholen 5801
wiederholte Beobachtung 5802
wiederholte Operation 5798
wiederholte Provokation 5689
Wiederholung 5800
Wiederholung 5807
Wiederholung der Auswertung 5719

wiederkehrend 5713
Wiederzulassung 5677
Wille 7447
Willenskraft 7448
Willkürmuskulatur 7372
Wimper 2478
Windel 1871
Winkel 285
Wirbel 7305
Wirbel- 7306
wirbellos 3596
wirbelloses Tier 3595
Wirbelsäule 6423
Wirbelsäule 7307
Wirbeltier 7308
Wirkmechanismus 4060
Wirkpotential 5269
wirksam 4671
wirksam 64
Wirksamkeit 2158
Wirksamkeitsprofil 2159
Wirksamkeitspunktzahl 2160
Wirksamkeitsvariable 2161
Wirkstoff 145
Wirkstoffdesign 2062
Wirkung 2152
Wirkung gegen Tumorwachstum, -ausbreitung 359
Wirkungsgrad 2162
wirkungslos 4481
Wirkungsprofil eines Medikaments 2070
Wirkungsweise 4060
Wirt 3140
Wirt-Parasit-Beziehungen 3143
Wirtschaft 2136
wirtschaftliche Konkurrenz 2135
wirtschaftlicher Wettbewerb 2135
Wirtschaftsanalyse 2134
Wirtsresistenz 3141
wischen 7450

Wissenschaft 6061
Wissenschaftler 6064
wissenschaftlich 6062
wissenschaftliche Arbeit 1957
wissenschaftlicher Fehltritt 6063
Witmaack-Ekbom-Syndrom 5861
Woche 7417
Wochenbett 3921
Wohl 7427
Wohlfahrt 7427
Wohn- 5333
Wohnheim 5831
Wohnung 3148
Wohnung 5831
Wort- 7298
wörtlich 7299
Wortschatz 7361
Wunde 7472
Wurf 3849
würgen 5875
Würgen 5876
Würgereflex 2760
Wurm 7469
wurmförmig 7302
Wurm mittel 315
Würze 2624
Wurzel 5956
Wurzelkanal 5657
Wut 5632
wütend 3624
wütend 5595
X-Achse 7462
X-Chromosom 7480
xanthomatöser Knoten 7481
Xanthopsie 7497
Y-Achse 7492
Y-Chromosom 7490
Z-Achse 7502
Z-Test 7510
zähflüssig 7344

Zähflüssigkeit 7343
Zahl 1544
Zahl 1900
Zahl 2589
Zahl 4566
zählen 1545
Zahlung 4941
Zählung 1544
Zählung 2963
Zahn 6991
zahn- und kieferregulierendes Gerät 4718
zahnärztlich 1794
zahnärztliche Praxis 1798
Zahnarzt 1801
Zahnbelag 5158
Zahncreme 6994
Zahnbürsten 6993
Zahnen 1803
Zahnfleisch 2850
Zahnfleisch 2932
Zahnformel 1803
Zahnfüllung 3451
Zahnheilkunde 1802
Zahnkrone 1596
Zahnpasta 6994
Zahnpflege 1796
Zahnprothese 1805
Zahnputzmittel 1799
Zahnschmelz 2247
Zahnschmerz 6992
Zahnstein 1795
Zäkum 1025
Zäpfchen 6696
Zäpfchen 7224
Zecke 6943
Zehe 6974
Zeichen 1608
Zeichen 6235
Zeichen 6746
Zeichen und Symptome 6244

**Japanese日本語**

617

628

# Japanese/日本語

632

**Japanese/日本語**

644

653

658

Japanese/日本語